Core Pathology

THIRD EDITION

Alan Stevens MB BS, FRCPath
Former Senior Lecturer in Histopathology
University of Nottingham Medical School
Former Honorary Consultant Histopathologist to Queen's Medical Centre
Nottingham University Hospitals NHS Trust
Nottingham, UK

James Lowe BMedSci, BM BS, DM, FRCPath
Professor of Neuropathology
University of Nottingham Medical School
Honorary Consultant Histopathologist to Queen's Medical Centre
Nottingham University Hospitals NHS Trust
Nottingham, UK

Ian Scott BSc, MB BS, MD, DPhil, FRCPath
Consultant Neuropathologist
Hull and East Yorkshire Hospitals NHS Trust
Honorary Clinical Senior Lecturer
Hull York Medical School
Hull, UK

USA Advisor:

Ivan Damjanov MD, PhD
Professor of Pathology
Department of Pathology and Laboratory Medicine
University of Kansas School of Medicine
Kansas City, Kansas, USA

MOSBY

ELSEVIER

MOSBY
ELSEVIER

an imprint of Elsevier Limited.

© 2009, Elsevier Limited. All rights reserved.

First edition 1995
Second edition 2000
Third edition 2009

The right of Alan Stevens, James Lowe and Ian Scott to be identified as authors of this work has been asserted by him/her/them in accordance with the Copyright, Designs and Patents Act 1988.

Main edition ISBN: 978-0-7234-3444-3
Reprinted 2009
International edition ISBN: 978-0-7234-3459-7

British Library Cataloguing in Publication Data
A catalogue record for this book is available from the British Library

Library of Congress Cataloging in Publication Data
A catalog record for this book is available from the Library of Congress

Notice
Medical knowledge is constantly changing. Standard safety precautions must be followed, but as new research and clinical experience broaden our knowledge, changes in treatment and drug therapy may become necessary or appropriate. Readers are advised to check the most current product information provided by the manufacturer of each drug to be administered to verify the recommended dose, the method and duration of administration, and contraindications. It is the responsibility of the practitioner, relying on experience and knowledge of the patient, to determine dosages and the best treatment for each individual patient. Neither the Publisher nor the author assume any liability for any injury and/or damage to persons or property arising from this publication.

The Publisher

ELSEVIER your source for books, journals and multimedia in the health sciences
www.elsevierhealth.com

Working together to grow
libraries in developing countries
www.elsevier.com | www.bookaid.org | www.sabre.org
ELSEVIER | BOOK AID International | Sabre Foundation

The publisher's policy is to use **paper manufactured from sustainable forests**

Printed in China

Last digit is the print number: 9 8 7 6 5 4 3 2

Core Pathology

This book is respectfully dedicated to the memory of

IAN GEOFFREY WILSON
(1954–2007)

From 1974 until his untimely death, a stalwart member of the Histopathology Department of University Hospital, Queen's Medical Centre, Nottingham, UK
Ian was a kindly gentle giant, generous to all with his time, knowledge, humour and wisdom – a true gentleman. He is sadly missed. The authors are privileged to have known him and worked with him.

Commissioning Editor: Kate Dimock
Development Editor: Louise Cook
Project Manager: Alan Nicholson
Design: Stewart Larking
Illustration Manager: Bruce Hogarth
Marketing Manager: Allan McKeown

Contents

Contents

Contents

Preface to the third edition

In the first edition of this book, the Preface took the form of a lengthy 'Credo' in which we stated the philosophy and principles on which we based the content and approach of the book. Our views about the inappropriately large size of the curriculum remain unchanged, so we have concentrated on presenting the core knowledge of the basic pathological processes as lucidly as we can, and, in the systemic pathology section, we aim to give the student a knowledge of which diseases exist, how they arise, their effects, and their usual (and sometimes unusual) outcomes. We place the greatest emphasis on the diseases that medical students might reasonably expect to encounter in their subsequent clinical practice, whether in hospital or community practice.

Our aim, as always, is to present the important pathology in as clear and concise a manner as we can, supplemented by carefully selected pictures and artworks, and relating the pathology to clinical medicine and surgery where relevant. To assist the student in assimilating the contents, we have used **telegraph headings** to provide a brief overview of the succeeding text, **blue boxes** which contain the important clinical aspects of disease, **pink boxes** dealing with more advanced information, often the cell biology and molecular genetics of the disease, and **key facts boxes** acting as summaries and revision aids. In addition there are some **data set boxes**, typically containing clinical chemistry profiles when abnormal biochemical parameters are an essential component of diagnosis.

Although the book has been written to aid students in traditional medical education courses, in this edition we have tried to assist students who are in problem-based learning courses by strengthening the clinical context within the book as well as providing some sample problem-based exercises at the end of each system pathology chapter. Brief answers to the problems are given at the end of the book, and more detailed answers, of greater educational value, are on the website. Of course, we have also updated the text, expanded some sections, and improved the quality of some illustrations.

Regular readers of our books will note that there is no dedication related to wine in this edition, as we wished instead to dedicate it to one of the kindest and finest men any of us have met, sadly taken from his friends, work colleagues and lovely family as we were beginning the preparation of this book. As a result, we have written it in a state of rather depressed sobriety; we hope that the quality of the writing has not deteriorated as a result.

Alan Stevens, James Lowe, Ian Scott
Nottingham 2008

A polemic from a retiring author

As this is the last book I shall write, I asked my fellow authors if they would permit me to write a personal note about something on which I have strong opinions. They agreed, provided it was in the form of a considered polemic rather than a hysterical rant. I ask you to give it consideration.

In over 40 years working as a histopathologist, I have met and worked with many histopathologists from many countries, and they have (with rare exceptions) been intelligent men and women, with logical thought processes and considerable common sense. Why then have we allowed sloppy nomenclatures and classifications to creep into our daily usage? I cite a few examples:

Hodgkins disease and Non-Hodgkins Lymphoma – Where is the intellectual rigour in defining a large group of important tumours of many different types by naming it according to what it is not? Imagine the furore and general dismay if anthropologists classified humankind into male humans and non-male humans. It is not as if we are now ignorant of the nature of the neoplastic cell in Hodgkins disease.

Small cell and non-small cell carcinoma of the lung – The above argument applies again, but there is the added stupidity of the nomenclature. When I first worked in histopathology, we had only routinely stained paraffin sections to work on; electron microscopes were research tools scarcely available for diagnostic histopathologists, and immunocytochemical techniques were undiscovered. In cases of undifferentiated or anaplastic tumours, we were compelled to use imprecise descriptive terms like 'spindle-cell sarcoma', 'small cell undifferentiated tumour', etc. Has 40 years of progress in laboratory technology been wasted? We know the cell of origin of 'small cell carcinoma of the lung' – why not use it? We know the cells of origin of all the tumours in the 'non-small cell carcinoma' group – why not use them? Let accurate pathological classifications, with a valid scientific basis, inform clinical prognosis and management decisions.

Invasive/in situ vulval carcinoma and NNED (non-neoplastic epithelial diseases) – This one makes me weep. I have tried to find a definition of NNED, but the closest I can find is its widespread use to avoid naming the precise vulval disease present, once it has been established that it is not an invasive or in situ squamous carcinoma. As such, it presumably contains contact dermatitis, lichen planus, lichen simplex chronicus, lichen sclerosus, psoriasis, vulval Candidosis, and about another dozen or so other inflammatory vulval diseases, most of which are much more common than invasive and in situ carcinoma. Where do malignant melanoma and epidermal cyst of the vulva fit into this schema?

There are many other examples of the sloppy use of words and glib empty phrases, for example, diseases being classified as 'of usual type', but I will stop now before I spontaneously combust. Although I disapprove of the above nomenclatures and classifications, and their like, we have felt obliged to use them in this book so as not to confuse the students, but I hope you can detect the undercurrent of derision in our treatment of them.

Alan Stevens
Nottingham 2008

Acknowledgments

The authors wish to thank many people who have helped in the preparation of this book and its previous editions, particularly the laboratory staff in the Nottingham University Hospitals NHS Trust who prepared the histological sections and electron micrographs from which the illustrations in the book are taken. We would also like to thank our colleagues who did some of our clinical and laboratory work for us on occasions when we were writing, particularly Dr. Keith Robson, Janet Palmer, Lianne Finnerty and Catherine Hills, and other colleagues in the Trust and outside who passed on to us suitable slides for photomicrography, and material for photomacrography. Those who supplied colour transparencies from their own collections are acknowledged separately in 'Illustration Acknowledgements'. We are grateful to Linda Dewdney and Irene Smith for their invaluable secretarial, administrative and word-processing assistance. We were fortunate to have the photographic skills of Anne Kane available to us; in addition to photographing new specimens and slides for this edition, she greatly improved the quality of many of the pictures used in previous editions by using computer wizardry. Finally, we would like to express our gratitude to Professor Ivan Damjanov, University of Kansas School of Medicine, who carefully read through the entire manuscript of the Second Edition, pointed out errors, and made many useful suggestions which we have incorporated in this edition. If there are any errors in this edition, it is our fault, not his.

We would also like to thank the staff at Elsevier (Kate Dimock, Louise Cook, Alan Nicholson) for their help in the preparation of this third edition.

Illustration acknowledgments

Many former and current colleagues in the Nottingham University Hospitals Trust kindly gave us pictures from their own collections. They are:

Dr. R. Allibone – Figs 11.16, 13.25, 17.36, 17.43b, 17.46, 19.20.

Dr. M. Anderson – Figs 19.13a, 19.22, 19.23a&b, 19.24a&c, 19.25, 19.28, 19.29a.

Dr. I. D. Ansell – Figs 17.12, 17.17b, 17.24b, 17.31, 17.40.

Mr. P. Bradley – Figs 12.34, 12.35, 12.37.

Dr. K. Dalziel – Figs 19.1, 19.2, 19.3, 19.5a.

Mr. R. Downes – Figs 22.3, 22.5.

Dr. R. Emerson – Fig. 23.31e.

Mr. I. Foster – Figs 24.22, 24.23.

Mr. K. Gibbin – Figs 5.29, 12.8, 12.9, 12.10a, 12.26, 12.27, 12.28, 12.29, 12.30a, 12.41, 12.42.

Dr. P. D. James – Fig. 11.5.

Dr. T. Jaspan – Fig. 16.2a.

Dr. I. Leach – Figs 10.5b, 10.7, 10.37, 10.38, 10.40, 10.41, 10.42a, 10.43, 10.45, 10.46, 10.48, 10.49, 10.51, 10.52, 18.8a.

Kate Martin – Fig. 16.24.

Dr. P. Small – Figs 4.9, 5.7, 12.21.

The late Dr. P. G. Smith – Figs 14.6, 16.13a, 16.15a.

Dr. J. Zuccollo – Figs 5.2, 5.3, 5.5, 5.6.

We are also grateful to the following for permission to use illustrations:

Dr. I. G. Barrison – Fig. 14.25a (from *Gastroenterology in Practice*, Gower Medical Publishing, 1992).

Dr. W. F. Jackson – Fig. 16.8a (from *Colour Atlas and Text of Clinical Medicine*, Mosby-Wolfe, London 1992).

Dr. R. Marakian – Fig. 7.12 (from *Clinical Immunology*, Gower Medical Publishing, London, 1991).

Dr. M. Thornhill – Figs 12.1a, 12.2, 12.3, 12.4, 12.5, 12.6, 12.17.

Profs. D. Ellison and S. Love (Eds) – Figs 21.1, 21.2b&c, 21.14, 21.15, 21.16, 21.29, 21.35. (from *Neuropathology*, Times Mirror Mosby, 1998.

Mr. W. G. J. Edwards, Keeper of the Gordon Museum, Guy's Hospital, London. – Fig. 8.12.

Pathology at the core of medicine

1

PATHOLOGY IS THE STUDY OF THE PATTERNS, CAUSES, MECHANISMS AND EFFECTS OF ILLNESS (DISEASE)

A thorough understanding of disease processes is essential if physicians and surgeons are to recognize, diagnose and treat all diseases with accuracy and competence. Pathology is therefore a vital component of medical education for all doctors, nurses and other health-care practitioners, greatly improving the skill and efficiency of all concerned.

For a doctor to be able to interpret the complaints of a patient (the **symptoms** of disease) and understand the abnormalities found on examination (the **signs** of disease), it is important to be familiar with the range of abnormalities possible in an organ or tissue. If such knowledge is supported by that of the potential **causes** of abnormality, it is possible to arrange investigations and, ultimately, to **treat** disease. Pathology is the bedrock of clinical medicine, and its study continues throughout clinical practice.

A knowledge of disease patterns forms the basis of a doctor's skill in diagnosis, which is rooted in listening to the patient's account of the features of the illness (the **clinical history**), and in simple **physical examination**.

Clinical symptoms

A man presents to the Emergency Room with sudden onset of severe, crushing, continuous central chest pain, radiating into the left side of the neck and down the left arm. The patient also mentions that he had previously transiently experienced similar, less severe, pain in his chest on physical exertion, but that the pain had gone away on resting. The latest episode is associated with severe breathlessness, and the patient feels very unwell. He has cold, clammy skin and low blood pressure.

Even without physical examination, the doctor can build up a picture of the most likely pathological processes at work, and will know what mechanisms are operating and what the causative factors and likely effects are. Thus, immediate, possibly life-saving, treatment can be instituted. From a knowledge of the range of diseases that can affect the heart, and their causes, the doctor deduces that the patient probably has severe disease affecting his coronary arteries, which have become partially blocked by a disease process called atheroma (see Chapter 10), and that this partial blockage has resulted in the heart muscle occasionally being short of oxygenated arterial blood during periods of strenuous physical activity, leading to heart muscle pain (angina) in the past.

The conclusion is that the most recent episode may have resulted from complete blockage of the artery, which has been made total by the development of a blood clot (thrombus). This has caused complete cessation of arterial blood supply to part of the muscular wall of the heart, and consequent death of the heart muscle cells due to loss of oxygen supply. The doctor will make a working diagnosis of myocardial infarction. Knowing the likely etiology of a disease allows rational planning of investigations to confirm the clinical diagnosis. In this instance an electrocardiogram (ECG) will show diagnostic changes, and levels of enzymes liberated from dead heart muscle will be elevated in the blood.

A knowledge of the mechanisms involved (pathogenesis) also allows implementation of treatment; in this instance administration of an agent to promote lysis of thrombus allows reperfusion of heart muscle and may limit the extent of damage.

The thoughts in the doctor's mind will be as illustrated in *Fig. 1.1.*

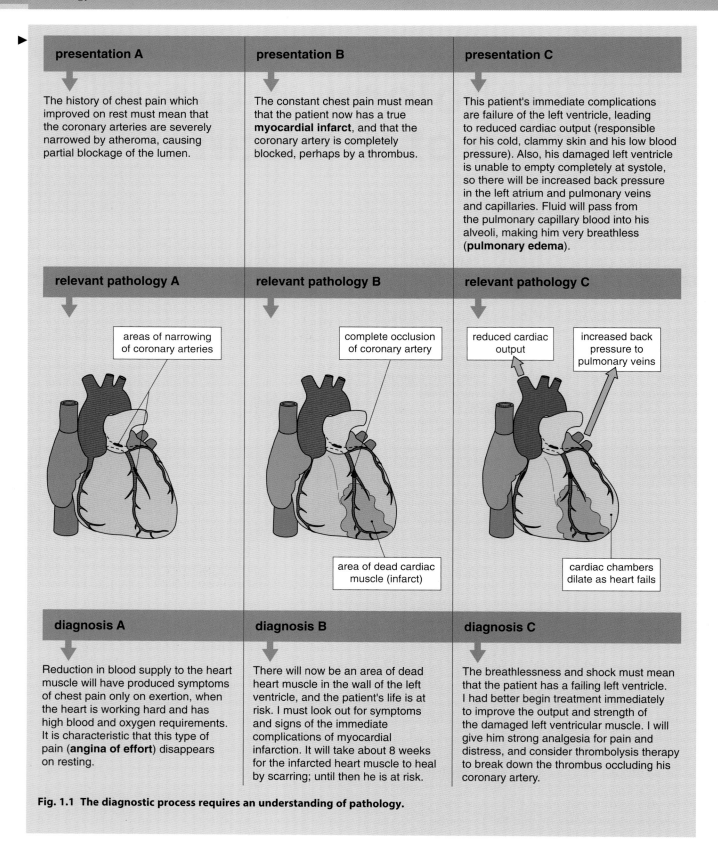

presentation A

The history of chest pain which improved on rest must mean that the coronary arteries are severely narrowed by atheroma, causing partial blockage of the lumen.

presentation B

The constant chest pain must mean that the patient now has a true **myocardial infarct**, and that the coronary artery is completely blocked, perhaps by a thrombus.

presentation C

This patient's immediate complications are failure of the left ventricle, leading to reduced cardiac output (responsible for his cold, clammy skin and his low blood pressure). Also, his damaged left ventricle is unable to empty completely at systole, so there will be increased back pressure in the left atrium and pulmonary veins and capillaries. Fluid will pass from the pulmonary capillary blood into his alveoli, making him very breathless (**pulmonary edema**).

relevant pathology A

areas of narrowing of coronary arteries

relevant pathology B

complete occlusion of coronary artery

area of dead cardiac muscle (infarct)

relevant pathology C

reduced cardiac output

increased back pressure to pulmonary veins

cardiac chambers dilate as heart fails

diagnosis A

Reduction in blood supply to the heart muscle will have produced symptoms of chest pain only on exertion, when the heart is working hard and has high blood and oxygen requirements. It is characteristic that this type of pain (**angina of effort**) disappears on resting.

diagnosis B

There will now be an area of dead heart muscle in the wall of the left ventricle, and the patient's life is at risk. I must look out for symptoms and signs of the immediate complications of myocardial infarction. It will take about 8 weeks for the infarcted heart muscle to heal by scarring; until then he is at risk.

diagnosis C

The breathlessness and shock must mean that the patient has a failing left ventricle. I had better begin treatment immediately to improve the output and strength of the damaged left ventricular muscle. I will give him strong analgesia for pain and distress, and consider thrombolysis therapy to break down the thrombus occluding his coronary artery.

Fig. 1.1 The diagnostic process requires an understanding of pathology.

Fig. 1.2 Common terms used in pathology

English	Pathology jargon	Explanations
Patterns of disease	Natural history	The natural history of a disease comprises many aspects, including its origins, initial effects, progress, late effects and outcome (prognosis). Many diseases can be diagnosed at an early stage by a doctor's awareness of their origins and initial effects.
Causative factor or factors	Etiology or etiological factors	Some diseases have a single, clearly defined cause, e.g. an infection. In others, many different etiological factors operate to induce disease, and there is no single cause.
Mechanisms of disease	Pathogenesis	The mechanisms whereby the initial disease process produces structural and functional abnormalities and, hence, symptoms and signs.
Effects of disease	Sequelae	The sequelae (or complications) of a disease are the secondary 'knock on' effects.

Pathology encompasses all aspects of disease

Special terms are used to refer to patterns, causes, mechanisms and effects of disease. These are given and explained in *Fig. 1.2*. Diseases can result from primary abnormalities at three levels:

- Genetic function.
- Physiological/biochemical function.
- Gross structural arrangement of cells, tissues and organs.

Many diseases reflect abnormalities at all three levels, since a genetic abnormality will induce a biochemical abnormality, and this can be manifest as a structural abnormality. An adequate understanding of pathology is therefore based on a sound grounding in normal cell biology, structure (histology and anatomy) and physiology. As most of this information is available in specialized texts relating to other aspects of human biology, extensive presentations of normal material are avoided here.

A limited number of tissue responses underlie all diseases

Cells and tissues respond to disease processes in a limited number of ways, which can be considered as **basic pathological responses**. The first part of this book is devoted to the principles of these responses. These include:

- Adaptation of cells to changes in their environment (Chapter 2).
- What happens to cells when they cannot adapt, and how cells die (Chapter 3).
- Disorders due to abnormal cell growth, for example cancer (Chapter 6).
- Tissue responses to injury, and how tissues heal (Chapter 4).

- Genetic and immune factors in disease (Chapters 5 and 7).
- Adverse environmental factors that cause disease (Chapter 9).

These basic pathological processes are illustrated by examples from medical practice.

A single disease process has different effects in different systems

As well as understanding the basic types of pathological process, it is necessary to know how they affect various tissues and organs. For example, although Chapter 6 covers the basic pathology of benign tumors and cancers, you will also need to know which tumors occur in which tissues and organs, and their natural history, particularly in terms of progress and final outcome. For example, one common form of cancer called squamous cell carcinoma can occur in many organs and tissues, including the skin, mouth, esophagus, anus, uterine cervix, and the bronchial tree. Although the tumor retains the same name wherever it arises, it behaves very differently in each different site. For example, a squamous cell carcinoma in the skin is slowly progressive, easily cured, and has a good outcome, rarely being life-threatening. Conversely, a squamous cell carcinoma in the esophagus or bronchial tree is more rapidly progressive, difficult to cure, and has a poor outcome, being life-threatening.

There is no short cut to this kind of knowledge, and it is necessary to be familiar with the details of the common pathology of the various organ systems. This approach is termed **systemic pathology** and is presented in Chapters 10 to 25. Full accounts of the pathology of each organ system are given, centered on the common and important diseases which, in our experience, it is essential to understand in some detail. For other less common or less important diseases, only the most significant facts are presented, often in an easily assimilable form such as a list or a table.

Pathology covers five main disciplines

Traditionally pathology has been subdivided into five main disciplines, reflecting the way in which clinical pathology is practiced in hospital centers.

Histopathology: the study of diseases from the perspective of structural, particularly histological, abnormalities of cells and tissues. Most of this book is about histopathology.

Hematology: the study of primary diseases of the blood, as well as the effects of other diseases on the blood.

Chemical pathology: the study of diseases from the perspective of biochemical abnormalities, both as primary disorders and as the effects of other diseases on biochemical parameters in the blood, urine and other tissues.

Microbiology: the study of diseases from the perspective of isolating, identifying and treating infections by bacteria, fungi, viruses and parasites. Microbiology is often further divided into virology, bacteriology, and parasitology.

Immunopathology: The study of diseases through analysis of immune function, particularly identifying primary diseases of the immune system, as well as the effects of other diseases on the immune system.

A reflection of modern developments in cell biology, the new discipline of **molecular pathology,** is now emerging. Many diseases can now be defined by detection of molecular, rather than structural, abnormalities.

As specialist books now deal with hematology, chemical pathology, microbiology and immunopathology in great detail, this text presents only relevant aspects of these subjects, integrated into other chapters.

PATHOLOGY IS THE BASIS OF CLINICAL LABORATORY MEDICINE

Disease processes can have many effects, some of which are manifest as alterations in the cellular and biochemical composition of the blood. Frequently, the first manifestation of a disease process is not at its primary site, but takes the form of secondary effects. For example, in diabetes mellitus, although there is a primary abnormality in the pancreas, the diagnosis can be made by analysis of blood and urine glucose levels. Detection and analysis of similar secondary effects are of immense value in deducing the nature and site of underlying disease processes, and make a vital contribution to patient care. This is the basis of **diagnostic pathology**, increasingly being termed **laboratory medicine**.

To confirm or screen for disease the physician or surgeon sends samples from the patient to the pathology laboratory and asks for an appropriate analysis. The results, taken in conjunction with other investigations such as radiological examination, can pinpoint the site and likely nature of the disease process. If necessary, a tissue sample can be obtained from a diseased organ, and an accurate diagnosis established by histological examination. Two illustrative examples are shown in *Figs 1.3* and *1.4.*

Laboratory medicine is vital in medical and surgical practice

An early responsibility in medical and surgical training is to request relevant laboratory investigations to clarify the nature of disease in patients under your care. These investigations cover the whole range of laboratory medicine disciplines, the most common sample required being blood.

The development of techniques whereby small tissue samples (**biopsies**) can be obtained easily and painlessly from almost all areas of the body has had a huge impact on clinical medicine. There is now increasing reliance upon direct histological examination of abnormal cells, tissues and organs in establishing a diagnosis. For many diseases, current medical practice now revolves around accurate localization of an abnormality, using modern imaging methods (computerized tomography, magnetic resonance imaging and ultrasound scans), followed by direct sampling of the abnormal tissue by a guided biopsy method; the sampled tissue can then be examined by microbiological, histological, immunological, or biochemical techniques.

Good clinical practice requires:

- A knowledge of the systems pathology of each organ so that the range of disease processes likely to be causing an abnormality can be considered.
- A knowledge of the underlying basic pathology of each disease process, so that appropriate samples can be taken and relevant tests requested.
- An understanding of investigative techniques so that laboratory medicine results can be interpreted and a diagnosis established.

Pathology and laboratory medicine underpins much of clinical medical practice. This text is an introduction to pathology and laboratory medicine from a histopathological perspective. It offers an insight into the underlying basic pathology of the main disease processes and, through discussion of the systems pathology of each organ, provides a sound basis for clinical practice.

Pathological investigation in diagnosis – Case 1

HEMATOLOGY DEPARTMENT, UNIVERSITY HOSPITAL

Consultant/General Practitioner and patient location	Surname		Report no.	
Clinical details Weakness,lethargy and pallor ?anemic ?type	Forename		Date received	
	Age 63	Sex M	Hospital no.	
Specimen Blood - full blood count please				

HEMOGLOBIN	W.B.C.	PLATELETS	M.C.V.	M.C.H.	R.B.C.	P.C.V.	
7.0	5.6	650.0	57	16.5	4.24	0.242	
M 13.0-18.0 F 11.5-16.5 g/dl	4.0-11.0×10⁹/1	150-400×10⁹/1	76.99 fl	27-32 pg	M 4.5-6.5 F 3.8-5.8 ×10¹²/1	M 0.40-0.54 F 0.37-0.47	

	NEUTROPHILS	LYMPHOCYTES	MONOCYTES	EOSINOPHILS	BASOPHILS	METAM'S BANDS	MYELOCYTES	PROM'CYTES	BLASTS	NUCLEATED RBC
×10⁹/1	2.11	2.99	0.31	0.13	0.06	<-(Cell counter estimates)				
%	37.7	53.4	5.5	2.3	1.1					
×10⁹/1	2.0-7.5	1.5-4.0	0.2-0.8	0.04-0.4	0.01-0.1	RETICULOCYTES (25-85)		E.S.R.		mm/1hr

Marked hypochromia & microcytosis 'Pencil cells' present
Iron deficiency anemia

(a) SNOP: HEMATOLOGY   Date of report

CHEMICAL PATHOLOGY DEPARTMENT, UNIVERSITY HOSPITAL

Consultant/GP and patient location	Surname		Report no.	
Clinical details Anemic, iron deficiency & blood loss ?bleeding from GI tract	Forename		Date received	
	Age 63	Sex M	Hospital no.	
Specimen Feces - for occult blood				

Occult blood - positive

(b) SNOP: CHEMICAL PATHOLOGY   Date of report

HISTOPATHOLOGY DEPARTMENT, UNIVERSITY HOSPITAL

Consultant/GP and patient location	Surname		Report no.	
Clinical details Iron deficiency anemia bleeding from gut. Colonoscopy - ulcer in gut. Biopsied	Forename		Date received	
	Age 63	Sex M	Hospital no.	
Specimen Fragments of cecal ulcer				

Histology - Biopsy of cecal ulcer shows invasive, poorly
differentiated adenocarcinoma

(c) SNOP: HISTOPATHOLOGY   Date of report

Fig. 1.3 (a) A 63-year-old man complains of increasing weakness and lethargy. On examination he appears very pale, suggesting that he is anemic. The physician takes a blood sample for hematological analysis. The hemoglobin level is low, the cells are small (low MCV), and each red cell contains reduced amount of hemoglobin (low MCH). Red cell numbers are also reduced (low RBC). The low packed cell volume (PCV) reflects the reduced number of small red cells. These are the typical features of an iron deficiency anemia, which could be due to either inadequate iron intake or excessive blood loss. The high platelet count suggests that there has been recent blood loss. An increased number of reticulocytes would have supported this diagnosis, but the estimation was not performed.

Fig. 1.3 (b) On further questioning the patient admits that he occasionally passes very dark feces. A fecal sample is sent to the chemical pathology laboratory for analysis.

Fig. 1.3 (c,d) The patient is bleeding into his bowel, but where? Radiological examination by barium enema suggests an abnormality in the cecum. Using a colonoscope, the surgeon examines the full length of the colon and finds an ulcer with raised edges at the site of radiological abnormality in the cecum. Some samples of tissue are taken from the edges and floor of the ulcer, and sent to the histopathology laboratory for histological examination.

(d)

The underlying disease (colon cancer) has been traced, and treatment can begin immediately. At the time of presentation the patient had no major complaints about his bowel, and the diagnosis was established by thorough investigation of a secondary effect.

Pathological investigation in diagnosis – Case 2

CHEMICAL PATHOLOGY DEPARTMENT, UNIVERSITY HOSPITAL

Consultant/General Practitioner and patient location	Surname		Report no.
Clinical details Urine thick & frothy ?proteinuria Edema - ?low serum albumin	Forename		Date received
	Age 47	Sex F	Hospital no.
Specimen (A) Urine - for protein (B) Blood - for albumin			

(A) Urine - protein - 14.70g/save. Volume 1.5 litre/save

(B) Blood - albumin - 18g/litre (N=24-48)

a SNOP:	**CHEMICAL PATHOLOGY**	Date of report

Fig. 1.4 (a) A 47-year-old woman is admitted because of weakness, lethargy and swelling of fingers and feet. She mentions that her urine has been unusually 'thick' and very frothy. Her physician sends samples of urine and blood to the chemical pathology laboratory for analysis.

HISTOPATHOLOGY DEPARTMENT, UNIVERSITY HOSPITAL

Consultant/GP and patient location	Surname		Report no.
Clinical details Edema, proteinuria & hypoalbuminemia Nephrotic syndrome ?cause	Forename		Date received
	Age 47	Sex F	Hospital no.
Specimen Needle biopsy of kidney			

Paraffin sections	- 5 glomeruli, all showing diffuse basement membrane thickening and mesangial increase
Electron microscopy	- immune complex deposition in subepithelial, subendothelial, intramembranous and mesangial locations
Immunofluorescence	- granular deposition of IgG, IgM, IgA, C_3 and C1q
Conclusion	- Lupus glomerulonephritis, with a membranous pattern

b SNOP:	**HISTOPATHOLOGY**	Date of report

Fig. 1.4 (b) Armed with this evidence of severe protein loss in the urine, and a low serum albumin level, taken in conjunction with the clinical features, the physician knows that the patient suffers from the **nephrotic syndrome**. The primary lesion will be in the kidney, and its true nature requires further investigation. Needle biopsy of the kidney is performed, and the small kidney samples are sent to the histopathology laboratory for histological and electron microscopic examination. The locations of the immune complexes, and the pattern of immunofluorescence (demonstrating three types of immunoglobulin and two types of complement) are typical of glomerular involvement in systemic lupus erythematosus.

IMMUNOPATHOLOGY DEPARTMENT, UNIVERSITY HOSPITAL

Consultant/GP and patient location	Surname		Report no.
Clinical details Nephrotic syndrome Renal biopsy histology suggests SLE nephritis	Forename		Date received
	Age 47	Sex F	Hospital no.
Specimen Blood			

C_3 - 0.40g/l (N=0.63-1.19)
C_4 - 0.07g/l (N=0.11-0.43)
C3dg - 25units/ml (n=5-12)-grossly elevated
ANA   - 1:1600 (IgG class)
ENA   - Sm-positive
        Ro-negative
        La-negative
ds DNA - Crythidia Lucilliae-positive 1:80
         ELISA 1048iu/L-strong positive

The autoantibody profile is highly suggestive of SLE, and the hypocomplementemia indicates active disease.

c SNOP:	**IMMUNOPATHOLOGY**	Date of report

Fig. 1.4 (c) The report suggests that the kidney disease is secondary to a widespread immunological disease, **systemic lupus erythematosus** (see Chapter 25). The physician therefore sends a further blood sample to the immunopathology laboratory for confirmation of the diagnosis. The positive titer for double-stranded DNA is strongly suggestive of the diagnosis.

Et voila! The diagnosis is established, and treatment of this life-threatening disease can begin.

Cellular adaptations to disease

2

CELLS AS ADAPTABLE UNITS

Cells are constantly exposed to changes in their environment

Cells are constantly exposed to changes in their local environment as a result of normal physiological processes as well as abnormal conditions encountered in a disease. If cells were static and rigid systems, these changes in the cellular environment would profoundly affect the function of tissues, but there are homeostatic mechanisms which allow cells and tissues to cope with such **physiological stimuli**. Importantly, these mechanisms are brought into play not only in physiological situations, but also to limit damage in response to disease processes. When environmental changes lie outside an acceptable range of normality they can be termed **pathological stimuli**. The main causes of disease that lead to changes in the environment of cells are listed in *Fig. 2.1*.

This chapter will illustrate how cells can become modified as adaptive responses in disease. If cells cannot adapt they become damaged and die, the subject of Chapter 3.

Cells adapt to acceptable changes in their environment by modifying metabolism or growth pattern

To maintain normal function, cells have a physiological ability to adapt to acceptable environmental changes. Many of these modifications are **physiological metabolic adaptations**, and represent fine regulation of metabolic function not reflected in easily detectable changes in structure. For example:

- During periods of fasting, fatty acids are mobilized from adipose tissue to supply energy.
- During periods of relative calcium lack, calcium is mobilized from bone matrix by the activity of osteoclasts under the influence of parahormone.
- Following the administration of certain drugs (e.g. rifampin, an antimicrobial agent), hepatic microsomal enzymes are induced in cells to facilitate drug metabolism.

Other cell adaptations to environmental change are **physiological structural adaptations** caused by a change in the normal pattern of growth accompanied by detectable structural changes. These normal adaptive structural changes can be divided into three broad types:

- **Increased cellular activity** (increase in size or number of cells) usually results from increased functional demands on a tissue or from an increase in hormonal stimulation.
- **Decreased cellular activity** (reduction in size or number of cells) usually results from a reduction in hormonal stimulation of a tissue or from a decrease in functional demands.
- **Alteration of cell morphology** (change in cell differentiation) occurs when changes in the cellular environment cause an alteration in cell structure.

These adaptive changes in cell growth are part of a process termed **tissue remodeling**. This is an important concept in understanding gross structural changes in organs and tissues and involves both cells and the extracellular matrix to which cells are anchored.

Fig. 2.1 Causes of pathological stimuli

Type	Examples
Genetic	Gene defects, chromosomal defects
Nutritional	Deficiency or excess of dietary substances, e.g. iron, vitamins
Immune	Damage caused by the immune system, e.g. autoimmunity
Endocrine	Deficient or excessive hormone activity
Physical agents	Mechanical trauma, thermal damage, irradiation
Chemical agents	Toxicity due to many agents, e.g. heavy metals, solvents, drugs
Infective	Infection by viruses, bacteria, parasites, fungi and other organisms
Anoxia	Most commonly due to abnormal respiratory or circulatory function

THE CELL STRESS RESPONSE TO INJURY

Damaged cells produce proteins which protect against further damage

In response to some pathological stimuli, cells exhibit a series of metabolic changes known as the **cell stress response**, which is an important basic cellular mechanism that enables cells to survive environmental insults. Stressed cells turn down the genes coding for normal structural proteins (**housekeeping genes**) and show high levels of expression of genes coding for a set of proteins which have cell-organizing and protective functions (**cell stress genes**). Many of the cell stress proteins were originally described in response to experimental heat shock, hence a major group is termed the heat shock proteins (HSPs). The general terms 'heat shock protein' and 'cell stress protein' are synonymous.

Cell stress proteins are vital for cell viability

The stress proteins are expressed at low levels in normal cells, where they have important roles, but levels increase following exposure to damaging stimuli. Experimentally, a cell stress response can be induced in response to stimuli as diverse as heat, hypoxia, heavy metals, irradiation and viral infection. An indication of the fundamental biological importance of this cellular response is that the stress proteins exhibit a very high degree of inter-species conservation, with many of the stress proteins among the most conserved gene products in evolution. This evolutionary conservation suggest that the cell stress proteins are essential to cell survival, and their increased production in a cell stress response provides the extra stress proteins needed in pathological conditions.

Cell stress proteins are cytoprotective

The members of the HSP group of cell stress proteins are named according to size.

- The small heat shock proteins act as molecular chaperones, associating transiently with normal or damaged proteins to protect them from damage.
- **Ubiquitin** is an abundant protein in normal cells and has a role in removing old or damaged proteins by acting as a co-factor for proteolysis. Once ubiquitylated, such damaged proteins are recognized and degraded by a protease complex termed the proteasome (*Fig. 2.2*).

In certain cells which undergo chronic stress, permanent aggregates of abnormal cell constituents and ubiquitin form visible masses known as **inclusion bodies** within the cytoplasm. One example of this phenomenon is when liver cells are chronically exposed to alcohol and form masses of the intermediate filament cytokeratin and ubiquitin, visible as pink-stained inclusion bodies. These are eponymously termed **Mallory's hyaline**. Another example is the **Lewy body** in nerve cells (see pages 472 and 474). The formation of an inclusion body is believed to be a cytoprotective response and has been termed the **aggresomal response**.

Production of the cell stress proteins following exposure to a damaging stimulus is a rapid response that minimizes cell damage and ensures cell viability. Cell stress proteins can only protect against certain levels of damage, more severe stimuli leading to cell degeneration or death (see Chapter 3).

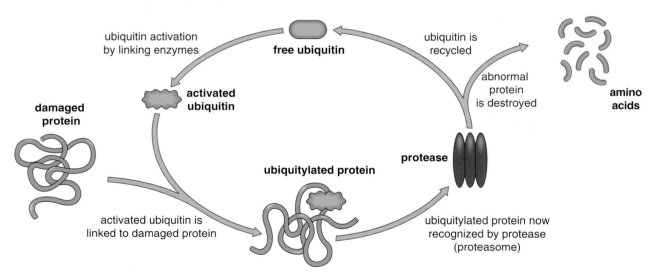

Fig. 2.2 The function of ubiquitin in cell stress. Damaged proteins are recognized by a series of enzymes which covalently link the damaged protein to ubiquitin to form a ubiquitylated protein. Ubiquitylation marks the protein for degradation into small peptides or amino acids by a cytosolic protease termed a proteasome.

ADAPTIVE RESPONSE IN DISEASE

Cells respond to damaging stimuli by extending adaptive processes

As well as mounting an immediate cell stress response, cells can adapt to damaging stimuli, becoming modified to achieve a new, steady state of metabolism and structure that better equips them for survival in the abnormal environment. Cells may adapt to a pathological (disease) stimulus by extending the three normal physiological adaptive responses:

- Increased cellular activity.
- Decreased cellular activity.
- Alteration of cell morphology.

Inability to adapt successfully to an environmental change leads to failure of cellular function and may result in sub-lethal cellular damage or cell death, as discussed in Chapter 3. This may be because the cell involved is particularly susceptible to the pathological stimulus, or because the stimulus is so severe that it overwhelms the cell stress response and other adaptive reactions.

Different cell types show different degrees of susceptibility to environmental changes. Some cells, such as cerebral neurons, are highly sensitive to changes in their environment and die rapidly when conditions are outside the physiological norm. Others, such as fibroblasts, are extremely resistant to damage and can survive severe metabolic change, for example complete deprivation of oxygen, for relatively long periods of time without apparent harm.

Change in cellular growth pattern is an adaptive response in disease

Cells can adapt to certain pathological stimuli by altering their pattern of growth. This may be reflected in changes in the size, number or differentiation of cells in affected tissue. The terms used to describe such changes are outlined in *Fig. 2.3*.

Increased functional demand on a tissue can be met by increase in cell number (hyperplasia) as well as by increase in cell size (hypertrophy)

Certain organs or tissues may adapt to a disease process by increasing functional cell mass. The effect of this is to increase the functional capacity of the organ. There are two mechanisms that lead to an increase in cell mass (*Fig. 2.4*).

Hyperplasia is an increase in the number of cells in a tissue caused by increased cell division. As this type of change can occur only in tissues that have the capacity for cell division, hyperplasia is not an adaptive response seen in skeletal muscle, cardiac muscle or nerve cells, which are non-dividing cell populations. Hormonal influences are important in this growth response.

Hypertrophy is an increase in the size of existing cells, accompanied by an increase in their functional capacity. Cell enlargement is brought about by increased synthesis of structural components, associated with accelerated activity of cellular metabolism and rises in levels of RNA and organelles required for protein synthesis. Hypertrophy is particularly seen as a response to increased demand in tissues composed of cells which are unable to divide (skeletal and cardiac muscle).

Although hypertrophy and hyperplasia may occur independently of each other, they are often seen together in an organ or tissue (combined hypertrophy and hyperplasia).

An organ or tissue that has undergone hypertrophy or hyperplasia is associated with an increase in its size and weight. This can be detected in some organs by noting a physical increase in size, either on physical examination or on imaging.

Increased cell mass in a tissue can result from physiological stimuli

An increase in functional cell mass through hypertrophy and hyperplasia may be physiological.

- The thyroid gland enlarges in pregnancy owing to the stimulus of pregnancy-associated high levels of thyroid-stimulating hormone (TSH) on thyroid epithelial cells (*hyperplasia*).
- In athletes, skeletal muscle fibers increase in size (*hypertrophy*) in response to exercise and increased metabolic demands (*Fig. 2.5*).
- Under the influence of endocrine stimulation in pregnancy, breast epithelial cells and myometrial smooth muscle cells both increase in size and number (*hypertrophy and hyperplasia*) (*Fig. 2.6*).
- Under the influence of ovarian endocrine stimulation in the menstrual cycle, endometrial glands increase in size as a result of proliferation of cells (*hyperplasia*) (*Fig. 2.7*).

Fig. 2.3 Changes in growth pattern of cells	
Change in size of cells	
Atrophy	Reduction in the size of cells
Hypertrophy	Increase in the size of cells
Change in number of cells	
Involution	Decrease in the number of cells
Hyperplasia	Increase in the number of cells
Change in differentiation of cells	
Metaplasia	Stable change to another cell type

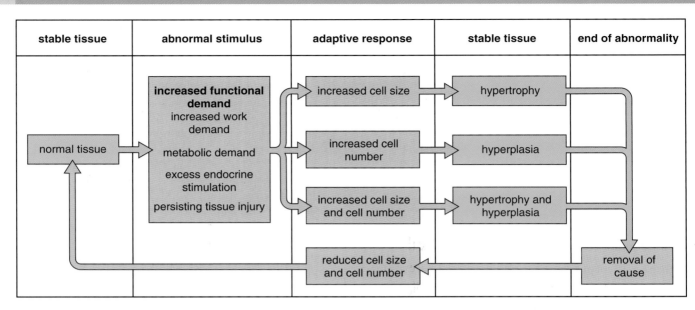

stable tissue	abnormal stimulus	adaptive response	stable tissue	end of abnormality
normal tissue	**increased functional demand** increased work demand metabolic demand excess endocrine stimulation persisting tissue injury	increased cell size	hypertrophy	
		increased cell number	hyperplasia	
		increased cell size and cell number	hypertrophy and hyperplasia	
		reduced cell size and cell number		removal of cause

Fig. 2.4 Adaptive responses resulting in increased tissue mass. Increased functional demand or endocrine stimulation are what usually cause hypertrophy and hyperplasia. These new patterns of growth are stable while the causative stimulus persists, but once it is removed the tissue returns to a normal pattern of growth.

Fig. 2.5 Hypertrophy of skeletal muscle in response to exercise. Hypertrophy in the absence of hyperplasia is typically seen in muscle where the stimulus is an increased demand for work. Taken at the same magnification, (a) shows muscle fibers in transverse section from the soleus muscle of a normal 50-year-old man, and (b) shows fibers from the same muscle in a veteran marathon runner. Note the dramatic increase in the size of the fibers in response to the demands of marathon running.

Increased cell mass in a tissue can result from pathological stimuli. Increased functional cell mass also occurs as a response in disease states.

- If the serum calcium is abnormally low, the parathyroid glands increase the number of parahormone-secreting cells (*hyperplasia*).
- If the aortic valve outflow is severely narrowed by disease (see pages 183 and 186), the muscle of the left ventricle of the heart responds with an increase in the size of cardiac muscle cells (*hypertrophy*) to overcome the resistance to flow and ensure an adequate blood pressure (*Fig. 2.8*). This is also seen in myocardial muscle when systemic hypertension causes an increased demand on cardiac function (see pages 10 and 11) such that left ventricular hypertrophy is a feature of hypertension.
- Obstruction of the colon by a tumor causes an increase in size (*hypertrophy*) of the smooth muscle cells of the bowel wall proximal to the obstruction.
- Estrogen produced by certain ovarian tumors causes abnormal proliferation of the endometrium (*hyperplasia*), which increases in bulk and leads to an abnormal pattern of menstrual bleeding.
- If a kidney is removed or ceases to function, the remaining healthy kidney increases in size and weight to compensate for the loss. The process of hyperplasia leads to enlargement of structures such as glomeruli, and is often termed **compensatory hyperplasia**.

Fig. 2.6 Hyperplasia and hypertrophy of myometrium in pregnancy. On the left is a normal uterus showing the normal mass of smooth muscle in its wall. On the right is a uterus from a recently pregnant woman, in which the striking increase in mass of smooth muscle is evident. At a cellular level, this is due to both hyperplasia and hypertrophy of uterine smooth muscle.

Fig. 2.7 Hyperplasia of endometrium in response to estrogen. (a) Early proliferative endometrium. (b) Secretory phase endometrium. Micrograph (a) shows endometrial glands following the menstrual phase. Micrograph (b) shows that in response to estrogen secreted as part of the normal menstrual cycle there has been an increase in the number of cells in each gland, resulting in a much higher volume fraction of gland relative to stroma. This is an example of physiological hyperplasia.

Fig. 2.8 Hypertrophy of cardiac muscle in response to valve disease. (a) Transverse slices of a normal heart and a heart with hypertrophy of the left ventricle. (b) Histology of cardiac muscle from a normal heart. (c) Histology of cardiac muscle from a hypertrophied heart. The upper macroscopic specimen (a) demonstrates the normal thickness of the left ventricular wall (L) for comparison with the greatly thickened wall (T) in the lower specimen, taken from a heart in which severe narrowing of the aortic valve caused resistance to systolic ventricular emptying. The increased mass of the left ventricle is due to enlargement of cardiac muscle cells as a result of hypertrophy. This can be seen by comparing the diameter of fibers from the normal heart (b) with those from the diseased heart (c). Note that the size of nuclei in the hypertrophied cardiac muscle is also increased; it has been found that such nuclei are frequently polyploid (i.e. contain several times the normal quantity of DNA).

Hyperplasia may not be uniform and sometimes occurs as nodules

Hyperplasia may not occur uniformly throughout a tissue; instead, nodules of excessive cell growth (hyperplastic nodules) develop between areas of normal tissue, giving rise to the term **nodular hyperplasia**. Most examples of nodular hyperplasia occur in tissues in which cells are responding to a trophic hormone. It is likely that the hyperplasia seen in these conditions is a result of a disturbance in the hormone responsiveness of the target tissue. Nodular hyperplasia is seen most commonly in the prostate gland (*Fig. 2.9*), thyroid gland, adrenal gland and the breast.

Hyperplasia or hypertrophy can revert to normal growth

A key feature of hyperplasia is that the altered pattern of growth ceases following removal of the causative stimulus, and the tissue reverts to its normal state. For example, if a person stops working out, their muscle mass returns to normal. If a diseased heart valve is replaced, a hypertrophied ventricle can return to a more normal size. This feature distinguishes hyperplasia from neoplasia (the formation of tumors such as cancer, which will be discussed in Chapter 6), in which there is excessive cell growth that does not regress on removal of the causal stimulus.

Reduced functional demand leads to reduction in cell number or cell size

When the mass of functioning cells in a tissue becomes reduced, the tissue is said to have undergone **atrophy**. There are two mechanisms of reduction (*Fig. 2.10*):

- **A reduction in the size and volume of individual cells**, associated with reduction in cellular metabolism and reduced synthesis of structural proteins. Physical reduction in the size of established cells is achieved through an increase in the catabolism of cytosolic structural proteins by the ubiquitin–proteosome

Fig. 2.9 Nodular hyperplasia of the prostate gland. (a) Normal prostate gland. (b) Nodular hyperplasia of prostate gland. These macroscopic specimens are transverse slices through the prostate gland. Note the nodules (N) in (b), which are the result of nodular hyperplasia. This is an extremely common condition in elderly men, resulting in compression of the prostatic urethra (U) and difficulty with micturition.

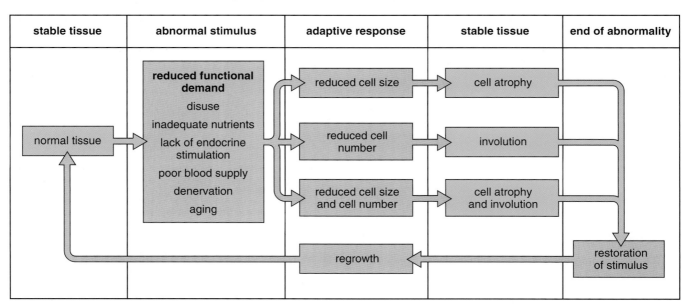

Fig. 2.10 Adaptive responses resulting in reduced tissue mass. Reduced functional demand, reduction in trophic stimuli, or reduction in nutrients are the usual stimuli that cause involution or cell atrophy. Atrophic or involuted tissues are stable patterns of growth that persist while the lack of stimulation or demand causing them remains. However, once appropriate stimulation or demand returns, the tissue reverts to a normal pattern of growth.

system, and by the removal of organelles by autophagy (*Fig. 2.11*).

- **Death of established cells** in an organ or tissue, causing a reduction in the number of functioning cells. This is brought about by the activation of specific cell systems which act to bring about cellular dissolution and elimination from tissues, sometimes called programmed cell death. The best studied example of this type of cell death is termed **apoptosis** (see *Fig. 3.12* and pages 28–34). **Involution** is a form of physiological atrophy involving apoptosis of cells.

In many tissues that have undergone cellular atrophy, a brown pigment called **lipofuscin** accumulates within the shrunken cells. This pigment, composed of degenerate lipid material in secondary lysosomes, is produced by breakdown of the cell membranes and organelles through autophagy (*Fig. 2.12*). Lipofuscin builds up, particularly in the atrophic myocardial fibers of elderly people, giving rise to macroscopically evident brown coloration of the myocardium (**brown atrophy**).

Atrophy is usually associated with a reduction in the size and weight of an organ or tissue. In some instances cell mass lost through cellular atrophy or involution is replaced by either adipose or fibrous tissue. This replacement tissue frequently appears as brightly eosinophilic material called **hyaline**. As a consequence of this replacement by support tissues, the macroscopic size of an organ or tissue may be preserved despite the loss of specialized parenchymal cells and hence of specialized function.

Autophagy and cell atrophy

Fig. 2.11 In cellular atrophy, structural proteins and organelles of a cell are destroyed, with a parallel reduction in the size and functional capacity of the cell. This is an adaptive response as it allows the cell to survive in adverse conditions by reducing its metabolic overheads. Cell constituents are eliminated by a process of autophagy: unwanted cell organelles become enwrapped by membrane derived from the endoplasmic reticulum (ER) (a), forming an autophagic body (b) which subsequently fuses with vesicles containing lysosomal acid hydrolases (c). The action of the hydrolases brings about degradation of the organelles. Cells that are actively undergoing atrophy can be seen ultrastructurally to contain numerous autophagic vacuoles. These bodies become electron dense, but have internal tubular or vesicular profiles (derived from membrane-fusion events) that have earned them the alternative name of tubulovesicular bodies (d). Late autophagic bodies (e) become more electron dense and may form residual bodies (f) containing lamellar undigested lipid-rich cell material called lipofuscin (see *Fig. 2.13*).

Fig. 2.12 Lipofuscin in cellular atrophy, seen in the cardiac muscle of an elderly patient. Cellular atrophy is associated with autophagy of cellular structural elements and a consequent reduction in size of the cell. One effect of this is that indigestible material, principally phospholipids, accumulates in lysosomal-derived bodies. This material can be seen on light microscopy as yellow-brown granules (L) called lipofuscin, here shown in the myocardium of a 90-year-old woman. Ultrastructural examination of lipofuscin reveals it to consist of electron-dense material within membrane-bound granules of varying size, which often have myelin-like figures. Lipofuscin commonly accompanies the cellular atrophy that occurs in many tissues with aging, and thus is often called **wear and tear pigment**.

Fig. 2.13 Involution of the thymus. (a) Thymus in a child. (b) Thymus in an adult. Micrograph (a) shows the dense cellularity of a child's thymus gland, heavily populated by lymphoid cells forming thymic cortex (C) and medulla (M) with dividing septa (S). In contrast, in the adult (b) the gland undergoes involution associated with a dramatic reduction in size and, as with many examples of involution, becomes largely replaced by adipose tissue (A).

Reduction in cell mass may be physiological

Many physiological processes require that a tissue response is switched off as part of a reduction in functional demand. This is seen particularly when the mass of a target organ is maintained by endocrine stimulation which becomes reduced, for example when the thyroid gland returns to its normal size after the physiological hyperplasia induced by puberty or pregnancy. In old age, a combination of factors such as reduced physical activity and changes in the pattern of endocrine secretion leads to reduced size (atrophy) of many organs and tissues. Examples of physiological atrophy or involution are:

* The thymus gland involutes after childhood (*Fig. 2.13*).
* The myometrium involutes post partum.
* With reduced activity in old age, skeletal muscle fibers decrease in size (*aging atrophy*).
* In the aging parathyroid gland, hormone-secreting cells diminish in number and are replaced by fat cells.
* The testis undergoes atrophy as a result of reduced gonadotrophic stimulation in old age.

Reduction in cell mass occurs in some pathological states

Many disease processes lead to a reduction in functional demand, hormonal or nervous stimulation, or nutrition of tissues; atrophy or involution occurs as an adaptive response.

* Skeletal muscle fibers in the leg undergo cellular atrophy if the leg is immobilized, for example when splinting is used in the treatment of a fracture (*disuse atrophy*).
* Gradual reduction in blood supply to a tissue results in loss of functional cells through involution, as well as through cellular atrophy (*ischemic atrophy*).

* Damage to axons supplying muscle causes atrophy of affected muscle fibers (*denervation atrophy*) (*Fig. 2.14*).
* After trauma to the spinal cord, skeletal muscle fibers supplied by affected spinal nerve roots undergo atrophy (*denervation atrophy*)
* Following ablation of the pituitary gland by surgery, the cells of the adrenal cortex decrease in size and number owing to lack of ACTH stimulation (*Fig. 2.15*).

Developmental causes of reduced cell mass are termed 'agenesis', 'aplasia' and 'hypoplasia'

Certain developmental defects result in abnormally small organs or complete failure of development of organs or tissues. Such examples must be distinguished from atrophy and involution, in which the tissue or organ had originally developed in a normal fashion (*Fig. 2.16*).

* Complete failure to produce the embryonic cell mass destined to form an organ is termed **agenesis**.
* Failure of a correctly formed embryonic cell mass to differentiate into a developed organ is termed **aplasia**.
* If organ-specific structures develop correctly but are abnormally small, the organ is termed **hypoplastic**.
* If organ-specific structures develop correctly but are histoanatomically abnormally configured, the organ is termed **dysgenetic**.

Tissues may adapt to environmental stimuli by a change in cell differentiation termed 'metaplasia'

Certain long-standing environmental stimuli render the environment unsuitable for some specialized cell types and, as an adaptive response, the proliferating cells change their pattern of differentiation. These cells can adapt to a change

Fig. 2.14 Atrophy of skeletal muscle with denervation. (a) Normal muscle. (b) Denervated muscle. Micrograph (a) shows normal skeletal muscle fibers. In micrograph (b) damage to many of the axons in the main nerve supplying the muscle has caused atrophy of fibers (A) which had been innervated by now-damaged axons. Fibers are small and angulated. With time, axon sprouting may reconnect some denervated fibers, which then return to normal size.

Fig. 2.15 Atrophy of the adrenal gland. (a) Normal adrenal. (b) Atrophic adrenal. Specimen (a) is a slice of normal gland, in which yellow cortex (**C**) can be distinguished from the small amount of grey medulla (**M**); (b) is from a patient who had surgical ablation of the pituitary gland, leading to lack of ACTH causing a reduction in the size of the adrenal gland, specifically affecting the cortex.

in environment by differentiating to a new, mature, stable type of cell, which better equips them to withstand an environmental stress. This process is termed **metaplasia**, and examples are summarized in *Fig. 2.17*.

- In the bronchi, under the influence of chronic irritation by cigarette smoke, the normal ciliated columnar mucus-secreting respiratory epithelium is replaced by squamous epithelium (*squamous metaplasia*).
- In the cervix the normal columnar epithelium of the lower endocervix changes to squamous epithelium in response to exposure to the acid vaginal environment (*squamous metaplasia*).
- In the urinary bladder the normal transitional epithelium may be replaced by squamous epithelium in response to chronic irritation by bladder calculi or infection (*squamous metaplasia*) (*Fig. 2.18*).
- The esophageal squamous epithelium is replaced by columnar epithelium in response to exposure to gastric acid in cases of gastric reflux (see page 249).

Metaplasia most commonly occurs in epithelial tissues, but may also be seen elsewhere. For example, areas of fibrous tissue exposed to chronic trauma may form bone (*osseous metaplasia*). In many settings, metaplasia coexists with hyperplasia; for example, the squamous epithelium that arises by metaplasia in response to calculi in the bladder may also be hyperplastic.

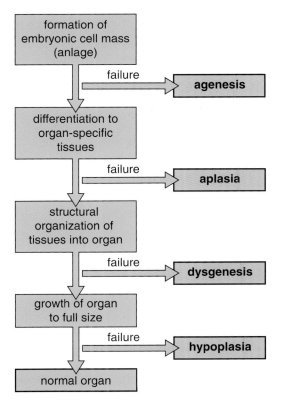

Fig. 2.16 Developmental causes of reduced cell mass.

Fig. 2.17 Examples of metaplasia

Original tissue	Stimulus	Metaplastic tissue
Ciliated columnar epithelium of bronchial tree	Cigarette smoke	Squamous epithelium
Transitional epithelium of bladder	Trauma of bladder calculus	Squamous epithelium
Columnar epithelium in gland ducts	Trauma of calculus	Squamous epithelium
Fibrocollagenous tissue	Chronic trauma	Bone (osseous) tissue
Esophageal squamous epithelium	Gastric acid	Columnar epithelium
Columnar glandular epithelium	Vitamin A deficiency	Squamous epithelium

Fig. 2.18 Squamous metaplasia in urinary bladder. The transitional epithelium of the urinary bladder (T) has become severely traumatized by a bladder stone (calculus), not seen in this micrograph. In response, squamous metaplasia has occurred, with replacement of the normal transitional epithelium (T) by stratified squamous epithelium (S). Squamous metaplasia also occurs in the bladder when there is chronic irritation by the parasitic infection schistosomiasis. In such cases the squamous epithelium is better suited to withstand the new environment than is the native transitional urothelial epithelium.

Adaptive responses in disease occur only with tolerable environmental changes

The adaptive responses of hyperplasia, hypertrophy, atrophy, involution and metaplasia occur only if the damaging stimulus is tolerable to the affected cells. Failure to adapt leads to cell damage and, if the stimulus is severe or prolonged, may result in cell death. The relationships between these outcomes are summarized diagrammatically in *Fig. 2.19.*

> ## Key Facts
> ### Cell adaptation
>
> - Cells are adaptable within physiological limits.
> - Cells can respond to injury by producing cell stress proteins, which protect from damage and help in recovery.
> - Increased demands are met by hypertrophy and hyperplasia.
> - Reduced demand is met by atrophy.
> - Cell loss from tissues can be achieved by programmed cell death (apoptosis).
> - Tissues can adapt to demand by a change in differentiation known as metaplasia.

CELL BIOLOGY OF GROWTH ADAPTATION

Cell adaptation is influenced by growth factors accompanied by altered gene expression

The molecular signaling pathways involved in the adaptive responses of hyperplasia, hypertrophy and metaplasia are gradually being understood, but as yet this understanding is incomplete. There is increasing recognition that cell growth is under the control of various **growth factors**, which act upon specific cell-surface receptors that are then linked to internal cell signaling pathways.

Growth factor receptors, many of which trigger secondary messenger systems through having tyrosine kinase activity, modulate transcription regulation and thereby directly affect the processes of gene regulation. Alterations in the relative concentrations of growth factors, in the expression of growth-factor receptors, in the activity of cell signaling

Fig. 2.19 Summary of tissue response to environmental change. Adaptive responses allow cells to survive in the face of a change in the cellular environment. Failure to adapt is associated with cell damage or cell death.

pathways or transcription regulatory systems can result in altered cell growth.

For example, hyperplasia may be caused by a local increase in the concentration of a growth factor, or by an increase in expression of growth-factor receptors on cells, or by upregulation of a cell signaling system. It is clear that these factors have synergistic actions in promoting or regulating growth. Factors that inhibit cell growth have also been recognized in animal models, but are less well characterized in humans.

Increasingly, such growth factors are being manufactured by recombinant genetic techniques, and attempts are being made to administer them therapeutically. The finding that ciliary neuronotropic growth factor can prevent the death of nerve cells in animal models of neurodegenerative disease offers the exciting prospect of preventing certain neurodegenerative diseases in humans. In cases where the bone marrow has been suppressed or deprived of normal levels of growth factor, the use of recombinant erythropoietin to induce hyperplasia of the red cell compartment of bone marrow has also achieved encouraging results, e.g. preventing anemia in chronic renal failure.

Colony-stimulating factors, involved in the control of cell growth of blood cells, are being used to help recovery of bone marrow function in patients who have received chemotherapy.

Unfortunately, important side-effects of systemic administration of some growth factors have included fever, loss of weight, loss of appetite, and hypotension – a reflection of the diverse effects of these factors, not limited to regulation of growth. It is likely that such systemic side effects will limit many of the hoped-for therapeutic applications for these factors.

The result of cellular activation by growth factors is the alteration of gene expression in cells. Many of the genes that are involved in control of cell growth and activated in cellular adaptive changes are also **proto-oncogenes**, and are implicated in the disorganization of cell growth that is the hallmark of neoplasia (development of cancer), discussed in Chapter 6.

Stem cells are probably involved in metaplasia

It is possible that one differentiated cell type directly turns into another mature type of cell leading to metaplasia, a process termed **transdifferentiation**. Although there are some arguments supporting the idea of transdifferentiation, more support lies with the idea that local stem cells that would normally form one cell type are instead stimulated to form another cell type.

Whether metaplasia develops through transdifferentiation or via stem cells, molecular systems must be activated that result in a change in cell fate.

At present it is unclear whether gene activation, gene silencing or a combination of the two is responsible for metaplasia in several examples that have been studied in detail. Those interested in this area should check the literature on one of the most studied forms of metaplasia, the formation of columnar epithelium in the esophagus in Barrett's esophagus. Understanding how cell populations regulate differentiation is becoming important in several diseases where one cell lineage appears to 'stop,' leading to deficiency of a specialized cell type within a tissue; for example, part of the conjunctiva of the eye may become deficient in mucus-secreting cells.

Models of metaplasia

There is interest in factors that regulate metaplasia. The pancreas has been studied in animal models seeking treatment for type I diabetes. Transdifferentiation patterns have been characterized and signalling pathways discovered. Dexamethasone induces pancreatic differentiation to hepatocytes, whereas epidermal growth factor induces exocrine–endocrine transdifferentiation.

Chronic obstructive pulmonary disease as a clinical example of hyperplasia and metaplasia

Chronic obstructive pulmonary disease (COPD) is a common condition and in the vast majority of cases is linked to cigarette smoking (see Chapter 11).

It has been proposed that a combination of toxic agents in cigarette smoke, cytokines secreted by local inflammatory cells, secretion of local proteases, and factors derived from local infecting organisms (bacterial and viral) stimulate cellular secondary messenger systems and lead to cell proliferation and changes in cell differentiation within the epithelium lining the airways.

In the lung airways, as in other tissues, epithelial cells are constantly being lost and replaced. New cells are derived from local adult stem cells that are capable of differentiating into adult cell types. Such adult stem cells have a restricted potential for differentiation and are not multipotential. The altered environment caused by cigarette smoking is believed to change the balance between cell loss, cell proliferation and cell differentiation at the level of the local stem cell populations in the airways. Some factors may also cause epigenetic changes to stem cells, resulting in an irreversible commitment to a new line of differentiation or pattern of growth.

The resulting structural changes seen in the airways in COPD include generalized epithelial hyperplasia, hyperplasia of mucous secretory cells, and squamous metaplasia of the normal columnar epithelium (*Fig. 20.20*).

- An important clinical effect of these changes is oversecretion of mucus, which is linked to the hyperplasia of mucus-secreting cells. Mucus becomes retained in the airways, partly because the proportion of cells bearing cilia is reduced, some lining cells now being metaplastic squamous cells. The mucus secretion gives rise to a defining clinical feature, seen in many patients with COPD, of a persistent cough, productive of mucus on most days of the year.
- Retention and stagnation of the abnormally produced mucus increases the risk of developing secondary bacterial infections of the lung, another feature of patients with COPD.
- Reduction in the effective lumen from increased wall thickness of airways (epithelial hyperplasia) and mucous plugging leads to functional airways obstruction that can be measured by a reduced peak flow or FEV_1/VC ratio on spirometry.

Fig. 2.20 Pathology of COPD. The normal airway is transformed in COPD by a combination of hyperplasia and metaplasia.

Cell injury and death 3

There is only a small number of stereotyped responses to cell injury

When exposed to injurious stimuli such as extremes of cold, heat, oxygen tension, changes in pH, or deprivation of vital nutrients, cells have only a limited repertoire of responses. One of the simplest of these is **cell shut-down**. This response is initiated rapidly (within a few minutes) after injury and is usually reversible once the injurious agent is removed or neutralized. Cell shut-down results in suppression of protein, RNA and DNA synthesis, and the inhibition of many enzyme-catalyzed reactions. Another potentially reversible response is activation of the **ubiquitin–proteasome system** (see page 8). This response leads to proteolytic digestion of cellular constituents and depletion of cytoplasmic volume, resulting in **cell atrophy**. A component part of proteasome activation involves the encapsulation of organelles and other cellular constituents within intracytoplasmic membranes that are subsequently fused with lysosomes, a process known as **autophagy** (see *Fig. 2.11*). This process relies on a functional microtubular transport system, defects in which can result in the accumulation of unwanted cellular debris.

Pathological cell death is due to irreversible cell injury

If the insult is more severe, exposure of cells to damaging stimuli often results in pathological cell death. Cell death can also occur as a response to exogenous agents such as ionizing radiation or exposure to toxins or drugs, the latter being referred to as **xenobiotics**. Cells can also be fatally injured as a consequence of infection, whether bacterial, fungal or viral.

Cell death may occur via two fundamentally different processes:

- Certain damaging stimuli, particularly those mediated by the immune system and cytokines, cause cell death by switching on **apoptosis** (see *Fig. 3.12*), a form of **programmed cell death**. This type of response is of great importance in disease and is discussed later in the chapter.
- Other types of damaging stimuli impair key cellular systems, causing dysfunction outside an adaptable range, after which cell death occurs by a process termed **necrosis**.

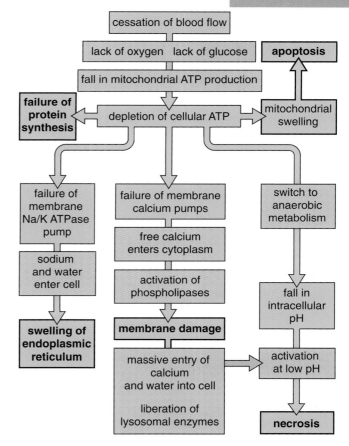

Fig. 3.1 Cellular response to ischemia. ATP production by mitochondria relies on an adequate supply of oxygen and of energy substrates such as glucose. Mitochondrial function is therefore compromised soon after failure of blood supply, resulting in failure of production of ATP. One consequence of lack of ATP is failure of ATP-dependent membrane pumps, which normally pump sodium (and with it water) out of cells. Failure of membrane ion pumps leads to accumulation of sodium and water in the cell cytoplasm, with disruption of internal membrane systems. Failure of internal membrane pumps also allows free calcium to enter the cytosol, where it activates many destructive enzyme systems. Structural damage to internal membranes and the cytoskeleton, coupled with lack of ATP, leads to impairment of key synthetic pathways, including those of protein synthesis. Rupture of lysosomes and intracellular liberation of powerful hydrolytic enzymes, active at a low pH, brings about further cellular dissolution.

Molecular mechanisms in damaged cells

ATP loss causes failure of biosynthesis and ion pumps

If cells become hypoxic or mitochondria are directly damaged, they cannot produce adequate ATP. The capacity of cells for anaerobic production of ATP is limited by accumulation of lactate and is usually soon exhausted. Lack of ATP causes failure of membrane pumps, probably contributing to swelling of internal membrane systems in cells, seen as so-called 'cloudy swelling.' There is also failure of many biosynthetic processes, most of which require ATP.

Cytosolic free calcium is a potent destructive agent

The normal concentration of calcium in the cytosol is very low and there are finely tuned regulatory systems to ensure that this is not disturbed. Free calcium is used by secondary messenger systems to activate a variety of cytosolic enzymes:

- Protein kinases which bring about phosphorylation of other proteins.
- Phospholipases, which can attack membrane lipids.
- Calpain, a protease which can cause disassembly of cytoskeletal proteins in cells.

Calcium is usually rapidly removed from the cytosol by ATP-dependent calcium pumps. In normal cells calcium is bound to buffering proteins, such as calbindin or parvalbumin, and is contained in the endoplasmic reticulum (ER) as well as in mitochondria. If there is abnormal permeability of calcium-ion channels, direct damage to membranes, depletion of ATP, or damage to mitochondria, calcium concentrations in the cytosol increase. If this cannot be buffered or pumped out of cells, uncontrolled enzyme activation takes place, with further damaging consequences. It has become evident that uncontrolled entry of calcium into the cytosol (*Fig. 3.2*) is an important final common pathway in many causes of cell death.

Reactive oxygen metabolites damage cells

In all cells, highly reactive oxygen metabolites are constantly generated. Because they are potentially damaging to cells, they are constantly scavenged by protective systems, the integrity of which, in turn, is dependent upon an adequate nutrient supply (*Fig. 3.3*).

Fig. 3.2 Cytosolic free calcium is a potent destructive agent.

Fig. 3.3 Reactive oxygen metabolites damage cells.

▶ The main scavenging systems are:

- Antioxidants such as vitamin E.
- Glutathione peroxidase.
- Superoxide dismutase.
- Catalase.

The most important of the reactive oxygen species are generated when oxygen is reduced to water, and most are created by systems involved in electron and oxygen transport:

- Superoxide anion (O_2^-).
- Hydroxyl radical (OH^-).
- Hydrogen peroxide (H_2O_2).

Certain generative reactions are catalyzed by the presence of free iron in cells, which is therefore potentially damaging.

Another important source of reactive oxygen species is xanthine, which accumulates in hypoxic tissues as a metabolite of ATP. In hypoxic conditions, accumulated xanthine can be oxidized by the enzyme xanthine oxidase to generate reactive oxygen species.

Reactive free radicals can also be produced as intermediates in the metabolism of certain toxins (e.g. carbon tetrachloride) and drugs (e.g. paracetamol/acetaminophen), by irradiation, and by neutrophil leukocytes as part of the mechanism for bacterial killing. These reactive species have several damaging effects:

- Peroxidation of lipids in cell membranes takes place, causing membrane permeability.
- Thiol groups in proteins are attacked. Certain critical proteins are then damaged, for example membrane Na/K ATPase pumps.
- DNA strands become fragmented.

- Mitochondria become depleted of NADPH and liberate free calcium into the cytosol.

Following ischemia, cells become depleted of energy, but reactive oxygen species do not develop as there is no oxygen in the tissues. If, as a consequence of re-establishing a blood supply, tissues are reperfused, huge amounts of reactive oxygen species are generated, both by mitochondria and by xanthine oxidase. Depleted energy-dependent scavenging mechanisms are overwhelmed, and extensive cell damage and death ensue.

This is the basis of so-called reperfusion necrosis: tissue necrosis takes place, not on cessation of blood supply, but on re-establishment. For this reason the xanthine oxidase inhibitor drug allopurinol has been used clinically in attempts to limit the extent of cardiac muscle necrosis following myocardial infarction, thought to be mediated by reactive oxygen species on reperfusion.

Membrane and cytoskeletal damage

The integrity of the cell membrane is essential for cell survival following damage. Direct damage to cell membranes is a primary event in immune-mediated injury, for example when complement activation leads to the formation of the membrane attack complex resulting in transmembrane pores, allowing influx of calcium into the target cell. In energy-depleted cells there is failure of biosynthesis of new membrane phospholipids; depletion of phospholipids also takes place when phospholipases are activated by free calcium, and membrane damage is inevitable. In addition, calcium-activated proteases destroy the cytoskeletal bracing of cell membranes by demolishing cytoskeletal link proteins, rendering cells abnormally fragile under contractile or osmotic stresses.

Key Facts
Cell injury

- The main targets for cell injury are cell membranes, mitochondria, cytoskeleton and cellular DNA.
- Because of interdependence, damage to one cellular system leads to secondary damage to others.
- Reactive oxygen metabolites are extremely harmful to cells and are produced on reperfusion after ischemia.

- ATP loss causes failure of biosynthesis and membrane pumps.
- Free calcium in the cytosol activates intracellular enzymes and may cause cell death.

Severe cell injury damages key cellular functions

Several interdependent cell components are primary targets for damaging stimuli:

- Cell membranes.
- Mitochondria.
- Cytoskeleton.
- Cellular DNA.

Because of interdependence, damage to one system leads to secondary damage to others, and ultimately, cell death occurs when a threshold of accumulated damage is passed. One example, which illustrates the concept of a cascade of accumulated damage, is seen in cells that are subject to lack of oxygen and nutrients owing to failure of blood supply (ischemia) (see *Fig. 3.1*).

- Primary impairment of mitochondrial energy production is due mainly to lack of oxygen (hypoxia) and glucose (hypoglycemia), but may also be caused by toxins, for example cyanide, which directly inhibit cytochrome oxidase.
- Primary cell membrane injury is due mainly to free radical-mediated damage, immune-mediated damage (particularly via the complement system), and direct actions of bacterial toxins.

Molecular mechanisms that are considered important in cell death are discussed in more detail in the pink box on page 20.

Cell response ranges from recoverable damage to instant death

If damage to a cell is minimal, the cell can recover following removal of the damaging stimulus. Damaged proteins and organelles are removed by a cell stress response and autophagy (see *Fig. 2.11*), with new structural components being synthesized. This is termed sublethal cell damage and is associated with recognizable structural changes.

In other situations a damaging stimulus may first cause sublethal damage and then, because the cell cannot recover, progress to cell death. There are two main structural routes of cell death that may occur after a lethal damaging stimulus: apoptosis (see page 28) and necrosis. It is becoming apparent that the magnitude and type of injurious stimulus can determine whether a cell undergoes death through apoptosis or necrosis: severe damaging stimuli tend to result in necrosis, and lower-grade damaging stimuli and stimuli from immune-mediated damage tend to cause apoptosis. A critical factor in the determination of whether a cell follows an apoptotic or a necrotic path to death seems to be how much cellular ATP is available after cell damage. In conditions where there is severe depletion of ATP, the necrotic pathway is followed.

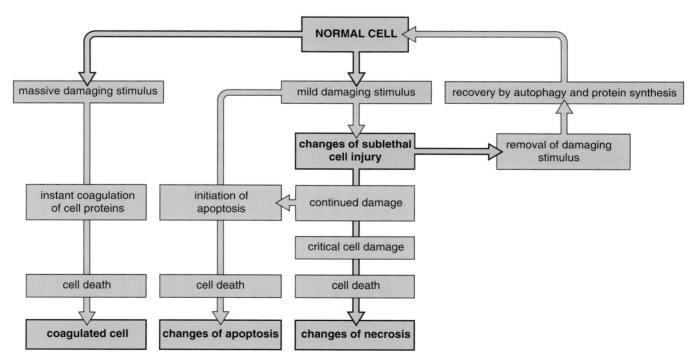

Fig. 3.4 Relationships between sublethal and lethal cell damage. Normal cells that are subject to a damaging stimulus may initiate apoptosis or may become sublethally damaged. If the stimulus abates, cells may recover by resynthesis of proteins and elimination of damaged components. If a damaging stimulus continues, either cells die through apoptosis or, when critical cell damage takes place, mainly through critical lack of ATP, cells die and undergo necrosis. Massively damaging stimuli, e.g. great heat or strong acids, cause immediate coagulation of proteins and death of cells (see *Fig. 2.12*).

Fig. 3.5 Relationships between sublethal and lethal cell damage. Following sublethal damage a cell may recover or, with persistence of the damaging stimulus, cell death may result. The sequential structural changes of cell death are termed 'necrosis'.

Mitochondrial damage can cause apoptosis

Fig. 3.6 After damage to mitochondrial membranes there is failure of ATP production and loss of the normal membrane potential of the mitochondrion. The mitochondrial membrane pores (PTPC *megachannels*) open and release proteins into the cytosol, which can cause apoptosis, as described below. If many mitochondria in a cell fail, causing a catastrophic reduction in ATP production, the cell will die by a non-apoptotic route.

In unusual circumstances, if the damaging stimulus to a cell is massive, the cell is killed immediately without passing through the stages of apoptosis or necrosis. This occurs most commonly with overwhelming physical agents such as severe heat or strong acids, both of which coagulate cell proteins. These relationships are summarized in *Figs 3.4* and *3.5*.

Sublethal damage is associated with reversible structural abnormalities

Sublethal damage can be identified from microscopic changes in affected cells. The first evidence of such damage is seen ultrastructurally as swelling of membrane-bound organelles, particularly endoplasmic reticulum and mitochondria.

- Mitochondrial swelling can be seen as an early event after cell damage. At first, spaces or vacuoles develop within the mitochondrion, distorting and separating the normally regular stacks of cristae. This change, termed **low-amplitude swelling**, is potentially reversible if the noxious stimulus is insufficient to cause cell death. Persistent insult leads to actual destruction of the cristae, the development of electron-dense aggregates in the mitochondrial stroma, and more severe swelling. At this stage, termed **high-amplitude swelling**, the changes are irreversible and the mitochondrion is permanently damaged. Proteins leak from mitochondria, leading to generation of apoptosis. Depletion of cellular ATP develops (*Fig. 3.6*).

- Swelling of endoplasmic reticulum (ER) is also seen early in the course of cell injury and is associated with loss of ribosomes attached to the rough endoplasmic reticulum (RER).

At the light microscopic level these reversible changes caused by organelle swelling are reflected in cellular swelling, paleness of the cytoplasm, and the development of small intracellular vacuoles, giving rise to the widely used descriptive terms **cloudy swelling** and **hydropic degeneration** (*Fig. 3.7a*).

Another manifestation of sublethal cell damage is impairment of fatty acid metabolism. Affected cells accumulate lipid within cytoplasmic vacuoles, giving rise to the term **fatty change**. This is seen particularly in cells that have a central role in fatty acid metabolism, especially hepatocytes (*Fig. 3.7b*). Mechanisms involved in fatty change are presented in *Fig. 3.8*.

Dead cells go through a series of structural changes termed necrosis

Lethal injury is followed by distinct structural changes in cells, which reflect disintegration of cellular structure due to activation of intracellular lysosomal enzymes. The dissolution of cells through the activity of intrinsic hydrolytic enzymes is termed **autolysis**. Autolysis brings about changes in both cytoplasm and nucleus during the evolution of a necrotic cell, as summarized in *Fig. 3.9*.

Fig. 3.7 Sublethal cell damage. (a) Hydropic degeneration. (b) Fatty change. Micrograph (a) shows a section of liver damaged by the poison paraquat. Normal liver cells (**N**) contrast with injured cells, which are swollen, pale and vacuolated (**H**). The normal cell cytoplasm is pink with a faint hint of purple, the purple coloration (basophilia) being due to ribosomes, mainly on the RER. With swelling of the ER, ribosomes become detached and reduced in number, so the normal purple cytoplasmic tint is reduced. Further cytoplasmic pallor is due to progressive swelling of the ER and mitochondria, known as **cloudy swelling** when mild, and **hydropic degeneration** when small, discrete vacuoles develop in the cytoplasm. Another example of sublethal damage is seen in micrograph (b), taken from the liver of an alcoholic patient. This shows extensive **fatty change** with large vacuoles (**V**) of fat within hepatocytes. As solvents used in conventional histological preparations dissolve out the fat to leave a clear space, lipid can be positively demonstrated only by using frozen sections.

Fatty change

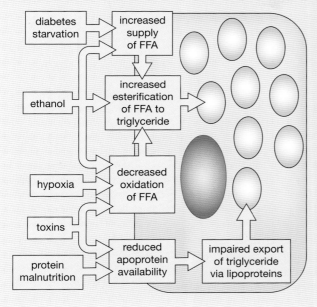

Fig. 3.8 Fatty change. This is a manifestation of sublethal metabolic derangement, seen in certain cells which have a high throughput of lipid as part of normal metabolic requirements. Such change is usually seen in the liver, but it also occurs less commonly in the myocardium and the kidney. Common causes of fatty change are toxins (particularly alcohol and halogenated hydrocarbons such as chloroform), chronic hypoxia and diabetes mellitus. Impaired metabolism of fatty acids leads to accumulation of triglycerides (fat), which form vacuoles in cells.

There are four main metabolic reasons for the accumulation of triglyceride in cells:

- Increased peripheral mobilization of free fatty acids (FFA) and uptake into cells (diabetes mellitus and nutritional deprivation).
- Increased conversion of fatty acids to triglycerides (alcohol).
- Reduced oxidation of triglycerides to acetyl-CoA (hypoxia and toxins including ethanol).
- Deficiency of lipid acceptor proteins, preventing export of formed triglycerides (carbon tetrachloride and protein malnutrition). Fatty change is reversible if the abnormality responsible is removed. It may be associated with other types of sublethal injury in cells.

 ## Key Facts
Sublethal damage

- Sublethal damage is recoverable, necrosis is not.
- The earliest visible sign of both lethal and sublethal damage is ultrastructural damage to mitochondria.
- Later sublethal damage can be seen as swelling of cellular organelles (hydropic degeneration).
- Fatty change is a manifestation of sublethal impairment of metabolism and is common in the liver.

Key Facts
Necrosis

- Intense eosinophilia of the dead cell is due to loss of RNA and coagulation of proteins.
- Nuclei undergo phases of pyknosis, karyorrhexis, and karyolysis, leaving a shrunken cell devoid of nucleus.
- Proteins may be liberated from the dead cells and be detected in the blood in diagnosis.

Several different patterns of necrosis are described

Several patterns of tissue necrosis have been traditionally described, reflecting the varying macroscopic appearances of the necrotic tissue.

- **Coagulative necrosis** describes dead tissue that appears firm and pale, as if cooked. In areas of coagulative necrosis, much of the cellular outline and tissue architecture can still be discerned histologically even though the cells are dead. It is likely that this type of response takes place because affected cells have relatively few lysosomes to bring about complete breakdown of cellular proteins. The most common cause of this pattern of necrosis is occlusion of the arterial supply to a tissue (*Fig. 3.10a*). Proteins liberated from dead cells can enter the blood (*Fig. 3.11*).
- **Liquefactive** or **colliquative necrosis** describes dead tissue that appears semi-liquid as a result of dissolution of tissue by the action of hydrolytic enzymes. The most common types of damage leading to the liquefactive pattern are necrosis in the brain owing to arterial occlusion (cerebral infarction, *Fig. 3.10b*), and necrosis caused by bacterial infections. In the brain, the huge lysosomal content of neurons, together with the relative lack of extracellular structural proteins (reticulin

a & b. With hematoxylin and eosin staining the normal cell has an open nucleus often with a visible nucleolus (**N**). The cytoplasm has a pale pink colour with a hint of purple from cellular RNA, mostly in rough endoplasmic reticulum. If there has been sublethal damage cytoplasmic vacuolation may be seen.

pyknotic nucleus

c & d. The early necrotic cell shows shrinkage and increased cytoplasmic eosinophilia (pink staining). There is a loss of cytoplasmic RNA resulting in lack of any purple tint to the cytoplasm. The nucleus (**N**) becomes small and intensely basophilic (purple staining), termed **pyknosis**, which indicates cessation of DNA transcription.

karyorrhexic fragments of nucleus

e & f. The process of necrosis continues with nucleases causing fragmentation of the nucleus into several small pieces (**K**) in a process termed **karyorrhexis**. The cell remains small and eosinophilic and may start to show irregularities in contour reflecting cell membrane breakdown.

g & h. Necrosis continues with complete dissolution of the nucleus termed **karyolysis** and leaves the necrotic cell as a mass of partly denatured protein still having the same rough outline as the normal cell. The cytoplasm is deeply eosinophilic and contrasts markedly with the normal cell shown in (a).

Fig. 3.9 Cellular events in necrosis. These sections are from the liver of a person poisoned by paracetamol (acetaminophen), a hepatic toxin. Many of the changes seen in necrosis are caused by the action of lysosomal hydrolases, which are released into the cell when cell membrane integrity is lost.

The nucleus of a necrotic cell first becomes small, condensed, and intensely stained with hematoxylin (basophilic). This appearance is termed pyknosis. Next, pyknotic nuclei become fragmented into several particles, a change known as karyorrhexis. Complete breakdown, or karyolysis, of the nucleus then takes place.

When tissue is damaged in this way, tissue defenses are activated to limit the damage and restore tissue function (see Chapter 4).

and collagen), leads to rapid loss of tissue architecture and liquefaction when lysosomal enzyme release takes place. In bacterial infection, microorganisms attract neutrophils into the area, which then release neutrophil hydrolases and cause liquefaction.

- **Caseous necrosis** describes dead tissue that is soft and white, resembling cream cheese. With this type of necrosis, dead cells form an amorphous proteinaceous mass but, in contrast to coagulative necrosis, no original architecture can be seen histologically. This pattern is invariably associated with tuberculosis (*Fig. 3.10c*).
- **Gummatous necrosis** describes dead tissue when it is firm and rubbery. As in caseous necrosis, the dead cells form an amorphous proteinaceous mass in which no

Key Facts
Patterns of necrosis

Several tissue patterns of necrosis are identifiable:

- The most common pattern is coagulative necrosis caused by occlusion of vascular supply.
- Liquefactive necrosis is seen in the brain and in infections.
- Caseous necrosis is seen in tuberculosis.
- Gummatous necrosis is seen in syphilis.
- Fibrinoid necrosis is seen in vessel walls in hypertension and vasculitis.

Fig. 3.10 Patterns of tissue necrosis. (a) Coagulative necrosis: kidney. (b) Liquefactive necrosis: brain. (c) Caseous necrosis: kidney. (d) Gummatous necrosis: liver. (e) Hemorrhagic necrosis: testis. (f) Fibrinoid necrosis: artery. Micrograph (a) is an example of coagulative necrosis in an area of kidney which has been killed by interruption of its blood supply (infarction). The outlines of a glomerulus (**G**) and surrounding tubules (**T**) are recognizable, despite the fact that all the cells are dead. Micrograph (b) shows liquefaction in a cerebral infarct. In contrast to (a), no residual tissue architecture has been preserved. The necrotic brain area has been transformed into a semi-fluid mass of protein with phagocytic macrophages. Micrograph (c) shows an area of caseous necrosis from a kidney infected by *Mycobacterium tuberculosis*. The necrotic area (**N**) is homogeneously pink and, compared to (a), has no semblance of underlying renal architecture. This pattern is also illustrated in Chapter 4.

Micrograph (d) shows an area of gummatous necrosis (**N**) in the liver of a patient with syphilis caused by long-standing infection by the spirochete *Treponema pallidum*. Micrograph (e) demonstrates an area of testicular hemorrhagic necrosis caused by torsion (twisting) of the testis on the end of the spermatic cord, such that the venous return is cut off. This leads to ischemia of the testis, as it becomes massively suffused with blood that cannot escape. Micrograph (f) shows a vessel that has undergone fibrinoid necrosis. The wall of the affected vessel is replaced by bright pink staining material (**F**). In this instance, damage to the vessels was due to severe hypertension.

Fig. 3.10 Patterns of tissue necrosis. (a) Coagulative necrosis: kidney. (b) Liquefactive necrosis: brain. (c) Caseous necrosis: kidney. (d) Gummatous necrosis: liver. (e) Hemorrhagic necrosis: testis. (f) Fibrinoid necrosis: artery. Micrograph (a) is an example of coagulative necrosis in an area of kidney which has been killed by interruption of its blood supply (infarction). The outlines of a glomerulus (**G**) and surrounding tubules (**T**) are recognizable, despite the fact that all the cells are dead. Micrograph (b) shows liquefaction in a cerebral infarct. In contrast to (a), no residual tissue architecture has been preserved. The necrotic brain area has been transformed into a semi-fluid mass of protein with phagocytic macrophages. Micrograph (c) shows an area of caseous necrosis from a kidney infected by *Mycobacterium tuberculosis*. The necrotic area (**N**) is homogeneously pink and, compared to (a), has no semblance of underlying renal architecture. This pattern is also illustrated in Chapter 4.

Micrograph (d) shows an area of gummatous necrosis (**N**) in the liver of a patient with syphilis caused by long-standing infection by the spirochete *Treponema pallidum*. Micrograph (e) demonstrates an area of testicular hemorrhagic necrosis caused by torsion (twisting) of the testis on the end of the spermatic cord, such that the venous return is cut off. This leads to ischemia of the testis, as it becomes massively suffused with blood that cannot escape. Micrograph (f) shows a vessel that has undergone fibrinoid necrosis. The wall of the affected vessel is replaced by bright pink staining material (**F**). In this instance, damage to the vessels was due to severe hypertension.

Fig. 3.12 Apoptosis. Apoptosis of cells is a programmed and energy-dependent process designed specifically to switch cells off and eliminate them. This controlled pattern of cell death, termed programmed cell death, is very different from that which occurs as a direct result of a severe, damaging stimulus to cells (discussed in Chapter 3).

integrated and, if death signals are dominant, molecular systems that trigger apoptosis are activated.

Importantly, cell survival is possible even in the face of signals that would normally cause death, provided that cell-survival signals have induced proteins with anti-apoptotic effects. The most studied of this class of anti-apoptotic proteins is termed Bcl-2 which, if present in high quantities, prevents a cell from committing itself to apoptotic death by inhibiting the mitochondrial activation complex. The activity of Bcl-2 is downregulated by the stress kinase pathway (Chapter 2),

which is one mechanism of regulating the threshold at which apoptosis is activated.

- **Effector phase:** a cell becomes committed to die through the activity of what has been termed a cell executioner pathway. This is the point of no return for the cell, after which it is irreversibly committed to die. Increasing evidence suggests that it is mitochondrial membrane permeability that acts as the decision-making factor in commitment to cell death. If the mitochondrial membrane becomes permeable, factors that cause apoptosis enter the cytosol from mitochondria.

Normal cells are arranged in close contact with each other and are united by cell junctions. Early in the process of apoptosis there is synthesis of enzymes needed to cause cell dissolution, but this is not associated with structural changes. During the signalling phase of apoptosis input from different pathways are integrated to decide a life/death fate for the cell.

In the execution phase of apoptosis proteases cause profound structural changes. The apoptotic cells lose surface specializations and junctions, shrinking in size. The nuclear chromatin condenses beneath the nuclear membrane. In contrast to necrosis (Chapter 3), cell organelles remain normal. Endonuclease enzymes cleave chromosomes into individual nucleosome fragments.

In the degradation phase there is splitting of the cell into several fragments known as **apoptotic bodies**. Nuclear fragmentation also occurs. Each fragment contains viable mitochondria and intact organelles. The process takes a few minutes only. The cell membrane shows changes in its lipid content and binds proteins to the outer surface.

In the phagocytic phase apoptotic fragments are recognized by adjacent cells, which ingest them by phagocytosis for destruction. Some fragments degenerate extracellularly, while others are ingested by local phagocytic cells, not shown on this diagram.

Labels: loss of microvilli and junctions; nuclear changes; apoptotic body; fragmentation; apoptotic body; phagocytosis

- **Degradation phase:** enzyme systems are activated which bring about the biochemical and structural features of apoptosis. The main enzymes involved are proteases called the caspases. The term caspase refers to the specificity of the proteases: 'c' refers to cysteine protease, 'asp' refers to cleavage after an aspartate residue in the target protein. The enzyme systems which are activated cleave or cross-link proteins, degrade DNA, expose phosphatidylserine on the outer cell membrane, and bring about morphological changes in the cell which are now regarded as classic for apoptotic cell death.

- **Phagocytic phase:** cell fragments produced by the apoptotic process are recognized by macrophagic and other phagocytic cells and are engulfed. The expression of phosphatidylserine on the outer cell membrane and the binding of thrombospondin on the cell surface both facilitate specific phagocytic recognition by other cells. This aspect of apoptosis allows the removal of dead cells without promoting an inflammatory response: dead cells are removed cleanly and with minimal disruption to adjacent cells.

Apoptosis may be started by activation of a surface receptor, cell membrane damage, direct mitochondrial damage, or irreparable DNA damage

There are four main systems which are believed to be specially relevant to the triggering of apoptotic cell death in human pathology (*Fig. 3.13*).

1. **Signal transduction pathway:** binding of specific ligands at cell surface receptors triggers a signal transduction cascade that activates initiating caspases. The receptors have cytoplasmic 'death recognition domains' that interact with homologous death domains on so-called adaptor proteins, carrying that signal to the initiating parts of the apoptotic pathway. Examples include:
   - Fas-Fas ligand-mediated apoptosis responsible for eliminating certain classes of lymphocyte from the immune system, as well as target-cell killing by cytotoxic T cells.
   - Cytokine-induced apoptosis of cells, as seen with tumor necrosis factor receptor (TNFR)-mediated apoptosis.

2. **Cell damage pathway:** cell damage initiates apoptosis by causing changes in mitochondrial membrane permeability, activating caspases and causing apoptosis. Examples include:
   - Free radical-mediated damage.
   - Cell anoxia.
   - High intracellular free calcium levels.
   - Perforin/granzyme-B-mediated cell death caused by cytotoxic T-lymphocyte-mediated cell death.

3. **DNA-damage/p53-p73 pathway:** damage to DNA results in accumulation of p53 protein in the cell, and this facilitates DNA repair. If this is not successful, the p53 system modulates transcription of factors that favor apoptosis. Examples include:
   - Apoptotic cell death after irradiation-induced DNA damage.

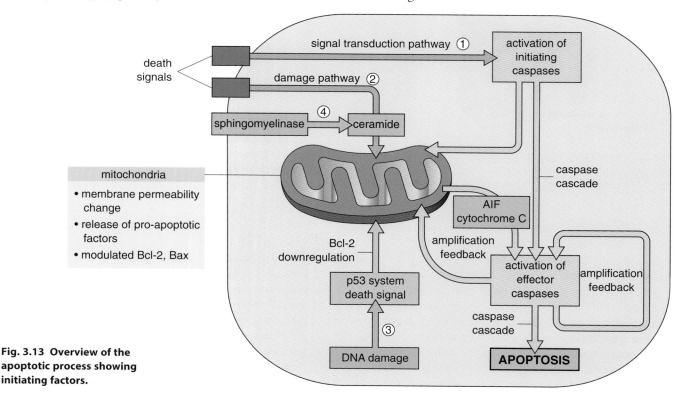

Fig. 3.13 Overview of the apoptotic process showing initiating factors.

- Apoptotic cell death induced by anti-tumor chemotherapeutic drugs.

4. **Cell membrane damage pathway:** damage to the cell membrane results in activation of the enzyme sphingomyelinase, generating ceramide. Ceramide then signals other intracellular events leading to apoptosis. Examples include:
   - Apoptotic cell death due to irradiation-induced cell damage.
   - Apoptotic cell death after free-radical-induced membrane damage.

The caspase enzymes involved in apoptosis can be divided into two groups: initiating and effector, analogous to executioner and executioner's sword

Caspases exist in an inactive form in the cytosol of most cells as procaspases and require cleavage for activation. Caspases may cause activation of other caspases, leading to the idea of a cascade of activation, analogous to that encountered in the blood coagulation cascade. The role of caspases is believed to be twofold:

- In certain situations, specific caspase activation is the signal that commits a cell to apoptotic cell death (acting as the executioner signal). These are called **initiating or 'upstream' caspases** (mainly caspases 2, 8, 9 and 10). Of these, the most studied is caspase 9. **Caspase 9** is activated on the mitochondrial surface as part of a protein complex that also involves the mitochondrial protein apoptosis activating factor 1 (**apaf-1**), and **cytochrome C** (see *Fig. 3.15*). **Caspase 8** is activated by signals from adjacent cytokine receptors that are in turn activated by binding substances such as **fas ligand** and tumor necrosis factor (**TNF**). Caspases 8 and 9 are involved in the activation of caspase 3.
- In all cases of apoptosis, specific caspases are the proteases that bring about structural degradation of the cell to give the classic morphological and biochemical features of apoptosis (acting as the executioner's sword). These are termed **effector or 'downstream' caspases** (caspases 3, 6 and 7). Activation of **caspase 3**, for example, degrades substrates such as cytoskeletal proteins, nuclear envelope proteins, cell signaling proteins and DNA repair enzymes. Thus, activation of caspase 3 by initiator caspases (such as caspase 8 or 9) results in dissolution of the nuclear membrane, cleavage of nuclear DNA, inhibition of inter- and intracellular communication, and finally engulfment of the cell (*Fig. 3.12*).

To further complicate matters, some caspases may be initiating proteases in some cell types, but effector proteases in other cell types.

Furthermore, in some systems some death-regulatory signals seem to act independently of caspase cascade activa-

Laboratory recognition of apoptosis is important in biological research

With a central role for apoptosis being found in so many disease processes, identifying apoptotic cells has become an important aspect in the investigation of the pathogenesis of disease. The recognition of apoptosis can be achieved by several techniques:

- Conventional morphology using light microscopy, or more specifically electron microscopy, will reveal characteristic structural features of apoptosis.
- If DNA is extracted from tissues and agarose gel electrophoresis performed, then a ladder pattern is seen corresponding to cleavage of DNA at nucleosomes by apoptosis-related endonucleases.
- Endonuclease activity results in breaks in double-stranded DNA. This can be detected in tissue sections by the tunel technique.
- Immunohistochemistry for transglutaminase can be used to identify cells in the effector stage of apoptosis.
- Immunohistochemistry for annexin-V on the cell surface can be used to identify cells that are in suspension, for example cells in culture using flow cytometry.
- Antibodies are now available for the majority of the caspase enzymes and activation of individual components of the apoptotic cascade can now be investigated by immunohistochemistry.
- Immunohistochemistry can also be used to detect activation of regulatory factors such as Bcl-2, Bax, Bad and Bcl-XL.

tion, committing cells to die in the absence of 'upstream' caspase activation. Although the executional 'upstream' signal is not caspases related, the executioner's sword is still enacted via 'downstream' effector caspase activation.

Mitochondrial damage may trigger the point of no return for apoptosis in many cell systems

It is now realized that proteins released from mitochondria are vital in the initiation of apoptosis. The integrity of the mitochondrial membrane systems has been proposed as the deciding factor in the fate of a cell: survival or death. In the study of apoptosis it has been found that the ability of mitochondria to maintain a transmembrane potential across their membrane systems becomes impaired before downstream, effector caspases are activated (*Fig. 3.14*).

The loss of mitochondrial potential is related to the opening of a huge composite ion channel that spans both inner and outer mitochondrial membranes, termed the **permeability transition pore complex** (PTPC), also referred to as the mitochondrial '*megachannel*'. This opening leads to the release of material from mitochondria into the cytosol.

Important molecules released include cytochrome C (activates downstream caspases by forming an apoptosome) and apoptosis-initiating factor (AIF) (a caspase-activating factor) (*Fig. 3.14*).

Importantly, certain proteins associated with mitochondria can regulate the process of apoptosis. Bcl-2 and Bcl-XL are proteins that prevent opening of the megachannel and stabilize proteins such as Apaf-1; hence, these proteins are protective against apoptosis. In contrast, mitochondrial-related proteins Bax and Bad serve to promote apoptosis by inducing opening of the megachannel.

There is the suggestion that some activated caspases may act to cause mitochondrial damage, thereby amplifying a cell-death cascade involving both signal-transduced caspase activation and mitochondrial–apoptosome caspase activation.

Direct mitochondrial damage, for example by toxins, free radicals or anoxia, can result in direct opening of the megachannel, releasing mitochondrial factors that activate apoptotic cell death. In this process, although effector (downstream) caspases are activated, the input of initiating (upstream) caspases is not required to trigger apoptotic cell death.

It therefore seems that factors which influence mitochondrial membrane permeability are important in regulating apoptosis in the cell. Pro-apoptotic factors increase permeability and allow the release of cytochrome C and apoptosis-initiating factor, whereas anti-apoptotic factors sequester vital proteins and preserve mitochondrial membrane integrity.

In cases of sublethal injury, mitochondria can either increase or decrease in number, as seen in tissue hypertrophy and atrophy, respectively; they can undergo changes in shape, an example being the megamitochondria seen in alcoholic liver disease; or they can develop ultrastructural abnormalities, such as the typical inclusions and abnormalities of the cristae seen in mitochondrial myopathies (see *Fig. 21.53*).

The executioner's sword of apoptosis can be activated by protein derived from disrupted mitochondria

Cytochrome C, and a protein called apoptosis-initiating factor (AIF), both derived from mitochondria, are powerful activators of the effector or 'downstream' caspases. Cytochrome C forms a complex with other proteins to form an important caspase cascade activator which has been called an **apoptosome**.

It seems that a crucial event in activating downstream caspases via formation of the apoptosome is the availability of cytochrome C in the cytosol. The Bcl-2 protein (an anti-apoptotic factor) sequesters cytochrome C and prevents it activating apoptosis via the apoptosome. This partly explains why high levels of expression of Bcl-2 protect cells from apoptotic cell death. Bcl-w probably also has anti-apoptotic effects by sequestering the pro-apoptotic protease-activating factor Apaf-1, stabilizing the mitochondrial membrane, and also by antagonizing opening of the mitochondrial megachannel.

Apoptotic fragments are recognized by receptors on phagocytic cells

The cell fragments generated by the apoptotic processes are characterized by a change in the lipid composition of the outer cell membrane, with flipping of phosphatidylserine from the inner leaflet to the outer surface.

Vitronectin and thrombospondin bind to the surface of apoptotic cells, and these proteins are recognized by phagocytic cells such as macrophages and lead to engulfment and elimination of apoptotic remnants. This mechanism of elimination does not induce proinflammatory mediators, and therefore does not produce an inflammatory response with the typical cellular infiltrate seen in areas of tissue necrosis.

Fig. 3.14 Mitochondrial integrity is a key factor in apoptosis.

The apoptosis signaling pathways are characterized by several branching and convergence points

Fig. 3.15 summarizes the events in apoptosis. It can be seen that there are several branching and convergence points in the four main pathways involved in this process. Importantly, mitochondrial factors, caspases, ceramide, and free radicals are involved at several points.

- The signal transduction pathway, activated by binding a ligand at a cell surface receptor, induces apoptosis by direct activation of initiating caspases and also acts by modulating pro-apoptotic and anti-apoptotic factors of the Bcl-2 family.
- DNA damage activates the p53 system, and this regulates the balance between pro-apoptotic and anti-apoptotic factors to cause cell death. This system is important, as it eliminates cells that have irreparable DNA damage. Failure of this system leads to the generation of tumors (Chapter 6).
- Direct damage to cells via a variety of mechanisms, especially related to the generation of free radicals, induces apoptosis by increasing the permeability of mitochondria and liberating pro-apoptotic factors into the cell that activate the effector arm of the apoptotic caspase enzyme system.

- Plasma membrane damage from a variety of stimuli, including irradiation, activates sphingomyelinase to generate ceramide from membrane lipids. Ceramide is then capable of initiating apoptosis.

Damage to DNA causes sublethal damage long after the event

Certain damaging agents, most notably irradiation, injure the genetic apparatus of cells, resulting in abnormal genetic functioning. This may not be manifest as immediate cellular dysfunction, but may predispose affected cells to later problems.

- Cell division to repair damage may not be effective, leading to poor healing in damaged tissues (see Chapter 4).
- Mutations in DNA may predispose to the development of tumors such as cancers (see Chapter 6).
- Cells with irradiation-induced DNA damage may be triggered to enter the apoptotic pathway of cell death.

Some cells are sensitive to damage whereas others are robust

Not all cells are equally susceptible to damaging agents. This is illustrated by the range of sensitivity exhibited by cells following cessation of oxygenation (hypoxia) to the whole body, as might happen after a cardiac arrest.

Fig. 3.15 Summary overview of the apoptotic process.

- The most sensitive cells are the large neurons of the hippocampus and cerebellum, which die after only 2–5 minutes without oxygen. More prolonged hypoxia causes damage to the majority of pyramidal cells in the cerebral cortex.
- The most robust cells are fibroblasts. These remain in an area of tissue damage even after all specialized parenchymal cells have been destroyed. It is possible to culture fibroblasts from the tissues of a person who has been declared somatically dead for many hours.

The reason why some cells are more sensitive to hypoxia than others lies in the varying metabolic capacities of the different cell types to survive ATP depletion and calcium influx, and to buffer free radical-induced damage. Apparently similar cells also have differing metabolic capabilities. For example, hepatocytes in the periportal region of the liver have low levels of enzymes that generate toxic metabolites from paracetamol (acetaminophen), whereas centrilobular hepatocytes have high levels. This explains why liver necrosis following paracetamol toxicity is limited to centrilobular hepatocytes.

Aging is a form of cell degeneration that is not understood

Aging is associated with degeneration and loss of function of many cellular systems. With increasing age the incidence of many important diseases increases, some of which are probably due to a cumulative environmental exposure to a causative agent. However, others are due to the process of biological aging itself. Several theories seek to explain aging at a molecular level, but none entirely explains aging as a single biological phenomenon.

Somatic death is followed by autolysis and putrefaction

Death of cells and tissues does not result in the inevitable death of the individual. However, if physiological functions are critically impaired through tissue damage, for example respiration or cardiac output, death of the individual (known as **somatic death**) occurs. Following somatic death there is death of all cells in the body, and the release of lysosomal enzymes causes decomposition of tissues through **autolysis**, being similar to the events of necrosis. Microorganisms, for example from the gut, also invade tissues and cause further putrefaction.

Postmortem colonization of tissues by microorganisms can be differentiated from infection occurring in life by the absence of an inflammatory response in the former.

The processes of autolysis and bacterial decomposition can be slowed by refrigeration or by preservation in preservative solutions. This is the main reason for fixation of surgically resected organs and tissues in preservatives such as formaldehyde solution (formalin); morphology is thus preserved and autolysis prevented.

Cell biology of aging

- **Programmed aging.** It has been proposed that cells have a programmed capacity for a limited number of divisions (the Hayflick Limit), after which cells are not replaced and atrophy ensues, with loss of function.
- **Telomere shortening.** As cells divide, the chromosome ends become progressively shortened owing to incomplete replication of the telomeres, eventually inducing senescence. Some cancers seem to reactivate telomerase, allowing unlimited cell division and virtual immortality.
- **DNA repair defects.** It has been suggested that aging is merely the result of the known inefficiencies in DNA repair, which occur at a low level in normal people. With time the proportion of cells carrying abnormal DNA increases and tissue function is impaired. This applies not only to nuclear DNA but also to mitochondrial DNA, which has much less effective systems for repairing damage. Defects in these systems are illustrated by progeria syndromes such as Werner's.

- **Degeneration in extracellular matrix materials**, through protein cross-linking, modification such as glycosylation, and oxidation, has been proposed as a mechanism that impairs function of the specialized parenchymal cells, leading to cell dysfunction with age.
- **Free radical damage.** Decrease in the availability of free radical scavenging systems is a possible mechanism whereby free radical-mediated damage becomes more significant with age and begins to cause cellular dysfunction and death. This would also cause damage to DNA, as well as to proteins.
- **Protein catabolic inefficiency.** All cells depend for survival on efficient systems for eliminating damaged or effete constituents. It has been suggested that a major contributor to aging is inefficiency in such systems, leading to cellular dysfunction and death.
- **Cumulative injury theories** propose that aging is the result of all cellular impairments sustained throughout life, whether through DNA damage, protein modification, free radical damage, or disease.

Tissue responses to damage

4

OVERVIEW OF TISSUE RESPONSES TO INJURY

When tissue is damaged and cells die, more than one outcome is possible, as summarized in *Fig. 4.1.*

The damaged area may be replaced by organized tissue identical in structure and function to that originally present.

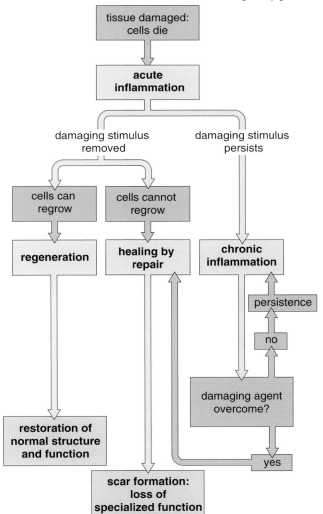

Fig. 4.1 Overview of tissue responses to injury.

Termed restitution, this is the ideal outcome. It can take place only if the damaging agent is removed, the cell debris is cleared from the site, and the specialized cells that have been destroyed have the capacity to regrow or **regenerate**.

If damaged cells cannot regrow, or local damage is so severe that tissue architecture is entirely destroyed, complete restitution of a damaged area is not always possible. In this case, the tissue response is to heal the damaged area by replacing it with non-specialized **scar tissue**, a process termed **fibrous repair**. This is the most frequent outcome of substantial tissue damage.

If the damaging agent persists (particularly if it involves infection), continuing tissue destruction, attempts to heal by fibrous repair, and immune responses occur concurrently, a process known as **chronic inflammation**.

Irrespective of the ultimate outcome of tissue damage, the initial response of the tissue is termed **acute inflammation** or the **acute inflammatory reaction**. This response is relatively non-specific, its main roles being to clear away dead tissues, protect against local infection, and allow the immune system access to the damaged area.

Acute inflammation is the most common early tissue response to tissue damage and destruction

The acute inflammatory response has three main functions:

1. The affected area is occupied by a transient material called the **acute inflammatory exudate**. The exudate carries proteins, fluid, and cells from local blood vessels into the damaged area to mediate local defenses.
2. If an infective causative agent (e.g. bacteria) is present in the damaged area, it can be destroyed and eliminated by components of the exudate.
3. The damaged tissue can be broken down and partly liquefied, and the debris removed from the site of damage.

The acute inflammatory response is controlled by the production and diffusion of chemical messengers derived both from damaged tissues and from the acute inflammatory exudate. These **mediators of acute inflammation** are discussed in a later section (see pages 36–44), after the features of acute inflammation have been presented.

The acute inflammatory exudate is derived from local vessels

The acute inflammatory exudate is composed of:

- **Fluid** containing salts and a high concentration of proteins including immunoglobulins.
- **Fibrin**, a high molecular weight, filamentous, insoluble protein.
- Many **neutrophil polymorphs**, from the blood white cell population.
- A few **macrophages**, phagocytic cells derived from blood monocytes.
- A few **lymphocytes**.

All of these components are derived from the blood as a result of changes that occur in blood vessels in the surviving tissue around the area of damage. These changes, the vascular and cellular responses of acute inflammation, are illustrated diagrammatically in *Fig. 4.2*. Briefly, the steps are:

1. Small blood vessels adjacent to the area of tissue damage initially become dilated with increased blood flow, then flow along them slows down.
2. Endothelial cells swell and partially retract, so that they no longer form a completely intact internal lining.
3. The vessels become leaky, permitting the passage of water, salts, and some small proteins from the plasma into the damaged area (**exudation**). One of the main proteins to leak out is the small soluble molecule fibrinogen.
4. Circulating neutrophil polymorphs initially adhere to the swollen endothelial cells (**margination**), then

actively migrate through the vessel basement membrane (**emigration**), passing into the area of tissue damage.
5. Later, small numbers of blood monocytes (macrophages) migrate in a similar way, as do lymphocytes.

Local vascular flow and permeability alter in acute inflammation

The main vascular changes that arise in acute inflammation are slowing of flow and dilatation of vessels, and an increase

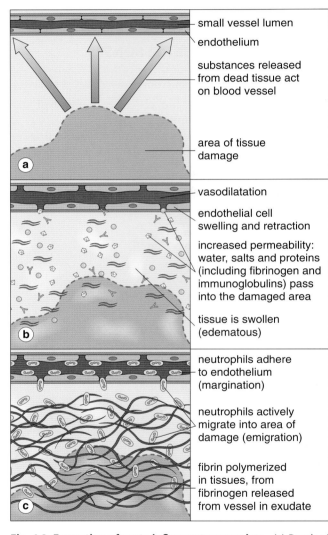

small vessel lumen

endothelium

substances released from dead tissue act on blood vessel

area of tissue damage

(a)

vasodilatation

endothelial cell swelling and retraction

increased permeability: water, salts and proteins (including fibrinogen and immunoglobulins) pass into the damaged area

tissue is swollen (edematous)

(b)

neutrophils adhere to endothelium (margination)

neutrophils actively migrate into area of damage (emigration)

fibrin polymerized in tissues, from fibrinogen released from vessel in exudate

(c)

Fig. 4.2 Formation of acute inflammatory exudate. (a) Death of tissue leads to the release of substances (chemical mediators) that act on nearby blood vessels. (b) Mediators produce: (i) persistent vasodilatation and loss of axial flow; (ii) endothelial cell swelling and separation; (iii) increased permeability, with exudation of water, salts and small proteins, including fibrinogen. Fibrinogen is converted to fibrin. (c) Mediators cause neutrophils to adhere to endothelium (margination), and move through vessel walls into damaged tissue (emigration). Blood monocytes/macrophages also emigrate by a similar mechanism slightly later. The damaged area becomes progressively replaced by the components of the exudate.

Clinical effects of acute inflammation

The four cardinal effects of acute inflammation were described nearly 2000 years ago by Celsus:

Rubor (redness)   **Dolor (pain)**
Calor (heat)   **Tumor (swelling)**

The redness and heat of acute inflammation are the result of vessel dilatation and increased blood flow to the inflamed part, and the swelling is caused by accumulation of exudate, particularly the fluid component. The pain is due to a combination of factors, including pressure on nerve endings from swelling, and a direct effect of certain chemical factors which are released to mediate the response.

When swelling and pain are marked, there is loss of function, either partial or complete, of the inflamed structure.

in the permeability of their walls, allowing diffusion of large proteins and fluid. The main structural changes in the vessel walls, and the factors that mediate increased permeability, are described in the later section on chemical mediators of acute inflammation (see pages 42–44).

Fibrin in the acute inflammatory exudate may have a role in allowing cell movement

Fibrin is a long, insoluble, filamentous protein formed by the polymerization of numerous molecules of the smaller, soluble, precursor plasma protein **fibrinogen**. The fibrinogen passes out from vessels with the fluid and salts, polymerizing into insoluble fibrin threads once outside the vessel lumen, by activation of the blood coagulation cascade.

It is widely speculated that the network of fibrin threads prevents the migration of microorganisms and produces a scaffold that might assist the migration of neutrophils and macrophages through the damaged area. However, there is no real proof that these are the precise functions of the network.

Fluid in the acute inflammatory exudate carries nutrients, mediators and immunoglobulins

It is logical to assume that the presence of fluids and salts may dilute or buffer any locally produced toxins in an area of tissue damage, but little more is known about their precise functions in the acute inflammatory reaction. Glucose and oxygen can diffuse into the area of inflammation to support macrophages. Fluid also allows diffusion of mediators of the inflammatory process, particularly plasma-derived precursors (see pages 42–5).

If immunity to an invading organism already exists, immunoglobulins in the exudate act as opsonins for neutrophil phagocytosis (see below).

The fluid in the exudate is not static but is constantly circulating from local vessels, through the extracellular space of the damaged tissue, to be reabsorbed by lymphatics. This increased flow of lymph takes antigens to the local nodes and assists in the later development of a specific immune response.

Cellular reactions are also needed in acute inflammation

The main cellular events in acute inflammation, all of which are caused by chemical mediators, are as follows:

- The normally pathologically quiescent endothelium has to be activated to allow adhesion of neutrophils.
- Normally inactive neutrophils have to be activated to enhance their capacity for phagocytosis, bacterial killing, and the generation of inflammatory mediators.
- Neutrophils have to develop the ability to move actively, in a directional fashion, from vessels towards the area of tissue damage.

Neutrophils are the main effector cells in acute inflammation

The neutrophil is the main cell that mediates the effects of acute inflammation. If tissue damage is slight, an adequate supply is derived from normal numbers circulating in blood. If tissue damage is extensive, stores of neutrophils, including some immature forms, are released from bone marrow to increase the absolute count of neutrophils in the blood. To maintain the supply of neutrophils, growth factors derived from the inflammatory process stimulate division of myeloid precursors in the bone marrow, thereby increasing the number of developing neutrophils.

Neutrophils adhere to endothelial cells prior to emigration

The adhesion of neutrophils to endothelium causes them to aggregate along the vessel walls in a process termed **margination**. There are three stages to this process (*Fig. 4.3*) mediated by different cell adhesion mechanisms:

- **Rolling** – neutrophils roll along the endothelium in close contact.
- **Adhesion** – neutrophils adhere firmly to the endothelium.
- **Aggregation** – adjacent neutrophils adhere to each other and undergo shape changes.

Neutrophils actively emigrate from vessels into tissues down a concentration gradient of chemotactic factors (*Fig. 4.4a*).

Key Facts
Neutrophils

- Produced by maturation of precursor cells in bone marrow.
- Most numerous white cell in blood, increasing in number in acute inflammation.
- Short lifespan once activated in tissues.
- Motile (ameboid) and able to move from vessels into tissues.
- Movement can be directional, attracted by chemotaxins (see *Fig. 4.4*).
- Actively phagocytic (see *Fig. 4.6*).
- Contain granules rich in a variety of proteases.
- Generated free radicals kill phagocytosed bacteria.
- Are a source of arachidonic acid to facilitate prostaglandin production.
- Increased neutrophil production by bone marrow is caused by cytokines generated in the inflammatory response.

Stages that precede neutrophil emigration

rolling	adhesion	aggregation	emigration
sLe^x	β_2 integrins	CD11b/CD18 (Mac-1)	β_2 integrins
L-selectin	VLA-4 ($\alpha_4\beta_1$), ICAM-1,	CD11a/CD18 (Mac-1)	ICAM-1
P-selectin	VCAM-1, $\alpha_4\beta_7$ integrin,	P-selectin	VCAM-1
E-selectin	MAdCAM-1		PECAM-1

Fig. 4.3 Cell binding is mediated by different molecules at each stage.

Fig. 4.4 Neutrophil emigration in acute inflammation. (a) Margination, emigration and migration of neutrophils (arrows). (b) Neutrophils marginated along vessel wall. (c) Neutrophils (arrows) emigrating into damaged tissue from vessel (V).

Activation of endothelium is a key process in acute inflammation

Endothelium in local vessels is activated both by products of tissue damage and by cytokines. This induces the expression of surface cell adhesion molecules, which interact with complementary molecules in the neutrophil cell membrane.

Some of the factors involved in the activation of endothelial cells, together with its role in neutrophil rolling and adhesion, are summarized in the pink box. The endothelium is modified to become sticky for neutrophils, to secrete factors mediating vasodilatation, and to promote platelet adhesion and aggregation.

Endothelial activation in acute inflammation

The endothelium plays a vital role as a physical barrier against diffusion of plasma outside vessels, as well as being the source of many regulatory molecules. Because of its extent and its constant secretion of messenger substances, the endothelium has been called the largest endocrine organ in the body.

The main factors secreted by the endothelium are:

- **Nitric oxide** and **prostacyclin**, which induce vascular relaxation and inhibit platelet aggregation.
- **Endothelin, thromboxane A2**, and **angiotensin II**, which cause vascular constriction.
- Growth factor **PDGF**, which promotes inhibitors, e.g. heparin-like substances.
- **Chemokines**.

In the normal state the endothelium provides a surface that prevents platelet aggregation and degranulation. The balance of secreted factors is a major determinant in control of regional blood flow. In acute inflammation this balance is changed and there is increased synthesis of a lipid-derived molecule known as **platelet-activating factor** (PAF), which increases vascular permeability; increased synthesis of nitric oxide, which promotes vascular dilatation; and more cell adhesion molecules are expressed, which allows neutrophil adhesion. In addition to modulation of secreted factors, the surface properties of the endothelium are altered in acute inflammation (*Fig. 4.5*).

- IL-1, TNF and chemokines increase the expression of adhesion molecules on the endothelium, especially **selectins,** which cause rolling of neutrophils.
- Chemokines on the endothelial surface bind to receptors on neutrophils and signal the expression of leukocyte **integrins**.
- Intercellular adhesion molecule 1 (ICAM-1) promotes adhesion of neutrophils and lymphoid cells.
- Vascular cell adhesion molecule 1 (VCAM-1) promotes adhesion of lymphoid and monocyte cells.

At the same time, other mediators of inflammation, particularly the **C5a** fragment of complement, induce increased expression of complementary cell adhesion molecules on neutrophils (β_2 **integrins**). The endothelium in acute inflammation is therefore metabolically altered to produce vasoactive factors (particularly PAF and nitric oxide) as well as to be sticky for neutrophils.

Fig. 4.5 Cell adhesion molecules involved in neutrophil adhesion. IL-1 interleukin-1, **TNF** tumor necrosis factor, **LTB$_4$** leukotriene B$_4$.

Systemic inflammatory response syndrome

This is an acute illness, the main features of which are caused by systemic activation of endothelium. This leads to generalized vasodilatation, platelet aggregation and widespread secondary organ dysfunction, particularly in the kidneys, liver, lungs, and heart.

The main clinical situation in which this syndrome occurs is septicemia from Gram-negative bacteria. The pathogenesis is due to inappropriate endothelial activation mediated by cytokines.

As more is understood about the pathogenesis of this syndrome, treatment by attempted blockade of IL-1 receptors or by administration of TNF-neutralizing antibodies is under trial.

Neutrophils are attracted to the area of tissue damage by chemical mediators

The movement of neutrophils from the vessel lumen into a damaged area is mediated by substances known as chemotactic factors, which diffuse from the area of tissue damage. The main neutrophil chemotactic factors are listed in the Key Facts on mediators (see page 45). These factors bind to receptors on the surface of neutrophils and activate secondary messenger systems, stimulating increased cytosolic calcium, with resulting assembly of cytoskeletal specializations involved in motility.

Neutrophils kill microorganisms and break down damaged tissue

The neutrophil polymorph is packed with large numbers of lysosomal cytoplasmic granules that are rich in proteolytic enzymes capable of breaking down both cells and extracellular matrix materials. Neutrophils also have great phagocytic potential and can actively ingest pathogens, which are then destroyed both by lysosomal enzymes and by mechanisms that generate toxic free radicals. Neutrophil phagocytosis is illustrated in *Fig. 4.6.*

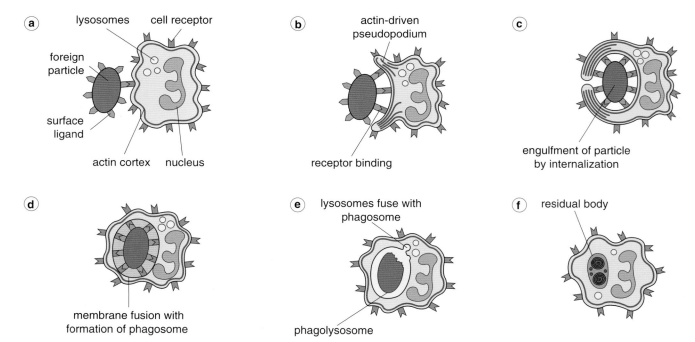

Fig. 4.6 Neutrophil phagocytosis. (a) Neutrophils have membrane receptors for the Fc portion of antibodies, complement factors bound to foreign particles, and bacterial polysaccharides. Neutrophils do not phagocytose material to which they do not bind. (b) As the first step in phagocytosis, the neutrophil binds to the abnormal particle by its specific receptors. The cell pushes out pseudopodia to surround the particle, driven by assembly and disassembly of actin filaments. (c) The pseudopodia fuse to enclose the abnormal particle completely, forming an endocytic vesicle. Special proteins probably allow final sealing of the membrane. (d) The internalized particle in the endocytic vesicle is called a phagosome. (e) The phagosome fuses with neutrophil granules, particularly primary granules, which discharge their contents, exposing the particle to a potent mixture of lysosomal enzymes. If the particle is a bacterium, killing is enhanced by hydrogen peroxide and superoxide, which are generated by the enzymatic reduction of oxygen by respiratory burst oxidases (RBOs) (membrane enzymes). (f) Foreign particle destruction is associated with the formation of a residual body containing degraded material.

Neutrophils are short-lived phagocytic cells

The disadvantage of neutrophils is that they are short-lived, surviving only a few hours once in the tissues. Consequently, the supply of neutrophils to a damaged area needs to be constantly replenished.

Any area of tissue damage will contain large numbers of viable, actively phagocytosing neutrophils, which are mixed with the remnants of dead neutrophils. As neutrophils die they release some of their lysosomal enzymes into the surrounding tissue, and these enzymes may continue to act outside the cell, breaking down structural proteins and partly liquefying the tissue.

Neutrophils are stimulated to emigrate in their greatest numbers where the tissue damage is caused by bacterial invasion, as many bacterial products are potent chemoattractants. This large-scale emigration is particularly beneficial because neutrophils not only break down and eradicate the damaged tissue, but also phagocytose and kill the causative bacteria. Where there has been massive emigration associated with tissue breakdown, a thick, liquid substance called **pus** is formed, containing necrotic cell debris, live and dead neutrophils and, sometimes, microorganisms.

Macrophages play a small part in acute inflammation

A minor component of the acute inflammatory exudate is formed by macrophages derived from monocytes in the circulating blood, which migrate into the damaged area later than neutrophils. They are present in very small numbers early in the course of acute inflammation, but with time increase in numbers to facilitate elimination of dead material. They are actively phagocytic and have powerful systems for bacterial killing. Because of a capacity for oxidative metabolism, they survive very much longer than neutrophils.

In addition to their phagocytic function macrophages have secretory roles, producing growth factors and cytokines, which mediate some of the events in the inflammatory response. They also assist in repair following tissue damage. Macrophages have more important roles in chronic inflammation (see pages 50–1).

The acute inflammatory exudate varies in its composition

The components of the acute inflammatory response may vary in their relative proportions depending on the site and cause of the inflammatory response.

- When neutrophils dominate the composition, and material is liquefied to form pus, the exudate is termed **purulent**.
- If fibrin is abundant, as often seen in relation to serosal surfaces (e.g. surface of the pericardium, lung or peritoneum), the exudate is termed **fibrinous**.

- When fluid is the major component the exudate is termed **serous**.

Examples of purulent, fibrinous, and serous exudates are illustrated in *Figs 4.7, 4.8* and *4.9*.

An abscess results from local tissue breakdown

If an area of tissue necrosis is extensive, and the cause is a pus-forming (pyogenic) bacterium, an acute abscess may form. An abscess is a mass of necrotic tissue, with dead and viable neutrophils, suspended in the fluid products of tissue breakdown by neutrophil enzymes. In its early stages it is surrounded by a layer of acute inflammatory exudate and is called an **acute abscess** (*Fig. 4.11*). At this stage, if the bacteria are able to survive, proliferate, and cause necrosis, it may continue to enlarge.

If the acute abscess enlarges only slowly or not at all, the acute inflammatory exudate forming the wall of the abscess

Acute inflammation may be harmful

It is paradoxical that the acute inflammatory process, which is meant to be protective and reparative, often produces severe illness and even death. To illustrate: in the two examples of common conditions given below the symptoms and complications of the disease are the result of the acute inflammatory process.

- In **acute epiglottitis**, infection of the upper airway by *Haemophilus* bacteria causes acute inflammation. The extensive outpouring of exudate into the soft tissues of the laryngeal submucosa can lead to such severe narrowing of the airway that respiration is compromised. Ultimately, the acute inflammatory response to infection can result in death through asphyxia.
- In **acute meningitis** (*Fig. 4.7*), infection of the leptomeninges by bacteria induces an acute inflammatory response. Although the bacteria may be of low pathogenicity and in themselves cause little tissue damage, the acute inflammatory response causes thrombosis of local blood vessels and prevents perfusion to the cerebral cortex, leading to severe brain damage. In this way, the acute inflammatory response to the infection produces more damage than the infective organism it is attempting to combat. Many other examples, and their clinical implications, are presented later in this book.

Fig. 4.7 Purulent exudate in the brain in meningitis. (a) Macroscopic specimen. (b) Histological section. In (a), which shows a child's brain, a thick, creamy exudate is visible beneath the arachnoid, most prominent in the frontal and temporal areas. This creamy appearance is due to the predominance of neutrophil polymorphs in the exudate, as illustrated in (b). The diagnosis of purulent meningitis can be made by the identification of large numbers of neutrophils (N) in a sample of cerebrospinal fluid removed by lumbar puncture; the causative bacterium can sometimes be seen in such samples, and the specimen should be sent for microbiological culture to identify the specific organism.

Fig. 4.8 Fibrinous exudate in the pericardium. (a) Macroscopic specimen. (b) Histological section. In (a) a 'shaggy' exudate covers the entire surface of both the visceral and the parietal pericardium, seen through a window cut in the parietal pericardium. This shaggy appearance is due to the predominance of fibrin (F) in the exudate, as seen in (b). The exudate destroys the normal, smooth surfaces of the pericardial cavity, and its presence can be detected clinically on auscultation, when a scratching noise can be heard with every heartbeat (pericardial friction rub).

is gradually replaced by granulation tissue and scar tissue. The central area of damaged tissue is not eradicated, and the central debris still contains viable proliferating bacteria, which remain capable of causing tissue damage; this is a **chronic abscess**.

Acute inflammation is orchestrated by chemical mediators

Many factors that mediate and orchestrate the events of acute inflammation have been documented. These chemical mediators of inflammation are important, as the process can be modified by drug therapy to minimize unwanted and potentially damaging effects. The mediators either come from cells or are plasma derived (*Fig. 4.10*). Plasma-derived mediators gain entry to the damaged area via the inflammatory exudate. They are mostly precursor proteins, which are activated by proteolytic enzymes and, once activated, generally have short half-lives. Once in tissues, they are rapidly inactivated by a variety of enzymatic or scavenging systems.

Histamine is the main preformed mediator of inflammation. Released from mast cells, basophils and platelets, it causes transient dilatation of arterioles, increases permeability in venules, and is the primary cause of increased vascular permeability in the first hour after injury.

Both prostaglandins and leukotrienes are derived by local synthesis from arachidonic acid. This long-chain fatty acid

Fig. 4.9 Serous pericardial effusion. Serous effusions are important only when they occur within a confined space, e.g. in the pericardial cavity. This echocardiogram shows a typical pericardial effusion greatly distending the pericardial sac (**PE**). The clinical problems arise because the substantially increased pressure in the pericardial cavity interferes with atrial filling.

Fig. 4.10 Main groups of mediators involved in acute inflammation

Cellular mediators of acute inflammation

Stored	Active synthesis
Histamine	Prostaglandins
	Leukotrienes
	Platelet-activating factor
	Cytokines
	Nitric oxide
	Chemokines

Plasma-derived mediators of acute inflammation

Kinin system	– Bradykinin
Clotting pathway	– Activated Hageman factor
Thrombolytic system	– Plasmin
Complement pathway	– C3a, C3b and C5a

Fig. 4.11 Acute abscess. Lung showing multiple acute abscesses (**A**) due to staphylococcal infection.

is liberated from cell membranes by activation of the enzyme, phospholipase A_2. There are two main pathways in arachidonic acid metabolism:

1. The **cyclo-oxygenase pathway** produces: thromboxane A_2 (TXA_2), which aggregates platelets and causes vascular constriction; prostacyclin (PGI_2), which inhibits platelet aggregation and dilates vessels; and stable prostaglandins (PGE_2, $PGF_{2\alpha}$, PGD_2), which cause vasodilatation and increase vascular permeability. PGE_2 also causes pain. There are two forms of cyclo-oxygenase, termed COX-1 and COX-2. COX-1 is normally present in cells as a constitutively expressed enzyme, whereas COX-2 is specially induced in cells where it plays a role in inflammation.

2. The **lipoxygenase pathway** produces leukotrienes (LTC_4, LTD_4, LTE_4), which cause vasoconstriction and increase permeability in venules. Leukotriene LTB_4 stimulates leukocyte adhesion to endothelium.

Platelet-activating factor (PAF) is synthesized by mast cells/basophils and can be stimulated by IgE-mediated release. Also synthesized by platelets, neutrophils, monocytes, and endothelium, it is a specialized phospholipid compound that causes vasoconstriction, increased vascular permeability, and platelet aggregation, and is at least 1000 times more potent than histamine. It also stimulates the synthesis of arachidonic acid metabolites.

Cytokines are polypeptide products of activated lymphocytes and monocytes. The main cytokines participating in acute inflammation are interleukin (IL)-1, IL-8, and tumor necrosis factor α (TNFα). These are responsible for:

• Induction of cell adhesion molecules on endothelium.
• Induction of PGI_2 (prostacyclin) synthesis.
• Induction of PAF synthesis.
• Fever, anorexia, and stimulation of acute-phase protein synthesis by the liver.
• Stimulation of fibroblast proliferation and secretory activity.
• Attraction of neutrophils into damaged area (IL-8).

The chemokines are a family of factors secreted by leukocytes and endothelial cells in response to tissue damage and to other inflammatory mediators. They are locally bound to the extracellular matrix and heparin-sulphate proteoglycans of cells, and establish a concentration gradient away from the focus of inflammation. Neutrophil rolling causes neutrophils to encounter chemokines bound to proteoglycans on endothelial cells. Specific chemokine receptors are activated, and this signals for activation of leukocyte integrins, mediating adhesion and emigration (see pages 38–9). Chemokines are removed from the circulation by the Duffy antigen receptor for chemokines (DARC) expressed on red cells.

Nitric oxide is a small molecule that is locally synthesized by endothelium and macrophages through the activity of the enzyme nitric oxide synthase. It is a powerful cause of vascular dilatation, and increases vascular permeability. As an important reactive oxygen intermediary it can also mediate cell and bacterial killing.

The complement system comprises a set of plasma proteins with important roles in immunity and inflammation. There is a cascade of activation, with production of numerous intermediary activated peptides. The main products with roles in acute inflammation are as follows:

- C3a increases vascular permeability by liberating histamine from mast cells/platelets.
- C5a increases vascular permeability by liberating histamine from mast cells/platelets, is chemotactic to neutrophils, and induces endothelial cell adhesion molecules.
- C345 complex is chemoattractive to neutrophils.
- C3b opsonizes bacteria and facilitates neutrophil phagocytosis.

The **kinins** are small peptides derived from plasma precursors by proteolytic cleavage. The system is activated by one of the coagulation proteins, activated **Hageman factor** (**Factor XII**); this cleaves the peptide prekallikrein to kallikrein. Kallikrein stimulates a high molecular weight kininogen to form bradykinin, which is a powerful mediator of increased vascular permeability, causes pain, and activates the complement system.

The **clotting pathway** is responsible for coagulation of blood by formation of fibrin from fibrinogen. Factor XII (Hageman factor) is activated in the inflammatory exudate when it comes into contact with collagen outside the vessel. It then stimulates the deposition of fibrin, activates the kinin system, and also stimulates the thrombolytic system. When fibrinogen is converted to fibrin, fibrinopeptides are formed. These cause increased vascular permeability, as well as being chemotactic for neutrophils.

The **thrombolytic pathway.** The enzyme plasmin (generated by plasminogen activator derived from endothelium by the action of bradykinin) is a proteolytic enzyme with several roles in inflammation.

Plasmin:

- activates the complement system.
- activates Hageman factor.
- lyses fibrin to form fibrin degradation products, which increase the permeability of vessels.

In acute inflammation these factors act in concert to bring about the structural and functional changes.

OUTCOME OF THE ACUTE INFLAMMATORY REACTION

Under favorable circumstances the acute inflammatory reaction is adequate to deal with a damaging event and to prepare the ground for healing. The outcome of the reaction depends on the removal of the inflammatory exudate, and its replacement either by regenerated cells of the original type (restitution) or by scar tissue (fibrous repair). The possible end-results are summarized in *Fig. 4.13*.

Resolution occurs where there has been minimal damage to the tissue architecture and cells can regrow

In some circumstances, although there may be extensive destruction of cells, damage to the support tissues is minimal. An acute inflammatory exudate forms which, on resolution, leaves the supporting stroma undamaged, and the only deficiency is in epithelial cells. The exudate can be

 Laboratory medicine

Clinical indications of an acute inflammatory process include:

- General malaise.
- Fever.
- Pain, often localized to the inflamed area, e.g. the right iliac fossa in acute appendicitis.
- Rapid pulse rate.

Laboratory investigations usually reveal:

- A raised neutrophil count in the peripheral blood.
- An increased erythrocyte sedimentation rate (ESR).
- An increase in the concentration of **acute-phase proteins** in the blood. These are normally present in small concentrations, but increase dramatically in response to acute inflammation. Produced by the liver, they are induced by circulating IL-1. Specific examples, the most common being **C-reactive protein**, may be measured in blood to monitor inflammatory processes.

Drug therapy of acute inflammation

The acute inflammatory response can be treated with anti-inflammatory drugs, which prevent the production of key mediators of inflammation.

- Phospholipase A_2 activity is inhibited by steroids, thereby limiting the production of arachidonic acid and its metabolites.
- Aspirin inhibits the cyclo-oxygenase pathway and prevents the synthesis of prostaglandins and thromboxane A_2.
- NSAIDS inhibit the fatty acid cyclo-oxygenase COX-2. COX-2 initiates the biosynthesis of prostaglandins and thromboxanes.

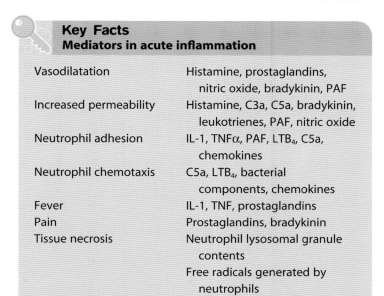

Key Facts
Mediators in acute inflammation

Vasodilatation	Histamine, prostaglandins, nitric oxide, bradykinin, PAF
Increased permeability	Histamine, C3a, C5a, bradykinin, leukotrienes, PAF, nitric oxide
Neutrophil adhesion	IL-1, TNFα, PAF, LTB_4, C5a, chemokines
Neutrophil chemotaxis	C5a, LTB_4, bacterial components, chemokines
Fever	IL-1, TNF, prostaglandins
Pain	Prostaglandins, bradykinin
Tissue necrosis	Neutrophil lysosomal granule contents
	Free radicals generated by neutrophils

Factors involved in vascular permeability in acute inflammation

There are two mechanisms for increased permeability of small vessels following tissue damage (*Fig. 4.12*):

- Toxins and physical agents may cause necrosis of vascular endothelium, leading to abnormal leakage (non-mediated vascular leakage).
- Chemical mediators of acute inflammation may cause retraction of endothelial cells, leaving intercellular gaps (mediated vascular leakage).

Experimental work has isolated three patterns of increased leakage of fluid from vessels, which occur at different times following injury:

1. An immediate response that is transient, lasts for 30–60 minutes, and is mediated by histamine acting on endothelium.
2. A delayed response that starts 2–3 hours after injury and lasts for up to 8 hours. This is mediated by factors synthesized by local cells, e.g. bradykinin, factors derived from complement, and factors released from dead neutrophils in the exudate.
3. An immediate response that is prolonged for over 24 hours and is seen if there has been direct necrosis of endothelium, e.g. in a burn or by a chemical toxin.

In disease it is likely that all three responses are activated, with an immediate prolonged response close to the centre of damage, and mediated responses at the interface between the damaged and healthy tissues.

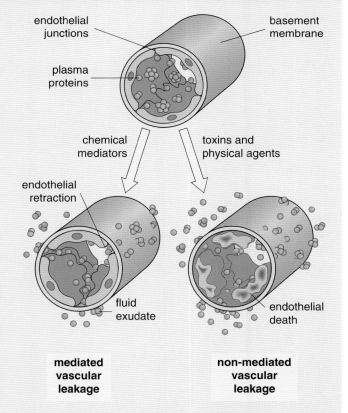

Fig. 4.12 The two main mechanisms for increase in vascular permeability.

removed from the inflamed area by a combination of liquefaction by neutrophil enzymes (with reabsorption of the fluid into lymphatics), and phagocytosis of particulate debris by macrophages.

Damaged cells regenerate, leaving the structure virtually as before, and normal function can be regained. This process, termed **resolution**, is obviously the best possible outcome, but unfortunately is not common. In most instances the support stroma is damaged and healing is by scar formation.

Regeneration of cells is limited to certain types. Nerve cells and cardiac muscle cells cannot divide, so any loss is permanent. Cells of liver and kidney do not normally divide, but following damage can divide to replace cells that have been lost. Other cells, such as surface epithelia, are constantly dividing and have a large capacity for regeneration following damage.

Organization and repair of acute inflammation lead to healing by collagenous scar

When there has been substantial structural damage to the tissue stroma, healing occurs not through resolution of the exudate, but by a process known as organization and repair, which eventually leads to the formation of a scar. The sequence of changes, shown diagrammatically and histologically in *Fig. 4.15* is as follows:

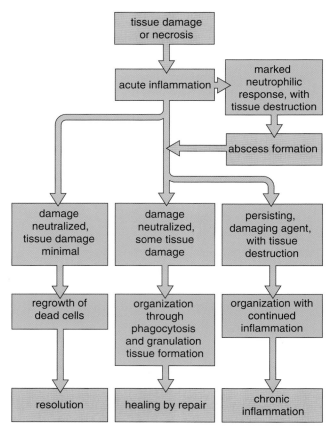

Fig. 4.13 **Flow diagram of outcomes of acute inflammation.**

Lobar pneumonia as an example of resolution of an exudate

Lobar pneumonia is a type of acute inflammation of the lung. It results from damage caused by certain types of pathogenic bacteria within the alveolar air sacs. The presence of the bacteria and their excreted toxins causes the death of epithelial cells (type 1 and type 2 pneumocytes) lining the alveolar spaces. The body's response is to produce an acute inflammatory exudate, the components of which (fluids, salts, fibrinogen/fibrin, other proteins, neutrophils and macrophages) pass out from the network of capillaries lining the alveolar sacs into the alveolar lumen.

As the infection develops, the air in a large number of alveoli is replaced by exudate (see *Fig. 4.14a*). This change tends to spread rapidly throughout all of the air sacs of a particular lobe of the lung (hence 'lobar' pneumonia), and a considerable proportion of the patient's gaseous exchange capacity is lost. Importantly, although cells lining alveoli die, the support stroma and vascular structure of the lung remain intact. Under favorable conditions, especially if the patient is treated with antibiotics, the neutrophils in the exudate phagocytose and destroy all of the causative bacteria, at which point the process of resolution can begin.

Enzymes released by neutrophils break up structural proteins (e.g. the fibrin) and remnants of dead cells, rendering the exudate highly liquid. Some of it is coughed up in sputum, but much of it can be reabsorbed into the alveolar capillary network or the pulmonary lymphatic system. Macrophages phagocytose any residual undigested debris, pass into the lymphatic system, and are transmitted to regional lymph nodes.

At the same time, remnant epithelial stem cells divide to reline the alveolar air spaces, differentiating into new type 1 and type 2 alveolar lining cells. Resolution can take place only if the damaged cells can divide and repopulate the injured area. Once the exudate is removed from the alveolar air spaces and epithelial cells are regenerated, gaseous exchange can begin again. If this process of resolution of an inflammatory exudate

(see *Fig. 4.14b*) does not take place, usually because of more severe structural damage to the supporting stroma, an area of scar tissue will eventually form in the lung.

Fig. 4.14 Resolution of acute inflammatory exudate in lobar pneumonia. In (a) the photomicrograph shows the fully formed exudate, rich in neutrophils and fibrin, filling all the alveolar spaces between alveolar walls. In (b) the exudate is in the process of resolution. The alveolar spaces largely contain fluid (which will be reabsorbed) and some residual macrophages (which will re-enter the blood or lymphatic circulations).

- Pre-existing capillaries in the undamaged tissue form new capillaries by budding into the damaged area, which is also infiltrated by macrophages, fibroblasts, and myofibroblasts. Macrophages phagocytose inflammatory exudate and dead tissue. **Vascular granulation tissue**, a fragile complex of interconnecting capillaries, macrophages and support cells, replaces the area of tissue damage (*Figs 4.15b* and *c*).
- There is progressive growth of fibroblasts and myofibroblasts, and the tissue defect is filled with the complex capillary network, proliferating fibroblasts, and a few residual macrophages (**fibrovascular granulation tissue**) (*Figs 4.15d* and *e*). With continued proliferation of the fibroblasts, and active collagen synthesis, many of the newly formed capillaries regress until a comparatively small number of vascular channels remain, connecting the damaged area of tissue to the normal undamaged area around it, and providing nutrients for the fibroblasts. Some of the persisting vessels acquire smooth muscle in their walls, and remain as functioning venules and arterioles.
- The intervening spaces between the vessels become progressively filled with fibroblasts synthesizing collagen (**fibrous granulation tissue**). The fibroblasts align themselves so that they deposit collagen in a mainly uniform pattern, running in a direction that provides maximum strength in the face of the physical stresses encountered. Contraction of the area of granulation tissue frequently occurs, partly through the contractile effects of the myofibroblasts. The size of the damaged area is thus reduced.

- Production of dense collagen by the fibroblasts forms a **collagenous scar**.
- Once the fibroblasts have synthesized sufficient collagen to fill the defect, they assume a resting status, in which they exhibit scanty cytoplasm and an elongated spindle-shaped nucleus (*Figs 4.15f* and *g*). These inactive fibroblasts are known as fibrocytes.

The process whereby the inflammatory exudate is replaced by granulation tissue is called **organization of the exudate**; that by which the granulation tissue is subsequently replaced by fibrous scar is called **fibrous repair**.

Local and systemic factors influence healing

Many factors, whether encountered in the course of inflammation or during wound healing, impair organization and repair processes:

- Inadequate nutrition impairs repair. Protein is required for collagen synthesis, as are vitamin C and zinc.
- Ischemia to tissues markedly impairs repair.
- Infection of tissues causes continued tissue damage, promoting a continued acute inflammatory response.
- Foreign material (including large areas of dead tissue) retained in an area of tissue damage acts as a nidus for infection, promoting inflammation. This is the rationale behind surgical debridement of necrotic material from large wounds.
- Steroids hinder the formation of granulation tissue, and their immunosuppressive effects may predispose to local infection.

vessel
endothelium

macrophages emigrate into the area of damage

area becomes semi-liquid

(a)

vascular granulation tissue

capillary buds grow into damaged area to form network

macrophages secrete fibrogenic and angiogenic factors

fibroblasts/ myofibroblasts

(b)

fibrovascular granulation tissue

fibroblasts proliferate and begin to deposit collagen

(d)

collagenous scar

collagen is dense

fibroblasts become inactive (fibrocytes)

vascularity is reduced

(f)

Fig. 4.15 Organization and repair. (a) Removal of debris by macrophages. (b) Vascular granulation tissue. (c) Vascular granulation tissue. This photomicrograph shows the abundant thin-walled vessels of vascular granulation tissue. The intervening tissue contains residual macrophages. (d) Fibrovascular granulation tissue. (e) Fibrovascular granulation tissue. This photomicrograph shows the tissue between the vascular networks becoming filled with proliferating fibroblasts, which are already tending to align themselves in the direction of tensile stress. (f) Collagenous scar formation. (g) Early collagenous scar. This photomicrograph shows the nuclei of the fibroblasts becoming compressed. The formerly active fibroblasts have become inactive resting fibrocytes.

(c)

(e)

(g)

- Radiation exposure reduces a damaged area's capacity for repair, e.g. a wound in an area of previous radiotherapy will heal poorly.
- Diabetes is associated with poor wound healing for several reasons, including susceptibility to vascular disease and ischemia, and increased susceptibility to infection.
- Denervation of an area impairs healing.

Healing is promoted by:

- Removal of dead tissues to allow apposition of healthy tissues.
- Administration of appropriate antibiotics in cases of infection.

Healing of wounds is also achieved by organization, repair and scar formation

The healing of tissue wounds, including those caused by surgical procedures, also occurs through the processes of organization and formation of granulation and scar tissue.

The ideal situation for healing is of a surgical wound in which adjacent surfaces are closely apposed and held together by suture material. The classic example of a sutured skin wound is given in *Fig. 4.16*. The key feature of this type of healing is that there is only a narrow space between the adjacent tissues, with a minimal amount of dead tissue limited to the very edges of the wound.

Where there has been extensive loss of cells a large tissue defect results, which has to be filled by granulation tissue. Examples include large surface ulcers or open wounds that cannot be sutured. Because the damage is extensive, the inflammatory response at the edges of the wound is usually intense, and the large amount of granulation tissue required means that healing takes a long time. However, the ultimate size of the collagenous scar is reduced by shrinkage of the healing wound. Myofibroblasts contract at the stage of granulation tissue formation, and this process, termed **wound contraction**, can reduce the surface area of an open wound to 10% of its original size.

Healing of closely apposed surfaces has been termed healing by **primary intention**; the healing of open wounds is sometimes termed healing by **secondary intention**. The differences between the two relate to the amount of infill required to bridge the tissue defect, rather than any special mechanistic differences.

Fig. 4.16 Stages in the healing of a sutured skin wound	
Day 1	Neutrophils appear at margins of incision and there is an acute inflammatory response on each side of the narrow incisional space, leading to swelling, redness, and pain at the wound site. Epithelial cells at edge of wound undergo mitosis and begin to migrate across wound.
Day 2	Macrophages begin to infiltrate the incisional space and to demolish fibrin. Surface epithelial continuity is re-established in the form of a thin surface layer.
Day 3	Granulation tissue begins to invade tissue space. Surface epithelial continuity is reinforced by thickening of epithelial layer.
Day 5	Incisional space is filled with vascular granulation tissue: collagen is progressively deposited. Surface epithelium achieves normal thickness. Acute inflammatory response at wound margins begins to subside, and swelling and redness of adjacent tissues is reduced.
Day 7	Sutures commonly removed from skin wounds. Wound has approximately 10% of tensile strength of normal skin.
Day 10	Further fibroblast proliferation and collagen deposition occur in granulation tissue in the incisional space, adding to strength of wound.
Day 15	Collagen deposition follows the lines of tissue stress. Granulation tissue loses some of its vascularity, but still appears pinker than adjacent tissues.
Day 30	Wound now has 50% of tensile strength of normal skin.
3 months	Wound achieves maximal 80% of tensile strength of normal skin. It now appears only marginally more vascular than adjacent skin. Complete blanching of scar takes several more months.

Damaged brain heals by growth of astrocytes rather than by formation of collagenous scars

Brain damage is generally not repaired through proliferation of fibroblasts, but through proliferation of the support cells of the brain, the astrocytes. The necrotic tissue is removed and replaced by fluid, which forms a cystic lesion. Surrounded by compacted glial fibers produced by astrocytes, this is termed a glial scar or astrocytic gliosis. The changes that follow damage to brain tissue are described in more detail in Chapter 21.

A fibrous scar is an inadequate end-result in bone healing

When bone is damaged, most commonly by fracture, collagenous scarring alone is insufficiently strong to repair the bone. Although bone fracture undergoes the same processes of organization, granulation tissue formation and fibroblast ingrowth, an additional proliferation of osteoblasts produces the highly specialized collagen extracellular matrix known as osteoid, which is then mineralized to form bone. The mixture of fibrous granulation tissue and developing new bone, which is called callus, bridges the defect between the broken bone ends. At a later stage the callus is refashioned to re-establish the normal structure of the bone prior to fracture. The details of fracture healing are given in Chapter 24.

CHRONIC INFLAMMATION

When a damaging stimulus persists, complete healing cannot occur, and chronic inflammation ensues

The sequence of **tissue damage → acute inflammation → exudate → organization of exudate → granulation tissue → fibrous scar** occurs only when the damaging stimulus is of short duration and does not persist. In such cases the changes leading to scar formation are consecutive.

If the damaging stimulus persists, the processes of continuing tissue necrosis, organization and repair all occur **concurrently**. In addition to acute inflammation, the specific defenses of the **immune system** are activated around the area of damage, and tissues are infiltrated by activated lymphoid cells. Histological examination of an affected area will show necrotic cell debris, acute inflammatory exudate, vascular and fibrous granulation tissue, lymphoid cells, macrophages and collagenous scar. This state, termed **chronic inflammation**, will persist until the damaging stimulus is removed or neutralized.

Chronic inflammation is a balance between repair and continued tissue damage

Chronic inflammation is the result of a balance between continuing tissue damage on the one hand, and eradication of the damaging stimulus, followed by healing and scar formation, on the other (*Fig. 4.17*).

- If the damaging stimulus is neutralized or eradicated, further tissue necrosis does not occur

Cellular events in wound healing

There are five key events in healing by organization and repair.

Local vessels:

1. Are stimulated to form outgrowths (**angiogenesis**).

Local support cells:

2. Divide to form fibroblasts and myofibroblasts (**mitogenesis**).
3. Migrate towards the area of tissue damage (**chemotaxis** and **motility**).
4. Secrete collagen (**fibrogenesis**).
5. Produce collagen-degrading enzymes (**remodelling**).

Peptide growth factors stimulate angiogenesis, promote cell division and migration, and stimulate collagen secretion. The main examples are platelet-derived growth factor (mitogenesis and chemotaxis), basic fibroblast growth factor (angiogenesis, mitogenesis, chemotaxis), transforming growth factor (fibrogenesis), IL-1 and tumor necrosis factor (fibrogenesis).

Molecules in the extracellular matrix facilitate adhesion of cells and act as signals, affecting differentiation and growth, e.g. fibronectin increases in tissues during healing, and mediates adhesion of growing capillaries and fibroblasts, as well as enhancing their response to basic fibroblast growth factor.

As part of the increase in the strength of a wound, the secreted collagen undergoes maturation. The molecular basis of this involves degradation as well as increased cross-linking. Degradation involves secretion of metalloproteinases by support cells that degrade collagen. The molecular type of collagen secreted early in granulation tissue formation is type III, which is later replaced by degradation and secretion of type I collagen.

and the repair response progresses to complete scarring.

- If the damaging stimulus cannot be eradicated or neutralized, the balance between tissue damage and tissue repair is maintained in a kind of stalemate and a state of chronic inflammation will persist, often for many years. During this time the balance may alter, often because of changing local or systemic factors in the patient.

Some of the possible outcomes are presented in relation to the example of chronic acid-induced ulceration of the stomach and duodenum (chronic peptic ulcer), illustrated in *Fig. 4.18*.

Immune mechanisms dominate the cellular responses in chronic inflammation

Although neutrophils are the key effector cells in acute inflammation, those in chronic inflammation are lymphoid cells and macrophages, a reflection of a tissue-based immune response to the damaging agent.

In chronic inflammation, macrophages not only act as phagocytic cells (removing and destroying cell debris) but become activated to fulfill other immunological and secretory functions.

Because lymphocytes, plasma cells and macrophages are invariably present in chronic inflammatory reactions, they are sometimes referred to as chronic inflammatory cells (*Fig. 4.19*).

The macrophage is a main effector cell in chronic inflammation

Macrophages are among the main effector cells in chronic inflammation, and have several roles. They are converted from inactive monocytes to functioning macrophages by trophic signals, the best characterized being γ-interferon.

The morphology of activated macrophages changes, particularly as the subcellular apparatus for protein synthesis develops. Such cells develop voluminous cytoplasm, at which stage they are known as epithelioid cells. In addition, fusion of activated macrophages is a common event, whereby multinucleate histiocytic giant cells are formed.

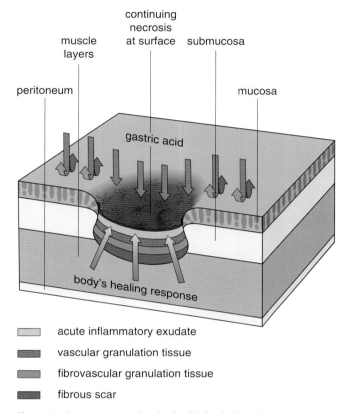

acute inflammatory exudate

vascular granulation tissue

fibrovascular granulation tissue

fibrous scar

Fig. 4.17 Factors operating in the biological stalemate of an active chronic peptic ulcer.

Chronic peptic ulcer illustrates the basic principles of chronic inflammation

The lining of the upper alimentary tract is normally protected from the adverse effects of the dilute hydrochloric acid and proteolytic enzymes produced in the stomach mucosa for food digestion. If the protective mechanisms break down, the acid and enzymes destroy the epithelium and supporting stroma (cause ulceration) of the wall of the alimentary tract, usually affecting the stomach or duodenum. This damaging stimulus is persistent, as the stomach is always producing acid and enzymes. Tissue damage stimulates an acute inflammatory reaction, with the formation of exudate close to the damaging acid in the stomach lumen. In the depths of the ulcer, furthest away from the acid, attempts are made to organize the exudate, and granulation tissue forms, which then progresses to collagenous scar.

In an established ulcer, all of these processes are occurring at the same time. A chronic peptic ulcer is therefore an example of chronic inflammation caused by the persistence of the damaging stimulus.

Fig. 4.17 shows diagrammatically the factors operating in a chronic peptic ulcer. *Fig. 4.18* shows the possible outcomes of such an ulcer, which depend on whether reparative responses are vigorous, or whether destructive responses cause progressive damage. The aim of treatment in peptic ulcer is to facilitate healing by removing or greatly reducing the damaging stimulus, i.e. the acid and enzymes secreted.

Outcomes of peptic ulcer

Fig. 4.18 Possible outcomes of peptic ulcer. (a) **Healing**. The damaging stimulus is overcome by the healing process, usually because gastric acid secretion is reduced or neutralized. The defect becomes filled with fibrous scar and is re-covered with gastric mucosa. **The ulcer heals completely**.

(b) **Perforation**. The healing and repair process is overwhelmed by continuing damage caused by increased levels of gastric acid. The process of ulceration continues, penetrating the full thickness of the wall leading to **perforation**.

(c) **Chronicity**. The damage caused by acid is counterbalanced – but not overcome – by the body's healing response. This stalemate situation leads to chronic gastric ulcer, which may persist for many years. Any change in the balance of the conflicting factors may lead to (a) or (b) above.

Once activated, macrophages have both a phagocytic and a major secretory role in defense against injurious agents, and are important in cell-mediated immunity, e.g. antigen presentation. They secrete:

- Mediators of acute inflammation, particularly platelet-activating factor and arachidonic acid metabolites.
- Highly reactive oxygen metabolites, which participate in bacterial and cell killing.
- Proteases and hydrolytic enzymes, which cause dissolution of extracellular material. This is particularly relevant to the role of macrophages in removing damaged material from areas of injury.
- Cytokines, IL-1, and TNFα. These stimulate fibroblast proliferation and collagen synthesis, which are important in any reparative response.
- Growth factors (PDGF, EGF, FGF). These stimulate growth of blood vessels, and division and migration of fibroblasts.

Fig. 4.19 Chronic inflammatory cells. Photomicrograph showing the lymphocytes, macrophages and plasma cells commonly found in areas of chronic inflammation, mainly the result of the immune responses involved in chronicity.

Granulomatous inflammatory reactions occur when neutrophil phagocytosis is inadequate to neutralize the causative agent

In certain diseases the acute inflammatory response, dominated by neutrophils, is transient and quickly replaced by an immune-based cellular reaction, which is characterized by aggregations of macrophages and lymphocytes. The macrophages often form discrete clusters called **granulomata**. A pattern of this kind is therefore frequently called **granulomatous inflammation**. It is an example of a chronic inflammatory response, as persistence of the damaging agent leads to concurrent tissue damage, inflammation and repair.

Damaging stimuli which provoke a granulomatous inflammatory response include:

- **Microorganisms which are of low inherent pathogenicity but which excite an immune response**. The most important group are the mycobacteria, which are intracellular pathogens with a resistant lipoprotein coating to the cell membrane. The most important mycobacteria in human disease are *Mycobacterium tuberculosis* (responsible for **tuberculosis**) and *M. leprae* (responsible for **leprosy**). Other organisms include *Trepomema pallidum*, which induces 'syphilitic gummata' and *Bartonella henselae*, which induces the granulomatous response seen in 'cat scratch disease.'
- Granulomata are produced in response to **helminth infection,** for example the eosinophil-rich schistosome egg granuloma seen typically in the liver.
- **Non-living foreign material deposited in tissues**. As the material is non-viable, neutrophil enzymes are powerless to destroy it and the material remains as a constant irritant within the tissues. Examples include both exogenous materials, which gain access to the tissues (e.g. inhaled inorganic dust such as **silicone** and **beryllium** in the lungs), and endogenous materials, which become misplaced or deposited in large quantities (e.g. precipitated urate crystals in gout) (see page 551), and keratin that has escaped from traumatized epidermoid cysts).
- Certain fungi cannot be dealt with adequately by neutrophils, and thus excite granulomatous reactions.
- **Crohn's disease** of the gastrointestinal tract (see page 260) is typified by a granulomatous response to an unknown antigen.
- Unknown factors, e.g. in the disease 'sarcoid' (see pages 212 and 567).

Tuberculosis is an example of granulomatous inflammation

The most common pattern of human tuberculosis (TB) is pulmonary. The *M. tuberculosis* organism is inhaled into the alveolar spaces of the lung, but other tissues are also affected, as described in the **systems pathology** later in the book.

Key Facts
Granulomatous inflammation

- Formed by aggregated of activated macrophages that have an epithelioid morphology.
- Often seen as a consequence of type IV hypersensitivity reactions.
- Granulomata frequently have a necrotic centre surrounded by a macrophage/epithelioid cell zone that is in turn surrounded by a cuff of lymphocytes.
- The inflammatory reaction is driven by cytokines, including IFNγ, lymphotoxin, IL-3, GM-CSF and IL-12.
- IL-12 shifts the response towards a Th1-driven cell mediated response rather than an antibody (Th2)-dominated reaction.
- Granulomata fail to develop in the absence of TNF secreted by activated macrophages.
- The response is modified in immunodeficiency states due to alterations in the Th1/Th2 profile.

Once in the lung the mycobacteria excite a transient but marked immune-mediated response, manifest by sensitization of T cells to produce cytokines (see Key Facts box). Neutrophils are inadequate to deal with the organisms, the cell walls of which are resistant to degradation, and after 3 weeks or so the initial acute inflammatory response is replaced by a chronic inflammatory pattern dominated by aggregates of macrophages, recruited and activated by T cell-derived cytokines. IL-12, released from antigen-presenting cells (APCs), drives the differentiation of CD4+ Th1 cells, which in turn release TNF, IL-2 and IFNγ. IFNγ is a potent activator of macrophages and also increases macrophage production of IL-12; thus, the macrophage activation loop by Th1 cells and APCs is autocatalytic. Activated macrophages also upregulate MHC class II, leading to their increased efficiency as antigen-presenting cells. Under the influence of cytokines such as IFNγ the epithelioid cells can fuse to form **multinucleated giant cells,** which in tuberculosis infection are known as **Langhans' cells**. The structure of a typical tuberculous granuloma is shown in *Fig. 4.20*. The type of immune response caused by TB is termed type IV hypersensitivity.

The histological appearances are modified in immunosuppressed patients

The central role of the CD4+ Th-1 cell in granulomatous inflammation is illustrated by cases of immunosuppression, for example HIV, where the CD4+ response is impaired. In these cases, granulomata do not form, the macrophages remain unactivated, and are not capable of containing the primary focus. This condition is known as progressive primary tuberculosis.

Fig. 4.20 A tuberculous granuloma. In (a) the typical structure of a tubercle is shown diagrammatically. A central area of amorphous caseous necrosis is surrounded by a zone of activated macrophages, in which multinucleate macrophages (Langhans' giant cells) are present. There are outer layers of lymphocytes and fibroblasts. The low-power photomicrograph (b) shows a tubercle in the lung, demonstrating the features illustrated in (a). The medium-power photomicrograph (c) shows greater detail of the edge of the tubercle.

The clinical presentation in leprosy varies from a Th1-dominated response to one dominated by a Th2 cytokine profile

Clinically, leprosy is divided into three main groups: tuberculoid, borderline and lepromatous. The tuberculoid pattern shows a Th1-driven cell-mediated response similar to that seen in tuberculosis, having an intense lymphocytic and macrophage infiltrate with few organisms being detected. Lepromatous leprosy shows a weak macrophage response, with few lymphocytes, and a failure to contain organisms – characteristic of a Th2-driven antibody-mediated response. Borderline leprosy shows an intermediate response. Thus, the clinical picture is dictated by the cytokine profile released in response to infection.

OTHER CAUSES OF GRANULOMATOUS INFLAMMATION

Sarcoidosis is a granulomatous disease of unknown cause

In sarcoidosis, discrete granulomata with histiocytic giant cells form, mainly in lymph nodes, lungs, liver, spleen and skin, although other organs (e.g. brain and bone) are occasionally affected. Histologically, the granulomata resemble those of TB, although there is never any true caseation and the granulomata are frequently accompanied by fibrosis. The granulomata are multiple and slowly increase in size, often becoming confluent. The cause of the disease is unknown. Affected patients most commonly present with clinical disease related to lung involvement, or with evidence of bilateral hilar lymph node enlargement. The multinucleate giant cells in sarcoidosis occasionally contain laminated calcific spherical concretions (**Schaumann bodies** or **asteroid bodies**).

Although the cause of the disease is unknown, the cellular reaction is driven by CD4+ T cells similar to that in tuberculous granulomata. There is also an increase in Th1 cytokines such as IL-2 and IFNγ, resulting in T-cell expansion and macrophage activation. In addition, there are systemic immunological abnormalities in patients with sarcoidosis, some of which suggest abnormalities in the function of helper and regulatory T cells (T_{reg}, Th3), the latter type being of major importance in the induction of T-cell tolerance and modulation of immune responses.

The disease is slowly progressive but frequently burns itself out, the formerly cellular granulomata becoming progressively smaller and more collagenized. Where there has been significant lung involvement, this healing phase may produce widespread pulmonary fibrosis. This is discussed in Chapter 25.

Developmental and genetic diseases

5

DEVELOPMENTAL DISORDERS

Factors that induce abnormal embryological development are known as 'teratogens'

Most teratogens induce abnormal development only if the mother and embryo are exposed to them at a particular stage of embryological development, often during the first 3 months (trimester) of fetal development, which is the period when there is most active embryological change. The likelihood of abnormality depends on:

- Dose and duration of exposure.
- Time of exposure.
- Individual susceptibility.

Many factors have been shown to be teratogenic in experimental animals, but largely harmless in humans. However, because for some factors the reverse is true, species specificity renders testing for drug teratogenicity using experimental animals something of a lottery.

The most important teratogenic factors recognized in humans are:

- Drugs and chemicals, e.g. thalidomide, alcohol.
- Ionizing radiations, e.g. X-rays.
- Maternal infections, e.g. toxoplasmosis, rubella, herpes simplex, syphilis.
- Genetic/chromosomal abnormalities, e.g. Down's syndrome, Turner's syndrome.

Failure of normal embryological development is usually evident at birth

In many cases the embryological error is so great that the embryo cannot survive and dies soon after fertilization.

Less severe abnormalities permit the embryo to develop to a later stage, but the fetus dies late in the pregnancy or shortly after birth; an example is bilateral renal dysplasia.

Some embryological abnormalities are not immediately lethal but produce disease in later life. For example, there are many embryological disorders that affect the final proper development of the heart; in some, the abnormality is not immediately fatal but produces severe illness (e.g. Fallot's tetralogy), whereas others are so mild that they are compatible with a normal existence (e.g. a small atrial or ventricular septal defect). Some of the more common and important congenital diseases of the heart are discussed in Chapter 10.

Examples of abnormal embryological development affecting the various systems are examined in the relevant chapters later in the book. The most important patterns of embryological maldevelopment are detailed in *Fig. 5.1*.

GENETIC FACTORS IN DISEASE

Three levels in the development of human genetics are now recognized: **classic genetics**, **cytogenetics**, and **molecular genetics**.

A full description of genetics, together with the detailed mechanisms of genetic and chromosomal disorders, is beyond the scope of this book. Readers are referred to one of the excellent student texts on clinical genetics.

A major advance in the application of genetics to disease has been the availability of high-throughput laboratory methods which allow the detection of chromosomal changes or mutations in specific genes. Students are also advised to consult specialist textbooks to understand the principles behind modern molecular genetic investigative techniques.

In addition to an application to the diseases which are generally classed as developmental and genetic, modern genetic investigation is transforming the understanding and investigation of neoplastic diseases. It is becoming increasingly realized that acquired genetic changes are responsible for the development of neoplastic diseases. The genetics and mechanisms involved in neoplasia are discussed in Chapter 6.

Throughout medicine, genetic susceptibility traits are being revealed that make a contribution to the understanding of disease.

Classic genetics is based on analysis of pedigrees and patterns of inheritance

Clinical analysis of inherited diseases has allowed the delineation of several distinct patterns. Although many diseases follow mendelian genetic principles of dominant, recessive, and sex-linked patterns, others are suggestive of a polygenic or multifactorial pattern. Forms of maternal inheritance are seen which can be explained by inheritance through mitochondrial, rather than nuclear, DNA.

The importance of classic genetics is that it allows counseling of families, based on the statistical chances of inheriting a disease. The recent developments in molecular genetic techniques can frequently reinforce such analysis by enabling precise diagnosis of disease, based on the identification of abnormal genes. Prenatal diagnosis and confident prediction of whether a fetus has inherited abnormal genes from the parents are now possible. Until all genes related to disease are identified, classic genetics, and counseling based on statistical risk, remain important parts of clinical practice.

Fig. 5.1 Patterns of embryological maldevelopment

Pattern	Mechanism	Common examples
Complete failure of organ development (agenesis)	Early failure of development of all or part of organ primordium	Renal agenesis (see *Fig. 5.2*)
Incomplete organ development (hypoplasia)	Probably due to influence of external teratogen during organ growth phase	Microcephaly (e.g. alcohol teratogenicity) Phocomelia (e.g. thalidomide teratogenicity, see *Fig. 5.3*)
Abnormal tissue organization (dysplasia)	Failure of organized tissue differentiation and maturation	Renal dysplasia (see *Fig. 5.4*)
Failure of embryological fusion (dysraphism)	Defects arise by failure of complete fusion of embryological primordia	Myelomeningocele (see *Fig. 5.5*) 'Ectopia vesicae'
Failure of involution	Temporary embryological structures that normally involute by apoptosis fail to do so	Persistent urachus Persistent thyroglossal duct Syndactyly (see *Fig 5.6*)
Failure of lumen formation (atresia)	Solid cylinders of cells fail to undergo central programed cell death to create a lumen	Esophageal atresia (see *Fig 5.7*) Biliary atresia
Organ or tissue displacement (ectopia)	Failure of normal migration of cells during embryological development	Maldescent of testes

Examples of common patterns of embryological maldevelopment

Fig. 5.2 Renal agenesis: an example of complete failure of organ development.
This fetus shows total failure of kidney development. The masses located at the site normally occupied by the kidneys are large fetal adrenals (**A**).

Fig. 5.3 Phocomelia: an example of incomplete organ development.
This fetus shows incomplete development of the arm (phocomelia). This congenital malformation may occur spontaneously, but is particularly associated with the chemical teratogen thalidomide.

Fig. 5.4 Renal dysplasia: an example of abnormal tissue organization. This child died shortly after birth, without passing urine. The kidneys show dysplasia, and are being converted into a connected mass of cysts.

Fig. 5.5 Myelomeningocele: an example of failure of embryological fusion. This common congenital malformation is known as 'spina bifida.'

Fig. 5.6 Syndactyly: an example of failure of involution by apoptosis. Fusion of digits is a common congenital malformation, and is the result of failure of the tissues between the digits to involute through apoptosis during development.

Fig. 5.7 Esophageal atresia: an example of failure of lumen formation. In this radiograph, injection of radio-opaque medium into the upper esophagus of a newborn infant demonstrates the failure of the lumen to develop by apoptosis.

Cytogenetics is based on analysis of chromosomal abnormalities

The production of chromosomal spreads and the staining of chromosomes to show bands have allowed direct observation of abnormalities of chromosomes (*Fig. 5.8*). The two principal types of abnormality apparent using these techniques are:

• Abnormalities in the number of individual chromosomes.
• Structural abnormalities in individual chromosomes.

Such cytogenetic analyses are an important aspect of medical investigation (see pages 59–63 and 88), and identification of carrier states allows genetic counselling to be given to at-risk families. Moreover, identification of specific forms of chromosomal abnormality provides an insight into the prognosis of certain types of tumor, particularly leukemias.

Knowledge of how gross changes in chromosomal material lead to abnormal phenotypes is growing through the application of molecular genetic techniques. Until the precise genes responsible for all such disorders are defined, cytogenetic methods remain important clinical and research tools.

Certain genetic disorders can be identified by detection of abnormal gene products

For many years, several genetic abnormalities have been confidently diagnosed by the identification of abnormal gene products. Some of these conditions have been diagnosed in utero, using prenatal tests based on identification of the abnormal product or the lack of a specific enzyme activity. Examples include the identification of abnormal hemoglobins in the hemoglobinopathies (e.g. sickle-cell disease), identification of children affected by phenylketonuria (PKU), and demonstration of the loss of specific enzyme activities in many of the metabolic diseases leading to storage of abnormal metabolites (e.g. the glycogenoses).

Interestingly, molecular genetic techniques have shown several types of genetic abnormality to underlie single apparently well-defined conditions (molecular genetic heterogeneity), which goes some way to explaining the variation seen in clinical expression of disease.

Genetic disorders are now identifiable by molecular genetic techniques

Recombinant DNA technology has revolutionized the diagnosis and investigation of genetic diseases. The main techniques enable individual genes to be identified and sequenced, and probes can be created for use in molecular genetic diagnosis of disease. The use of specific restriction enzymes, together with Southern blotting to separate DNA fragments, allows the identification of the linkage between specific chromosomal areas and disease, so that such regions may be searched to locate specific genes.

Karyotype Analysis

Fig. 5.8 Chromosome spread.

CYTOGENETIC ABNORMALITIES AND DISEASE

A normal haploid gamete has 22 autosomes and 1 sex chromosome

The normal (diploid) chromosome complement of the human somatic cell consists of 46 paired chromosomes, with 44 autosomes and two sex chromosomes (XX in females and XY in males); one half is contributed by the haploid maternal ovum, the other by the haploid paternal spermatozoon. Thus, after meiosis, the haploid maternal ovum will contain 22 autosomes and an X chromosome.

Similarly, the fertilizing paternal spermatozoon will contain either 22 autosomes and an X chromosome, or 22 autosomes and a Y chromosome, the sex of the embryo

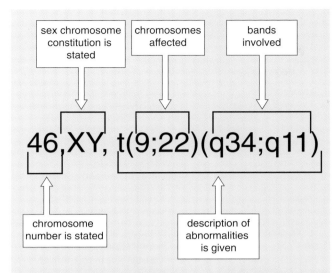

46,XY, t(9;22)(q34;q11)

- sex chromosome constitution is stated
- chromosomes affected
- bands involved
- chromosome number is stated
- description of abnormalities is given

Additional whole chromosomes are listed as '+' followed by the number, e.g. +21 for trisomy 21.

Abnormalities such as deletions, inversions, translocations (t) and fragile sites are denoted by an abbreviation (see *Fig. 5.11*), located to specific chromosome areas according to the following scheme:

- The short arm of a chromosome is termed 'p'.

- The long arm of a chromosome is termed 'q'.

- Chromosome regions are defined as numbered regions from the centromere outwards.

- Within each region, individual bands are given a number.

Fig. 5.9 Nomenclature and notation of karyotype analysis. The above example is a male with a translocation between chromosomes 9 and 22, both involving the long arm. This is the Philadelphia chromosome, seen in certain forms of leukemia (Chapter 15).

depending on which type of spermatozoon fertilizes the ovum. For successful blending of chromosomes, it is vital that the meiotic division in both ova and spermatozoa be faultless. However, abnormal chromosome separation during meiosis may result in deletion, non-disjunction or translocation of chromosomal material in either autosomes or sex chromosomes.

The convention used for describing the chromosomal complement of a cell on karyotype analysis is given in *Fig. 5.9*.

Abnormalities of chromosomes are a common cause of congenital abnormality

Abnormal chromosome numbers usually result from non-disjunction (i.e. failure of paired chromosomes to separate properly during cell division), and can occur in meiotic or mitotic divisions.

Gametes with only one of a pair of autosomes (monosomy) do not usually survive, and the majority of autosomal number disorders are due to extra chromosomal material, particularly trisomies (three copies).

Breaking and rejoining leads to structural chromosomal abnormalities

If there is a break in chromosomal material, the break can be rejoined. If a segment is involved, material may be lost (deletion), transposed into another chromosome (translocation), or abnormally inserted (inversion), as illustrated diagrammatically in *Fig. 5.10*.

The symbols used to describe the main structural abnormalities of chromosomes are listed in *Fig. 5.11*.

Translocation of one part of a chromosome to another is caused by breaking and rejoining (*Fig. 5.10a*). Translocation of chromosomal material is frequently reciprocal, thus there is no overall loss or gain of genetic material in the carrier, who is phenotypically normal. The problem with this type of abnormality is that when segregation takes place, two sets of material from one chromosome may end up in one gamete. For example, a translocation of chromosome 21 onto chromosome 14 may be present in the mother. An ovum may be then be produced with the normal chromosome 21, together with the abnormal chromosome 14 carrying the additional chromosome 21 material. If the gamete is then fertilized by a normal haploid sperm, three copies of chromosome 21 material are contained in the gamete.

Robertsonian translocation describes a special situation in which chromosome breaks occur close to the centromere of two chromosomes, resulting in one very large chromosome and one very small chromosome, which is frequently lost (*Fig. 5.10b*). Affected individuals appear to have 45 chromosomes on karyotype analysis. As with other forms of translocation, problems arise in gametogenesis, with the formation of unbalanced gametes containing both copies of the chromosomal material.

Ring chromosomes are associated with loss of genetic material. They are a special form of deletion in which a chromosome, having lost material from both ends, rejoins in a closed circle (*Fig. 5.10c*).

Inversions occur when two breaks in a chromosome take place. The resulting fragment is turned 180° and is reunited in the same chromosome.

The most common **deletion** syndrome is the *cri du chat* syndrome, caused by deletion of part of chromosome 5 (*Fig. 5.10d*). Microcephaly, muscular hypotonia and mental retardation are associated, and the affected infant has a characteristic shrill cry (hence *cri du chat*).

Abnormal chromosomes resulting from translocation are rare. They cause 'functional' trisomy syndromes, the most common leading to Down's, Edwards' and Patau's syndromes. Translocations may cause abnormal gene expression, resulting in tumor formation (see Chapter 6).

translocation

(a)

Robertsonian
(pericentromeric)
translocation

lost

(b)

ring chromosome

lost

(c)

deletion

lost

(d)

Fig. 5.10 Structural abnormalities of chromosomes. (a) Translocation. (b) Robertsonian translocation. (c) Ring chromosome. (d) Deletion.

Fig. 5.11 Main structural changes of chromosomes

Type	Symbol	Nature
Translocation	t	Two chromosomes break, rejoin, and exchange segments
Deletion	del	A segment of chromosome is lost
Inversion	inv	Two breaks occur; the middle piece is rotated and rejoins
Fragile site	fra	A chromosomal site with a tendency to break
Heterochromic site	h	Chromosomal region that stains differently from the rest, often of variable size in the normal population
Duplication	dup	Duplication of a segment of chromosome
Ring	r	Arises from breaks in both arms, with loss of both ends to form a ring

From observations after the nuclear explosions in Hiroshima and Nagasaki, exposure to ionizing radiations is known to be a causative factor in spontaneous mutations. Chemical agents and some viruses induce genetic abnormalities in cells in tissue culture, but there is no incontrovertible evidence that they have this effect in humans in vivo, although they can induce congenital malformations through interfering with embryological development.

It is known that some fetal chromosomal abnormalities, particularly those of chromosome number, become more common with increasing maternal age.

An abnormality in a haploid gamete is transmitted to all its daughter cells

An abnormality of chromosome segregation during meiosis gives rise to haploid gametes containing an abnormal chromosome complement. If the gamete goes on to form a cell by fertilization, all daughter cells will be affected.

Fortunately, many such abnormal gametes are probably incapable of participating in fertilization and, if fertilization does occur, the fetus usually dies in utero. (A high proportion of fetuses that spontaneously abort in early pregnancy have chromosomal abnormalities.)

However, a few fetuses with an abnormal chromosome complement survive in utero, growing to reproductive maturity. As all of their cells have the chromosomal abnormality, the gametes will be abnormal, and the chromosomal

Most new genetic and chromosomal abnormalities have no identifiable cause

As the reason for the development of most new genetic aberrations is unknown, they are referred to as 'spontaneous.'

disorder is thus passed on to the next generation. The various patterns of inheritance are discussed below.

MOSAICISM is caused by a chromosomal abnormality that develops during mitotic division AFTER fertilization

A problem in chromosome separation that originates in the embryo after fertilization is transmitted only to daughter cells formed after the defect has occurred. Non-disjunction is the most important chromosomal abnormality, producing the most common mosaic syndromes. The resulting embryo therefore contains at least two cell lines and is described as a **mosaic**.

Mosaicism may involve abnormalities in the autosomes, e.g. Down's syndrome (see below), or the sex chromosomes, e.g. Turner's syndrome (see page 63).

Genomic imprinting is the differential expression of a gene, depending on whether it is inherited from the mother or the father

In normal mendelian inheritance, genes inherited from either parent would be expected to have an identical and equal effect. Genomic imprinting describes the situation where the allele that is functionally expressed is determined by which parent contributes it. Imprinting is an example of an **epigenetic modification**, implying change in the structure but not the sequence of a gene. The two main mechanisms involved are DNA methylation and histone modification, which cause gene silencing.

The best-known example of diseases resulting from abnormal genomic imprinting is in the two quite distinct diseases Prader–Willi syndrome and Angelman's syndrome (*Fig. 5.12*). Both are due to a loss of function of a gene on chromosome 15 (15q11–13), termed the PWS/AS region coding a ubiquitin-ligase. Absence of the paternally derived region leads to Prader–Willi syndrome, whereas loss of the maternally derived region leads to Angelman's syndrome.

Uniparental disomy is a rare cause of non-mendelian inheritance

In uniparental disomy both chromosomes are inherited from the same parent. For example, a percentage of cases of Prader–Willi syndrome do not have abnormal imprinting with loss of one (paternal) chromosome 15: rather, both relevant chromosomes 15 regions are derived entirely from the mother, without deletion (two alleles are present).

The cause of uniparental trisomy is not known, but it may follow a trisomy in which one of the three chromosomes is lost. As well as Prader–Willi syndrome, uniparental disomy is rarely the cause of anomalous inheritance patterns, for example a hemophiliac father having an affected son.

Fig. 5.12 Summary of clinical features of Prader–Willi and Angelman syndromes

Prader–Willi syndrome	Angelman's syndrome
Neonatal hypotonia ('floppy baby')	Microcephaly
Mental retardation and learning difficulties	Severe mental retardation
Initial failure to thrive	Ataxic gait
Uncontrollable appetite & obesity	Epilepsy
Hypogonadism, small hands and feet	Absent speech
Characteristic facies	Characteristic 'happy face'

The most important abnormalities of autosomal numbers are the TRISOMIES

A trisomy is a situation in which there are three chromosomes of a particular type, rather than the normal pair. The most common example is trisomy 21, which produces Down's syndrome (*Fig. 5.13*).

In Down's syndrome, the additional chromosome 21 is usually the result of non-disjunction (failure of separation during meiosis) of chromosome 21 during formation of the haploid maternal ovum. The incidence of this disorder rises with increasing maternal age (1 in 3000 when the maternal age is below 30, 1 in about 300 in women aged 35–40, and about 1 in 30 in women over 45). In a small percentage of cases Down's syndrome is due either to translocation or to mosaicism. The likelihood of Down's syndrome occurring in a subsequent pregnancy depends on whether the abnormality has arisen by meiotic non-disjunction (relatively low), maternal translocation (high) or mitotic mosaicism (relatively low); this is important in genetic counselling.

Non-disjunction is responsible for 95% of cases, which have a recurrence risk of approximately 1%.

About 4% of cases are due to translocations:

- Robertsonian translocation 14;21. Recurrence is 15% if the mother is the carrier, and 1% if the father is the carrier.
- Translocation 21;22. Recurrence is 10% if mother is the carrier, and 5% if father is the carrier.

Other autosomal trisomies are much rarer (*Fig. 5.14*), accounting for 1% of cases.

In perinatal pathology, screening for abnormalities of autosomal number is routine in cases of fetal abnormality, to allow parental counselling.

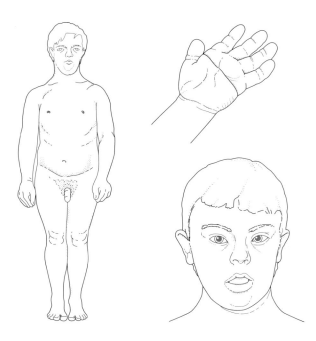

- Characteristic facies (flat facial profile, oblique palpebral fissures, low-bridged nose, epicanthal fold, open mouth, enlarged protruding tongue).

- Short stature (long bones of limbs are short).

- Short middle phalanx of little fingers.

- Horizontal palmar crease in short, broad hands.

- Hyperflexibility of joints.

- Poor muscle tone.

- Pelvic abnormalities.

- Congenital heart disease.

- Mental retardation.

- Alzheimer's disease beyond age of 40.

Fig. 5.13 Features of Down's syndrome.

Fig. 5.14 Rarer autosomal trisomies		
Name	**Chromosomal abnormality**	**Features**
Patau's syndrome	Trisomy 13	Mental retardation Microcephaly and microphthalmos Hair lip and cleft palate Cardiac abnormalities, e.g. ventricular septal defect (VSD) Abnormal feet ('rocker bottom') Polydactyly
Edwards' syndrome	Trisomy 18	Mental retardation Hypotonia/hypertonia Flexion deformities of fingers Cardiac abnormalities, e.g. VSD Abnormal feet ('rocker bottom') Abnormal head shape (prominent occiput) Low-set abnormal ears

Disorders of sex chromosome number arise by non-disjunction

The most important abnormalities of sex chromosome number arise from non-disjunction of chromosomes during meiotic division of male and female gametes.

- Meiotic division in female gametogenesis should produce two cells (ova), each with a single X chromosome. Non-disjunction may produce one cell with two X chromosomes (XX), and one with no sex chromosome at all (−).

- Meiotic division in male gametogenesis should produce two cells (spermatozoa), one with a single X chromosome, the other with a single Y chromosome. Non-disjunction may provide one with both X and Y chromosomes, and one with no sex chromosomes (−).

The most important syndromes produced by non-disjunction affecting sex chromosomes are:

- Turner's syndrome (mainly X-) (*Fig. 5.15*).
- Klinefelter's syndrome (mainly XXY) (*Fig. 5.16*).

- Infantile genitalia (even when adult).
- Widely spaced nipples.
- Micrognathia and prominent ears.
- Short stature.
- Redundant skin of neck (webbing).
- Primary amenorrhea.
- Cubitus valgus (wide carrying angle).
- Short fourth metacarpal bone.
- Congenital renal and aortic abnormalities.

Fig. 5.15 Turner's syndrome. Turner's syndrome is mainly due to non-disjunction in the meiotic division of gamete formation, but non-disjunction in mitotic division in the early embryo may produce Turner mosaics. About 20% of spontaneously aborted fetuses show the Turner chromosome pattern (X–).

- Tall stature with long arms and legs.
- Testes and penis small.
- Gynecomastia.*
- Female pubic hair profile.*
- High pitched voice.*
- Reduced facial and body hair.*

*feminization features

Fig. 5.16 Klinefelter's syndrome. Men with XXY Klinefelter's syndrome have greatly reduced fertility, but patients with mosaic types may be fertile. Other Klinefelter patterns include XXXY and XXXXY, with which mental retardation may be associated.

Laboratory medicine

Karyotype analysis of chromosomes is usually performed for prenatal diagnosis, or for investigation of conditions in postnatal life.

In postnatal diagnosis cells are derived from blood lymphocytes, or from biopsy of skin to obtain fibroblasts. In prenatal diagnosis, cells are derived from amniocentesis or chorionic villus biopsy.

Cells are cultured and a chromosome preparation is made. Chromosomes can be specially stained by a variety of methods which produce a banding pattern, the most common being Giemsa staining (G-banding). Increasingly, specific DNA probes are being used to analyze the presence of specific chromosomes or chromosome regions.

The main clinical situations in which it is useful to examine for chromosomal abnormalities are:

- Pediatric practice
  - Congenital abnormalities or dysmorphic state.
  - Mental handicap or learning difficulty.
  - Growth retardation.
  - Failure of sexual development at puberty.
- Obstetric practice
  - Infertility.
  - Recurrent spontaneous abortions.
  - Pregnancies in older women.
- Oncology
  - Malignancies, particularly leukemias.

GENE DEFECTS AND DISEASE

Many important diseases are due to abnormalities in single genes or small gene clusters, the chromosome numbers being normal. Such defects either may be expressed as dominant or recessive disorders with a mendelian inheritance pattern, or may require the coexistence of environmental factors before producing the disease (polygenic or multifactorial inheritance, see page 70).

Single gene defects are of varied mendelian pattern

Single gene defect diseases can be classified according to two criteria:

- Whether the abnormal gene is located on one of the 22 autosome pairs (autosomal) or on the sex chromosomes (sex-linked).

- Whether the disease is produced only when the abnormal gene is present on both members of the chromosome pair (homozygote), or can occur when the abnormal gene is present on only one member of the chromosome pair (heterozygote).

The following mendelian patterns of inheritance of single gene defects occur:

- **Autosomal dominant inheritance** (expressed in heterozygotes).
- **Autosomal recessive inheritance** (expressed in homozygotes).
- **Sex-linked recessive inheritance**. Virtually all sex-linked abnormalities are associated with genes on the X chromosome, and are therefore expressed mainly in males who only have one copy and cannot compensate with a normal X chromosome as in females. They are not usually expressed in heterozygous females, who have one normal and one abnormal X chromosome, but 'manifesting carriers' can occur in some X-linked disorders, e.g. Duchenne's muscular dystrophy (see page 489).

Sex-linked dominant inheritance is very rare.

In autosomal dominant inheritance the abnormal gene produces disease in heterozygotes, where a normal allele is also present

Theoretically, in autosomal dominant inheritance the gene can produce disease either in homozygotes, i.e. when the abnormal gene is present in both members of a chromosome pair, or in heterozygotes, when only one member of the chromosome pair has the abnormal gene. Because homozygous affected individuals are very rare, the usual mating is between a homozygous normal individual and a heterozygous affected individual.

Each affected individual is a heterozygote for the disease and will have a genotype **Aa** for the relevant gene (**A** is the abnormal gene, **a** its normal allele); unaffected individuals

Key Facts
Autosomal dominant inheritance

- Homozygotes and heterozygotes manifest the disease, but the great majority are heterozygotes (i. e. all affected individuals in *Fig. 5.17*).
- Both males and females are affected, e.g. **III**, 4 and 5.
- Only affected individuals can pass on the disease to their children; clinically unaffected individuals do not pass on the disease (e.g. **II**, 1).
- The disease is therefore passed on (on average) to only half of their children.
- The disease appears in every generation.

will have the genotype **aa**. The gametes produced by the affected male in the first generation (**I**) will be **A** and **a**, and the non-affected female will produce **a** and **a** gametes. Thus, the possible combinations after fertilization are as shown in *Fig. 5.18*.

The affected progeny (approximately 50%) are heterozygotes (**Aa**) like the affected parent. Affected homozygotes (in this case, **AA**) are rare, since they can only arise from matings between two affected heterozygotes. This is unlikely where the gene abnormality is rare, but the chances are greater when parents are related. The common autosomal dominant disorders are listed in *Fig. 5.19*.

As a result of a new mutation or non-penetrance, autosomal dominant disease may affect offspring of clinically unaffected parents

Spontaneous mutation is a common event in certain diseases that subsequently show an autosomal dominant inheritance, although the rate varies greatly from disease to

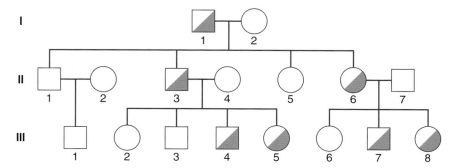

Fig. 5.17 A typical pedigree in autosomal dominant inheritance

	A	a
a	Aa (affected)	aa (normal)
a	Aa (affected)	aa (normal)

Fig. 5.18 Punnett square for autosomal dominant inheritance

Fig. 5.19 Common and important autosomal dominant diseases

Achondroplasia	Dwarfism due to short limb bones	see page 557
Adult polycystic disease	Enlarging cysts replacing kidney	see page 390
Neurofibromatosis 1	Multiple nerve sheath tumors	see page 479
Neurofibromatosis 2	Acoustic neuromas	
Familial polyposis coli	Multiple colonic adenomata and carcinomas	see page 264
Hereditary spherocytosis	Spherical red cells with short lifespan	see page 321
Huntington's disease**	Progressive neuronal degeneration	see page 473
Myotonic dystrophy**	Muscle weakness and wasting	see page 489
Familial hypercholesterolemia	Increased cholesterol levels	see page 162
Osteogenesis imperfecta	Brittle bones, fracturing with minimal trauma	see page 557
Marfan's syndromes	Abnormal elastic tissues – skeletal, cardiovascular and ocular disease	see page 163
Some Ehlers–Danlos syndromes*	Abnormal collagen – skin, joint and vascular effects	see page 163
Retinoblastoma	Malignant tumor of eye	see page 500

*Other Ehlers–Danlos syndromes show autosomal or sex-linked recessive inheritance.
**These neurological disorders are known to be the result of inserts of multiple triplet repeats.

disease. It is believed that new mutations are responsible for approximately 50% of cases of neurofibromatosis, and 80% of cases of achondroplasia.

Non-penetrance is where the abnormal genotype is not manifest in the form of disease. The phenotype appears normal, and there is no clinical expression of the disease (*Fig. 5.20b*).

The identification of specific gene abnormalities for several of the autosomal dominant conditions now allows molecular diagnostic evaluation using specific gene probes.

Unstable tandem trinucleotide repeat sequences underlie several major diseases

Molecular genetic analysis of several dominantly heritable diseases has revealed a common factor in the underlying genetic abnormality.

Myotonic dystrophy, Huntington's disease, Kennedy's syndrome, fragile-X syndrome, and several spinocerebellar ataxias have all been shown to have expansion of tandem repeats of three nucleotides. In patients with Huntington's disease there are as many as 100 triplet repeats in the gene, whereas normally these areas contain 9–34 repeats. There is commonly an inverse correlation between the length of the repeat sequence, the age of onset and the clinical severity of the disease.

This finding provides an explanation for the clinical phenomenon of 'anticipation,' whereby a dominantly inherited disease becomes more severe with each generation. As the repeat enlarges, the disease worsens clinically and has an earlier onset. Recent findings have also suggested that apparently unaffected parents may have repeats at the upper limit of normal, suggesting that the mutational event is amplification of the gene.

Fragile-X syndrome, the most common cause of mental retardation (1 in 2000 births), is also due to an expanded trinucleotide repeat at the fragile site on the X chromosome. This abnormality can be demonstrated in karyotype analysis as a discontinuity of staining at the end of the long arm of the X chromosome.

Autosomal recessive disorders produce clinical disease in homozygotes

In autosomal recessive inheritance the disease is manifest only by homozygotes who have received one abnormal gene from each unaffected parent, the parents being heterozygotes for the abnormal gene. A typical pedigree is shown in *Fig. 5.21*. The incidence of the autosomal recessive disease state will depend on the number of heterozygotes in the general population, i.e. the gene frequency. If the abnormal gene is rare in the general population, the chances of a mating between two non-affected heterozy-

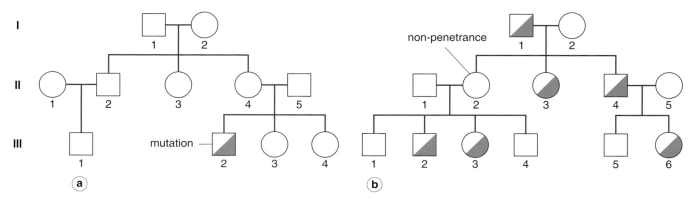

Fig. 5.20 **Autosomal dominant pedigree with mutation and non-penetrance.**

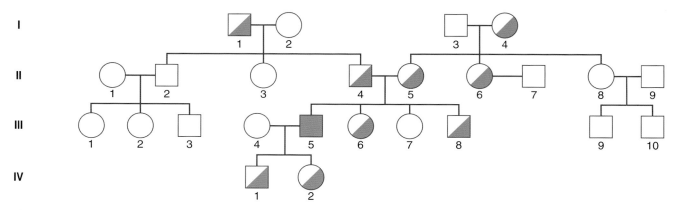

Fig. 5.21 **Typical pedigree in autosomal recessive inheritance (see *Fig. 5.22* for Punnett squares).**

gotes are low. If the gene is common, the chances are accordingly greater, and the disease incidence will be high. Thus, mating between close relatives increases the incidence of disease. Some autosomal recessive genes have a high frequency in certain races, e.g. the gene frequency for cystic fibrosis is high in Caucasians (1 in 25 are heterozygotes), and the gene for sickle-cell disease (*Fig. 5.23*) is common in those of native African origin (approximately 1 in 12).

Note that, with small average family sizes in western society, the incidence of most clinically apparent autosomal recessive diseases is low; it is therefore tempting to consider each new case as a new spontaneous mutation, as any heterozygote carriers are usually asymptomatic (see *Fig. 5.22*). However, for genetic counseling purposes it is vital to try to identify all related non-affected heterozygotes. Fortunately, in many of the diseases it is possible to identify heterozygotes. For example, where the homozygous state is associated with complete absence of a particular enzyme, the heterozygotes have a reduced level of the enzyme, lying somewhere between normal levels and complete absence.

Similarly, heterozygotes for the hemoglobinopathies have a mixture of normal and abnormal hemoglobins.

The identification of specific gene abnormalities for several of these conditions now allows molecular diagnostic evaluation using specific gene probes. This has opened the way both for population screening for carrier states in heterozygotes, and for confident genetic counseling in cases of prenatal diagnosis.

Cystic fibrosis is a very common autosomal recessive disorder, with a frequency of 0.5–0.6 per 1000 live births.

Disease is caused by mutations in the gene coding for a chloride transporter called the cystic fibrosis transmembrane conductance regulator (CFTR). A genetic test is available to detect individuals who carry a mutant gene (heterozygotes), and there is debate as to the ethical and cost–benefit issues of implementing any population-wide screening program.

It has been advised that genetic testing for CF should be offered to adults with a positive family history, to partners of people with CF, to couples currently planning a pregnancy, and to couples seeking prenatal care.

	B	b
B	BB (homozygote normal)	Bb (heterozygote carrier)
b	Bb (heterozygote carrier)	bb (homozygote affected)

	B	b
b	Bb (heterozygote carrier)	bb (homozygote affected)
b	Bb (heterozygote carrier)	bb (homozygote affected)

	B	B
b	Bb	Bb
b	Bb	Bb
	(all heterozygote carriers)	

	B	B
B	BB (homozygote normal)	BB (homozygote normal)
b	Bb (heterozygote carrier)	Bb (heterozygote carrier)

Fig. 5.22 Punnett squares for autosomal recessive inheritance (see also Fig. 5.21).

Fig. 5.23 Common and important autosomal recessive diseases

Disease	Biochemical effect	Notes
Cystic fibrosis	Abnormal transport protein	see page 221
Sickle-cell anemia	Abnormal hemoglobin	see page 322
Thalassemias	Abnormal hemoglobin	see page 321
Glycogenoses	Enzyme deficiency	see Chapter 25
Mucopolysaccharidoses	Enzyme deficiency	
Lipidoses	Enzyme deficiency	
Phenylketonuria	Enzyme deficiency	
Wilson's disease	Copper accumulation	see page 146

Key Facts
Autosomal recessive inheritance

From the typical pedigree shown in *Fig. 5.21*, it can be seen that autosomal recessive diseases show the following characteristics:

- Affected individuals are homozygotes (see **III**, 5).
- Inheritance of clinical disease is from two unaffected heterozygous parents (see **II**, 4 and 5).
- Both males and females are affected.
- There is a 25% chance of two unaffected heterozygous ('carrier') parents producing an affected homozygous child (see **III**, 5).
- There is a 50% chance of two unaffected heterozygous parents producing an unaffected heterozygous child (carrier) (see **III**, 6 and 8).
- There is a 25% chance of two unaffected heterozygous (carrier) parents producing an unaffected non-carrier child with normal genes (see **III**, 7).
- All offspring of an affected homozygote and a normal non-affected homozygous individual will be unaffected heterozygous (carrier) children (see **IV**, 1 and 2).
- The disease is not manifest in every generation. In the pedigree shown, the disease is manifest only in generation **III**, although there are non-affected (carrier) heterozygotes in generations **I, II, III** and **IV**.

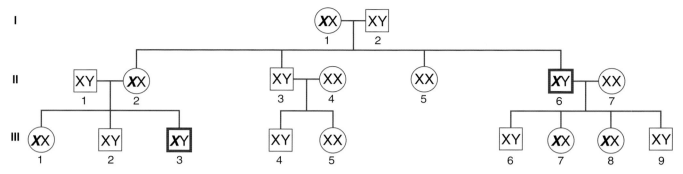

Fig. 5.24 Typical pedigree for X-linked recessive inheritance.

	X	Y
X	**X**X (carrier female)	**X**Y (affected male)
X	XX (normal female)	XY (normal male)

	X	Y
X	**X**X (carrier female)	XY (normal male)
X	**X**X (carrier female)	XY (normal male)

	X	Y
X	**XX** (affected homo-zygous female)	**X**Y (affected male)
X	**X**X (carrier female)	XY (normal male)

Fig. 5.25 Inheritance possibilities in X-linked recessive inheritance (Punnett squares).

Sex-linked disorders are almost entirely due to abnormalities of the X chromosome

Most diseases associated with abnormal genes on the sex chromosomes are due to mutant genes on the X chromosome and show recessive inheritance (X-linked or sex-linked recessive; *Fig. 5.26*).

In the female, the abnormal gene on one X chromosome is balanced by the possession of a normal allele on the other, so the abnormal gene is not manifest. The female

From the pedigree shown in *Fig. 5.24* it can be seen that X-linked recessive disorders show the following characteristics:

- The abnormal gene is on an X chromosome (**X**).
- The disease affects males (**II**, 6 and **III**, 3).
- The disease is transmitted by heterozygous females who are unaffected (**I**, 1 and **II**, 2).
- Unaffected males do not carry or transmit the gene (e.g. **II**, 3).
- Each male offspring of a heterozygous female carrier has a 50% chance of being affected (e.g. **II**, 3 and **II**, 6; **III**, 2 and **III**, 3).
- Both affected males and unaffected heterozygous females can transmit to produce unaffected heterozygous female carriers (e.g. **III**, 1, **III**, 7 and **III**, 8).

shows no features of the disease, but is a carrier. In the male, the abnormal gene on the sole X chromosome is not balanced, as there is no normal allele on the Y chromosome; the abnormal gene is therefore expressed, and males will display the disease.

Fig. 5.24 shows a typical pedigree for an X-linked recessive disorder. The mating combination shown in the third example in *Fig. 5.25* is extremely unlikely in most X-linked recessive disorders, but may occur where the gene frequency of the abnormal X-linked gene is fairly high. For example, in some Afro-Caribbean communities the X-linked gene that produces one type of glucose-6-phosphate dehydrogenase deficiency is about 1 in 10 males, with a relatively high percentage of heterozygous females. In these circumstances it is not rare to find a homozygous (XX) female with clinical manifestations of the enzyme defect (see third pattern in *Fig. 5.25* (*)).

Fig. 5.26 Common and important X-linked recessive diseases

Hemophilia A	Bleeding tendency due to clotting factor VIII deficiency	
Hemophilia B	Bleeding tendency due to clotting factor X deficiency	
G6PD deficiency	Attacks of hemolytic anemia after certain drugs	
Duchenne muscular dystrophy	Progressive muscle weakness due to dystrophin deficiency	see page 489
Becker muscular dystrophy	Relative dystrophin deficiency	see page 489
X-linked (Bruton's) agammaglobulinemia	Decreased gamma globulins due to B-cell maturation failure	see page 97
X-linked ichthyosis	Permanently thick, scaly skin due to steroid sulphatase deficiency	

X-linked dominant inheritance diseases are very rare

One example of an X-linked dominant inheritance disease is hypophosphatemic osteomalacia (vitamin D-resistant rickets), in which failure of proper mineralization of bone results from excessive phosphate loss in the urine and low blood phosphate levels. The abnormal dominant gene is on the X chromosome, and is expressed in both males (X Y) and females (X X) who have received an abnormal X chromosome from an affected heterozygous mother (X X). Affected fathers (X Y) transmit the gene only to their daughters.

Several mitochondrial proteins are encoded by mitochondrial DNA

Although most genetic material is located in the cell nucleus, DNA is also found in mitochondria. This type of DNA is transmitted to offspring by maternal inheritance to both male and female, and thus defects can be passed on to the offspring (**mitochondrial inheritance**). A typical pedigree is shown in *Fig. 5.27*.

Key Facts
Mitochondrial inheritance

See *Fig. 5.27*.

- Inheritance is only through maternal lines, as mitochondria in the embryo are derived from the ovum.
- All children of an affected mother receive a dose of abnormal mitochondria in the ovum (e.g. **II**, 1, 3 and 5; **III**, 1–5 and 8; **IV**, 1–4).
- If an affected male has children, his progeny are unaffected (e.g. **II**, 5, **III**, 8).
- The severity of disease may vary, as the dose of abnormal mitochondria may vary in different tissues. A mixture of genetically normal and abnormal mitochondria in tissues is termed **heteroplasmy**.

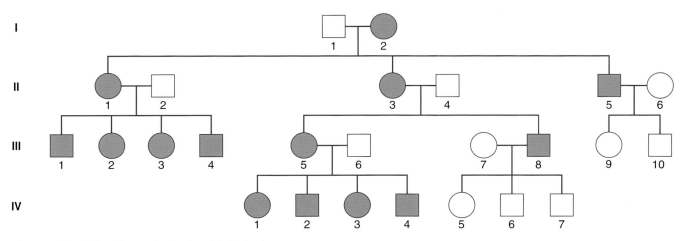

Fig. 5.27 Typical pedigree of mitochondrial inheritance.

Fig. 5.28 Mitochondrial cytopathies – clinical features

Skeletal muscle weakness: myopathy with abnormal mitochondria in skeletal muscle fibres
Eye movement disorder: external ophthalmoplegia. Extraocular muscles show abnormal mitochondria within fibres
Deafness: sensorineural pattern of deafness associated with loss of nerves in the vestibulocochlear structures
Cardiac muscle disease: abnormal mitochondria within cardiac muscle cells leads to heart failure
Myoclonic epilepsy: an unusual pattern of epileptic seizure activity sometimes associated with metabolic causations.
Lactic acidosis: impaired respiratory chain function leads to defective processing in the Krebs cycle
Stroke: cerebral vascular abnormality leads to recurrent strokes.

Although both males and females are affected, only affected females can transmit to offspring. The most important group of diseases inherited in this way are the mitochondrial cytopathies, which commonly present as progressive disease involving skeletal and cardiac muscle or brain in adult life. Associated with deficiencies in a number of mitochondrial respiratory enzymes, some are characterized by the presence of large abnormal mitochondria, often containing large inclusions, beneath the sarcolemma. The clinical features that might suggest a mitochondrial cytopathy are presented in *Fig. 5.28*.

A proportion of mitochondrial proteins are coded for by nuclear genes, and so a clinical phenotype characterized by abnormal mitochondrial function may be inherited through an autosomal route.

There are many disorders in which genetic factors play only a partial role

The terms **polygenic** and **multifactorial** are often used synonymously when describing inheritance. However:

- Polygenic diseases result from the interaction of a number of scattered genes, each of which has a slight effect on the phenotype. The final clinical picture is a summation of each of the individual gene effects.
- Multifactorial diseases result from a combination of genetic (often polygenic) and environmental factors. Genetic make-up is believed to produce predisposition to a disease, environmental factors acting as the trigger.

Many diseases observed to have a high incidence within families but with no evidence of a recognizable inheritance pattern (**familial tendency**) are diseases with polygenic or multifactorial inheritance. Such diseases are common, and include congenital malformations present at birth (e.g. hare lip, cleft palate; *Fig. 5.29*), some congenital heart malformations, and diseases which manifest themselves in childhood, adolescence and adult life (e.g. psoriasis, see page 510), diabetes mellitus (see pages 569–72), hypertension (see pages 164–6), atopic diseases, schizophrenia, manic depressive psychosis, rheumatoid arthritis (see pages 549–50 and 566–7), and gout (see pages 551–2). In most cases the nature and location of the abnormal genes are not known.

Fig. 5.29 Cleft palate.

MOLECULAR GENETICS AND DISEASE

Molecular biology techniques have made investigative genetics possible

Modern molecular genetics, using DNA isolation, fragmentation with restriction enzymes, and probes to specific genes, have a wide application to clinical medicine. If the gene for a disease is known, abnormalities in gene structure can be determined in individuals and the presence of a mutation established. In cases of familial disease in which the genetic abnormality is not known, linkage analysis of the disease to specific chromosome regions is possible, with ultimate isolation of the gene responsible.

The ultimate aim of molecular genetic approaches to disease is to develop techniques of gene therapy to repair or complement the defective gene, thereby preventing disease.

Other approaches using molecular genetic profiling are to determine specific subtypes of polygenic disease and use this information to predict response to different available drugs (personalized medicine).

Neoplasia 6

INTRODUCTION

A key characteristic of the adaptive responses of cells, as discussed in Chapter 2, is that if the stimulus is removed, any alteration in cell growth reverts to normal. In contrast to these reversible adaptive responses, certain stimuli cause changes in genetic material that result in a permanent alteration of the normal cellular growth pattern. Such altered cells, which are termed neoplastic, fail to respond normally to signals controlling cell growth. They proliferate excessively in a poorly regulated manner, forming a lump or tissue mass called a neoplasm (literally, new growth).

This chapter considers the nature of neoplasia, the clinical study of which is termed oncology, and the classification and diagnosis of tumors. Causes of neoplasia are discussed, and the basic science relating to properties of neoplastic cells reviewed.

CHARACTERISTICS AND TERMINOLOGY OF NEOPLASTIC DISEASES

Terms used to describe neoplastic diseases

By convention, a neoplastic mass of cells is known as a tumor. The Latin derivation was originally used to refer to any tissue swelling, although this literal use has largely gone out of fashion. The term **cancer** is frequently in lay use and is equated with any malignant neoplasm. The name is derived from the Latin word for a crab, as such tumors were perceived to seize upon adjacent tissues with pincer-like outgrowths. Study of different tumors reveals that cancers originating from different tissues display varying degrees of aggressiveness: some are slow-growing and indolent, whereas others spread rapidly to many parts of the body and rapidly cause death. The generic term cancer is not, therefore, always suitable for professional use, as it conveys no information about the likely biological behaviour of a tumor.

A neoplasm is composed of cells that grow in a poorly regulated manner

In a neoplastic state, cellular proliferation and growth occur in the absence of any continuing external stimulus. The term neoplasia therefore describes a state of poorly regulated cell growth, in which the neoplastic cells are said to be transformed. In neoplastic cells and tissues there is a failure of the normal mechanisms that control cellular proliferation and maturation. The molecular nature of these events is part of the study of carcinogenesis, reviewed towards the end of this chapter.

Each neoplastic cell has an alteration in its genome, responsible for abnormal growth

The state of neoplasia arises out of changes in genetic material, which are then transmitted to each new generation of cells within the neoplasm. Neoplastic growth contrasts with hyperplasia (discussed in Chapter 2) in that although there is abnormal proliferation of cells in the latter, this ceases with removal of the causative stimulus. Recent molecular genetic study has shown that an alteration in the key genes controlling cell growth underlies the majority of tumors (*Fig. 6.1*). Such genes are termed oncogenes, and examples are discussed in the later section on carcinogenesis (see page 88).

There are two main types of neoplasm: benign and malignant

Early in the study of tumors, clinical observation identified two main patterns of neoplastic growth:

- If the margins of the tumor were well defined and the tumor grew only locally, the neoplasm was termed benign.
- If the margins of the tumor were poorly defined and the neoplastic cells were growing into and destroying the surrounding tissues, the neoplasm was termed malignant.

Benign tumors generally have a very good prognosis and only rarely lead to death. In contrast, malignant tumors are a major cause of morbidity and mortality.

FAILURE TO ACHIEVE CELLULAR DIFFERENTIATION IS A PARTICULAR FEATURE OF MALIGNANT NEOPLASMS

Following cell division from a precursor or stem cell, normal cells assume a specific function, which involves the develop-

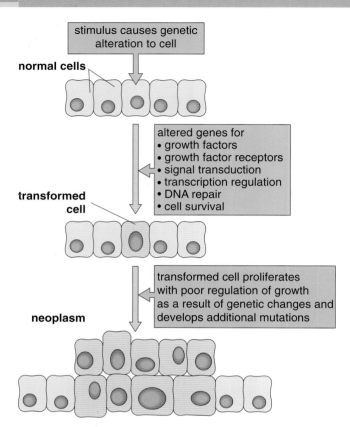

Fig. 6.1 Events in neoplastic transformation. Normal cells develop abnormalities in key genes regulating growth and are transformed into neoplastic cells.

The boxes in the figure read:

stimulus causes genetic alteration to cell

normal cells

altered genes for
• growth factors
• growth factor receptors
• signal transduction
• transcription regulation
• DNA repair
• cell survival

transformed cell

transformed cell proliferates with poor regulation of growth as a result of genetic changes and develops additional mutations

neoplasm

ment of specialized structures such as mucin vacuoles, microvilli or cilia, known as differentiation. Whereas stem cells can be said to be relatively undifferentiated, the fully mature cell of any particular cell line is said to be highly differentiated. In association with loss of regulation of cell growth, neoplastic cells commonly fail to achieve a highly differentiated state. Histological features associated with this are shown in *Fig. 6.2*.

In general the cells of benign neoplasms are differentiated to a degree which corresponds fairly closely to that of the cells from which they were derived (*Fig. 6.2b*). This differentiation frequently extends to the retention of the functional attributes of the tissue of origin. For example, benign tumors of endocrine tissues frequently secrete hormones and may have endocrinological effects.

In the case of malignant neoplasms, variable degrees of differentiation may be seen.

• When the constituent cells closely resemble the tissue of origin the tumor is termed a well-differentiated malignant neoplasm (*Fig. 6.2c*).
• When tumor cells show only a passing resemblance to the tissue of origin the neoplasm is termed a poorly differentiated malignant neoplasm (*Fig. 6.2d*).
• When, because of failure of differentiation, it is not possible to identify the cell of origin on morphological

observation, the growth is termed an anaplastic malignant neoplasm (*Fig. 6.2e*).

The degree of differentiation of a neoplasm is generally related to its behaviour. A poorly differentiated neoplasm tends to be more aggressive than a well differentiated one.

Along with failure of differentiation in neoplasia, cells are said to show atypical cytology. The associated features are:

• Increased variation in the shape and size of cells (cellular pleomorphism).
• Increased variation in the shape and size of nuclei (nuclear pleomorphism).
• Increase in the density of staining of nuclei (nuclear hyperchromatism).
• Disproportionately large increase in the size of nuclei, relative to the size of the cell cytoplasm (increased nuclear: cytoplasmic ratio).

Fig. 6.2e shows how the cytological features of neoplasia become more marked with loss of differentiation.

Benign tumors grow locally, are generally slow growing, and compress adjacent tissues

Benign tumors, the cells of which closely resemble the tissue of origin, generally do not have highly abnormal dysregulation of growth. Such tumors grow locally, and generally have a very slow pace of growth. Two main factors influence the effects of such tumors:

• As a benign tumor grows, it causes compression of adjacent tissues. This may have adverse effects if the resulting mass causes blockage of a lumen, e.g. gut or airway.
• If a benign tumor has an endocrine function, it may cause disease due to uncontrolled secretion of hormone.

An example of a benign tumor of the thyroid gland is illustrated in *Fig. 6.3*.

Malignant tumors grow into adjacent tissues and can spread to other parts of the body

The most significant property of malignant neoplasms is that growth is not confined to the site of origin of the tumor, i.e. the primary tumor. Control of cell growth becomes so abnormal that cells can grow into adjacent local tissues, in a process termed invasion (*Fig. 6.4*). As neoplastic cells invade they usually do so at the expense of the local tissues, causing damage and destruction.

The most sinister property of malignant neoplasms is that cells from the primary tumor can become detached, move to a different part of the body, and grow as a separate mass of tumor. This process is known as metastasis, and the resulting detached masses of cells are termed metastases or secondary tumors. As with the malignant primary tumor, metastases grow at the expense of local tissues and usually result in tissue destruction.

The ways in which benign and malignant tumors differ are shown in *Fig. 6.5*.

Fig. 6.2 Histological features of loss of differentiation. (a) Normal colonic epithelium. (b) Benign neoplasm of colon. (c) Well-differentiated malignant neoplasm of colon. (d) Poorly differentiated malignant neoplasm of colon. (e) Anaplastic malignant neoplasm of colon. (f) Benign neoplasm of smooth muscle. The cells of a benign neoplasm (b) resemble those of the normal epithelium (a), in that they are columnar and have an orderly arrangement. Loss of some degree of differentiation is evident in that the neoplastic cells do not show mucin vacuolation. The cells of the benign neoplasm of smooth muscle (f) closely resemble normal muscle cells. Cells of the well differentiated malignant neoplasm (c) have a haphazard arrangement and, although gland lumina (**G**) are formed, they are architecturally abnormal and irregular. Nuclei vary in shape and size. Cells in the poorly differentiated malignant neoplasm (d) have an even more haphazard arrangement, with very poor formation of gland lumina (**G**). Nuclei show greater variation in shape and size than in (c).

Cells in anaplastic malignant neoplasm (e) bear no relation to the normal, with no attempt at gland formation. There is tremendous variation in the size of cells and of nuclei, with very intense staining (nuclear hyperchromatism) of the latter. Without knowing the site of origin it would be impossible to tell what sort of tumor this was by histology. Well-differentiated tumors of support cells resemble their cell of origin, as shown in this example of a benign tumor of smooth muscle (f). In a poorly differentiated malignant neoplasm of smooth muscle, cells show marked variation in size and shape of nuclei, with hyperchromatism and numerous mitoses. A smooth muscle origin can then be established only by the use of electron microscopy or immunohistochemistry.

Fig. 6.3 Benign neoplasm of thyroid gland. This low-power micrograph shows the features of a benign epithelial neoplasm. The tumor is very well circumscribed, and although it compresses adjacent tissue it does not grow into it.

Fig. 6.4 Edge of malignant tumor of breast showing invasion. Islands of neoplastic cells can be seen extending into adjacent adipose tissue (**A**) by invasion. The edge of the tumor is therefore not well circumscribed, in contrast to a benign lesion.

Fig. 6.5 Histological features of neoplasms

	Benign	Malignant
Behavior	Expansile growth only; grows locally	Expansile and invasive growth; may metastasize
Histology	Resembles cell of origin (well differentiated)	Shows failure of cellular differentiation
	Few mitoses	Many mitoses, some of which are abnormal forms
	Normal or slight increases in nuclear/cytoplasmic ratio	High nuclear/cytoplasmic ratio
	Cells are uniform throughout the tumor	Cells vary in shape and size (cellular pleomorphism) and/or nuclei vary in shape and size (nuclear pleomorphism)

A neoplasm must develop stromal support components if it is to grow

If neoplastic cells are to grow, they must obtain adequate nutrients by developing an appropriate set of support tissues, particularly an adequate vascular supply. Just as normal cells interact with support tissues and induce stroma formation, neoplastic cells also retain this ability. Tumors develop a vascular stroma by secretion of **angiogenesis factors**. The ability of a tumor to induce and maintain a vascular supply is a key factor in its growth (see pink box). A tumor mass therefore contains the genetically abnormal neoplastic cells and a component of normal support tissues.

In well differentiated lesions the induction of stroma is usually well developed and the neoplastic cells grow without problems. In less well differentiated neoplasms the induction of stroma may be poor and outstripped by proliferation of neoplastic cells. This may limit the speed of growth of a tumor and frequently leads to death of cells in the centre of a tumor mass. Certain tumors induce a stromal response that is disproportionate to the number of tumor cells. Such tumors are often termed desmoplastic.

The growth rate of a neoplasm is determined by several factors

Different tumors grow at different rates. In general terms, benign tumors and well-differentiated malignant tumors grow more slowly than poorly differentiated lesions, although there are many exceptions.

The rate of growth of a tumor depends on many factors:

- The proportion of cells which are in the cell cycle as opposed to those that have differentiated and entered the G0 (non-proliferating) part of the cell cycle.

Tumor angiogenesis is controlled by positive and negative regulatory factors

If tumor cells fail to recruit an adequate blood supply they will not grow. Additionally, a vascular network is required by tumors for spread by metastasis: studies have shown a good correlation between the density of vessels in certain tumors and the probability of spread by metastasis.

The two most important angiogenesis factors secreted by cells, including tumor cells, are:

- Vascular endothelial growth factor (VEGF): secreted by many cell types and acts on receptors expressed on endothelial cells to induce endothelial cell growth, migration, and vessel formation (see *Fig. 6.6*).
- Basic fibroblast growth factor (bFGF): induces endothelial cell growth and migration.

Angiogenesis is also modulated by proteins termed angiopoietins (Ang), which interact with endothelial cell receptors:

- Ang1 promotes stabilization and growth of vessels from capillary types to larger types by recruiting periendothelial cells.
- Ang2 promotes remodeling and maturation of developing vascular networks.

Anti-angiogenesis factors are normally produced by cells to prevent angiogenesis and include:

- Thrombospondin (platelet factor 4).
- Angiostatin: cleavage product of plasminogen.
- Endostatin: cleavage product of collagen type XVIII.
- Vasostatin: cleavage product of calreticulin.

A key molecular event in some tumors may be failure of production of anti-angiogenic factors. Therapeutic trials are currently under way to see whether endostatin can inhibit tumor growth, already suggested in some experimental tumors in mice. The drug thalidomide has anti-angiogenic effects and is being used in clinical trials for some tumors, including brain tumours in children.

angioblast	Angioblasts proliferate under influence of VEGF acting on VEGF-R2 receptors. VEGF is secreted by local cells. bFGF also promotes growth.
endothelial cell	Lumen formation and inhibition of growth of endothelial cells.
support cell	VEGF acting on VEGF-R1 receptors mediates endothelial tube formation.
	Ang1 binding to endothelial cells recruits support cells around endothelial tubes.
mature vessel	Maturation and stabilization with remodeling of vessels occurs under the influence of Ang2 and local growth factors.

Fig. 6.6 Angiogenesis.

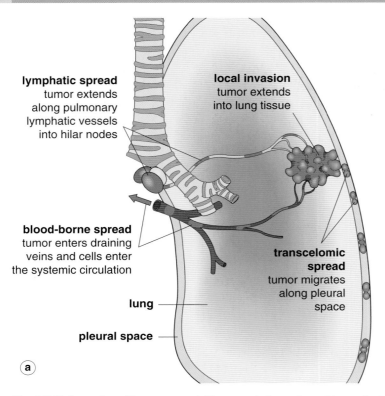

lymphatic spread tumor extends along pulmonary lymphatic vessels into hilar nodes

local invasion tumor extends into lung tissue

blood-borne spread tumor enters draining veins and cells enter the systemic circulation

transcelomic spread tumor migrates along pleural space

lung

pleural space

(a)

(b)

Fig. 6.7 Main routes of tumor spread. The spread of a malignant tumor is shown diagrammatically (a) and in a real specimen (b) for a carcinoma of the lung. The four main routes, i.e. local, lymphatic, blood-borne and transcelomic, are shown. In (b) the malignant neoplasm originated in a bronchus (**B**) and spread locally into adjacent lung (arrow). Tumor has also spread via lymphatics and is evident as white deposits in hilar lymph nodes (**N**), which also contain carbon pigment.

Fig. 6.8 Local invasion in malignant neoplasm of colon. This low-power micrograph shows purple-stained malignant tumor (**T**) extending through submucosa (**S**) and muscle (**M**) of the colon wall by local invasion. Via this route, neoplastic cells may invade adjacent organs such as the bladder.

Fig. 6.9 Lymphatic invasion by tumor. (a) Histology of invasion of lymphatic vessel. (b) Tumor in para-aortic lymph nodes. Micrograph (a) shows malignant cells (**M**) in a small lymphatic vessel. Cells break off from the primary tumor, enter small lymphatics and are carried to lymph nodes, where they frequently grow as metastases. The macroscopic appearance of tumor in nodes is shown in (b); the nodes (**N**) are enlarged and replaced by tumor which, in this instance, originated from the testis.

- The death rate of cells in the tumor. Tumor cells are particularly prone to programmed cell death by the process of apoptosis (see *Fig. 2.21*). Tumors that develop genetic changes which allow them to escape from growth control by apoptosis tend to become rapidly growing.
- The adequacy of supply of nutrients to the tumor, derived from induction of a stroma by the neoplastic cells.

If cell proliferation greatly exceeds cell death in the tumor, it will grow in size rapidly.

Malignant neoplasms spread to other sites by four main routes

Spread of a malignant tumor from its primary site (metastasis) is by four main routes (*Fig. 6.7*):

- **Local invasion**. The most common pattern of spread of malignant tumors is by direct growth into adjacent tissues (*Fig. 6.8*). Tumors may also spread along natural tissue planes, e.g. along nerves.
- **Lymphatic spread**. Tumor cells frequently spread via draining lymphatic vessels and are conducted to local lymph nodes, where they grow as secondary tumors (*Fig. 6.9*).
- **Vascular spread**. Tumor cells can spread via the veins draining the primary lesion. Gastrointestinal tumors are frequently conducted via the portal vein, giving rise to metastases in the liver. Tumor cells that enter systemic veins most frequently form metastases in the lung, bone marrow, brain and adrenal glands (*Fig. 6.10*).
- **Transcelomic spread**. Primary tumors in the abdominal cavity or the thorax can spread directly across celomic spaces, e.g. the peritoneal or pleural cavities, by seeding cells which then migrate to the surface of other organs.

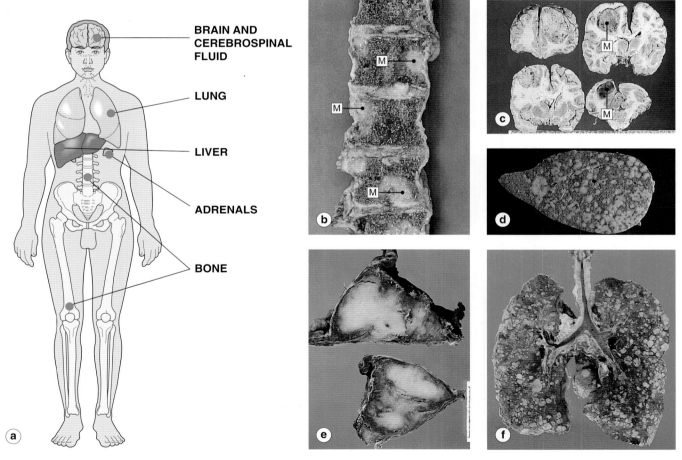

Fig. 6.10 Main sites of blood-borne metastasis. (a) Sites of hematogenous metastasis. (b) Metastasis in bone. (c) Metastasis in brain. (d) Metastasis in liver. (e) Metastasis in adrenals. (f) Metastasis in lungs. Blood-borne tumor metastasis leads to growth of secondary tumors in several main sites. The macroscopic appearances of bone metastasis are shown in (b), where lesions are seen in vertebrae (**M**). Numerous metastases from a neoplasm of the stomach (**M**) are seen in the brain in (c). The liver is the most common site for metastases from tumors in the gastrointestinal tract, as seen in (d), which arose from a colonic neoplasm. In (e) metastatic tumor has replaced both adrenal glands, as is commonly seen with spread from lung and breast tumors. The lung (f) is the most common site for bloodborne metastases from tumors outside the gastrointestinal tract, particularly mesenchymal tumors.

BRAIN AND CEREBROSPINAL FLUID

LUNG

LIVER

ADRENALS

BONE

For invasion and metastasis to occur, neoplastic cells have to acquire special attributes

Neoplastic cells have to develop several attributes in order to metastasize, as summarized in *Fig. 6.11*. Within any primary tumor it is likely that only a proportion of cells acquire these attributes by developing additional genetic mutations as part of further abnormalities in cell growth.

To grow through basement membrane into the extracellular matrix and then enter a vessel, neoplastic cells must express surface molecules for adhesion (particularly specific integrins that bind to laminin and fibronectin). To grow into adjacent tissues or vessels, cells must also be motile and capable of migration.

The production of enzymes that degrade extracellular matrix appears to be an important factor in metastasis, one of the most studied being the matrix metalloproteinases, which degrade the type IV collagen in basement membranes.

Whether, once in the circulation, a cell establishes a metastasis in a particular organ is probably determined by many factors. It is likely that both tumor cell and host organ tissues must express complementary cell adhesion molecules. The host organ should also have an appropriate environment, including the absence of protease inhibitors and the presence of appropriate growth factors.

The specific requirements for individual tumors and target organs are, as yet, poorly understood. However, they continue to represent an important research area, as understanding why tumors metastasize opens the way for direct therapeutic intervention.

Despite the uncertainties surrounding metastatic potential of tumors, there are recognizable patterns or 'fingerprints' of metastasis, which relate to the site and histological type of tumors. For example, certain tumors frequently spread to bone (kidney, lung, thyroid, prostate, breast), whereas other types, such as melanoma, have a much greater latitude and can invade and grow in a wide range of foreign tissues.

Lysis of basement membrane takes place by secretion of proteases, as well as inhibition of protease inhibitors

Migration of cell is stimulated by self-secreted motility factor and anchorage of cell to molecules in extracellular matrix

Fig. 6.11 Cellular events needed for metastasis. Neoplastic cells have to develop special attributes of altered growth in order to metastasize. In order to escape the confines of the basement membrane (a), cells secrete proteases. As these can normally be inactivated by inhibitors secreted by stromal cells, inhibition of this process is required to allow disruption of basement membrane. Once the basement membrane is breached, cells must acquire receptors that can anchor them to the extracellular matrix (b) and must develop motility.

Neoplasms are frequently associated with systemic effects

Patients with a neoplasm frequently have systemic symptoms, the most frequent being:

- Weight loss.
- Loss of appetite.
- Fever.
- General malaise.
- Anemia.

In many cases the cause of these constitutional symptoms is uncertain, but they are most probably due to effects of secreted cytokines such as tumor necrosis factor and IL-1. These are released from inflammatory cells present in areas of tumor.

Some tumors, whether benign or malignant, retain the function of their organ of origin; if this happens to be an endocrine function, the tumor may exert harmful effects by secretion of excess hormone.

Paraneoplastic syndromes are also frequently recognized in association with tumors. These are syndromes that are not the result of direct effects of the tumor or metastases. For instance, certain tumors derived from non-endocrine cells can secrete hormones (ectopic hormone secretion); lung tumors derived from squamous epithelium can secrete a parathormone-related product, resulting in hypercalcemia. Other tumors are associated with weakness of muscle (myopathy), malfunction of peripheral nerves (neuropathy), or cerebellar ataxia.

Increasingly, it is being shown that these syndromes are due to autoantibodies generated to tumor cells, which cross-react with normal tissues and cause immune-mediated damage.

Both benign and malignant neoplasms can cause death

Malignant tumors, once disseminated, often lead to the death of a patient, the main reasons being:

- Cachexia and the development of poor nutrition from the effects of widespread tumor metastases. Progressive weakness and death result, often from a secondary infection such as a pneumonia. Tumor cachexia is believed to be mediated by activation of cytokines from tumor and inflammatory cells responding to the tumor.
- Obliteration of a vital organ or system by either primary or metastatic tumor.

Most benign tumors will behave in a relatively innocuous manner and, for the most part, are not life-threatening.

However, although the main problems caused by the presence of a mass lesion are amenable to surgical resection, the location of a benign tumor may be important in influencing the outcome; for example, a benign tumor of the brain stem may lead to rapid death because of its critical site.

Histological assessment of neoplasms allows prediction of likely tumor behavior

Examination of the pathological features of a neoplasm provides a useful guide to its likely behavior. Two main assessments are made: analysis of the degree of differentiation and growth pattern of the tumor, and evaluation of how far a tumor has spread. In addition, special techniques may be used to obtain further prognostic information. These are listed towards the end of the chapter, where diagnosis of neoplasia is discussed.

Grading of tumors is performed by looking at cellular cytology

To allocate a grade to a tumor the following cellular features are assessed:

- The degree of differentiation of tumor cells, with reference to the tissue of origin.
- Variation in size and shape of constituent cells of the tumor. The degree of variation (**pleomorphism**) increases with failure of differentiation, and a high degree of variability is seen in malignant tumors (see *Fig. 6.2d*).
- The number of cells containing mitotic figures. Known as the mitotic index, this provides a crude indication of the rate of cell proliferation. The index is generally high in more malignant tumors and low in benign tumors.

As an example, a well-differentiated malignant tumor of the breast epithelium (carcinoma of the breast) would be expected to show structures that resemble small ducts or gland-like spaces, whereas a poorly differentiated malignant tumor of the breast epithelium would not show any attempt to form a glandular pattern. Similarly, mitoses would be expected to be in small numbers in the well-differentiated tumor but numerous in a poorly differentiated tumor (*Fig. 6.12*).

Staging of a tumor offers an indication of how far it has spread

The size of a primary tumor, the degree to which it has invaded locally, and the extent to which it has spread, ultimately determine the chances of survival once a neoplasm has been diagnosed. Assessment of such factors is termed tumor staging. There are several schemes for standardized staging of individual tumors, one of the most frequently applied being the Dukes' staging for neoplasms of the rectum (page 265). The TNM system is based upon extent of local tumor spread, regional lymph node involvement and the presence of distant metastases (*Fig. 6.13*). It can be

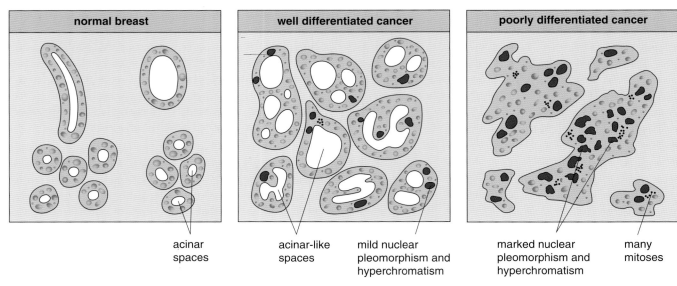

normal breast	well differentiated cancer	poorly differentiated cancer

acinar spaces

acinar-like spaces

mild nuclear pleomorphism and hyperchromatism

marked nuclear pleomorphism and hyperchromatism

many mitoses

Fig. 6.12 Grading of tumors. Distinction between a well differentiated and a poorly differentiated tumor is assessed by grading. In this example the well differentiated tumor resembles its normal counterpart but shows some architectural and cytological abnormality. In a poorly differentiated tumor there is little architectural resemblance to the tissue of origin, and cells show more pronounced cytological abnormalities.

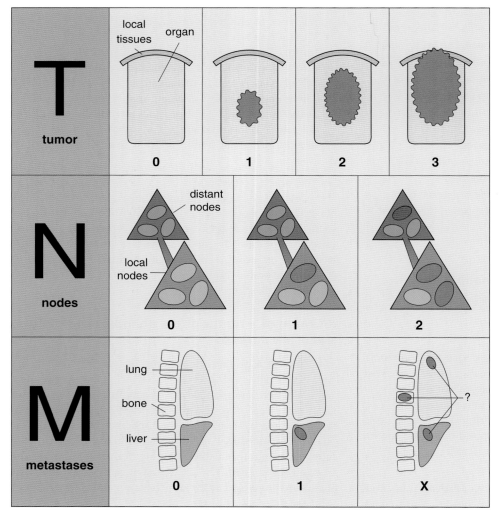

T tumor — local tissues, organ — 0 1 2 3

N nodes — distant nodes, local nodes — 0 1 2

M metastases — lung, bone, liver — 0 1 X

Fig. 6.13 Staging of carcinoma by TNM system. The general principles of TNM staging are as follows:

T refers to primary tumor. The accompanying number denotes the size of tumor and its local extent. The number varies according to site.

N refers to lymph node involvement, and a high number denotes increasing extent of involvement.

M refers to the extent of distant metastases.

As an example, the TNM system for staging malignant neoplasms of the breast is:

T0 = breast free of tumor
T1 = lesion <2 cm in size
T2 = lesion 2–5 cm
T3 = skin and/or chest wall involved by invasion

N0 = no axillary nodes involved
N1 = mobile nodes involved
N2 = fixed nodes involved

M0 = no metastases
M1 = demonstrable metastases
MX = suspected metastases

applied to many different types of tumor, although the criteria are different for each tumor site.

The stage of a tumor is generally the most important indicator of likely prognosis and of appropriate therapy; tumors at an advanced stage (extensive spread) may require aggressive treatment, whereas early-stage tumors (localized) may be treatable by relatively conservative measures.

In situ neoplasia is a stage of neoplasia prior to the development of invasion

Although an epithelial neoplasm may show the cytological features of malignancy, i.e. cellular pleomorphism and increased mitotic activity, it may not be invasive on histological examination. This phenomenon, termed carcinoma in situ, represents a very early stage of neoplasia. In molecular terms it is probable that the genetic abnormalities allowing metastasis (see *Fig. 6.11*) have not yet developed.

Neoplasms of this type are most commonly encountered in epithelial tissues, for example squamous epithelium of the cervix (see page 420), skin, and breast, where cytologically malignant cells may be confined within ducts (intraductal carcinoma) or within lobules (intralobular carcinoma, see pages 444 and 446).

The diagnosis of tumors at the stage of in situ neoplasia is clearly important as, if left, such lesions would progress to become invasive, whereas early detection and treatment at this pre-invasive stage is often completely curative.

Dysplasia is a histological term applied to cells that have some of the cytological features of neoplasia

The term dysplasia is used to describe the histological appearance of cells that show an increased rate of cell division, coupled with incomplete maturation. Like neoplastic cells, dysplastic cells tend to exhibit a high nuclear to cytoplasmic ratio and there is an increased number of mitoses. Dysplastic tissues may also show loss of the normal architectural relationships between cells.

Dysplasia most frequently arises in epithelial tissues that have been subject to chronic irritation. In these instances there is usually evidence of an associated inflammatory response. However, dysplasia can occur in the absence of obvious tissue damage or repair, and in such cases the cytological features of the dysplastic tissue may merge with those described in early neoplasia. It is important to identify dysplasia, as in some circumstances true neoplastic change follows after a period of time, and can develop over many years. A sequence from dysplasia through in situ neoplasia to invasive neoplasia is now well recognized in several tissues (*Fig. 6.14*).

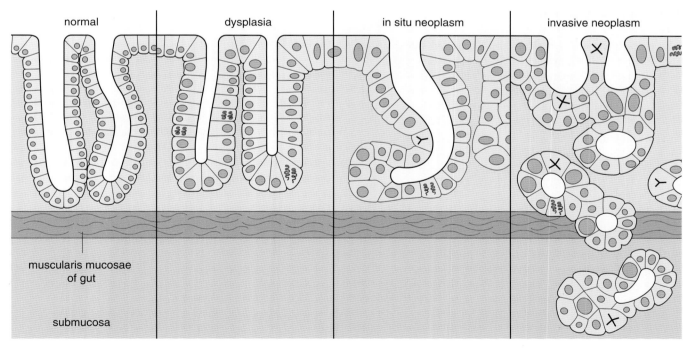

Fig. 6.14 Progression of dysplasia to neoplasia. A sequence of progression from dysplasia through in situ neoplasia to invasive neoplasia is often seen in several tissues. In the diagram, as in real life, the distinction between dysplasia and in situ neoplasia is difficult and emphasis is placed on loss of normal tissue architecture to signify the development of neoplasia. The main areas in which this situation develops are: squamous epithelium at the squamocolumnar junction of the uterine cervix; epidermis of sun-exposed skin; colonic mucosa after long-standing chronic colitis; and gastric mucosa after long-standing chronic gastritis. The altered cell turnover in dysplasia probably allows local environmental factors to cause genetic abnormalities leading to neoplasia.

Premalignant lesions can be treated to prevent later development of invasive neoplasia

Certain lesions, including some benign neoplasms, are known to progress, with time, to invasive neoplasia. The recognized progression from dysplasia through carcinoma in situ to invasive neoplasia has already been mentioned. Important conditions which can be treated in their premalignant stage are:

- Adenomatous polyps of the colon.
- Cervical epithelial in situ neoplasia.
- Dysplasia of the colon in long-standing ulcerative colitis.
- Dysplasia of the stomach epithelium.

The dysplasia is not, in itself, a neoplastic condition, and removal of the adverse environmental stimulus responsible often allows restoration of the normal cell growth pattern.

Dysplastic conditions are often treated by surgical removal or ablation of affected tissue to minimize the risk of subsequent malignancy.

TUMOR NOMENCLATURE AND CLASSIFICATION

The name given to a tumor should provide information about its cell of origin and its likely behavior (benign or malignant). Unfortunately, as with many areas of medicine, the classification and nomenclature of tumors has evolved over many years and is full of inconsistencies. Some tumors are named on the basis of a macroscopic feature, or histological and behavioral observation. Others are given eponymous or semi-descriptive names, which were coined when there was poor understanding of histogenesis but have been retained because they have been in use for so long. It is not unusual for a single tumor to have many synonyms.

Nomenclature of tumors of epithelial origin

Some benign neoplasms of surface epithelia, e.g. skin, are known as **papillomata** (singular: **papilloma**) because they form frond-like growths. This is prefixed by the cell of origin, e.g. squamous cell papilloma of skin.

Benign neoplasms, of both solid and surface epithelium, are termed **adenomata** (singular: **adenoma**), and are also prefixed by the tissue of origin, e.g. thyroid adenoma, renal adenoma, adrenal adenoma, colonic adenoma.

A malignant tumor of any epithelial origin is termed a **carcinoma**. Tumors of glandular epithelium (including that lining the gut) are termed **adenocarcinomas**. Tumors of other epithelia are prefixed by the cell type of origin, e.g.

Fig. 6.15 Nomenclature of tumors of support cells and muscle

Tissue of origin	Benign	Malignant
Fibrous	Fibroma	Fibrosarcoma
Bone	Osteoma	Osteosarcoma
Cartilage	Chondroma	Chondrosarcoma
Adipose	Lipoma	Liposarcoma
Smooth muscle	Leiomyoma	Leiomyosarcoma
Skeletal muscle	Rhabdomyoma	Rhabdomyosarcoma

squamous cell carcinoma, transitional cell carcinoma, hepatocellular carcinoma. To classify a carcinoma further, the tissue of origin is added, e.g. adenocarcinoma of prostate, adenocarcinoma of breast, squamous carcinoma of larynx.

Nomenclature of tumors of mesenchymal tissues

For tumors composed of mesenchymal tissues (support cells or muscle) the nomenclature is more consistent than that for epithelial types. The tissue of origin takes the suffix -**oma** if the tumor is benign, or -**sarcoma** if it is malignant. For example, a benign tumor of cartilage is termed a chondroma, and a malignant tumor is termed a chondrosarcoma. A summary of nomenclature of other tumors of support cells is shown in *Fig. 6.15*.

Nomenclature of other tumors

Neoplasms that do not fit into either the epithelial or the support cell categories are named according to their tissue of origin (histogenetic nomenclature). The main categories are as follows.

Lymphomas. These tumors of the lymphoid system are composed of neoplastic lymphocytes, and vary in grade of malignancy from slow-growing to highly aggressive (see Chapter 15).

Malignant melanoma. Highly malignant tumors derived from melanocytes, usually identifiable by their melanin content.

Leukemias. Malignant tumors derived from hemopoietic elements in bone marrow which circulate in the blood (see Chapter 15).

Embryonal tumors. A group of malignant tumors seen mainly in childhood, derived from primitive embryonal blastic tissue; the most common types are nephroblastoma of the kidney (see *Fig. 17.26*) and neuroblastoma of the adrenal medulla (see *Fig. 16.23*).

Gliomas. Tumors derived from the non-neural support tissues of the brain are named according to the cell of origin, e.g. astrocytoma, oligodendroglioma (see Chapter 21).

Germ cell tumors. Tumors derived from germ cells in the gonads, but also rarely arising in non-gonadal sites (Chapters 18 and 19).

Teratomas. A type of germ cell tumor which differentiates to form elements of all three embryological germ cell layers: ectoderm, endoderm, and mesoderm. Teratomas may be benign or malignant, and as well as arising in the gonads they also occur in non-gonadal sites in young people, particularly in the sacrum and mediastinum.

Neuroendocrine tumors. Tumors of neuroendocrine cells which secrete polypeptide hormones or biologically active amines. Examples include pheochromocytoma of the adrenal medulla (see page 346), carcinoid tumor of the appendix (page 270) and medullary carcinoma of the thyroid (page 340). Some tumors are given functional names, e.g. insulinoma, prolactinoma, glucagonoma, and VIPoma. Clinical syndromes may result from the excessive hormone secretion by the tumor.

Hamartomas. Non-neoplastic overgrowths of tissues that would normally occur in the site in question. Although they are developmental abnormalities rather than true neoplasms, they are often grouped with neoplasms because they appear as localized tissue masses. Common examples are hemangiomas (see page 170), and melanocytic nevi (moles).

Choristomas. Non-neoplastic overgrowths of tissues that would not normally occur in those sites. Although developmental, like hamartomas, they are considered alongside tumors because they present as a mass of tissue.

Tumors with eponymous names

Many tumors continue to be named after the person who recognized or popularized them. The most common examples are:

Ewing's sarcoma. A malignant tumor of bone seen in young people, probably derived from primitive neuroendocrine cells.

Hodgkin's disease. A malignant proliferation of lymphoid tissues, classified as a subgroup of the lymphomas.

Kaposi's sarcoma. A malignant tumor thought to be derived from endothelium and driven by infection with herpes virus-8, now often seen in association with AIDS.

Burkitt's lymphoma. A form of lymphoma derived from B cells, in which Epstein–Barr virus has a causative role.

BIOLOGY OF NEOPLASIA

Carcinogenesis is the train of biological events that underlies the development of neoplasia. At the cellular level, neoplasms are ultimately caused by genetic mutations, resulting in abnormal control of growth. There is now much evidence to suggest that this genetic damage is a multistep development, requiring the interaction of several processes, often over a period of many years.

Abnormalities in genes regulating cell proliferation underlie neoplastic transformation

Four main genetic mechanisms are thought to have a role in the development of most human neoplasms:

- Expression of genes resulting in inappropriate activity of products which, under normal circumstances, stimulate growth. Such genes are termed oncogenes and act in a dominant fashion. (Phenotype is affected even if one allele is present, which abnormally stimulates growth.)
- Loss of activity of genes which, under normal circumstances, produce products that inhibit cell growth. Such genes are termed **tumor suppressor genes** or **anti-oncogenes**. They can rarely act in a dominant manner to cause benign tumors (heterozygotes with one abnormal gene), but generally act in a recessive manner to produce malignant tumors. (Malignant phenotype only develops if both alleles fail to suppress growth.)
- Over-expression of genes which, under normal circumstances, produce products that prevent normal cell death. Failure to eliminate genetically damaged cells allows continued growth of tumors.
- Loss of activity of gene products which, under normal circumstances, would repair damaged DNA. Loss of activity leads to a state of DNA instability with the development of somatic mutations in oncogenes or tumor suppressor genes.

The genetic reason for neoplastic transformation is variable:

- Point mutations in oncogene causing production of abnormally functioning product or loss of a suppressor.
- Gene amplification causing excessive production of oncoprotein product.
- Chromosomal rearrangements whereby an oncogene is activated inappropriately by another promoter region.

It is now recognized that tumors normally have several genetic aberrations, the sum of which results in neoplastic transformation of cells. A tumor may develop additional oncogene abnormalities with time, resulting in a more aggressive growth pattern. The mechanisms by which oncogenes act are summarized in *Fig. 6.16*.

Growth factors regulate cell division

Cells are induced to proliferate by specific growth signals from a variety of growth factors, which include hormones, cytokines and classic growth factors. These bind to cell surface receptors which are virtually all transmembrane proteins having a cytosolic domain with tyrosine kinase activity. In response to a positive growth signal cells undergo internal reorganization of actin-dependent adhesion mechanisms, show an increase in intracellular calcium, and following activation and nuclear translocation of transcription factors, the cell cycle is entered.

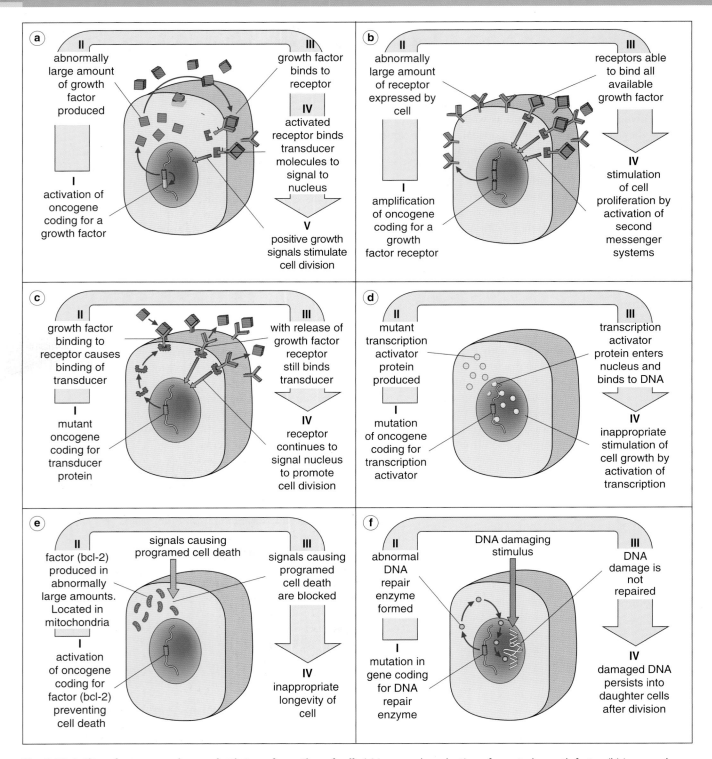

Fig. 6.16 Action of oncogenes in neoplastic transformation of cells (a) Increased production of secreted growth factor. (b) Increased expression of growth factor receptors. (c) Mutation in transducer protein gene. (d) Mutant transcription factor production. (e) Overproduction of factor that prevents cell death. (f) Loss of activity in DNA repair systems.

The cell cycle is controlled at several points

The cell cycle is controlled by complexes of cyclins and cyclin-dependent kinases

Cells which are in an active state of proliferation are said to be in the cell cycle (*Fig. 6.17*).

Progression of a cell through this cycle is controlled by the synthesis, degradation and state of phosphorylation of proteins called cyclins (cyclins A, B, D, E). The cyclins form complexes with cyclin-dependent kinases (CDKs), and these complexes control progress through the cell cycle by activating a variety of proteins by phosphorylation. A variety of cyclin-dependent kinase inhibitors (CDKIs) are also present which modulate the activity of the cell cycle.

- p21, p27 and p57 have broad activity as inhibitors of CDK activity.
- p15, p16, p18 and p19 (INK4 proteins) in**hibit** CD**K4** and CDK6.

Cell cycle checkpoints make sure that only normal cells complete replication

There are important checkpoints in the cell cycle which are policed by surveillance systems in the cell nucleus designed to prevent cells replicating if they become damaged, especially if there is existing DNA damage. A cell which has been halted in its progression through the cell cycle can either activate DNA repair mechanisms or, if these fail, switch on apoptosis to eliminate itself.

- The transition from the G1 to the S phase of the cell cycle can only happen when a transcription factor called E2F is free in the nucleus. During G1, E2F is normally bound to Rb protein and must be released to allow movement through G1 to S phase, past a point late in G1 called the restriction point. This is achieved by the phosphorylation of Rb, releasing E2F. Phosphorylation of Rb is achieved by synthesis of cyclin D, which forms a complex with CDK4 and 6, and then the formation of a cyclin E–CDK2 complex. If a cell has an abnormal Rb that overexpress CDK4 or cyclin D will also functionally fail to prevent checkpoint arrest after G1, as Rb will tend to be phosphorylated.
- The transition between the G2 and the M phases is regulated by the formation of the CDK1–cyclin B complex. After entry to M phase, cyclin B is rapidly destroyed by the ubiquitin–proteasome system.

Fig. 6.17 Cell cycle. Following the M (mitosis) phase cells can either enter a non-dividing state, termed G0, or continue through the cell cycle. Phases G1, S and G2 constitute so-called interphase cells. During S phase, cells replicate DNA. Three of the important cell cycle checkpoints are shown (black wedges): the G1/S restriction point (R) is regulated by the state of phosphorylation of Rb. On phosphorylation of Rb, the E2F transcription factor is liberated allowing progression into S phase. The other major checkpoints are the intra-S checkpoint that monitors errors in transcription forks, and the G2/M checkpoint that monitors assembly of the mitotic spindle apparatus. These are regulated by Cdk/cyclin complexes as shown. If replication errors cannot be corrected at these checkpoints, the cells enter the apoptotic pathway.

- The gene coding for p53 protein is activated in the presence of DNA damage and causes an increase in the cyclin-dependent kinase inhibitor (CDKI) p21 protein termed WAF1. This inhibitor prevents phosphorylation of cyclins and hence arrests the cell in its progression through the cycle. If a cell has an abnormal form of p53 protein then this regulatory function will be impaired, and so cells with damaged DNA may complete mitosis, thereby propagating a mutation.

Oncogenes are central to the development of tumors

Oncogenes were originally isolated from tumor-forming RNA retroviruses (v-onc).

Viral concogenes (*v-oncs*): genes within a virus that code for a protein involved in the development of neoplasia.

Cellular oncogenes (*c-oncs*): genes that code for proteins in the development of neoplasia.

Proto-oncogenes (*p-oncs*): genes that code for proteins involved in the control of cell growth.

A proto-oncogene can lead to the development of a tumor by three main mechanisms:

- Mutation – leading to a mutant protein product.
- Gene amplification – leading to excess protein product.
- Abnormal gene promotion – the oncogene is driven by an abnormal promoter:
  ○ Host derived: usually in association with a chromosome translocation.
  ○ Virus derived: in the setting of a retroviral infection.

Oncogene products, all key molecules in signal transduction and control of normal cell growth are referred to by the abbreviated name of the tumor virus or system in which they were discovered. For example, *ras*, found in rat sarcoma virus, is a protein that acts on the GTP intracellular second messenger system.

In humans, abnormalities of oncogenes are found in tumors, and are thought to be primary events in malignant transformation. Usually, multiple oncogene abnormalities are seen in a single tumor.

Fig. 6.18 summarizes the important oncoproteins, giving examples of associated tumors and the respective reasons for their activation.

Absence of tumor suppressor genes promotes neoplasia

The first suppressor gene to be discovered was found in a malignant tumor of the retina in childhood, known as a retinoblastoma. The gene is located on chromosome 13 and is termed Rb. Familial forms of disease are inherited as an autosomal dominant trait, in which affected children have one mutant gene (inactive) and one normal gene (active). To develop a retinoblastoma, the second gene must undergo a somatic mutation in the child. In sporadic retinoblastoma both genes must undergo mutation, a chance event which means that sporadic tumors are rare. Since the discovery of the Rb gene's absence in retinoblastoma, its absence has been established in many other tumors.

Located on chromosome 17, another suppressor gene, p53, has been found to be lost in so many types of tumor that it has been proposed as the most common genetic abnormality in neoplasia. In a normal cell p53 is activated in response to DNA damage, activating systems that bring about DNA repair and arresting the cell cycle. In cells where repair is not achieved, p53 can cause the cell to enter the apoptotic pathway of cell death, eliminating the possi-

Fig. 6.18 Main oncogene products and mechanisms of abnormal regulation

Proto-oncogene	Function	Oncogene type	Reason for activation
ras	GTP binding	Signal transduction	Point mutation
myc	Transcription activator	Nuclear regulator	Translocation
n-*myc*	Transcription activator	Nuclear regulator	Translocation
erb-B1	EGF receptor	Growth factor receptor	Amplification
erb-B2 (neu)	EGF-like receptor	Growth factor receptor	Amplification
bcl-2	Mitochondrial protein	Inhibit apoptosis	Translocation
abl	Tyrosine kinase	Signal transduction	Translocation
sis	PDGF β chain	Growth factor	Over-expression

EGF – epidermal growth factor   PGDF – platelet derived growth factor   GTP – guanosine triphosphate bility of division of a cell with damaged DNA. Loss of activity of p53 in a cell allows the proliferation of cells with DNA damage.

The absence of APC, another tumor suppressor gene, is responsible for the development of familial adenomatous polyposis coli. People who inherit a single inactive copy of the gene develop multiple benign adenomata of the large bowel (see page 263). If cells develop a second mutation of the normal inherited gene on the other allele, it leads to development of carcinoma of the colon. The molecular basis of defective APC function has been determined. In normal cells, APC protein binds another protein termed α-catenin and brings about its degradation. α-Catenin is a transcription factor, and if APC function is defective through mutation, raised levels of α-catenin occur in the cell, driving cell proliferation.

Many of the tumor suppressor genes have been called 'gatekeeper' genes, in that they normally directly control the proliferation of cells, and a loss of function allows a cell to enter a state that leads to fully developed neoplasia.

Damage to genes that regulate DNA repair predisposes to neoplasia

Cells are constantly exposed to stimuli that cause damage to DNA, and there is a well developed system for detection and repair of DNA, including the action of p53 discussed above.

Mutation in DNA repair genes allows the proliferation of cells with DNA mutations, so-called replication error-positive phenotype (RER+). This state can be assessed by looking at microsatellite sequences (tandem repeated DNA sequences) in cells, which normally remain constant. With DNA repair errors, cells develop changes in the repeat length of microsatellite DNA, a condition termed microsatellite instability.

Several genes have been characterized that code for DNA repair elements (*hMSH2*, *hMLH1*, *hPMS1*, *hPMS2*).

Mutations in such genes are found in those patients who have an inherited predisposition to colonic carcinoma not linked to the APC gene. Development of a replication error-positive phenotype is also encountered in many sporadic tumors as a result of a somatic mutation in DNA repair genes. The genes coding for DNA repair systems are sometimes called 'caretaker' genes, in that they look after the DNA, defective function leading to genetic instability in which there is an overall increased risk of a cell developing a mutation in any gene, including a proto-oncogene.

Tumors are composed of several genetic clones derived by acquired mutations

It is widely recognized that tumors become less well differentiated and more aggressive with time. This property, termed progression, is due to the emergence of subpopulations of cells with new genetic abnormalities that make growth control more abnormal and facilitate metastasis. Any large tumor is therefore composed of a whole set of slightly different cells (tumor heterogeneity) as a result of further acquired somatic mutations (*Fig. 6.19*). Any mutations that favour tumor survival or spread are chosen by a form of natural selection.

Fig. 6.19 Tumor progression and genetic heterogeneity. As tumors develop they undergo further somatic mutation, which causes abnormalities in other oncogenes. Mutations may also lead to cell death. A mutation that puts a cell at a survival disadvantage will cause that clone to be eliminated. A tumor will ultimately consist of many different subclones of cells, those with greater growth potential gradually coming to dominate the lesion.

This is an important concept, as it explains how a primary tumor may respond to therapy whereas metastatic lesions do not, as they are composed of cells with properties allowing invasion, motility, and growth in another site. It also explains how, after apparent clinical response, a tumor may re-emerge as resistant to chemotherapeutic drugs: resistant cells are selected and eventually come to dominate the tumor.

Cytogenetic studies have documented a mixture of molecular genetic and cytogenetic features that accompany clinical and histological evidence of tumor progression. As research continues, it is hoped that the precise gene abnormalities underlying the cytogenetic abnormalities will be identified, allowing a molecular assessment of the likely biological behaviour of a neoplasm.

Recurring cytogenetic abnormalities are seen in some tumors

Cytogenetic examination of the chromosomal complement of cells has identified several recurring chromosomal abnormalities in specific tumors.

More recent molecular biological investigation has demonstrated some of the genetic effects of these structural abnormalities. In most instances this takes the form of overexpression of an oncogene or deletion of a suppressor gene. The most important abnormalities are listed in *Fig. 6.20*. Detection of these cytogenetic abnormalities in tumor samples is not only useful in determining either diagnosis

Techniques for detecting cytogenetic changes in tumors

Traditional karyotypic analysis is performed on metaphase spreads and requires viable tumor maintained in culture for a short time. Technical limitations mean that it only works for solid tumors in about 40% of cases, and can only detect relatively large changes.

Structural changes for which sequence data are available, for example certain translocations producing fusion oncogenes, can be detected by FISH (fluorescence in situ hybridization) or RT-PCR (reverse transcriptase polymerase chain reaction). Spectral karyotyping (SKY) allows simultaneous labeling of all chromosomes by fluorescent probes and permits the detection of complex and small chromosomal abnormalities.

or prognosis, but also important because they are ultimately related to abnormal gene expression.

Chemical carcinogens have a role in several human tumors

Many chemical carcinogens have been identified, and their effects documented in experiments in which animals

---

Fig. 6.20 Cytogenetic abnormalities in human neoplasms

Tumor	Cytogenetic abnormality	Effects
Chronic myeloid leukemia	t(9;22)(q34;q11) (Philadelphia chromosome)	Fusion oncogene bcr-abl leads to protein with tyrosine kinase activity
Follicular lymphoma	t(14;18)(q32;q21)	*IgH* gene from chr14 fused to *Bcl-2* gene on chr21 leading to prevention of apoptosis
Ewing's sarcoma	t(11;22)(q24;q12)	Fusion of the *FLT-1* gene from chr11 with the *EWS* gene on chr22 leading to a fusion protein with high transcription activator activity
Alveolar rhabdomyosarcoma	t(2;13)(q35;q14)	*PAX3* gene from chr2 is fused with the *FKHR* gene on chr13 leading to a fusion protein with transcription factor activity
Synovial sarcoma	t(X;18) (p11;q11)	*SYT* gene from chr18 is fused to *SSX1 SSX2* gene on X chromosome. Possible ectopic expression of SSX1/2 products
Neuroblastoma	Homogeneous staining regions and double minute chromosomes	Amplification of *n-myc*
Burkitt's lymphoma	t(8;14)(q24;q32)	Fusion of *c-myc* on chr8 with *IgH* from chr14 leading to *c-myc* expression

exposed to the agents develop neoplasia. The main groups of relevance to human disease are:

- Polycyclic hydrocarbons, found in tars, are among the potent agents in cigarette smoke that cause lung cancer.
- Aromatic amines are mainly encountered through industrial exposure (e.g. rubber or dye industry) and are converted to active agents in the liver. They become concentrated by excretion in the urine, and so have their main effect on the urothelium, where cancers develop.
- Nitrosamines have been shown to be potent carcinogens in animals, and in humans there is a pathway for conversion of dietary nitrites and nitrates to nitrosamines by gut bacteria. These agents are thought to cause cancer in the stomach and gastrointestinal tract.
- Alkylating agents can bind directly to DNA and are directly mutagenic. They are rare in the environment, but examples are used in cancer chemotherapy (e.g. cyclophosphamide), raising the possibility that the use of such agents to treat one tumor may predispose a patient to the development of another.

There are three main groups of chemical carcinogen

Chemical carcinogens may cause the development of neoplasia either directly or indirectly. They can be grouped into three classes according to the mechanism by which they stimulate the development of neoplasia:

Genotoxic: cause direct damage to DNA leading to mutations. The abnormal areas of DNA are prone to further damage in replication, and are resistant to normal DNA repair mechanisms.

Mitogenic: bind to receptors on or in cells and stimulate cell division without causing direct DNA damage. In experimental skin carcinogenesis such agents have been shown to bind to and activate protein kinase C, causing sustained epidermal hyperplasia.

Cytotoxic: produce tissue damage and lead to hyperplasia with cycles of tissue regeneration and damage. In some cases it is believed that cytokines generated in response to tissue damage act as mitogenic factors.

Chemical carcinogens can be further divided into two groups:

Direct acting: the agent is capable of directly causing neoplasia.

Procarcinogens: the agent requires conversion to an active carcinogen. This conversion takes place by normal metabolic pathways.

In procarcinogens the cytochrome P450 oxygenase system plays an important role in conversion in many instances. Detoxification reactions also occur, the accumulation of carcinogen being determined by a balance between:

- Dose of procarcinogen.
- Rate of detoxification and elimination.
- Rate of conversion to the active form.

Chemical carcinogens can be divided into initiating and promoting agents

The original concepts of chemical carcinogenesis were largely derived from work on experimental induction of malignant skin tumors in mice. It was found that some agents, such as polycyclic aromatic hydrocarbons, could cause cancer of the skin if they were painted onto mice in high doses. In low dosage they would not cause cancer but would render the skin susceptible to developing cancer on exposure to another agent which, on its own, would not induce cancer. From this work it was possible to define two types of chemical carcinogen (*Fig. 6.21*).

Initiating agents

- Exposure of cells to an initiating agent does not directly cause neoplasia but renders cells susceptible to developing neoplasia if they are later exposed to certain other agents.
- The initiating agent causes genetic abnormality of exposed cells. The genetic damage will cause an abnormality which is not in itself sufficient to result in abnormal cell growth.
- Most initiating agents are examples of genotoxic carcinogens.

Promoting agents

- Exposure of normal cells to a promoting agent causes no abnormality.
- Prolonged exposure of initiated cells to a promoting agent causes the development of neoplasia.
- Transient exposure of initiated cells to a promoting agent will also not result in the development of neoplasia.
- The promoting agent causes increased cell turnover (inducing cell proliferation). With continued exposure to the promoting agent, cells that have a genetic abnormality (caused by the initiating agent) develop

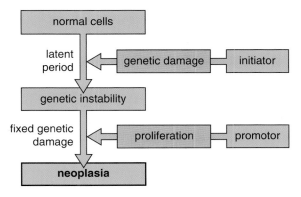

Fig. 6.21 Action of initiating and promoting carcinogens

Predicting the carcinogenicity of chemical agents

Important emphasis has been placed on the determination of whether an agent is a carcinogen. Two types of test can be used.

- **Mutagenicity studies.** Strains of *Salmonella typhimurium* which are unable to synthesize histidine are mixed with a microsomal fraction from rodent liver and a test chemical. The microsomes enable conversion of a procarcinogen to an active form. If the chemical is a mutagen then some bacteria undergo mutation and acquire the ability to make histidine. This is detected by plating out the test bacteria on a

medium which is deficient in histidine. This type of test (the Ames test) will detect genotoxic chemical carcinogens but is insensitive to cytotoxic or mitogenic types.
- **Carcinogenicity studies.** Chemical agents are administered to rodents at high doses and the incidence of tumors is evaluated on pathological and histological examination after near lifelong exposure. This approach appears valid for genotoxic carcinogens but may not be appropriate for non-genotoxic agents because of dose considerations and species specificities.

secondary genetic abnormalities in key genes regulating cell growth (oncogenes).
- With increased cell proliferation, clones of cells develop which have loss of growth control and the characteristics of a neoplasm.
- Many promoting agents are examples of mitogenic carcinogens.

Three stages have been defined in chemical carcinogenesis

From experimental work three stages of chemical carcinogenesis have been defined:

Initiation: induction of genetic changes in cells. The nature of the initial changes in cells is still uncertain. In experimental chemical carcinogenesis in skin, the Harvey *ras* gene has been identified as being frequently mutated. This gene is involved in epidermal proliferation, and when it becomes abnormal epidermal cells are less responsive to signals that normally cause terminal differentiation. Only relatively few genes have been identified as being mutated in other animal models of chemical carcinogenesis.

Promotion: induction of cell proliferation. In this phase of carcinogenesis a promoting agent, either a mitogen or a cytotoxic agent, brings about increased cell proliferation. Promotion is initially reversible if the promoting agent is withdrawn.

Progression: If there is persistent cell proliferation, initiated cells acquire secondary genetic abnormalities in oncogenes which first lead to dysregulation and eventually to autonomous cell growth. The ultimate end-point of progression is the development of an invasive neoplasm.

Although many environmental agents fit into the categories of initiating and promoting agents, some can act as both initiator and promoter (complete carcinogens).

Study of chemical carcinogenesis is relevant to the treatment of human disease

The understanding of molecular aspects of chemical carcinogenesis has led to the development of the concept of chemoprevention. This proposes strategies for intervention at the phase of premalignancy using drugs to reverse or halt the process of carcinogenesis. Drugs that are under investigation include:

- Tamoxifen in breast carcinoma.
- Retinoids and β-carotene in head, neck and lung tumors.

Key Facts
Chemical carcinogenesis

- Most work on chemical carcinogenesis has been developed in experimental animal studies.
- Following exposure to a carcinogenic agent there is a long latent period before a neoplasm develops. It is thought that altered cells are primed but require a second change to bring about molecular genetic changes expressed as neoplasia.
- From the evidence supplied by animal models, carcinogenesis is a multistage process:
  - **Initiation**: an event that alters the genome.
  - **Promotion**: an event that causes proliferation of the transformed cell takes place, giving rise to a neoplasm.
  - **Progression**: new genetic mutations occur, with the development of subclones of neoplastic cells.

Only a few infections are implicated in human neoplasia

Based on the fact that viruses are known to be directly responsible for some neoplasms in animals, it is not unreasonable to assume that similar viruses cause certain human neoplasias; however, relatively few viruses have been implicated, as summarized in *Fig. 6.22*. Two types of viral carcinogenesis have been described related to activation of oncogenes:

- Slow-transforming viruses insert virus-derived DNA into the genome randomly. If chance dictates that the viral DNA is integrated next to a proto-oncogene, then the viral DNA causes abnormal promotion of the proto-oncogene, leading to neoplasia.
- Acute-transforming viruses contain a viral oncogene, and when virus-derived DNA is inserted into the host genome the transcribed viral oncogene is expressed, leading to neoplasia.

The precise molecular mechanisms whereby viruses cause neoplastic transformation are beginning to be determined, e.g. papilloma viruses produce proteins that inactivate certain products made by tumor suppressor genes (see pages 83 and 86–7), thereby allowing cells to escape normal regulation of growth. Bacteria have been implicated in neoplasia. The development of gastric lymphoma has been directly related to infection by *Helicobacter pylori*.

Irradiation is a potent cause of neoplastic transformation

An increased incidence of neoplasia following exposure to ionizing radiation has long been documented and is due to a direct increase in DNA damage. There are two main effects of DNA damage through irradiation:

- Formation of DNA breaks.
- Development of DNA instability.

Direct exposure to ionizing radiation, for example repeated exposure to X-rays, increases the risk of tumors in bone marrow and in the skin of exposed areas. Exposure to radioactive material in the environment is a more complex issue, as the type of tumor is related to the type of exposure and to possible incorporation of radioactive material in body tissues. For example:

- Inhalation of radioactive dust or gas (e.g. radon) increases the risk of carcinoma of the lung.
- Ingestion of radioactive iodine increases the risk of carcinoma of the thyroid.
- Incorporation of radioactive metals into bone increases the risk of tumors of bone marrow and bone.

A frequently overlooked source of radiation which is a major cause of neoplasia is UV light in sunlight (see Chapter 9). This is known to increase the risk of development of many types of malignant skin tumor (see pages 521–7).

Fig. 6.22 Viruses implicated in human neoplasia

Virus	Neoplasm
Epstein–Barr	Burkitt's lymphoma Nasopharyngeal carcinoma B-cell lymphomas and some cases of Hodgkin's disease
Hepatitis B	Hepatocellular carcinoma
Human papillomavirus	Cervical carcinoma Some carcinomas of the skin
HTLV-1	T-cell leukemia/lymphoma
HHV-8	Kaposi's sarcoma

Biological agents such as hormones play a role in tumor growth

In some circumstances hormones are thought to contribute to the etiology or growth of neoplasia:

- Hormones may be required to promote tumor growth. Estrogens stimulate the proliferation of breast and endometrial tissue and can predispose to the development of carcinoma of the breast and endometrium in animal models. Certain tumors depend on hormones for continued growth.
- Carcinomas of the breast that express estrogen receptors can be treated by anti-estrogen drugs, and this often causes regression of tumor.
- Carcinoma of the prostate can be treated by removal of testosterone stimulation by orchidectomy or the administration of estrogenic drugs.
- In a unique situation, children of women treated during pregnancy with the synthetic estrogen diethylstilboestrol develop carcinoma of the vagina. This is an example of an agent acting in utero causing neoplasia in later life.

Cytokines may also be involved in the control of growth of neoplastic cells. For example, one form of tumor of white blood cells, termed hairy-cell leukemia, can be treated with interferon.

Asbestos is an example of a physical agent that causes neoplasia

Asbestos fibers (see page 211) which are inhaled are a potent cause of neoplasia in the lung and pleura. This is often after a long period of latency following exposure. The association with primary malignant tumors arising in the pleura is particularly strong, as in the absence of previous asbestos exposure they are extremely rare (see page 220). The precise mechanism whereby asbestos fibers cause neoplasia is unresolved.

Many dietary factors are implicated in neoplasia but their role is uncertain

A variety of dietary substances have been implicated in the cause of neoplasia, particularly neoplasia in the gut. A diet high in fat is associated with a higher risk of development of carcinoma of the breast and colon compared to populations with a low-fat diet. A diet low in fiber is associated with an increased incidence of carcinoma of the colon compared to populations with a high-fiber diet. High levels of nitrates or nitrites in the diet are associated with an increased risk of development of carcinoma of the stomach.

Preneoplastic conditions are diseases associated with an increased risk of developing tumors

Certain non-neoplastic diseases are known to carry an increased risk of later development of neoplasia and are termed preneoplastic conditions.

Hyperplasia is one such condition; endometrial hyperplasia and hyperplasia of the epithelium of breast lobules and ducts both predispose to the development of carcinoma.

In some instances a chronic increased proliferation of cells results in **dysplasia**, which then progresses to carcinoma. For example:

- Chronic gastritis predisposes to the development of carcinoma of the stomach.
- Chronic colitis predisposes to the development of carcinoma of the colon.
- Hepatic cirrhosis predisposes to development of liver cell carcinoma.

Chronic autoimmune diseases are associated with the development of localized neoplastic transformation of lymphoid cells to form a lymphoma. For example:

- Celiac disease predisposes to the later development of gut lymphoma.
- Autoimmune thyroiditis predisposes to the development of thyroid lymphoma.

Immune responses are being explored to combat established human tumors

Neoplastic transformation results in an abnormal phenotype of cells and may be associated with the development of abnormal antigens. Although immune responses to tumors are evident, they seem weak and, in human disease, do not normally appear to contribute significantly to the response to an established tumor.

There are two main classes of tumor-related antigen:

- Tumor-specific antigens are present only on tumor cells. These are well established in animal models, but their role in human tumors is uncertain at present. The presence of a significant lymphoid infiltrate, including cytotoxic lymphocytes in certain tumors, suggests that an immune response to tumor-specific antigens may be taking place. Clinical observations have indicated that patients with tumors having a lymphoid infiltrate have a better prognosis than those without an infiltrate. This has prompted treatment protocols whereby lymphocytes are harvested from surgically excised tumors, cloned in culture to produce killer cells, and transfused back to the patient in an attempt to enhance any tumor-related immune response. Great interest is being shown in developing tumor vaccines against tumor-specific antigens. For example, MAGE proteins are normally expressed in germ cells in the absence of class II antigen and hence cannot be recognized by the immune system. MAGE proteins are also expressed on several tumors with class II antigens, so it is possible that vaccination against MAGE proteins could be used to combat certain tumors. The identification of similar novel tumor antigens with a view to developing a vaccine is an active research area.
- Tumor-associated antigens are present on both tumor cells and some normal cells. Included in this group are the oncofetal antigens, which are normally expressed in development but become re-expressed in the neoplastic cells. For example, α-fetoprotein (AFP) is expressed in hepatocellular cancer, and carcinoembryonic antigen (CEA) is expressed in cancers of the gastrointestinal tract.

EPIDEMIOLOGY OF NEOPLASTIC DISEASE

In humans there is an association between the incidence and types of cancer encountered and age, as summarized in *Fig. 6.23*.

There is a small number of tumors of childhood. These are distinct from those that occur in adult life, being mainly tumors recapitulating embryonal tissues ('blastomas') and leukemias.

Tumors in early adult life are uncommon, being mainly tumors of bone, lymphomas, and germ cell tumors. These lesions may well be precipitated by an abnormal response to normal growth and endocrine stimuli.

An increasing incidence of a wide range of epithelial neoplasms is seen with age in later adult life. This is probably the result of an accumulation of events required for a multi-step causation of neoplasia. The incidence of the most common neoplasms is shown in *Fig. 6.24*.

Epidemiological studies are important in the search for etiological factors in the development of a wide range of neoplastic diseases. The observation of 'clustering' of cases of a certain type of cancer in a particular geographical location may provide a pointer to an environmental etiological factor.

Key Facts
Cancer epidemiology

- Cancer is the second most common cause of death (after ischemic heart disease) in most developed countries, accounting for about 23% of all mortality.
- The incidence of the different histological types of cancer varies greatly between populations, and is attributable to occupational, social and geographic factors.
- The incidence of lung cancer is increasing rapidly in women as a result of cigarette smoking. It now exceeds breast cancer as the leading cause of cancer death (as opposed to incidence).
- The incidence of malignant melanoma of the skin is increasing among Caucasians in many countries. This is the result of exposure to UV radiation because of the fashion for suntanning.

- There is a high incidence of stomach cancer in Japan compared to other countries, which has been attributed to dietary factors (particularly smoked, raw fish).
- The survival rate for many tumors has been greatly increased over the past two decades as a result of advances in, and the greater availability of, treatment.
- Cancer prevention strategies depend for the most part on the elimination of causative factors, largely identified through epidemiology.
- Cancer detection strategies depend on screening populations for early forms of neoplasia at an early stage of development, e.g. cervical carcinoma and breast carcinoma.

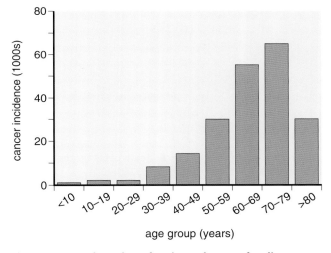

Fig. 6.23 Annual number of registered cases of malignant neoplasia, by age group, in the UK. The number of reported cases of malignancy increases markedly after the age of 50. The reduction in cases after the age of 79 is because there are few individuals alive and at risk in this age range. In addition, case ascertainment is probably less robust in this age group.

Heritable neoplastic conditions have revealed genetic abnormalities important in neoplasia

Several neoplastic conditions are heritable, and genetic analysis has led to the identification of several of the molecular genetic abnormalities underlying neoplasia discussed earlier. The most important heritable neoplastic syndromes are given in *Fig. 6.25*.

Detailed studies of family groups in which there has been a high incidence of either a single type of cancer or a particular group of cancers has led to the understanding that certain families have a genetic predisposition to develop cancers of a particular type. Often, in these 'familial tendency' cancers, the tumors that occur tend to be atypical in some way. Most commonly, the tumors present at an earlier age than is usual for that specific tumor, and may be of an unusual histological type.

The best-known example is in colorectal carcinoma. The role of the autosomal dominant disorder, familial polyposis coli, in the development of colorectal carcinoma has long been known, but recent studies in families with a high incidence of colorectal carcinoma have pointed to another, much larger, group in which a gene disorder predisposes to the development of colorectal carcinoma. The tumors typically occur a decade or two before the usual age for the development of colorectal carcinoma. This is dealt with in more detail in Chapter 13, pages 262–5.

A similar genetic basis for malignant tumor has been found in families with a high incidence of adenocarcinoma of the breast (see Chapter 20, pages 445).

The importance of these findings is twofold. First, it enables the gene defect specific to the affected family members to be identified, with the eventual potential for more widespread screening tests applied to the population as a whole, but particularly in the members of the affected family. Second, it allows early screening of family members with the gene defect before the tumor has developed; for example, in the colorectal cancer group, regular colonoscopies are performed to detect and treat the developing tumors at an early stage when there is every chance of successful surgical treatment.

Estimated 10 leading sites of cancer leading to death, grouped by sex, as a percentage of all cancer death (United States 2002)*

Prostate	30
Lung and bronchus	14
Colon and rectum	11
Urinary bladder	7
Melanoma of the skin	5
Non-Hodgkin's lymphoma	4
Kidney and renal pelvis	3
Oral cavity	3
Leukemia	3
Pancreas	2
All other sites	19

31	Breast
12	Lung and bronchus
12	Colon and rectum
6	Uterine corpus
4	Non-Hodgkin's lymphoma
4	Melanoma of skin
4	Ovary
2	Pancreas
2	Thyroid
2	Urinary bladder
20	All other sites

Estimated 10 leading sites of new cancer cases grouped by sex, as a percentage of all new cancer cases (United States 2002)*

Lung and bronchus	31
Prostate	11
Colon and rectum	10
Pancreas	5
Non-Hodgkin's lymphoma	5
Leukemia	4
Esophagus	3
Liver and intrahepatic bile duct	3
Urinary bladder	3
Kidney	3
All other sites	22

25	Lung and bronchus
15	Breast
11	Colon and rectum
6	Pancreas
5	Ovary
4	Non-Hodgkin's lymphoma
4	Leukemia
2	Uterus
2	Brain and other nervous system
2	Multiple myeloma
23	All other sites

Fig. 6.24 (a) Estimated new cancer cases for the 10 leading sites by sex, USA, 2002. (b) Estimated cancer death cases for the 10 leading sites by sex, USA, 2002. Data derived from Jemal A, et al. Cancer Statistics, 2002. CA Cancer J Clin 2002; 52:23.

Fig. 6.25 Characterized heritable neoplasia syndromes

Syndrome	Tumor caused	Defect
MEN syndromes	Multiple tumors in endocrine organs	Mutations on chromosomes 10 and 11
Polyposis coli	Adenomata and carcinomas of the colon	Absent tumor suppressor gene *APC*
Li–Fraumeni	Breast cancer and sarcomas	Mutated tumor suppressor gene *TP53*
Xeroderma pigmentosum	Skin cancer	Abnormal DNA repair
Familial retinoblastoma	Malignant tumor of the retina	Absent tumor suppressor gene *Rb*
Neurofibromatosis type 1	Benign and malignant tumors of peripheral nerves	Abnormal tumor suppressor gene *NFI*

DIAGNOSIS OF NEOPLASIA

The diagnosis of neoplasia is based on clinical investigation, imaging, and laboratory testing, which will ultimately involve histological examination of suspect tissue. It is now common for oncology services to work as a team, the pathological diagnosis being made only after detailed consultation over clinical features and imaging. Precision in diagnosis is particularly important, as chemotherapy regimens are now closely matched to specific tumor types.

There are several techniques for obtaining tissue from a suspected neoplastic lesion.

Biopsy of tissues can be performed by several techniques (*Fig. 6.26*), and material processed for histology. Samples can also be assessed by electron microscopy.

Cytology can be performed on many types of tissue sample to look for neoplastic cells (*Fig. 6.27*). Increasingly, diagnoses of deep-seated solid tumors are being made by aspiration of cells, using a fine needle placed in the tumor under radiological control.

Cytological sampling of cells from some epithelial surfaces can be done without radiological control, and in some cases can be carried out in family practices without hospital admission. For example, cells from the surfaces of the cervix can be obtained easily by family practitioners, smeared onto microscopic slides, placed in fixative, and transported to a local laboratory for staining and microscopic examination.

This technique not only identifies established malignant change in the epithelia, it also detects early dysplastic abnormalities in the epithelial cells that might indicate a premalignant change, so that full investigation can be performed and the abnormal area treated or removed before full malignant change supervenes (see page 420).

Fig. 6.27 Methods of obtaining cells for cytological examination

Cells shed naturally into body fluids

Sputum, urine, CSF, fluid in pleural or peritoneal cavities

Cells obtained by exfoliation

Scrape smear of cervix
Brush cytology of lesions in gastrointestinal tract by endoscopy

Cells aspirated by needle

Blood and bone marrow
Needle aspiration of solid tumors (breast, thyroid, pancreas)

Tumor markers

Certain tumors liberate products that can be detected in blood, thereby acting as tumor markers. These may aid diagnosis, but may also be used to follow up therapy when blood levels become increased, often before imaging can detect tumor recurrence (*Fig. 6.28*).

Fig. 6.28 Examples of tumor markers

Tumor marker	Tumor
α-Fetoprotein (AFP)	Hepatocellular carcinoma Germ cell tumors
Human chorionic gonadotropin (hCG)	Trophoblastic tumors
Acid phosphatase	Prostatic carcinoma
Carcinoembryonic antigen (CEA)	Gastrointestinal tract neoplasia
Hormone products	Endocrine tumors

Fig. 6.26 Techniques for obtaining tissue samples by biopsy

Needle biopsy

Uses cutting needle to sample tumor
Sample is a core of tissue 1–2 mm wide and 2 cm long
Small size can make histological interpretation difficult
Can be applied to any lesion, including those in brain

Endoscopic biopsy

Uses small forceps to sample lesions seen at endoscopy
Samples are fragments 2–3 mm in size
Small size can make histological interpretation difficult
Applied to lesions in GI, respiratory, genital and urinary tracts

Incision biopsy

Scalpel used to remove sample of lesion
Sample is variable in size depending on nature of lesion
Applied to surgically accessible lesions only

Excision biopsy

Whole abnormal lesion surgically removed
Sample is variable in size depending on nature of lesion
Applied to surgically accessible lesions only

Advances in molecular pathology have allowed the development of novel anticancer drugs

Recently, several new drugs have been developed that inhibit specific proteins involved in cell cycle entry and progression or target specific secondary messenger pathways in tumor cells. A few of these are listed below to illustrate how molecular pathology can be used to detect the specific target by screening patients prior to treatment.

Cancer	Drug (screening target)	Mechanism of action
Breast cancer	Herceptin (trastuzumab) (HER-2)	Herceptin is a monoclonal antibody that binds to HER2, a member of the EGF-receptor family of proteins. Binding of Herceptin reduces the activation of the HER2-linked tyrosine kinase and induces activation of the cell cycle inhibitors p21 and p27.
Gastrointestinal stromal tumors (GIST)	Glivec (imatinib) (c-kit mutation)	Glivec is an inhibitor of the receptor tyrosine kinases for PDGF and stem cell factor (SCF), c-kit and inhibits PDGF- and SCF-mediated cellular events. In vitro, imatinib inhibits proliferation and induces apoptosis in GIST cells, which express an activating c-kit mutation.
Glioblastomas	Temodal (temozolamide) (MGMT Activity)	O6-methylguanine-DNA methyltransferase (MGMT) confers resistance to therapeutic methylating and chloroethylating agents in human brain tumours. Therefore, assay for MGMT activity can predict the response of tumours to agents such as temozolamide.
Pediatric gliomas	Rapamycin (cyclin D, caspase 3, Bcl-2)	Rapamycin blocks mTOR (mammalian target of rapamycin) functions in a variety of malignancies. Molecular characterization of upstream and downstream mTOR signaling pathways is thought to allow a better selection of rapamycin-sensitive tumors.

Survival rates vary greatly between the different types of tumor

The length of survival following a diagnosis of neoplasia varies according to the biological nature of the tumor, how far it has spread, and whether any effective therapy can be given. One of the most useful facts to remember for each of the tumor types is the average 5-year survival rate, as this allows the disease to be put into perspective during discussion with a patient. *Fig. 6.29* shows the current 5-year survival for a range of common tumors.

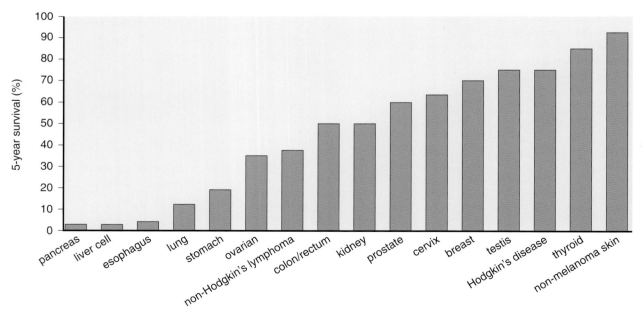

Fig. 6.29 Average 5-year survival rates for common neoplasms. The chances of surviving for 5 years after diagnosis vary greatly according to the type of neoplasm.

Basic immunopathology

IMMUNOLOGICAL FACTORS IN DISEASE

Designed to combat the effects of invasion by adverse environmental factors such as microorganisms and toxic chemical agents, the immune response is a normal defense mechanism. It usually works effectively, but illness may result from:

- Inadequate immune response.
- Excessive immune response.
- Unwanted or inappropriate immune response.

It is not our intention to present the various components and mechanisms of immune responses in disease, as these are covered in standard immunology texts, but rather to give a succinct outline of clinically relevant immunopathology.

INADEQUATE IMMUNE RESPONSES

Inadequate immune responses can result from immunodeficiency states. There are two classes of immunodeficiency syndrome:

- Primary immunodeficiency, which is present at birth and often the result of a genetic disorder (*Fig. 7.1*).
- Secondary immunodeficiency, which is acquired secondary to drug treatment or disease process (*Fig. 7.2*).

X-linked agammaglobulinemia (Bruton's) is associated with few or absent B cells and low levels of IgG

This occurs in male infants and is a panhypoglobulinemia. The levels of IgG are greatly reduced and other immunoglobulin levels are very low or absent. Although B lymphocytes are greatly reduced or almost absent, cellular immunity is intact, as T cells are not involved. The infant presents with recurrent pyogenic infections which characteristically begin sometime after about 6 months of age, when all the maternal transplacental antibodies have disappeared. Common sites for infection are the lungs and bones and the most common infecting bacteria are streptococci, pneu-

mococci and *Haemophilus influenzi*. Maturation of B cells is halted at the pre-B cell stage, and no mature B cells or plasma cells can be formed, so there is almost complete lack of humoral immunity. The defect is in mutations of a gene on the X chromosome (called the BTK gene – for Bruton's or B-cell tyrosine kinase), the tyrosine kinase being essential for transducing signals to the pre-B cell receptors to stimulate further maturation. Over 300 mutations in BTK have been found. In patients with this disorder about 50% have a family history, the other 50% representing new mutations.

Isolated IgA deficiency is a very common primary immunodeficiency but is usually asymptomatic

In this condition there is a marked reduction in the level of serum IgA, but other immunoglobulins are normal. Lymphocytes responsible for producing IgA fail to mature into secreting IgA plasma cells. In most cases this isolated IgA deficiency is detected by accident, but some patients have an increased tendency to respiratory and other infections. Occasionally the isolated IgA deficiency is associated

Fig. 7.1 Primary immunodeficiency states

Abnormal component of immune system	Example
Antibodies	X-linked hypogammaglobulinemia (Bruton's disease: X-linked recessive) Isolated IgA deficiency
T cells	Thymic aplasia (DiGeorge syndrome)
B and T cells	Severe combined immunodeficiency • Swiss type (autosomal recessive) • Adenosine deaminase deficiency (autosomal recessive) • X-linked recessive
Phagocytes	Chronic granulomatous disease
Complement	C2, C4 deficiency

with a partial deficiency of other immunoglobulins, particularly IgG, and these patients have a greater incidence of recurrent infections.

Common variable immunodeficiency is a bit of a mixed bag

Patients with this disorder are predisposed to the development of recurrent infections. It occurs equally in men and women, and the onset of the recurrent infections usually begins in the second or third decade of life. Patients are found to have markedly low immunoglobulin and antibody levels. It can be distinguished from X-linked Bruton's agammaglobulinemia by the fact that normal numbers of B-cells are present, although their function appears disordered, in some cases associated with impaired T-cell signaling. Sometimes there is an excess of T-suppressor cell activity or inadequate T-helper cell activity. Some cases are associated with intrinsic failure of pre-B cells to mature. Patients with this condition have a high associated incidence of the common autoimmune disorders, including Hashimoto's disease and rheumatoid arthritis.

The most important failure of T-cells is DiGeorge syndrome

In these infants there is partial or complete failure of T cells to form, associated with hypoplasia of the thymus gland. This failure is the result of failure of development of the third and fourth pharyngeal pouches, and therefore the parathyroid glands are also absent. Affected infants have a characteristic facial appearance, with midline facial clefts, mainly cleft palate, a small receding mandible and low-set ears. There is a high incidence of congenital cardiac malformations and the absence of the parathyroid glands leads to hypocalcemia.

Onset of recurrent infections begins soon after birth and the infant is particularly vulnerable to infections by viruses and intracellular bacteria. If a child has some thymic remnant and survives the early years, then T cells may increase in number and the efficiency of cell-mediated immunity may be almost normal by the age of 5 years. The prognosis is often associated more with the severity of the cardiac defect than with the immunological defect. The underlying genetic abnormality is deletion of part of chromosome 22; less than 10% of patients have an inherited deletion, and so in more than 90% of cases the disease is due to a new deletion.

The most common combined primary immunodeficiency of B- and T-cell function is called 'severe combined immune deficiency'

This condition may be inherited in either an autosomal recessive (Swiss type) or an X-linked recessive pattern. Some of the autosomal recessive types are associated with adenosine diaminase deficiency. In the X-linked type there is a mutation in the interleukin-2 receptor-γ gene (IL2RG). In the autosomal recessive pattern associated with adenosine deaminase deficiency the gene defect is on chromosome 20; it is thought that the enzyme deficiency leads to accumulation of substrate in cells, and the substrate is particularly toxic to immature lymphoid cells of the developing immune system.

The condition is due to a failure of the development of both B- and T-cell precursors from the primitive stem cell. As a result of B- and T-cell failure the thymus is small or absent, and lymphoid tissue in lymph nodes and the gut is also greatly reduced.

Children present early in life with recurrent infections, including candidal thrush, pneumonia and diarrhea. There is a very low blood lymphocyte count and low blood immunoglobulin levels. Without treatment (usually bone marrow transplantation), death occurs within the first 2 or 3 years of life. One of the most common fatal infections is *Pneumocystis pneumonia*, see pages 101 and 124).

Ataxia–telangiectasia and the Wiskott–Aldrich syndrome are very rare forms of combined immunodeficiency

Ataxia–telangiectasia is inherited as an autosomal recessive disorder and the syndrome comprises a predisposition to infection associated with low IgE and IgA levels and depressed cell-mediated immunity, cerebellar degeneration and atrophy of the spinocerebellar tracts, and peculiar areas of telangiectatic blood vessels in the conjunctiva and on the flexor aspects of the forearm. The commonest site for recurrent infections is the upper respiratory tract, including the nasal sinuses, and severe bronchiectasis is a long-term complication. The neurological manifestations become apparent when the child begins to walk, and progressive mental retardation may occur. There may also be associated endocrine abnormalities, including gonadal dysgenesis.

The responsible gene (ATM gene) is located on chromosome 11. The cells are oversensitive to X-rays, leading to frequent chromosome and chromatid breaks; chromosomes 7 and 11 are especially vulnerable, particularly at sites which are known to be related to T-cell receptor function, coding for immunoglobulin heavy chains and for hematological malignancies. This may explain the immune defects and the high incidence of malignancy, particularly lymphomas, leukemias and brain tumors.

Wiskott–Aldrich syndrome presents clinically with eczema, recurrent infections and a low platelet count, and is an X-linked recessive disease affecting male infants. The earliest manifestations are usually due to the low platelet count and include hemorrhagic episodes, often from the alimentary tract. Recurrent respiratory infections develop later, and children who survive to the age of 8 or more have a very high incidence of malignant lymphoma and acute lymphoblastic leukemia. Immunologically there is a low IgM level, but the IgA and IgE levels are usually raised. Hematologically these children have small platelets, and at least part of the reduction in number is due to increased destruction of circulating platelets by the spleen. Splenectomy may lead to a rise in platelet numbers. Bone marrow transplantation is the treatment of choice.

The responsible gene is called Wiskott–Aldrich syndrome protein (**WASp**) and is located on the X chromosome. Its expression seems largely confined to hemopoietic and lymphoid cells, and appears to be related to the movement of actin filaments in the cytoskeleton of these cells, particularly B and T cells, dendritic cells, neutrophils and platelets.

The most important primary abnormality of phagocytic cells is called 'chronic granulomatous disease'

This disease mainly occurs in boys and is due to an X-linked recessive inheritance pattern; a small proportion of cases show an autosomal recessive pattern. Blood and marrow neutrophils are deficient in the nicotinamide adenine dinucleotide phosphate (NADPH) oxidase system and are unable to produce hydrogen peroxide and superoxide, which destroys their bactericidal killing ability, leading to foci of persisting infection, particularly in the skin, bones, lung and lymph nodes. The infecting bacteria are often unusual organisms which are not usually severely pathogenic. The neutrophils are able to respond to infection by migrating to the site and are able to phagocytose the bacteria. However, once phagocytosed, the neutrophils are unable to kill the bacteria. As a result there is often a secondary macrophagic response in the area of infection, producing histiocytic granulomas.

Secondary immunodeficiency is much more common than primary immunodeficiency

In general the immune system does not work well in early infancy and old age, although infants are partly protected by the presence of maternal antibodies that have crossed the placenta. On a worldwide scale severe malnutrition is an important cause of an impaired immune response. An increasingly common and important cause of secondary immunodeficiency is drug therapy, either corticosteroid therapy for a wide range of diseases, or the specific immunosuppressive therapy given in transplantation to prevent

---

Fig. 7.2 Main causes of secondary immunodeficiency

Old age
Chronic malnutrition
Widespread malignancy
Metabolic diseases (diabetes, chronic liver failure, chronic renal failure)
Drug therapy (cytotoxic therapy, steroid therapy)
Splenectomy (pneumococcal septicemia)
AIDS (acquired immunodeficiency syndrome)

---

rejection and as part of a cytotoxic chemotherapy regimen for the treatment of malignant disease.

HIV-AIDS is an important cause of secondary immunodeficiency

HIV-AIDS (acquired immune deficiency syndrome) caused by human immunodeficiency virus (HIV) leads to severe impairment of the cell-mediated immunity system. It affects 40 million people in the world, with an estimated 5 million new cases and 3 million deaths worldwide in 2004. In brief, HIV infection leads to destruction of CD4 lymphocytes and a decreased helper/suppressor T-cell ratio in the blood. The virus gains entry to T cells by attaching to surface CD4 molecules via chemokine receptors and causes cell death. The virus has several key protein components that can be used in diagnosis.

An immune response to virally infected cells develops, with both humoral and cell-mediated components. This initially contains the infection but, importantly, does not eliminate it. After several years, this immune response fails to control infection due to antigenic variation in virus proteins. (The median time from infection with HIV to development of clinical AIDS in transfusion cases is 4.5 years. For other groups the timescale is less certain.) As the virus proliferates, there is depletion of CD4 cells, leading to severe immunosuppression.

Most disease is caused by RNA retrovirus HIV-1, but HIV-2 also causes AIDS and is most common in West Africa. Transmission is by sexual contact, blood transfusion, intravenous drug abuse, and vertically from mother to child.

There are four clinical phases of HIV infection

1. Primary infection. The HIV virus has a strong affinity for CCR5+ CD4+ effector memory T lymphocytes, macrophages and dendritic cells of the immune system, and attaches to these cells in mucosal surfaces (e.g. in sexual transmission) and blood (in intravenous and transplacental transmission). Viruses gain entry into cells via chemokine receptors and viral replication takes place. A general viremia develops, with viral nucleic acid and the HIV p24 antigen detectable in blood, peaking at about 6 weeks. There is an acute, massive loss of CCR5+ CD4+ T cells from mucosal sites. At this time, antibodies to HIV start to be detected in ▶

► the blood (seroconversion). About 50% of patients develop an influenza-like illness, rashes or lymphadenopathy at this time, associated with a transient fall in CD4 lymphocytes (seroconversion illness). Antibody tests for HIV become positive around 6 weeks after infection.

2. **Asymptomatic phase (CDC* category A disease).** Individuals have antibodies to HIV in blood, but are otherwise asymptomatic. They are infective and can transmit the disease. The duration of this phase is variable but is typically 5–8 years. About 5% of patients remain asymptomatic for several decades. There is a polyclonal hypergammaglobulinemia, and CD8 cells directed against viral antigens are increased in number in blood; numbers of CD4 cells remain within the normal range.

Symptoms relating to loss of immune regulation may become evident, such as worsening of existing psoriasis, folliculitis or eczema, or the development of immune thrombocytopenia.

3. **AIDS-related complex (CDC category B disease).** In this phase of HIV infection the proportion of CD4 infected cells increases and numbers in blood fall to around 350/μL. Patients develop general malaise, fever lasting longer than 3 months, night sweats, weight loss and diarrhea. Generalized lymphadenopathy is common (persistent generalized lymphadenopathy), with evidence of impaired cell-mediated immunity and reduced T-cell numbers.

Superficial fungal infections are frequent and infections with pathogens such as *Salmonella* and *Haemophilus* are severe. The incidence of cervical intraepithelial neoplasia (see page 419) is increased because of greater susceptibility to genital human papilloma virus infection.

4. **AIDS (CDC category C disease).** As CD4 counts fall below 200/μL there is fully developed immunodeficiency, with complications of opportunistic infection, the development of HIV infection of the central nervous system and the development of neoplastic disease. In addition, infections with non-opportunistic organisms occur more frequently and with greater clinical severity. CD8-positive cells reacting against HIV become virtually undetectable in blood. The type of opportunistic infections that develop can be related to the degree of loss of CD4 cells, as summarized in *Fig. 7.3*.

The development of neoplastic disease is a common feature of late HIV infection.

- Kaposi's sarcoma caused by human herpes virus-8 typically occurs in the skin (see page 528).
- High-grade lymphomas are common, including primary lymphomas of the nervous system (see page 484).
- Invasive carcinomas of the cervix may develop as a result of human papillomavirus infection (see page 418).

Since the introduction of highly active antiretroviral therapy (HAART), there has been an 80% reduction in mortality in treated populations.

Lipodystrophy develops in about 25% of patients, with typical thinning of the face due to loss of subcutaneous fat (lipoatrophy). The cause is believed to be multifactorial, including effects from drug therapy.

*CDC = Center for Disease Control (USA)

Fig. 7.3 Opportunistic infections in AIDS

CD4⁺ cells in blood (normal lower limit 450–500/μL)	Increased risk for opportunistic infection
Fewer than 350 cells/μL	Tuberculosis and syphilis may become reactivated. Herpes zoster. Oral candidiasis
Fewer than 200 cells/μL	*Pneumocystis jirovecii* pneumonia Systemic fungal infections including cryptococcal meningitis and histoplasmosis Parasitic infestations of the gut such as *Cryptosporidium*
Fewer than 100 cells/μL	Cerebral toxoplasmosis Progressive multifocal leukoencephalopathy due to papovavirus infection of CNS Cytomegalovirus infection of retina, CNS or gut. *Mycobacterium avium intracellulare* infections

Children with AIDS show clinical differences from adults

Children with vertical transmission of HIV show certain clinical differences from adult cases. About 25% of affected children die in the first year of life, with rapid development of immunosuppression, usually from *Pneumocystis* pneumonia. The 75% with a longer course of disease develop severe bacterial infections, with both routine pathogens and a range of opportunistic infections similar to those seen in adults.

Lymphocytic interstitial pneumonia occurs in 50% of affected children. CNS infection is manifest by developmental delay and progressive motor abnormalities.

EXCESSIVE IMMUNE RESPONSES

Excessive immune responses can cause 'hypersensitivity' reactions

Although immune mechanisms have a protective role in eliminating damaging agents, they may be abnormally amplified so that the response is damaging rather than beneficial. Such an excessive immune response can produce a severe and damaging reaction in a person exposed to a 'routine' antigen, and is termed a **hypersensitivity reaction**.

Hypersensitivity reactions have been divided into four types, I, II, III and IV. It is important to realize that more than one immunological mechanism may be involved in a single disease. Although it is possible to identify a predominant hypersensitivity response underlying an immune-related disease, other aspects of the immune response network are nearly always operating. Examples of diseases caused by hypersensitivity responses are presented in the systems chapters in this book (Chapters 10–25).

Type I hypersensitivity reactions are due to an excessive response of IgE to the presence of an allergen (antigen)

In this type of response (also known as immediate hypersensitivity or anaphylactic sensitivity) an often harmless antigen reacts with specific IgE antibodies located on membrane Fc receptors on mast cells (*Fig. 7.4*). The IgE is initially produced by specific B cells, driven by T-helper cells stimulated by exposure to antigen. This initial exposure also stimulates local recruitment of eosinophils in tissues. On re-exposure, antigen now binds to the specific IgE on mast cells and causes rapid release of preformed chemical mediators from the mast cell (*Fig. 7.5*). These mediators produce marked vasodilatation, smooth muscle spasm, increased permeability of small blood vessels, and excessive secretion in epithelial glandular tissues. Local eosinophil activation and release of mediators also contributes to the response. A group of patients who are particularly prone to develop type I hypersensitivity reactions are those who produce excessive amounts of IgE (**atopic** tendency) and can suffer from a wide range of clinical manifestations. Many of these

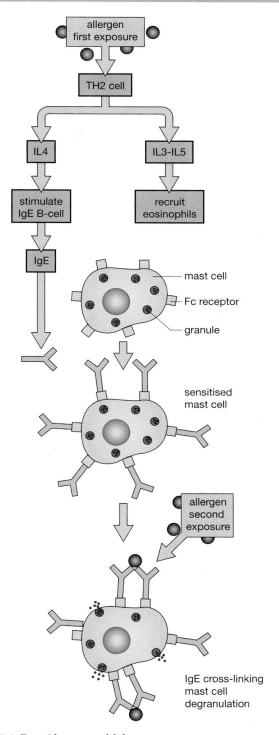

Fig. 7.4 Type I hypersensitivity response.

conditions are discussed elsewhere in this book. The commonest and most important are:

- Atopic dermatitis (acute eczema).
- Allergic rhinitis (hay fever), often associated with:
  - Atopic conjunctivitis.
  - Extrinsic allergic asthma.
  - Food allergies.

Fig. 7.5 Mediators released from mast cells in type I hypersensitivity

Mediator	Effects
From mast cell granules	
Histamine	Increased vessel permeability, smooth muscle spasm, increased secretion by epithelial glands
Enzymes – proteases (e.g. tryptase) and acid hydrolases	Direct tissue damage, production of kinins, activation of complement
From arachidonic acid pathway	
Leukotrienes C4, D4 and E4	Increased vascular permeability, smooth muscle spasm, particularly bronchial
Leukotriene B_4	Attractant for neutrophils and eosinophils
Prostaglandin D_2	Smooth muscle spasm, particularly bronchial

Anaphylaxis is a severe manifestation of type I hypersensitivity

Anaphylaxis is an acute IgE-mediated systemic reaction occurring in a person who is exposed to an antigen to which they have previously been sensitized. Important causative antigens include insect stings, drugs (particularly antibiotics), transfused blood products, and some food items, for example peanuts. The onset of symptoms is rapid, with palpitations, tingling sensations, itching of the skin and difficulty breathing. They develop urticaria in the skin and larynx, and often develop bronchospasm. If untreated they may develop shock, with cardiovascular collapse leading to death.

Type II hypersensitivity reactions result from circulating antibodies binding to cellular antigens

In this response, preformed circulating antibody binds to some antigen as part of a tissue component, and this is followed by damage or death to the cells bearing the antigenic epitope. The antibody-coated cells may be killed either as a result of lysis of the cell membrane following activation of the complement system, or by killer cells directed against the antibody-coated cell. The target cells may be phagocytosed by macrophages. Important clinical examples include:

• Immune hemolytic anemia. Common and important examples include hemolytic disease of the newborn, autoimmune hemolytic anemia and incompatible blood transfusion.
• Antibody-induced thrombocytopenic purpura and neutropenia.
• Pemphigus and pemphigoid. In pemphigus there is an antibody to an antigen in the intracellular cement of the keratinocytes in the epidermis, mainly in the prickle

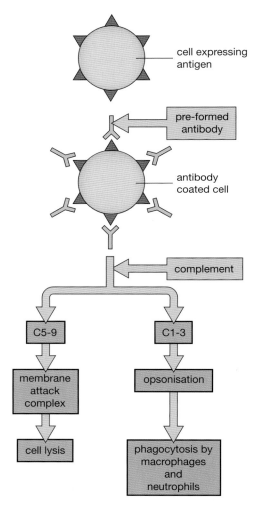

Fig. 7.6 Type II hypersensitivity response.

cell layer. In pemphigoid the antibody is to an antigen situated in the epidermodermal basement membrane (see pages 227 and 516).

- Goodpasture's syndrome. This is due to a reaction between an antibody and the basement membrane of glomerular capillaries in the kidney and the alveolar capillaries in the lung (pages 209, 305, 365 and 375).
- Hyperacute graft rejection of a renal transplant (see page 385).

Type III hypersensitivity reactions are due to the deposition of soluble circulating antigen–antibody complexes in vessel walls or other tissues

After deposition the immune complexes cause damage by complement activation (*Fig. 7.7*). Complexes may also bind to mast cells and cause mast cell degranulation. The attraction of neutrophils to the site releases lysosomal enzymes that further mediate tissue damage. Cell death may be augmented by the formation of occlusive platelet aggregates within the lumina of very small blood vessels, leading to ischemia. Type III hypersensitivity reactions often show a vasculitis in affected tissues involving fibrinoid necrosis of small blood vessel walls. This type of response is characteristic of so-called serum sickness, is seen in certain forms of glomerulonephritis (see page 375), and is also seen in the autoimmune disease systemic lupus erythematosus (SLE). The main tissues involved are the renal glomerulus, skin, and joints.

Type IV hypersensitivity reactions do not involve antibodies but are cell mediated and caused by sensitized T lymphocytes

In type IV reactions, antigen-presenting cells lead to Th1 lymphocyte expansion and secretion of proinflammatory cytokines (*Fig. 7.8*). Cytokine release influences the activity of neutrophils, macrophages and cytotoxic lymphocytes. Some type IV reactions are characterized by the presence of large numbers of lymphocytes and macrophages, sometimes with macrophage accumulation to produce **granulomas**. There are three main patterns of type IV hypersensitivity:

- Reactions stimulated by microorganisms, particularly certain bacteria (tuberculosis and leprosy), some fungi (histoplasmosis, chronic candidiasis) and some viruses (see pages 109 and 117).
- Contact dermatitis due to a reaction between sensitized T lymphocytes and a complex antigen produced by a foreign substance and a carrier protein in the skin, such as in contact hypersensitivity to nickel or poison ivy.
- Rejection of tissue or organ grafts, discussed further on page 106.

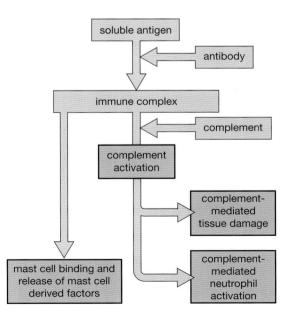

Fig. 7.7 Type III hypersensitivity response.

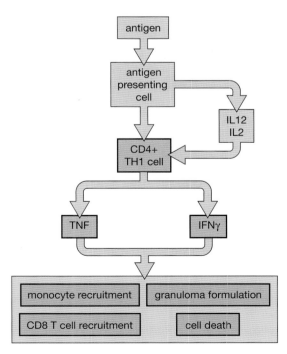

Fig. 7.8 Type IV hypersensitivity response.

INAPPROPRIATE IMMUNE RESPONSES

The most important inappropriate immune responses produce autoimmune diseases

Autoimmune diseases are the result of the body producing an immune response against its own tissues or individual tissue components. Sometimes the immune response is an antibody response (autoantibodies), sometimes it is cell-mediated. In many instances cell damage is by a cell-mediated cytotoxic response, and abnormal antibodies are generated to internal cell constituents, which are not, in themselves, damaging to cells. Such autoantibodies are useful in diagnosis and typing of certain immune-mediated diseases.

In autoimmune diseases it is recognized that the normal mechanisms that ensuring tolerance for self-antigens have broken down. It is known that some autoimmune diseases have a genetic component, e.g. certain diseases are associated with particular HLA histocompatibility types. In other situations an autoimmune disease can be triggered by a microbial infection, although the mechanisms underlying this are uncertain.

Autoimmune diseases may either be organ specific or affect many tissues

In some cases an autoimmune response is directed against a single component of a single tissue (**organ-specific auto-immune disease**), but more often it is against a tissue component present in many tissues and organs throughout the body (**non-organ-specific autoimmune disease**).

The most important **non-organ-specific autoimmune diseases** are summarized in *Fig. 7.9*, and each is discussed in greater detail in other chapters. Many of these diseases are autoimmune rheumatic diseases. These are extremely common and together account for a large health burden.

In these conditions, multiorgan involvement is frequently caused by secondary damage due to circulating immune complexes. For example, in SLE there are autoantibodies against components of cell nuclei, particularly double-stranded DNA, which are not, in themselves, damaging to cells. Immune complexes form and are deposited in blood vessels, glomerular capillaries, skin, joints, skeletal muscle and brain, leading to tissue damage. This group of disorders is often collectively called the 'connective tissue diseases,' as they have a major impact on blood vessels and support tissues throughout the body.

The organ-specific autoimmune diseases are listed in *Fig. 7.10*, each being discussed in more detail in the relevant later chapters. There is a tendency for several organs to be involved in affected individuals, suggesting that there is a general autoimmune predisposition for this group of diseases.

Autoantibodies directed against the diseased tissue are often found in the blood (*Fig 7.11*). In many cases it is uncertain whether the antibodies are pathogenic. It is known that healthy individuals produce small amounts of antibody against certain tissue components, but no harm ensues. For example, many people may have small titers of antibodies against nuclear DNA, but this is not associated with tissue damage. High titers of autoantibodies are nearly always associated with disease.

The systemic vasculitides are examples of autoimmune diseases

A series of inflammatory diseases of blood vessels are grouped together as the systemic vasculitides. These can be classified according to the size of vessel involved into small, medium and large vessel vasculitis. In this group of conditions immune-mediated inflammatory responses are responsible for damage to blood vessels. Specific autoantibodies are found in some of these conditions. The pathology and

Fig. 7.9 Non-organ-specific autoimmune disease

Disease	Main organs involved	Page reference
Systemic lupus erythematosus	Skin, kidney, joints, heart, lung	see page 561
Progressive systemic sclerosis and variants	Skin, gut, lung	see page 564
Polymyositis and dermatomyositis	Skeletal muscle, skin	see page 490
Rheumatoid disease	Joints, lungs, systemic vessels	see page 566

classification of this group of autoimmune diseases is presented on page 167.

Autoinflammatory diseases are related to inappropriate response to cytokines

Many of the responses of the immune system are mediated through cytokines acting through cytokine receptors. An uncommon group of disorders is now recognized where the response to cytokines is abnormal, usually because of mutation in a gene coding for a cytokine receptor. Although these diseases are very uncommon, they illustrate a general concept of importance in understanding disease pathogenesis.

The main diseases coming into the category of autoinflammatory diseases are the familial periodic fevers such as familial Mediterranean fever and TNF receptor-associated periodic syndrome (TRAPS). Patients show recurrent attacks of inflammation and fever in the absence of an obvious conventional precipitating cause. Molecular investigation has shown that these diseases are related to mutation in genes coding for molecules involved with innate immune cell function. Key cytokine pathways that include TNF, IL-1 and proteins associated with bacterial sensing have all been associated with this class of disease. Several conditions have been linked to mutations in the pyrin and tumor necrosis factor receptor superfamilies. Key inflammatory-regulating pathways become abnormally active, such that cytokine signaling is inappropriately amplified and prolonged, leading to inflammatory-mediated tissue damage.

Therapeutic targets

Initial approaches to therapy for autoimmune diseases involved the administration of corticosteroids or agents that non-specifically suppressed the immune response, with significant side effects. Better understanding of pathogenesis and the ability to manufacture biological modifying drugs as monoclonal antibodies that specifically bind to receptors, has led to a new group of disease-modifying drugs:

Cytokine pathway blockade for autoinflammatory disease

- TRAPS: etanercept.
- Ankylosing spondylitis and psoriatic arthritis: anti-TNF therapies.

Blockade of B and T lymphocytes for autoimmunity

- SLE: mycophenolate mofetil, rituximab.

Blockade of cytokines or adaptive immune responses

- Rheumatoid disease: anti-TNF therapy and rituximab.
- Psoriasis: anti-TNF therapy and efalizumab or alefacept.

Fig. 7.10 Organ-specific autoimmune disease.

Organ	Disease	Associated autoantibody	Comment
Skin	Vitiligo	Antityrosinase antibodies	Hypopigmentation
Thyroid	Graves' disease	Thyroid-stimulating antibodies Thyroid growth-stimulating antibodies	Hyperthyroidism caused by type III stimulatory hypersensitivity response
Thyroid	Hashimoto's disease	Anti-thyroid specific antibodies	Hypothyroidism
Adrenal cortex	Addison's disease	Anti-adrenal antibodies	Hypoadrenocorticalism
Stomach	Autoimmune (type A) gastritis	Anti-intrinsic factor and parietal cell antibodies	Pernicious anemia
Pancreatic islet cells (insulin-producing)	Type I diabetes mellitus	Anti-islet β-cell (insulin) antibody	Diabetes mellitus due to cell-mediated cytotoxicity to pancreatic β cells
Skeletal muscle	Myasthenia gravis	Antibody to acetylcholine receptors	Muscle fatigue due to type III inhibitory hypersensitivity response

Immune responses prevent transplantation of organs from one individual to another

Organ transplantation is increasingly being used to treat irreversible diseases of the kidney, liver, heart, lung, and bone marrow. Unfortunately, the action of the immune system can lead to the transplanted tissue being destroyed, a process termed **transplant rejection**. For the best chance of survival, antigens in the graft and recipient must be alike.

After blood group identity, the most important set of antigens in transplantation immunology are the histocompatibility antigens, human leukocyte associated antigens (**HLA antigens**). The endothelial cells that line the blood vessels of the graft are particularly rich in both HLA antigens and blood group antigens, and so blood vessels are an important target of the host's immune response to a transplanted allograft. The effects of transplant rejection are discussed in relation to the transplanted kidney (see page 385), heart (see page 184) and bone marrow (see page 329).

There are three patterns of rejection seen in transplanted organs

The patterns of rejection seen in post-transplant organs are:

- Hyperacute – due to preformed host antibodies reacting with HLA antigens in the donor organ.
- Acute – associated with necrosis of vessels in the graft (acute vascular rejection) and an infiltration of the graft tissues by CD4-positive T lymphocytes (acute cellular rejection).
- Chronic – slowly progressive destruction of graft structure and function, mainly as a result of vascular occlusion, with an infiltrate of lymphocytes, plasma cells and eosinophils

The most detailed work, and the greatest experience, has been obtained by observation in kidney transplantation (see page 385), but bone marrow, liver, heart and lung transplants are now not uncommon.

Laboratory medicine

Fig. 7.11 Autoantibodies used in the diagnosis of disease

Disease	Autoantibody correlating with disease diagnosis
Hashimoto's disease	Anti-microsomal, anti-thyroglobulin
Graves' disease	Anti-TSH receptor
Diabetes mellitus type I	Anti-islet cell
Pernicious anemia	Anti-parietal cell, anti-intrinsic factor
Chronic active hepatitis	Anti-smooth muscle
Primary biliary cirrhosis	Anti-mitochondrial
Autoimmune thrombocytopenia	Anti-platelet
SLE	Anti-double-stranded DNA
Sjögren's syndrome	Anti-ribonucleoprotein
Scleroderma	Anti-centromeric
Rheumatoid disease	Rheumatoid factor (anti-IgG)

Autoantibodies can be detected in the blood in many diseases (see *Fig. 7.11*). Although it is not always certain that they are responsible for initiating the tissue damage, their detection in high titers provides a useful pointer to the diagnosis of some of these diseases (see *Fig. 7.10*). The autoantibodies listed in the right hand column of *Fig. 7.11* have a high correlation for the diseases indicated. However, it is not uncommon to have several positive autoantibodies and, for some diseases, to have clinical and pathological overlap.

Fig. 7.12 Hashimoto's thyroiditis. Unfixed cryostat section of human thyroid stained with fluorescein labeled serum from a Hashimoto's patient.

Introduction to infectious diseases

This is not a microbiology book

In this chapter we present an overview of the way in which common and important microorganisms and other parasites produce pathological lesions, and hence disease, when they gain access to the human body. No comprehensive details are given of the taxonomy, cultural characteristics and other laboratory identification methods, or of treatment. If you really need these, you must consult a microbiology textbook.

Infection is prevented by both specific and non-specific defense mechanisms

The body has both non-specific and specific defense mechanisms, both of which serve to prevent organisms gaining access to tissues and causing infection.

Non-specific defense mechanisms play an important role in preventing infection, and the main ways in which these are breached are summarized in *Fig. 8.1*.

The acute inflammatory response (see Chapter 4) is able to immobilize and kill many types of infective organism in a non-specific manner. The immune system is able to mount a response against infections by both humoral and cell-mediated mechanisms, different organisms being neutralized by different mechanisms (see Chapter 7).

Fig. 8.1 Barriers to bacterial invasion

Barriers to invasion	Predisposition to infection
Keratin layers of skin	Wounds, insect bites
Glandular secretions and IgA e.g. in gut and lungs	Reduced in isolated IgA deficiency
Secretion currents e.g. in respiratory tract	Reduced by cigarette smoking Reduced in cystic fibrosis (see page 221) Reduced in immotile cilia syndromes (see page 220)
Bacterial commensals e.g. in vagina and gut	Changed by antibiotic therapy

Spread of infection can be by several routes

Once an infective organism has gained entry to the body, it seldom remains localized but spreads to other tissues via several possible routes:

- **Local spread**. This route is facilitated by destruction of local tissues, especially if exotoxins are produced by the organism.
- **Lymphatic spread**. Organisms may be taken in macrophages to lymph nodes, or may gain access to lymphatic fluid. Enlargement of lymph nodes may be due to the generation of an immune response, but may also be as a result of infection by the organism.
- **Hematogenous spread**. Organisms may travel freely in plasma (e.g. many bacteria and hepatitis B virus) or within cells such as monocytes (herpes, cytomegalovirus, HIV, mycobacteria). There are several terms used to describe bloodborne spread of an infecting agent. Viremia and bacteremia are used to describe passive carriage of viruses and bacteria respectively, without growth in the bloodstream. The term 'septicemia' is used when there is severe systemic manifestation of bacteremia, with growth of bacteria in the bloodstream. This commonly leads to toxic shock syndrome (see pages 111 and 417).
- **Spread in tissue fluids**. This takes place in pleural and abdominal cavities, and is an important feature of peritonitis and pleural infections.
- **Neural spread**. The rabies virus and the varicella zoster virus produce infection by traveling along nerves.

In this chapter we outline the common and important infections and infestations

They are divided into:

- **Bacteria** – pages 108–21
- **Fungi** – pages 122–4
- **Viruses** – pages 124–8
- **Prions** – page 128
- **Protozoa** – pages 129–34
- **Flukes (Trematodes)** – pages 134–5
- **Tapeworms (Cestodes)** – pages 135–6
- **Roundworms (Nematodes)** – pages 137–8

BACTERIAL INFECTIONS

Bacterial pathogenicity is due to factors in the organisms as well as the host response

Pathogenicity is the capacity of an organism to cause disease. Pathogenic bacteria can cause damage in several main ways:

- Bacteria can produce **exotoxins** that directly lead to cell and tissue damage.
- Bacteria can liberate **endotoxins** that cause systemic disease (see *Fig. 8.2*).

- Bacteria can produce toxins that functionally impair cells without cell death.
- Bacterial products may directly excite an acute inflammatory reaction.
- Antigens from the bacteria stimulate a type III hypersensitivity reaction by the host.
- Bacterial antigens excite a chronic inflammatory response by stimulating a type IV hypersensitivity reaction.

There is frequently overlap between these factors, and one organism may cause damage via several mechanisms.

Endotoxic shock syndrome

Bacterial endotoxins are derived from the lipopolysaccharide (LPS) component of the outer bacterial cell wall. The most important endotoxins are those produced by Gram-negative organisms such as *Escherichia coli*, *Proteus* and *Pseudomonas aeruginosa*. They produce local effects, but the most important disorders are those associated with a Gram-negative septicemia in which the release of large amounts of endotoxin in the bloodstream produces endotoxic shock syndrome. The consequences are summarized in *Fig. 8.2*.

- Macrophages are stimulated to produce TNF-α.
- Neutrophils become activated and adhere to endothelium.
- The endothelium is activated, and releases nitric oxide, producing vasodilatation.
- Factor XII is activated by LPS and causes secondary activation of the coagulation/fibrinolytic system, kinin system, and complement system.

The major clinical features are profound hypotension, respiratory difficulty, tissue hypoxia, and systemic acidosis. The syndrome may cause death within hours of onset and is complicated by secondary changes in the lungs, termed 'adult respiratory distress syndrome' (ARDS) (see pages 206–7). If the patient survives, renal and liver failure commonly develop. The generalized activation of mediators of inflammation throughout the circulatory system has led to coinage of the term 'systemic inflammatory response syndrome' (SIRS).

Recently, monoclonal antibodies directed against LPS have been used therapeutically to block its effects in septicemic states. Additionally, monoclonal antibodies have been used to neutralize circulating IL-1 and TNF, thereby preventing secondary damaging effects.

Fig. 8.2 Pathogenesis of endotoxic shock syndrome.

Some bacteria have a propensity to produce pus and are termed 'pyogenic'

Some bacteria produce a particularly vigorous acute inflammatory reaction, leading to local tissue necrosis. The reason for this is the presence of chemical factors in the bacterial walls which are chemoattractants for neutrophils. The infected necrotic area is liquefied by the effects of enzymes released by dying neutrophils, and is converted to a homogeneous semi-liquid material composed of dead host tissue, live and dead neutrophils, and live and dead bacteria, all suspended in the fluid component of the exudate.

The combination of necrotic tissue, acute inflammatory exudate and bacteria produces a semi-liquid material known as **pus**. For this reason, causative organisms are termed **pyogenic bacteria**.

Some bacteria produce a chronic granulomatous inflammatory response

Some organisms fail to excite an acute inflammatory response. Instead, the body mounts a type IV hypersensitivity reaction, and the resulting tissue response is in the form of granulomatous inflammation (see pages 53–4), as exemplified by pulmonary TB (see pages 53–4 and 195). The main organisms that excite a granulomatous response to infection are:

- TB, caused by *Mycobacterium tuberculosis.*
- Leprosy, caused by *Mycobacterium leprae.*
- Other mycobacterial infections.
- Syphilis (*Fig. 8.4*) and other spirochetal infections.
- *Yersinia enterocolitica* infection.
- Organism of cat-scratch disease (see page 121).

Syphilis causes chronic inflammation with type IV hypersensitivity

Syphilis is caused by a spirochete, *Treponema pallidum*, which is transmitted mainly by sexual contact. The organisms gain access at the site of inoculation, usually the genitalia, and produce the primary lesion, known as a **chancre**. The organism is then disseminated throughout many organs from the site of inoculation. An immune response develops and the primary infection heals, but thereafter the disease becomes a chronic inflammatory condition, affecting many organs. Serological tests can be performed to detect infection.

Syphilitic infection is traditionally divided into four stages, primary, secondary, latent and tertiary, with a further congenital pattern. The effectiveness of treatment with penicillin and other antibiotics has largely eliminated tertiary syphilis, but the disease in its primary, secondary and latent patterns remains an important sexually transmitted disease worldwide.

1. **Primary syphilis.** A chronic inflammatory nodule (called a **chancre**) forms in the skin or mucosa at the site of entry of the organisms during sexual activity (typically penis, vulva or cervix, less commonly oral or anal mucosa). There is a heavy infiltrate of chronic inflammatory cells, particularly lymphocytes and plasma cells, in the dermis or submucosa at the site of entry, becoming apparent as a raised nodule 1–12 weeks after exposure. The chancre ulcerates, and often then becomes secondarily infected by other bacteria (see *Fig. 8.3*), and there may be painless enlargement of regional lymph nodes. Many spirochetes are present in the chancre, which is highly infectious. Long before the primary chancre has developed, spirochetes have migrated to regional lymph nodes and throughout the body via the bloodstream.

Fig. 8.3 Syphilitic primary chancre. The skin of the penile shaft shows a shallow ulcer that had begun as a raised hard skin nodule, which had quickly ulcerated to form the large lesion seen here. Enlargement is due to secondary infection by other bacteria.

2. **Secondary syphilis.** This stage typically occurs 1–3 months after onset of the infection, resulting from spread of the organism to many sites in the body. The most obvious manifestations are: any of a number of **skin rashes** (most frequently a coppery brown, diffuse, macular rash); mucosal involvement, with the formation of ulceration in the buccal mucosa (**snail-track ulcers**); shallow ulcers in the genital mucosa; and, often, the formation of warty growths around the genitalia (**condylomata lata**). Not only is this secondary stage the most infective, with large numbers of organisms in the ulcerated and warty mucosal lesions, but the organism is also most likely to be transmitted to another person at this point. Generalized enlargement of the lymph nodes may also occur, and organisms are numerous in the lymph nodes. This stage typically lasts 4–12 weeks.

▶

► 3. **Latent syphilis**. This is a stage in which an infected person is asymptomatic but still harbors the infection. There may be recurrence of secondary syphilis during this period.

4. **Tertiary syphilis**. This occurs after a period of latency, typically 3–30 years. It affects about one-third of patients who have untreated syphilis. There are two main histological patterns of disease:

   • Small vessels develop proliferation of their intimal lining, with surrounding plasma cell infiltration (endarteritis obliterans). This leads to tissue damage because of poor blood supply. The main consequence is the development of **thoracic aortic aneurysm**.

   • A type IV cell-mediated immune response causes areas of necrosis to develop in several tissues. These areas, known as '**gummas**' (see *Fig. 8.5*) are surrounded by activated macrophages, fibroblasts, and lymphoid cells, including plasma cells.

The main effects of tertiary syphilis are summarized in *Fig. 8.4*.

Fig. 8.5a&b Gummas in tertiary syphilis. (a) shows a liver containing several confluent areas of white gummatous necrosis, and (b) shows the histology of an active gumma, with a central area of necrosis **N** surrounded by a chronic inflammatory, partly granulomatous, reaction.

5. **Congenital syphilis** follows transmission of spirochetes across the placenta from an infected mother. Multiplication of the organisms in the fetus frequently leads to intrauterine death, and children who survive demonstrate the infantile pattern of congenital disease, namely a persistent nasal discharge ('sniffles'), a desquamative dermatitis (particularly of hands and feet), interstitial fibrosis in the lungs ('pneumonia alba') and liver ('congenital syphilitic hepatitis'; see *Fig. 8.6*), and osteochondritis and periostitis.

Infants who survive into childhood may demonstrate the late effects of the osteochondritis and periostitis, in the form of a collapsed nose bridge ('saddle-nose deformity') and bowing of the tibiae ('saber tibia') due to chronic periostitis. There may also be scarring at the corners of the mouth ('ragades'), notched incisor teeth ('Hutchinson's teeth'), blindness due to interstitial keratitis, and eighth cranial nerve deafness.

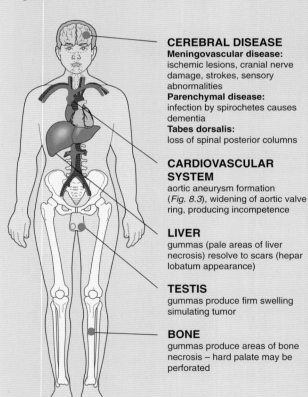

CEREBRAL DISEASE
Meningovascular disease:
ischemic lesions, cranial nerve damage, strokes, sensory abnormalities
Parenchymal disease:
infection by spirochetes causes dementia
Tabes dorsalis:
loss of spinal posterior columns

CARDIOVASCULAR SYSTEM
aortic aneurysm formation (*Fig. 8.3*), widening of aortic valve ring, producing incompetence

LIVER
gummas (pale areas of liver necrosis) resolve to scars (hepar lobatum appearance)

TESTIS
gummas produce firm swelling simulating tumor

BONE
gummas produce areas of bone necrosis – hard palate may be perforated

Fig. 8.4 Systemic involvement in tertiary syphilis. Syphilis has its main effects on blood vessels and the nervous system.

Fig. 8.6 Diffuse congenital syphilitic hepatitis. This infant's liver shows diffuse fine fibrosis and a chronic inflammatory cell infiltrate compressing and destroying the hepatocytes **H.**

BRIEF REVIEW OF COMMON BACTERIA AND THEIR DISEASES

In this section we give a brief summary of the more frequently encountered bacteria and the important diseases they cause. For fuller details of taxonomy, cultural characteristics and laboratory investigations, students should consult a medical microbiology textbook.

Staphylococci are pyogenic (pus-forming) bacteria which can also cause disease by the exotoxins they secrete

These are Gram-positive cocci which normally colonize human skin. There are three common species, *S. aureus*, *S. epidermidis* and *S. saprophyticus*, of which *S. aureus* is most commonly responsible for pyogenic infection and the enterotoxin-associated syndromes.

S. aureus is an important cause of common bacterial skin infections such as superficial folliculitis, boils, and particularly wound infections. It may also cause pneumonia and lung abscess (particularly in children), lactational breast abscess and osteomyelitis (children), all characterized by the production of tissue necrosis and pus-formation. Exotoxins secreted by *S. aureus* can produce a range of disorders, including an acute gastroenteritis (*Fig. 8.7*).

An important group of *S. aureus* spp. are those that have developed resistance to the potent antibiotic methicillin (**methicillin-resistant *Staphyloccus aureus* – MRSA**). This is an important cause of hospital-acquired infections.

S. epidermidis is less pathogenic than *S. aureus* but is a particularly important infecting organism of prostheses, such as prosthetic heart valves, ventriculoperitoneal shunts, and other long-term catheters, including indwelling urinary catheters. *S. saprophyticus* rarely causes post-coital urinary tract infection in women.

Streptococci of medical importance are mainly of the β- and α-hemolytic types

The β-**hemolytic streptococci** can be subdivided into various types by Lancefield grouping. The most important group in human infections is group A, *Streptococcus pyogenes*, which can cause disease either by direct infection, usually with pus formation, particularly in the skin and soft tissues, or by indirect systemic toxic or immunological effects. The major diseases resulting from *Streptococcus pyogenes* are summarized in *Fig. 8.9*, and an example is shown in *Fig. 8.8*.

The only significant group B organism is *Streptococcus agalactiae*, which can cause postpartum infection in both mother and baby. It produces a febrile illness in the mother, and may produce bacteremia, pneumonia or meningitis in the infant. The organism is a commensal in the vagina, and infection may occur during vaginal delivery.

The α-**hemolytic streptococci** are also known as the viridans streptococci, and cause important diseases such as lobar pneumonia, ear infections, and subacute bacterial endocarditis.

Fig. 8.8 Erysipelas of the face. Spreading acute inflammation of the dermis and subcutis due to infection by *Streptococcus pyogenes*.

Fig. 8.7 Important diseases caused by *Staphylococci*		
Toxin	**Disease**	**Clinical features**
Enterotoxins A and D	Acute gastroenteritis	Food poisoning, usually vomiting only, 3–6 h after ingestion Processed meats, dairy products
Toxic shock syndrome toxin	Toxic shock syndrome	Septicemia and toxemia, exfoliating rash on palms and soles *S. aureus*-colonized tampons a cause in women
Epidermolytic toxin ('exfoliatin')	Staphylococcal scalded skin syndrome	Usually infants. Toxin destroys intercellular connections between keratinocytes → blistering → desquamation/exfoliation

Fig. 8.9 Important diseases caused by *Streptococcus pyogenes*

Direct infection

Skin	Impetigo	Pustular infection of epidermis
Skin	Erysipelas	Spreading infection of dermis (see page 111 and Fig. 8.8)
Soft tissues	Cellulitis and necrotizing fasciitis	Severe spreading infection of subcutis and deeper tissues (see page 513)
Upper respiratory tract	Pharyngitis and tonsillitis	Bacterial sore throat
Uterus	Puerperal sepsis	From skin, nose or throat of medical attendants – now rare

Toxin/immunologic infection

Skin	Scarlet fever	Red rash due to erythrogenic toxins
Kidney	Acute glomerulonephritis	Immune reaction of streptococcal pharyngitis (see page 233)
Heart and other organs	Rheumatic fever	Immune reaction to cell wall component of *Streptococcus pyogenes* (see page 187)

The most important α-hemolytic streptococcus is *Streptococcus pneumoniae*

This organism (also called pneumococcus) colonizes the human respiratory tract in up to 5% of the normal population, rising particularly in winter and early spring to 40–50%. Spread is by droplet cross-infection. The most common infections are:

- Acute otitis media, particularly in infants and children (see pages 239, 241–2).
- Pneumonia, particularly of lobar pattern (see page 194).
- Acute purulent meningitis, particularly after otitis media, infection of paranasal sinuses, and pneumonia (see page 465).

In the early stages of acute pneumococcal infection there is frequently a transient bacteremia, and blood culture can be a useful investigation.

Other α-hemolytic streptococci are important causes of bacterial endocarditis

The α-hemolytic group of streptococci includes members such as *S. mutans, S. mitior and S. sanguis* which are important infectors of previously damaged heart valves. Although of low pathogenicity, the organisms can colonize thrombus on aortic and mitral valves which have been distorted and scarred by previous rheumatic heart disease (see page 182). The presence of the bacteria stimulates continuous thrombus formation, and fragments of thrombus break off, entering the circulation; this is the basis of the disease called **subacute bacterial endocarditis** (see page 183). The organisms gain access to the thrombotic material on the valves during a transient bacteremia, often arising when small numbers of bacteria pass into the bloodstream during trauma to a site where the streptococcus is a commensal, most commonly during dental extraction.

Neisseria are Gram-negative cocci which can produce gonorrhea or meningitis, and a particularly virulent form of septicemia

Neisseria gonorrhoeae ('gonococcus') is the bacterium responsible for the sexually transmitted disease gonorrhea, which infects the urethra, prostate, epididymis and testis in men, and the vagina, cervix, uterus and fallopian tubes in women (see pages 417 and 428). It can also produce a gonococcal bacteremia with pustular skin lesions and arthritis. In women the infection may lead to a salpingitis which, if severe, may proceed to pelvic inflammatory disease and infertility.

Neisseria meningitidis ('meningococcus') is carried in the pharynx of 5% of people and is an important cause of acute bacterial meningitis (see page 465), particularly in young children. It tends to occur in minor epidemics, mainly in closed or semi-closed institutions such as schools

Fig. 8.10 Skin rash in meningococcal septicemia. A widespread petechial rash (which does not blanch on pressure) is due to microthrombosis in skin blood vessels. Similar changes occur in all other organs, including the adrenals and brain, leading to sudden death in many cases.

and colleges. Acute meningococcal septicemia (which may occur without evidence of meningitis) is one of the septic shock syndromes. It is clinically characterized by rapid onset, circulatory collapse, multiorgan failure and widespread disseminated intravascular coagulation, with a high fatality rate. A rapidly spreading petechial rash in the skin (see *Fig. 8.10*) and bilateral hemorrhagic necrosis of the adrenals (see page 345) are characteristic.

Corynebacteria are mainly commensal, but one species causes diphtheria

Corynebacteria are widely distributed in nature and are mostly harmless. Diphtheria, however, is caused by certain toxigenic strains of *Corynebacterium diphtheriae*, normally located in the pharynx, nasopharynx or tonsils. Occasionally the primary focus is in the skin, usually an infected abrasion, cut, ulcer or burn. Local production of exotoxin produces necrosis and acute inflammation in adjacent cells and tissues, in the pharynx and tonsil producing the so-called 'diphtheric membrane' composed of necrotic mucosal cells, submucosa, and the associated acute inflammatory exudate.

Systemic distribution of the toxin may produce necrosis of myocardial fibres, cranial and peripheral nerves, and impaired kidney function due to interstitial nephritis. There is also generalized toxemia and prostration.

Diphtheria has been largely eradicated in many areas of the world as a result of childhood vaccination.

Clostridial diseases are mainly due to the effects of potent toxins

Clostridia are anaerobic bacilli which produce long-lived spores, which may be found in the soil and in the gut of humans and animals. There are four main types, each producing a different toxin-mediated disease (*Fig. 8.11*).

The genus *Bacillus* are soil organisms: one type produces food poisoning and the other causes anthrax

Bacillus cereus is an important cause of food poisoning with two different patterns, each due to different bacterial toxins. One toxin produces vomiting 1–4 hours after ingestion, and the other causes diarrhea about 12 hours after ingestion. The toxins are food-borne and are common on rice and other pulses. This form of food poisoning is most common after eating previously cooked rice which has been reheated.

Bacillus anthracis produces potent toxins and causes anthrax, a potentially fatal disease which is now rare. Anthrax is primarily a disease of herbivorous farm and domestic animals, and human disease is acquired by contact with the feces, urine or saliva of affected animals. Most commonly the anthrax spores enter through the skin and produce localized swelling and ulceration, the ulcer being covered by a characteristic black necrotic scab (cutaneous anthrax). In most cases the lesion and infection remain localized to the site of primary penetration, but in a small percentage of cases a severe septicaemia develops, which is usually fatal.

Inhalation of anthrax spores leads to the site of primary penetration being in the lung alveoli (inhalational or pulmonary anthrax), leading to pulmonary edema and hemorrhage, shock, and often death within a few days.

Direct infection from infected animals is now very rare except in the developing world, and occasional cases are still attributed to contact with animal products such as hides, skins, wool, etc. It is known that anthrax spores are very long-lived.

Fig. 8.11 Diseases due to clostridial toxins

Bacterium	Disease	Clinical data
Clostridium difficile	Pseudomembranous colitis	See page 257. Now an important hospital-acquired infection.
Clostridium perfringens	Gas gangrene	Infection of dirty (e.g. soil-containing) wounds Toxins lead to spreading destruction of tissue
Clostridium tetani	Tetanus (lockjaw)	Neurotoxin (tetanospasmin) causes muscle spasms and convulsions Frequently fatal Soil contamination of penetrating wound
Clostridium botulinum	Botulism	Ingestion of pre-formed neurotoxin in inadequately sterilized or processed food Muscle paralysis and death

Listeria monocytogenes causes meningitis in the newborn and elderly, and abortions or stillbirths in pregnant women

The organism *Listeria monocytogenes* is excreted in large amounts in cows' milk, and may therefore be present in unpasteurized dairy products. However, it is also an occasional component of the normal gut flora. Infection of neonates usually results from transplacental infection from an infected mother, and adults acquire the infection by ingestion of contaminated food. In many cases significant clinical infection is associated with an element of immune incompetence.

Escherichia coli is responsible for a wide range of diseases according to the type of virulence factor possessed by the particular pathogenic strain

E. coli is a normal commensal in the human gut, and all strains produce an endotoxin. Pathogenic varieties have additional virulence factors which produce different patterns of disease. One of the most important virulence factors is a group of enterotoxins that produce diarrheal disease, some varieties of which also induce the **hemolytic–uremic syndrome**, leading to acute renal failure and death. The important pathogenic elements of *E. coli* infection are:

- Urinary tract infection – local spread from anus.
- Neonatal meningitis – the virulence factor is the presence of a capsule (K1 capsular type) around the bacterium.
- Diarrheal diseases – often severe, watery and hemorrhagic, are associated with strains that produce potent enterotoxins. These are a common cause of 'traveller's diarrhea,' acquired through ingestion of contaminated food or water.

The strain known as *E. coli 0157:H7* (enterohemorrhagic) has a high mortality rate because it is complicated by hemolytic–uremic syndrome (see page 328 and 364). Most cases are associated with the ingestion of contaminated undercooked beef.

Proteus species are gut commensals which can also cause urinary tract infection

Like *E. coli*, this Gram-negative bacillus normally colonizes the colon, but can spread locally from the anus to produce urethritis, cystitis and pyelonephritis. It may also produce wound infections, particularly hospital-acquired.

Enterobacter, *Serratia* and *Klebsiella* are also Gram-negative rods commensal in the gut, and may cause lower urinary tract infections. These usually occur in the elderly who are in hospital or following catheterization. *Klebsiella* can produce a severe atypical hemorrhagic pneumonia, often with lung abscess, in vulnerable individuals such as the immunosuppressed, malnourished and diabetic.

Salmonella and *Shigella* species are not normally present as commensals in the gut, and cause diarrheal disease

The *Salmonella* group contains many members, most of which cause diarrheal disease that remains confined to the bowel with no spread of bacteria beyond. *Salmonella typhi* and *paratyphi* produce systemic diseases ('typhoid fever' and 'paratyphoid fever') in which bowel involvement is only part of a widespread symptomatic bacteremia. The organisms are ingested in contaminated water (in underdeveloped countries) or in food which has been contaminated during handling by someone who is a carrier of the organism. Asymptomatic carriers excrete *Salmonella typhi* in feces and urine. The onset is gradual, with non-specific malaise, fever and headache, sometimes with myalgia and arthralgia. This represents the stage when the organisms have entered via the gut and are being disseminated by lymphatics and thence to the bloodstream. The mucosa-associated lymphoid tissue in the gut, particularly the Peyer's patches in the small intestine, become enlarged and ulcerated (see *Fig. 8.12*), and often manifest as bloody diarrhea. Perforation through the necrotic Peyer's patches in terminal ileum may occur. Recovery and relapse are frequent, and after recovery the patient may become a chronic carrier and a potential source of infection to others.

The *Shigella* group comprises four important organisms responsible for bacillary dysentery. *Shigella dysenteriae* causes the most severe symptoms. There is sudden onset of watery and bloody diarrhea, often with abundant mucus, with severe dehydration (which may be fatal in children without proper medical care). The symptoms and outlook are generally most severe in children; adults may have a more gradual onset and milder symptoms. Infection is by the orofecal route from the feces of carriers or convalescents, and flies and food may be intermediate stepping stones. Pathologically, the colonic mucosa is hyperemic, acutely inflamed and focally ulcerated.

Fig. 8.12 Typhoid ulcers of ileum. This old museum specimen, from a man who died of typhoid fever in 1907, shows enlarged Peyer's patches, with ulceration and necrotic surface slough, characteristic of late-stage typhoid fever.

Pseudomonas is an important cause of hospital-acquired infection

Pseudomonas aeruginosa, a Gram-negative aerobic bacillus, is an important opportunistic pathogen in hospitalized patients, particularly those who are vulnerable because of some degree of immunosuppression (AIDS and cancer patients) and those in whom the normal barriers to bacterial invasion (see pages 140 and 222) are compromised. Common examples include people with severe burns and cystic fibrosis patients. It causes a wide range of infections, including:

- Respiratory infections (in cystic fibrosis and other chronic lung disease).
- Urinary tract infections (usually hospital-acquired following instrumentation of the bladder).
- Eye infections (producing destructive keratitis).
- Wound/skin infections (particularly in burns patients).

Bacteremia and septicemia may follow localized *Pseudomonas* infection in immunocompromised patients, particularly from urinary infections. Lung lesions in bacteremia (and in many primary lung infections) frequently show a bacterial vasculitis, with *Pseudomonas* bacilli in and around blood vessels in large numbers, often with associated thrombosis of the affected vessel. These vascular changes lead to multiple small white necrotic lesions, with a hyperemic or hemorrhagic rim (see *Fig. 8.13*).

Fig. 8.13 Lung in *Pseudomonas* septicemia. This lung, from a child who died following severe burns, shows the characteristic small white foci of necrotic infection with surrounding hyperemia.

Vibrio cholerae produces severe watery diarrhea, and leads to dehydration and electrolyte imbalance

The organism *Vibrio cholerae* is usually spread by the ingestion of water contaminated by the feces of an infected person, and is endemic in the summer months in areas of the world where public and personal sanitation is poor. In addition, small or large epidemics may occur at any time when there is a major breakdown in public sanitation, for example after severe flooding that destroys sewage systems and fresh water supplies.

The symptoms are due to an enterotoxins, and the organism has to be ingested in very large numbers to produce disease, as gastric acid destroys most of them. Any surviving bacteria pass into the small intestine which, if conditions are suitable for the organism, rapidly becomes colonized by adherence of the bacterium to the mucosal surface. The enterotoxin is produced in large quantities and leads to profuse outpouring of large quantities (up to 1 L every hour) of fluid, passed as a clear watery stool ('rice-water stool'). Loss of water and electrolytes leads to severe dehydration and metabolic disturbance (mainly hypokalemia and metabolic acidosis due to loss of bicarbonate). Unless the fluid and electrolyte imbalance is restored by intravenous fluid and electrolyte therapy, hypovolemic shock, cardiac irregularities and death will occur.

Yersinia enterocolitica produces an enterocolitis which can be clinically similar to acute appendicitis

Infection results from eating contaminated food of many types. During a subclinical incubation period of about a week, it is believed that the organism invades the epithelium of the small intestine and finds its way into the mucosa-associated lymphoid tissue, particularly the Peyer's patches, where it causes necrosis. Histologically, the foci of necrosis are surrounded by macrophages and giant cells to form granulomas, and may sometimes be difficult to distinguish from tuberculous infection and Crohn's disease. Mesenteric lymph nodes are enlarged and may contain granulomas. Clinically these developments are matched by abdominal pain, diarrhea and fever. The pain is often in the right iliac fossa, similar to acute appendicitis. The symptoms may last for some weeks.

Another Yersinia, *Y. parahaemolytica*, causes a more acute diarrheal illness, sometimes with vomiting and fever, following the ingestion of contaminated fish and shellfish. Symptoms begin any time from 12 to 48 hours after ingestion, and last for 24–48 hours.

Another Yersinia (*Y. pestis*) causes the historically famous disease called 'the plague'

Now rare, for hundreds of years the plague was a common epidemic illness in Europe, the Middle East and the Far East. Major epidemics in Europe in the 14th century (the 'Black Death') and in England in 1665 caused a significant reduction in population, estimated to be as high as 25% in some areas. Some small towns and villages, such as Eyam in Derbyshire, England, were almost completely wiped out in a matter of months. The organism causes mild infection in a variety of rodents, which form its natural reservoir. The major human epidemics are caused by transmission from rats to humans via bites from rat fleas, which become heavily infected by feeding on the blood of rats.

The bacteria proliferate and pass in lymphatics to the lymph nodes, which within a few days enlarge and become necrotic and hemorrhagic ('buboes'). From these the bacteria may pass in the bloodstream to the lungs to cause **pneumonic plague**, which is almost invariably fatal. Acute septicemia is associated with disseminated intravascular coagulation, which produces extensive internal hemorrhage and a confluent petechial and blue-black ecchymotic rash in the skin, the reason for the ancient name 'the Black Death.'

Campylobacter species are a common and important cause of diarrhea

The most common Campylobacter is *C. jejuni*, which is responsible for most cases of Campylobacter diarrhea. Clinically, the illness resembles Salmonella enteritis (see page 257) but may persist for longer, up to 3–4 weeks. In persistent disease the symptoms and signs may be difficult to distinguish from an attack of ulcerative colitis. Endoscopic examination of the colon may show inflamed and reddened mucosa, with focal superficial hemorrhage and ulceration; however, similar changes are also seen in the ileum and jejunum – not a feature of ulcerative colitis.

The organisms are widespread in many domestic animals, including cattle, sheep and poultry, and human infection is thought to be acquired through ingestion of contaminated food, particularly milk and poultry.

The organism formerly known as *Campylobacter pylori* associated with gastritis and duodenal ulcer has been reclassified and renamed *Helicobacter pylori* (see page 252).

Haemophilus influenzae causes a range of infections, including meningitis in children

Haemophilus species are common commensals in the upper respiratory tract, but only *Haemophilus influenzae* produces disease. It is responsible for acute exacerbations of chronic bronchitis in adults, but is mainly a disease of young children, causing acute tracheobronchitis and pneumonia, sinusitis, otitis media and epiglottitis. It was formerly an important cause of acute purulent meningitis in young children, but is becoming less so as a result of vaccination.

One of the most important virulence factors for *Haemophilus influenzae* is the possession of a capsule; non-capsulated forms are rarely pathogenic except as secondary invaders of the respiratory tract.

Haemophilus ducreyi causes the mainly tropical disease called chancroid, in which painful ulcers develop on the genitalia, often associated with inguinal lymph node enlargement.

Actinomyces israelii causes chronic suppurating abscesses in the neck, and less commonly in the appendix region

Actinomyces are common commensals in the mouth, particularly in the crypts of the tonsils and around the necks of the teeth. Occasionally the organism becomes pathogenic, with spread into the soft tissues of the neck to produce a lumpy swelling (*Figs 8.14* and *8.15*), which can discharge onto the surface through numerous sinuses. The discharge is a thin, watery fluid, within which can be seen small yellow fragments ('sulfur granules') – large aggregated colonies of the organism. The original source of the infection may be an infected tooth.

Actinomycosis may also occur in the abdomen, particularly in the right iliac fossa after appendix surgery.

Fig. 8.14 Actinomycosis of the neck. Actinomycotic abscess oozing clear fluid at its center, which will soon discharge to produce yellow 'sulfur' granules.

Fig. 8.15 Actinomycosis. A colony of *Actinomyces israelii* in a jaw abscess. The colony is surrounded by neutrophils. These colonies form the so-called 'sulfur granules' which are extruded when the abscess discharges.

Mycobacteria induce a chronic inflammatory granulomatous reaction

Mycobacteria are slender rod-shaped bacteria which are characterized by a waxy cell wall; this renders the organisms particularly resistant to adverse environmental conditions, such as dehydration and weak acids and alcohol. When they gain access to the body, the same wax coat makes the organisms resistant to destruction by neutrophils. Although the organisms can be phagocytosed by neutrophils in the normal way (see pages 40 and 53), the neutrophil enzymes are largely impotent against the mycobacteria because of the protective waxy wall, and the neutrophils die long before the organisms have been damaged; the bacteria emerge largely undamaged. Only macrophages, which are much longer-lived than neutrophils, can effectively phago-cytose and contain mycobacteria, although the organism has the capacity to initially proliferate within the macro-phages and resist destruction by blocking phagolysosome formation (see page 53). At this early stage of infection bacteria may escape from the macrophages to give a bacte-remia, with dispersal of organisms to many sites. Later, a T-helper cell response produces activated macrophages which can kill the organisms, recruits blood monocytes to the site of infection to become activated macrophages, and forms localized collections which attempt to contain and localize the infection. This localized collection of activated macrophages is the earliest step in the formation of a **tuber-culous granuloma.**

Thus, in summary, having gained access to the tissues, the mycobacteria excite a transient but ineffective neutro-phil response, followed by a marked immune-mediated response, manifest by sensitization of T-cells to produce cytokines which recruit and activate macrophages, the major cellular component of a chronic inflammatory granu-lomatous reaction. The type of immune response caused by mycobacteria is termed type IV hypersensitivity (see pages 103–4).

These changes are seen at their most classic in infection by *Mycobacterium tuberculosis*, the causative organism of tuberculosis (TB) in the lungs and elsewhere.

A granuloma in TB is termed a 'tubercle'

In the context of TB, aggregates of macrophages, i.e. the granulomas, are often called **tubercles.**

Each tubercle has an area of caseous tissue necrosis at its centre. This is characterized by its homogeneity, and no ghost pattern of the original tissue structure remains. Viable mycobacteria are present within the necrotic debris. To the naked eye, this necrotic tissue resembles cream cheese, hence its descriptive name **caseous necrosis**. The reason for the necrosis at the centre of tubercles is uncertain, as it is not seen in the centre of granulomas caused by other agents.

A tubercle is composed of activated macrophages with surrounding lymphoid cells and fibroblasts

The structure of a typical tuberculous granuloma is shown in *Figs 8.16 and 8.17*. Around the central area of caseous necrosis lies a collection of large, activated macrophages. Histologically, this functional activation is manifest by the presence of bulky pale-staining granular cytoplasm, which is rich in endoplasmic reticulum, with a prominent Golgi. Because of a minimal resemblance to some epithelial cells, the term **epithelioid cells** was originally coined for these macrophages.

Some of the activated macrophages cells fuse to form large multinucleate cells (macrophage polykaryons), with many nuclei arranged around the periphery and a large central cytoplasmic mass. In TB these giant macrophages are called **Langhans' cells.**

Around the zone of macrophages bordering the central caseous necrosis lies a collar of lymphocytes, reflecting the immunological response to the presence of mycobacteria.

As the tubercle persists, some fibroblasts appear within the lymphocyte collar and outside it. These are recruited by secretion of cytokines from the activated macrophages.

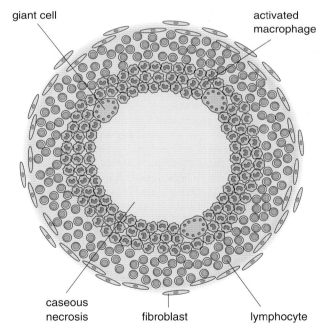

Fig. 8.16 A tuberculous granuloma (tubercle). This simple diagram shows the structure of an early tuberculous granuloma. There is a central area of amorphous necrotic debris (caseous necrosis) surrounded by a zone of activated macrophages. Within this zone are characteristic multinucleated macrophages with the cytoplasm in the center and the nuclei arranged peripherally (Langhans' giant cells). Outside the macrophage layer is a variable rim of lymphocytes, and outside that a layer of active fibroblasts, scanty in early granulomas but more substantial in older lesions.

Fig. 8.17a&b An early tuberculous granuloma. H&E. (a) shows a medium-power view of an entire early tuberculous granuloma. There is a central area of pink-staining amorphous caseous necrosis **C,** surrounded by a zone of activated macrophages **M**. Within the macrophage layer can be seen a typical Langhans' giant cell (**arrow**). Outside the layer of activated macrophages is a ring of lymphocytes **L**. In this very early tubercle, fibroblasts are very few and insignificant. (b) shows a higher-power view of that part of the tubercle containing the Langhans' giant cell (**arrow**); note its peripherally arranged nuclei and the amorphous nature of the caseous necrosis **C**.

The outcome of tubercle formation depends on the adequacy of the host immune response

Because *M. tuberculosis* is resistant to destruction, infections tend to be chronic and persistent, being difficult to eradicate by natural defence mechanisms. The outcome of tubercle formation depends on the balance between two conflicting sets of factors: those predisposing to extension of infection, and those predisposing to containment, or healing and eradication of infection.

Factors predisposing to extension of the infection include:

- Ingestion of large numbers of highly virulent organisms.

- Poor immune response, e.g. due to malnutrition, extreme youth, old age, intercurrent disease or immunosuppressive therapy.

Factors predisposing to containment or eradication include:

- Ingestion of small numbers of poorly virulent organisms.
- Good immune response, e.g. robust health, heightened immune status due to immunization.
- Administration of appropriate antibiotics.

Mycobacterium tuberculosis gains access to the lung by inhalation and causes pulmonary TB

The commonest pattern of mycobacterial infection is **pulmonary TB**, in which the organisms are inhaled by the victim in the droplets expectorated by someone with active pulmonary TB. The details of this disease and its various patterns and outcomes is given in Chapter 11, pages 195–197. The disease is still important in the malnourished in underdeveloped and poor nations, and is seen increasingly in the UK and USA in the immigrant populations and in the immunosuppressed (e.g. AIDS and transplant patients). New strains of *M. tuberculosis* are emerging which appear resistant to formerly successful antituberculous chemotherapy.

Mycobacterium tuberculosis infection by ingestion is now rare, but not completely eradicated

Drinking unpasteurized milk from cows suffering with bovine tuberculosis was once an important pattern of mycobacterial disease. Infection began in the tonsillar region, with a small focus of primary infection, often unrecognized. The tubercle bacilli then spread in lymphatics to the regional lymph nodes in the side of the neck, leading to tender lymphadenopathy; the lymph nodes often reached a large size and ulcerated through the skin, producing chronic discharging sinuses, a condition called **scrofula.** Sometimes the primary site was in the intestine, leading to tuberculous enlargement of mesenteric lymph nodes, with the risk of rupture into the peritoneum leading to **tuberculous peritonitis.**

Bovine patterns of tuberculosis have now been almost entirely eradicated in most countries as a result of tuberculin testing of cows and the slaughter of affected herds, combined with pasteurization of milk.

Infection with *Mycobacterium leprae* causes leprosy

Leprosy is a common and important disease in some areas of the world, such as the Indian subcontinent and sub-

Saharan Africa, and is mainly seen in the UK and USA in immigrants or visitors from those areas. It occurs in two main patterns, depending on the victim's immune response:

- **Lepromatous leprosy** mainly affects the skin, particularly of the periphery (e.g. feet, ears) in the form of irregular nodular thickening, usually with diminution or loss of sensation in the affected areas. The skin thickening is due to large collections of pale-staining macrophages (lepra cells) containing large numbers of organisms, in the layers of the dermis (see *Fig. 23.17*) the nodular thickenings may coalesce to produce great disfigurement.
- **Tuberculoid leprosy** which produces flat hyper- or hypopigmented skin lesions, but particularly affects nerves, with ill-formed granulomas around small and medium nerve twigs which are sometimes destroyed. This damage to nerves leads to patchy loss of sensation, predisposing to unrecognized trauma, persistent enlarging skin ulcers, and the risk of loss of digits, particularly fingers.

The difference between the two patterns is dependent on the T-helper cell response. In lepromatous leprosy there is an ineffective response, so bacteria are abundant in the lesions, and granulomas are not formed. In tuberculoid leprosy there is a good T-helper cell response, organisms are very scanty in the lesions, and granulomas are formed; it is the type IV hypersensitivity reaction itself that causes the tissue damage.

Treponema pallidum is a spiral bacterium which causes syphilis

The organism *Treponema pallidum* is very sensitive and is easily destroyed by heat and drying, so successful transmission is largely confined to intimate sexual contact between mucosal surfaces. The pathology of syphilis is illustrated and discussed on pages 109–110.

Other treponemes cause diseases which are not sexually transmitted, summarized in *Fig. 8.19*.

The *Treponema* species cannot be grown successfully in artificial culture media, so diagnosis is made on clinical features, microscopic examination of infected tissue and serology.

Leptospirosis is contracted by contact with rat urine in water

Leptospira are spiral bacteria which cause kidney infection in small mammals, particularly rats, which then pass the organism into rivers in their urine. Human infection can be by ingestion or penetration (e.g. through broken skin) of the organism, which passes into the bloodstream, the bacteremia being associated with a mild febrile illness which usually resolves with no further symptoms. In a small percentage of such cases rapid proliferation of the organism in the blood leads to septicemia, with kidney failure, jaundice, hemorrhage and liver failure due to leptospiral hepatitis (Weil's disease).

Fig. 8.18 Mycobacterial diseases other than tuberculosis and leprosy

Mycobacterium ulcerans	Chronic skin ulcerated nodule (Buruli ulcer)	Africa and Australia
Mycobacterium marinum	Chronic skin ulcerated nodules	From contaminated water, e.g. aquaria, swimming pools
Mycobacterium avium (intracellulare)	TB-like cervical lymphadenopathy or lung lesions Disseminated colonization of macrophages throughout body (AIDS-related)	Opportunistic infection in AIDS patients

Fig. 8.19 Other treponemal diseases

Endemic syphilis ('bejel')	West Africa Eastern Mediterranean	Nodular skin lesion Gummatous lesions later	*Treponema pallidum endemicum*
Yaws	Tropical equatorial	Nodule in skin at inoculation site, widespread skin granulomas, gummas, periostitis	*Treponema pallidum pertenue*
Pinta	Central and South America	Nodule at inoculation site becoming indurated plaques with depigmentation	*Treponema carateum*

Lyme disease is caused by a spirochete transmitted to humans through tick bites

The causative organism is *Borrelia burgdorferi*, a spirochetal bacterium which occurs in a wide range of mammals, but most human infections come from sheep, deer or dogs. The bacterium is transmitted to man through tick bites, the ticks jumping from the host mammal directly onto human skin, or more commonly from the grass on which the animals graze. The ticks are normally small and difficult to see until they have been attached to human skin for sufficient time to become distended with human blood (*Fig. 8.20*); the bacterium is transmitted to humans during this blood-sucking phase.

The usual first symptom of the disease is a red spot or patch of erythema at the site of the bite, the characteristic pattern of progression being the pattern known as **erythema migrans**, in which the red patch enlarges peripherally and shows central clearing. This is accompanied by systemic symptoms such as fever, lethargy, and muscle and joint pains. Later on most patients develop flitting and intermittent arthritis, particularly involving the knees, and these arthritic symptoms may occur on and off for months or even years. A few patients develop CNS symptoms, particularly meningoencephalitis and cranial nerve lesions.

Fig. 8.20 Deer tick attached to skin. This photomicrograph shows a deer tick **T** attached to skin. The tick was distended with blood which has been lost during processing. Note the inflammatory reaction **I** in the skin around the tick mouthparts.

Brucellosis is contracted by contact with infected animals or their products

The Brucella group are primary animal pathogens, and human infection is acquired by direct contact, ingestion (e.g. in infected milk) or inhalation. Organisms gain access to the bloodstream via lymphatics, and produce an illness characterized by malaise and fever with no localizing signs other than occasional lymphadenopathy. Histologically, the lymph nodes, liver, spleen and bone marrow may contain foci of granulomatous inflammation with central necrosis in some granulomas. The ill-defined symptoms may persist for weeks or months, and a few cases develop into chronic brucellosis, with the relapsing illness lasting for more than a year. There are three main pathogenic species, each with a different animal host:

- *Brucella abortus* (cow): worldwide, but most commercial herds are now Brucella-free.
- *Brucella melitensis* (sheep and goats): countries around the Mediterranean Sea, South America and Mexico.
- *Brucella suis* (pigs): southeast Asia, South America and the USA.

Legionella causes a severe atypical pneumonia known as Legionnaire's disease

Legionella is a recently discovered Gram-negative rod which is usually contracted by inhaling water droplets from contaminated water supplies, such as cooling towers, domestic and institutional shower systems and air-conditioning devices. There are about 20–30 species, but *Legionella pneumophila* is responsible for most cases. Inhalation may lead to:

- The development of anti-Legionella antibodies, but without the development of symptoms.
- A mild transient flu-like illness, called Pontiac fever.
- Full-blown Legionnaire's disease.

In Legionnaire's disease, an incubation period of 2–10 days, during which the patient may develop fever, malaise and flu-like symptoms, is followed by evidence of lung infection. This is signified by cough with mucoid sputum, high fever, and X-ray changes of patchy lung consolidation. There may also be diarrhea and mental confusion. The patchy lung consolidation spreads to become confluent and often bilateral, with rapidly deteriorating lung function. Even with early diagnosis and appropriate antibiotic therapy, the overall mortality rate is as high as 10–20%. In severe infections, investigations show evidence of impaired liver and kidney function. Legionella pneumonia is an important community- and hospital-acquired lung infection (see page 194).

Chlamydia are increasingly becoming recognized as associated with a wide range of diseases

Chlamydia are intracellular organisms, formerly thought to be viruses but now classified as small Gram-negative bacteria. There are three main groups. The commonest, *Chlamydia trachomatosis*, has many subtypes that give rise to a wide range of diseases.

C. trachomatosis subtypes **D–K** are the organisms responsible for a large number of sexually transmitted diseases, the most frequent of which are cervicitis, urethritis, salpingitis and pelvic inflammatory disease in women, and urethritis and epididymo-orchitis in men. It is a cause of Reiter's syndrome (see page 553). Members of this group may infect newborn infants on their passage through an infected maternal birth canal, particularly producing conjunctivitis.

C. trachomatosis **subtype L** produces the sexually transmitted disease lymphogranuloma venereum.

The other two main groups are **C. psittaci**, which causes the human pneumonitis psittacosis (see page 198), transmitted from birds, and **C. pneumoniae**, which causes atypical pneumonia, particularly in the young.

The most common disease caused by Bartonella is cat-scratch fever

Bartonella are small Gram-negative bacilli which are passed to humans by an insect vector from an animal reservoir. The most widespread organism is *Bartonella henselae* (formerly *Rochalimaea henselae*), which exists as a commensal in the tissues and blood of up to 50% of domestic cats.

The human illness cat-scratch disease is thought to result from the organism gaining access to the human skin by way of a scratch from the cat's claws, but many patients give no history of a scratch and have no evidence of a primary inflammatory skin lesion, so it is possible that in some cases the organism is transmitted via the cat flea. The main abnormality in the patient with cat-scratch disease is regional lymphadenopathy (see page 308), in which the histological features are characteristic and almost diagnostic (*Fig. 8.21*).

In AIDS patients severe systemic infections may cause a severe feverish illness, often associated with raised red polypoid lesions in the skin ('bacillary angiomatosis'), which may be clinically confused with the early lesions of Kaposi's sarcoma.

Other varieties of Bartonella cause 'trench fever', a feverish condition common in foot soldiers in both world wars, and a disease in the Andes known as 'Oroya fever'.

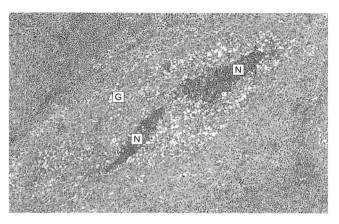

Fig. 8.21 Cat-scratch disease. In this condition, nodes show large histiocytic granulomas (**G**), which contain central necrosis and neutrophilic infiltrations (**N**). These are sometimes called 'suppurating granulomas'.

Rickettsial diseases are transmitted by insect vectors (usually ticks) and cause a range of febrile illnesses with headaches, rash and malaise

Rickettsiae are intracellular coccobacilli, usually transmitted to humans by tick bites from an animal reservoir which consists mainly of rodents of various types. There is significant geographical localization in most cases (*Fig. 8.22*).

The most severe rickettsial diseases are those that produce a spotted fever clinical picture; the rash is due to vascular leakage from rickettsial-damaged endothelial cells, and can lead to profound hypovolemic shock and death.

Fig. 8.22 Diseases due to rickettsial infection

Disease	Location	Organism	Host(s)	Transmitted by	Usual symptoms	Severe complications
Rocky Mountain spotted fever	USA	Rickettsia rickettsii	Small mammals, e.g. dog, rabbit	Ixodid ticks	Fever, headache, myalgia, hemorrhagic rash	Encephalitis, pneumonia, circulatory collapse
Epidemic typhus	Worldwide	Rickettsia prowazekii	Humans	Human body louse	Prolonged fever, headache, rash (often hemorrhagic)	Encephalitis, pneumonia, hypotension and renal failure
Endemic (murine) typhus	Worldwide (sporadic)	Rickettsia typhi	Rodents	Cat and rat fleas	Similar to epidemic typhus	Rare
Q fever	Worldwide	Rickettsia burnetii	Goats, sheep, cattle, rodents	In humans by inhalation or ingestion	Fever, headache, myalgia, pneumonia	Aortic valve endocarditis, granulomatous hepatitis Atypical lobar pneumonia
Scrub typhus (Tsutsugamushi disease)	Far East	Rickettsia tsutsugamushi	Rodents	Mite	Fever, headache, rash, ulcer at site of bite, lymphadenopathy	Severe pneumonitis Myocarditis

FUNGAL INFECTIONS

Fungi are ubiquitous in the environment. Many reside innocuously on the skin surface, some are commensals on the mucosal surfaces (e.g. the mouth and vagina), but very few are pathogenic. Pathogenic fungal infections can be divided according to the pattern of involvement:

- Superficial and deep fungal infections of the skin (see page 512).
- Infections of mucosal surfaces.
- Lung infections due to inhaled fungi (see page 198).
- Systemic bloodborne infections.

Immunosuppression is an important predisposing factor for fungal infections.

The main fungal infections of clinical significance are: dermatophytic fungi (skin), *Candida albicans* or thrush (mucosal and systemic), *Aspergillus* spp. (lung and systemic), zygomycoses (nasal sinuses), *Cryptococcus* (lung and brain), and *Histoplasma* (lung).

The reaction of tissues to fungi depends on the infection and site involved

The reactions seen to fungal infection are:

- **Minimal tissue reaction**. This is a particular feature of superficial skin infections by dermatophytic fungi. Histologically the tissue response is very low-key, with dilatation of dermal vessels and very minor neutrophil accumulation in the epidermis. *Cryptococcus neoformans* often shows minimal tissue reaction in the lungs and meninges, but this may be a manifestation of the patient's immunosuppressed state.
- **Acute inflammatory reaction**. This is seen mainly in primary mucosal fungal infections, such as oral, esophageal and vaginal Candida infections. There is vascular dilatation and a heavy neutrophil infiltration in the epithelium, often with ulceration. In the early stages of systemic bloodborne infection there is an acute inflammatory reaction, often followed by microabscess formation.
- **Granulomatous inflammatory reaction**. One of the characteristic tissue responses to fungi, particularly in deep subcutaneous and some systemic infection, is the so-called 'suppurating granuloma.' There is a central purulent neutrophil reaction, surrounded by a granulomatous histiocytic and giant-cell reaction. The fungi can usually be found within the purulent neutrophilic material. Some fungi, particularly yeasts (e.g. chromoblastomycosis), excite a purely histiocytic and giant-cell granulomatous reaction, without suppuration.

Dermatophytic fungi are common and cause a range of skin diseases

These fungi are located mainly on the skin surface, but hyphae insert themselves between epidermal keratinocytes. Both surface epidermis and the keratinocytes of hair follicles may be involved, as may finger and toe nails. Interference with the maturation of keratinocytes leads to surface scaliness of the skin, due to nucleated keratinocytes on the surface (parakeratosis) instead of anuclear keratin flakes (orthokeratosis), and there are reactive vascular and inflammatory changes in the dermis, manifest clinically as reddening of the skin. Involvement of the nail beds leads to thickening, opacity and discoloration of the nails. The clinical features depend on the fungus involved and the site of skin involvement. The details of the most common of these diseases (known collectively as the dermatophytoses, are shown on page 512 of Chapter 23. Involvement of hair follicles (fungal folliculitis), particularly by *Pityrosporum*, is one of the clinical features of AIDS.

Fungi may gain access to dermis and subcutis following penetrating injury

Although less common than bacterial causes, some fungi can infect the deep layers of skin to produce a chronic inflammatory suppurating mass which discharges pus onto the surface of the skin through numerous sinuses. Sometimes masses of fungal hyphae are discharged in the form of small granules within the pus from the deep abscesses (see *Fig. 8.23*). The most common site is the foot (see Chapter 23, page 512, for more details).

Fig. 8.23 Deep subcutaneous fungal infection of skin. This micrograph shows a chronic multilocular abscess in the deep tissues of the foot. Each locule contains pus **P**, within which are fungal colonies, some of which are forming compact 'granules' **C**. These may be discharged onto the skin surface, with the pus, through sinuses. The chronicity of the lesion is marked by the presence of fibrosis **F** around the abscesses.

***Candida albicans* is a normal commensal of the skin and alimentary tract, and superficial pathogenic infections are particularly common in orificial mucosa**

This organism occurs in both a yeast and a hyphal form. The commonest sites for infection are the mouth (oral thrush – see pages 225 and 228) and at the vulvovaginal orifice (see pages 416–7). In immunosuppressed individuals systemic bloodborne infection can occur, with small candidal abscesses in many organs. Intravenous drug abusers and patients with long-standing intravenous lines are particularly at risk; sometimes candidal endocarditis, with large mitral and aortic valve vegetations, is the basis of the widespread blood dissemination. In surface skin/mucosal lesions the hyphal forms predominate, with scanty yeast forms, whereas in endocarditis and the systemic microabscesses the yeast forms predominate.

***Aspergillus fumigatus* is an important opportunistic fungus in immunocompromised individuals**

This fungus is widely distributed in the environment and is usually non-pathogenic. In severely immunocompromised patients it may gain access to the lung periphery and proliferate rapidly (*Fig. 8.24*). An important feature of the organism is its ability to penetrate the walls of blood vessels, leading to thrombosis, vessel occlusion and tissue necrosis, particularly in the lung. Aspergillus lung disease is discussed and illustrated on pages 198–9. Although the main lesions are in the lung, Aspergillus can become systematized through the bloodstream to produce small lesions which are often necrotic or semi-cystic, owing to vessel occlusion by masses of hyphae and thrombus.

Aspergillus niger is a cause of otitis externa; the black fungus can be easily seen clinically in the external auditory canal.

***Cryptococcus neoformans* can cause pneumonia and meningitis**

This fungus exists only in the form of a spherical yeast, and has a thick capsule. It is common in bird droppings. Human infection occurs by inhalation of the yeast, particularly when it is airborne in dry dusty soils. In an immunocompetent individual the presence of Cryptococci inhaled into lung alveoli may be asymptomatic or associated with only a mild flu-like illness. The disease is at its worst in the immunocompromised individual, in whom the Cryptococci proliferate within the lung to produce pneumonic consolidation. The yeasts can spread to the meninges to give a meningitis (*Fig. 8.25*), and sometimes intracerebral accumulations of the capsulated yeast. There is often little or no inflammatory response of any type to the presence of the yeasts in either lungs or meninges, particularly in immunosuppressed patients, but a low-grade granulomatous reaction sometimes occurs.

***Histoplasma capsulatum* produces cavitating lung lesions, and can become disseminated in immunosuppressed individuals**

Like Cryptococcus, Histoplasma occurs in soil which is extensively contaminated by infected bird droppings. Human infection is by inhalation of dust containing the spores of the fungus. In healthy immunocompetent individuals symptoms are usually mild, with slight cough,

Fig. 8.24 Aspergillosis in the lung. Photomicrograph showing the branching system of *Aspergillus fumigatus* at the edge of an area of lung necrosis.

Fig. 8.25 Meningitis due to cryptococci. High-magnification photomicrograph showing a granulomatous inflammatory exudate in the meninges, with a piece of cerebral cortex (**C**). The cryptococcal yeast forms (arrowed) are present in the exudate, along with a few poorly formed giant cells.

malaise and occasionally fever ('acute primary histoplasmosis'); rarely, an acute pneumonia develops. Some patients, possibly slightly or moderately immune impaired, or repeatedly exposed to large quantities of spores, develop a chronic cavitating lung disease ('chronic cavitating histoplasmosis') which affects the apices of the upper lobes and therefore resembles adult-pattern tuberculosis (see page 195).

Disseminated systemic infection occurs in partly immunocompromised individuals, the fungus spreading from a lung lesion via the bloodstream to colonize lymph nodes, spleen, liver and bone marrow. The illness is chronic, with surprisingly mild non-specific symptoms. Severe symptoms may occur in patients with AIDS (for which it is one of the defining opportunistic infections), the disseminated systemic infection sometimes occurring many years after the initial exposure in an endemic area.

Histoplasmosis is uncommon in Europe, but endemic in parts of the central USA, mainly the Ohio and Mississippi river valleys.

Coccidiomycosis and blastomycosis cause lung lesions when the spores are inhaled

Coccidioidomycosis is endemic in southwestern USA. As with histoplasmosis, human infection is acquired by inhalation of dusty soil containing fungal spores, and a mild respiratory illness follows which resembles acute bronchitis. The tissue response in the lungs is the formation of a giant cell granulomatous reaction, which may enlarge and cavitate to produce radiologically obvious lesions. Healing is by fibrosis. In some cases the lung lesions fail to heal and organisms persist, occasionally becoming systematized. This may occur in individuals who are mildly or transiently immunocompromised, e.g. the elderly, malnourished, or on immunosuppressive therapy. AIDS patients may have particularly severe systemic lesions, involving the brain, bones, soft tissues and visceral organs. In this group the original pulmonary lesions frequently enlarge rapidly, with progressive respiratory impairment.

Blastomycosis is very similar in clinical and pathological features to coccidioidomycosis, with inhalation of soil dust-borne spores causing lung lesions characterized by a giant cell granulomatous reaction to the organism in the lungs, associated with trivial symptoms. Some patients have more severe pulmonary involvement with respiratory failure. It differs from coccidioidomycosis in that the main manifestation of systemic spread is the development of numerous enlarging and spreading skin lesions which undergo pustulation.

Pneumocystis carinii is an important cause of disease and death in immunosuppressed patients

Until recently this organism was regarded as a protozoan but has now, by some taxonomic sleight-of-hand, emerged

Fig. 8.26 Pneumocystis pneumonia. All lobes of the lung show consolidation as a result of the alveoli being filled with *Pneumocystis carinii* organisms and the associated reaction.

center-stage as a fungus. It is widespread and innocuous except in patients who have inadequate cellular immune mechanisms, and is particularly common in patients with AIDS and heavily immunosuppressed patients such as transplant recipients. Unless successfully treated it causes progressive pulmonary consolidation (*Fig. 8.26*), leading to respiratory failure and death.

VIRAL INFECTIONS

Three main outcomes of viral infection are cell death, cell proliferation, and latent infection

The most commonly seen viral diseases are manifest either by producing cell death or by stimulating cell proliferation.

Cell necrosis is the most common manifestation of viral infections. It may be due to a direct cytopathic effect of the virus, or may be the result of host immune defenses recognizing viral proteins in contact with class I antigen expression. For example, herpes and chickenpox produce skin blistering and mucosal lesions as a result of necrosis of epithelial cells, and influenza produces necrosis of the epithelial cells of the respiratory mucosa. With proliferation of poliovirus and rabies, neurons are killed, and liver cells are killed when infected with yellow fever virus.

Cell proliferation is stimulated by infections caused by variants of the human papillomavirus (HPV), responsible for warty overgrowth of the epidermal cells of the skin in viral warts, and overgrowth of the cervical epithelium in wart-virus infection of the cervical epithelium. This group is important because of the increasingly recognized link between HPV infection and the subsequent development of epithelial malignant tumors. HPV inactivates the product of p53 gene, which normally prevents cell division.

Latent infection is seen in several diseases when virus becomes integrated into the host genome. Reactivation of virus may then occur at a later date, causing episodes of cell necrosis. For example, herpes zoster may be latent in dorsal root ganglia, reactivating to cause shingles. Virus travels down axons to reach the skin, where productive infection leads to epithelial cell death and a painful blistering rash. Similarly, herpes simplex may be latent in epithelial cells, reactivating to cause cold sores, as well as active genital herpes.

Slow replication of virus inside the host cells may lead to persistent infection

In some situations virus may continue to replicate in host cells, evading immune responses and causing persistent infections. Such infections may be clinically asymptomatic and, because the individual is infective, are an important reservoir for disease spread. For example, human immuno-deficiency virus (HIV) is present at low levels as persistent infection in asymptomatic individuals, and hepatitis B virus can remain as a persistent active infection in certain cases.

Parvoviruses cause two important conditions, both in children

Parvoviruses are single-stranded DNA viruses which cause:

- 'Slapped cheek syndrome,' a febrile illness in children associated with a red maculopapular rash on the cheeks, due to parvovirus B19.
- Aplastic crises in children with sickle-cell anaemia.

Parvovirus may also cause arthritis in adults, and a form of summer diarrhea.

Papovaviruses include papilloma virus, polyomaviruses and simian vacuolating viruses

These are double-stranded DNA viruses with many sub-types, particularly in the papilloma virus group.

Papilloma viruses stimulate the proliferation of squamous epithelial cells to produce proliferating lesions called warts (hence often called 'wart virus'). They are transmitted from person to person by direct or indirect contact, and the virus persists in basal epithelial cells long after the original wart has clinically resolved, with potential for reactivation. Different subtypes of the virus are responsible for warts in different sites. Human papilloma virus (HPV) causes warts in:

- Skin – due to HPV1 and 2, with plantar warts mainly due to HPV1 (*Fig. 8.28*), and the rarer flat 'plane' wart due to HPV3. Warts in the skin around penis, vulva and anus may be due to HPV6, the genital wart virus.

- Anogenital skin – most are due to HPV6 and HPV11(see *Fig. 8.27*).
- Uterine cervix – mainly HPV16 and HPV18. These two subtypes are oncogenic, and infection is a factor predisposing to cervical intraepithelial neoplasia (CIN) and invasive malignancy.
- Larynx – 'juvenile papillomatosis' in young children. Where HPV is identified it is usually HPV6 and HPV11, the viruses responsible for anogenital warts. It is thought that infection is acquired during birth.

These conditions are discussed and illustrated in more detail on pages 270 and 419–20.

The polyoma viruses are two in number, called JC and BK. Although both are frequently present in the urinary tract and kidneys, they very rarely produce infective symptoms. In severely immunosuppressed patients JC virus causes progressive multifocal leukoencephalopathy (see page 471).

Fig. 8.27 Anogenital viral wart. This wart from the vulva shows the location of human papilloma virus (in this case HPV 6/11) in the infected epidermal layers of the warty fronds, using an in-situ hybridization method (location of the virus is shown black against a green counterstain).

Fig. 8.28 HPV in a plantar wart. EM showing numerous HPV1 particles in a keratinocyte from an active plantar wart (verruca).

Adenoviruses can cause epidemics of acute respiratory disease with pneumonia, conjunctivitis and infantile gastroenteritis

Adenoviruses are double-stranded DNA viruses, and there are over 40 types. Common conditions caused by this group are:

- A range of upper and lower respiratory tract infections, particularly in children, including pharyngitis (sore throat) and non-specific 'colds.' Atypical adenovirus pneumonia due to types 3, 4 and 7 can occur in young adults.
- Conjunctivitis associated with types 3, 7, 8 and 19.
- Acute diarrhea in children associated with types 40 and 41.

Hepadnaviruses cause hepatitis B

Hepadnaviruses are double-stranded DNA viruses with a circular shape. The only recognized pathogenic member is the hepatitis B virus, which causes hepatitis. This is discussed in detail in Chapter 14, page 284.

Herpes viruses are a large and important group, responsible for a wide range of diseases

Herpes viruses are double-stranded DNA viruses which cause many important acute and chronic human diseases. There are eight important types, numbered 1–8 (HHV1–8), but many have synonyms:

- HHV1 is also known as herpes simplex virus 1 (HSV1). It is the cause of cold sores around the mouth and gingivostomatitis (*Fig. 8.30*). Can also cause encephalitis (see page 468).
- HHV2 is also known as HSV2. It causes genital herpes and cutaneous herpes (see pages 411 and 511). This virus may rarely cause meningoencephalitis in the newborn and infants, possibly contracted during passage down the birth canal.
- HHV3 is also known as the varicella-zoster virus. This causes varicella (chickenpox) and zoster (shingles) – see *Fig. 8.29*.

Fig. 8.29 Herpes virus inclusions in skin. The keratinocytes in this skin biopsy from a chicken pox lesion show necrosis, and contain viral inclusions (**arrows**) due to HHV3.

Fig. 8.30 EMs showing HHV1 (herpes simplex virus) in the nucleus of a keratinocyte from an active cold sore in the mouth.

- HHV4 is also known as the Epstein–Barr virus (EBV). This causes infectious mononucleosis (glandular fever), but is also involved in Burkitt's lymphoma and nasopharyngeal carcinoma.
- HHV5 is also known as cytomegalovirus (CMV). It causes a wide range of diseases, including a mononucleosis syndrome resembling that due to HHV4, congenital infection, CMV pneumonitis and hepatitis. It is an important pathogen in the immunosuppressed, particularly AIDS patients.
- HHV6 and 7 have no synonyms. Both cause roseola infantum, a mild feverish illness in infants and young children, followed by a red maculopapular rash.
- HHV8 was recently shown to be present in Kaposi's sarcoma.

The poxvirus group cause a wide variety of skin lesions

The poxviruses are double-stranded DNA viruses and are the largest viruses. The most frequently occurring is *Molluscum contagiosum*, which is transmitted from human to human (see page 511). The others pass from animals to humans and include:

- Orf, contracted from sheep (blistering skin lesions).
- Cowpox, contracted from cows (blistering skin lesions on the hands of those milking infected cows).

The orthomyxoviruses cause influenza

These are single-stranded RNA viruses and there are three types, influenza A, influenza B and influenza C. The A and B types are the cause of influenza, and the emergence of new strains is fairly frequent, leading to epidemics and pandemics.

The new strains emerge as a result of either small mutations (antigenic drift) affecting the H (hemagglutinin) and N (neuraminidase) type-specific antigens in the viral envelope, or to a major change in the same antigens (antigenic shift). People with established immunity to previous strains of the virus have no resistance to the new strains. Influenza A also affects other animals, particularly birds, and new strains can develop in these animal reservoirs before infecting humans.

Avian influenza ('bird-flu') can cross the species barrier

Avian influenza is caused by certain type A strains of the virus, most of which produce only minor symptoms in affected birds, but the H5 and H7 strains are highly pathogenic. Of the many strains of avian influenza virus, only four (H5N1, H7N3, H7N7 and H9N2) have been known to cross the species barrier and infect humans, usually producing only minor symptoms. However, strain H5N1 can produce a rapidly progressive pneumonia in humans. It is thought that this strain of virus attaches directly to molecules lining the alveoli of the lungs, whereas most other avian and human influenza strains attach to molecules in the lining of the upper respiratory tract, mainly nose and pharynx.

Similarities in the clinical features have led to suggestions that the 1918 pandemic was due to a very similar avian influenza strain (H1N1) which had crossed the species barrier. There have been small outbreaks since 2004, largely in the Far East, but fortunately very little international spread.

Measles is caused by a paramyxovirus

Before vaccination, measles was a common childhood viral infection, usually presenting with prodromal malaise with cough, runny nose and eyes, and fever. After 2 or 3 days a red spotty or blotchy rash developed, initially on the face, but later spreading to the trunk and other sites, resolving slowly over the next couple of days. Complications, which can be fatal, include measles pneumonia (see *Fig. 8.31*) and post-infectious encephalitis (see page 466). In areas where vaccination is not available, measles is still an important cause of death in young children.

Fig. 8.31 Measles inclusion bodies. Giant cells from a case of fatal measles pneumonia in an immunosuppressed child. The giant cells contain intranuclear and cytoplasmic eosinophilic inclusions of the virus.

SARS (severe acute respiratory syndrome) is caused by a coronavirus

Coronaviruses are single-stranded RNA viruses which most commonly cause only minor upper respiratory symptoms, and coryza (the common cold). The coronavirus responsible for recent outbreaks of SARS has been named, with breathtaking originality, the SARS-associated coronavirus (SARS-CoV). In 2003 there was an outbreak which was first reported in the Far East, but which subsequently appeared in other parts of Asia, and in Europe, South America and North America. The disease presented with high fever, and the influenza-like symptoms of body aches, headaches and general malaise, but almost all patients developed severe pneumonia within 7 days.

Transmission is by close personal contact, largely through respiratory droplet spread. Mortality is about 10%, pneumonia being the major cause of death.

SARS-CoV is believed to be an animal virus that has recently crossed the species barrier by virus adaptation.

The only rhabdovirus of clinical significance is the rabies virus

The virus can infect all types of mammals, and human infection is usually acquired by a bite from an infected animal, most frequently a diseased dog (see *Fig. 21.25*).

The togaviruses cause rubella, hepatitis C, and a variety of severe feverish illnesses, including yellow fever

The following groups produce important diseases:

- Rubivirus causes rubella (German measles).
- Arbovirus is *ar*thropod-*bo*rne and causes a variety of serious encephalitic diseases, such as Eastern equine encephalitis and St Louis encephalitis, and diseases characterized by liver involvement and jaundice (yellow fever, dengue).
- Hepatitis C virus (see pages 286–7).

The arenaviruses mainly affect rodents, from whom humans become infected, usually via rodent urine or feces

Infection is followed by a febrile illness. In some cases the illness progresses to lymphocytic choriomeningitis (LCM) or one of the severe, often fatal, hemorrhagic fevers, such as Lassa fever.

The retroviruses are an important group because they include the AIDS virus and the oncoviruses HTLV1 and HTLV2

The human immunodeficiency virus (HIV) is the cause of AIDS (see page 467). HTLV1 is associated with T-cell leukemia, and HTLV2 with hairy cell leukemia (see page 326).

Histological diagnosis of viral infection

In addition to using microbiological techniques, it is possible to diagnose viral infection by histological examination of biopsy tissue. This is increasing in importance because severe viral infections become manifest as a result of immunosuppression states.

Intracellular inclusion bodies are produced in many infections, e.g. cytomegalovirus (*Fig. 8.32*), and can be recognized by light microscopy. The main inclusions of diagnostic use are given in *Fig. 8.33*.

Immunohistochemistry to detect specific viral proteins is now an important aid to diagnosis, e.g.

detection of herpes simplex in biopsy of necrotic tissue from brain can confirm a diagnosis of herpes encephalitis (see page 467).

In situ hybridization to detect viral genome is increasingly being used as an aid to diagnosis. Detection of different subtypes of HPV in skin and cervical lesions can be achieved in some cases.

Polymerase chain reaction (PCR) techniques, as with many areas of pathology, can also be used to detect small numbers of virus in biopsy material.

Fig. 8.32 Inclusion bodies in viral infection. These cells in the lung of a patient with immunosuppression show large intranuclear inclusions (**I**) caused by cytomegalovirus.

Fig. 8.33 Inclusion bodies of diagnostic use in viral infection

Virus	Inclusion body
Cytomegalovirus	Intranuclear inclusion surrounded by a halo
Rabies	Eosinophilic rounded cytoplasmic inclusions (Negri bodies)
Hepatitis B	Ground-glass cytoplasm in hepatocytes
Molluscum contagiosum	Eosinophilic cytoplasmic inclusions
Herpes simplex	Eosinophilic intranuclear inclusions
Papovavirus	Basophilic intranuclear inclusions

Prion diseases are caused by an infectious protein-only agent

Certain diseases of man and animals appear to be due to an infectious agent devoid of nucleic acid, composed only of protein called **prion protein**. The diseases include Creutzfeldt-Jakob disease (CJD), variant CJD (vCJD) and kuru in humans, scrapie in sheep, bovine spongiform encephalopathy (BSE) in cows and chronic wasting disease in deer, elk and moose. These are called the **transmissible spongiform encephalopathies** and involve degeneration and death of neurones in the brain (see *Fig. 21.26*).

A normal form of prion protein is found in cell membranes, but an 'infectious' form of the protein has a different structure and is resistant to breakdown by cell proteases. The normal form (called PrPC) has an alpha helical structure, whereas the 'infectious' form (called PrPSc) has a partly beta pleated sheet pattern. When PrPSc gains access to a neurone it triggers the conversion of normal cell prion

protein to the 'infectious' type. The cell accumulates the abnormal PrPSC and dies, releasing the abnormal protein into surrounding tissue to populate adjacent neurones, beginning the cycle all over again.

Most cases of disease are sporadic and of unknown origin. A small proportion of cases are genetic. A gene for the normal prion protein (PRPNP gene) has been identified, and mutations in this gene cause rare inherited prion diseases. Some cases of disease are transmitted either through surgical procedures or tissue transplantation. Transmission is also possible by ingestion. Ingested infectious prion protein can be absorbed via the mucosa-associated lymphoid tissue and then spread to other lymphoid organs, such as tonsils and spleen, where replication may occur. Spread to the brain is probably via nerves and the spinal cord. This may be the route by which human vCJD can be acquired from beef products infected with BSE. More details are given in Ch. 24.

PROTOZOAN AND METAZOAN (HELMINTHIC) PARASITES

Protozoa are unicellular eukaryotic organisms, whereas **metazoa** are multicellular eukaryotic orghanisms. The metazoa are subdivided into:

- **Nematodes** (roundworms).
- **Cestodes** (flatworms).
- **Trematodes** (flukes).

Diseases associated with protozoan and metazoan parasites are most common in tropical countries and in underdeveloped areas where public hygiene is poor, and where the insects which act as vectors in many of the diseases are abundant. However, with the increasing frequency and speed of international travel, many diseases that were previously rarely seen in Britain, Europe and North America are now becoming more common.

The main protozoan and metazoan parasitic infections of clinical significance are presented according to organ involvement in *Figs 8.34* and *8.48*.

DISEASES DUE TO PROTOZOA

The most important and severe protozoan diseases worldwide are:

- **Malaria** – caused by several types of *Plasmodium,* and transmitted to humans by mosquito bites. Parasites in red blood cells cause hemolysis and splenomegaly.
- **Amebiasis** – caused by *Entameba histolytica,* affects the colon producing ulcers and occasionally liver abscesses.
- **Trypanosomiasis** – caused by various members of the *Trypanosoma* family, can exist in two forms depending on the location and the trypanosome involved. African trypanosomiasis ('sleeping sickness') mainly affects the brain, whereas American trypanosomiasis can affect the heart, brain, esophagus and the immune system.
- **Leishmaniasis** – shows three distinct patterns depending on the species of *Leishmania* involved, but all are transmitted to humans by sandfly bites.

Protozoan diseases which are more common in temperate zones tend to be clinically less severe. They include:

- **Toxoplasmosis** – due to infection with *Toxoplasma gondii.*
- **Trichomoniasis** –due to *Trichomonas vaginalis.*
- **Giardiasis** – due to *Giardia lamblia.*
- **Cryptosporidiosis** – due to *Cryptosporidia* species.

Significantly, formerly clinically mild and transient diseases caused by protozoa are now becoming more important, occurring more frequently and with greater severity

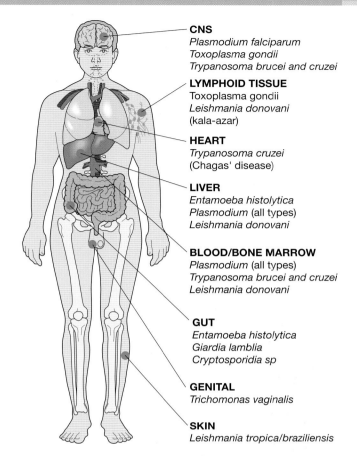

CNS
Plasmodium falciparum
Toxoplasma gondii
Trypanosoma brucei and cruzei

LYMPHOID TISSUE
Toxoplasma gondii
Leishmania donovani
(kala-azar)

HEART
Trypanosoma cruzei
(Chagas' disease)

LIVER
Entamoeba histolytica
Plasmodium (all types)
Leishmania donovani

BLOOD/BONE MARROW
Plasmodium (all types)
Trypanosoma brucei and cruzei
Leishmania donovani

GUT
Entamoeba histolytica
Giardia lamblia
Cryptosporidia sp

GENITAL
Trichomonas vaginalis

SKIN
Leishmania tropica/braziliensis

Fig. 8.34 Protozoan infections.

in the immunosuppressed population, e.g. transplant recipients, patients receiving immunosuppressive therapy, and AIDS patients.

The most important protozoal disease worldwide is malaria caused by the *Plasmodium* species

There are four species of Plasmodium involved (*P. vivax, P. falciparum, P. ovale* and *P. malariae*), but the complicated lifecycle of the parasite is much the same in all (*Fig. 8.34*).

In general, *Plasmodium vivax, Plasmodium ovale* and *Plasmodium malariae* produce a less severe illness than *Plasmodium falciparum.* All types show, to a greater or lesser extent, paroxysmal fevers, anaemia (mainly hemolytic in type), splenomegaly and hepatomegaly.

Plasmodium falciparum is the only type to cause cerebral malaria, and *Plasmodium malariae,* though generally causing a much milder disease than the others, may be complicated by the nephrotic syndrome (see Chapter 17, page 378).

The symptoms, signs and pathological changes in malaria are related to the sequelae of various aspects of the parasite's lifecycle in humans:

- Cyclical fever with rigors and sweats coincides with red cell rupture cycles at the release of merozoites. In *P. falciparum* the fever cycle is not always regular, owing to non-synchronous cycles, but occurs more frequently, usually daily.
- Severe anemia, due mainly to excessive red cell destruction, but marrow suppression may play a part.

- Hepatosplenomegaly due to excessive sequestration of red cells and red cell debris in spleen and hepatic Kupffer cells.
- Cerebral malaria occurs only in *Plasmodium falciparum*. There is rapid onset of severe headache and often convulsions, followed by coma and death. It is usually rapidly fatal. In *falciparum* malaria there is a very high level of parasitemia, so that vast numbers of red cells contain parasites, and the infected red cells are markedly adherent to capillary endothelial cells and to each other. In cerebral malaria, these changes lead to

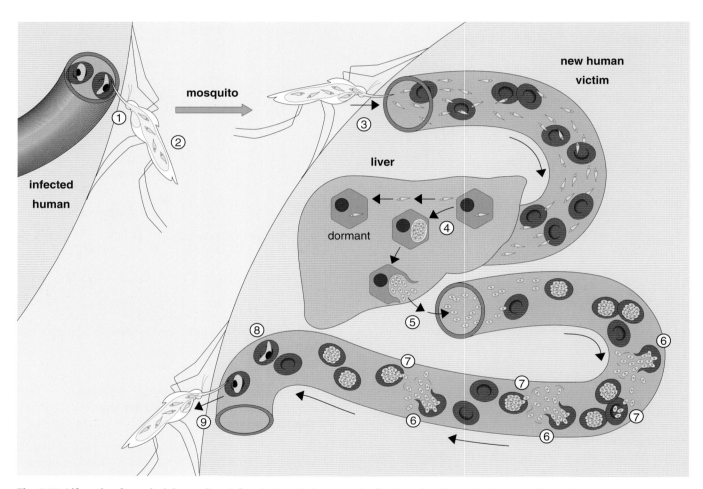

Fig. 8.35 Lifecycle of a malarial parasite. A female *Anopheles* mosquito feeds on the blood of a human suffering from malaria and ingests red blood cells containing male and female *Plasmodium* gametocytes (1). In the gut of the mosquito, the gametocytes reproduce sexually to produce infective sporozoites (2), some of which enter the mosquito salivary glands to be injected into the next human victim the mosquito bites (3). In the human, the parasites pass in the bloodstream to the liver, where they mature and reproduce asexually within hepatocytes to produce many thousands of merozoites (4), which are released into the bloodstream when the affected hepatocytes rupture and die (5). The merozoites invade human red cells and transform into trophozoites, which grow and then divide asexually to produce even more merozoites, which are released when the affected red cell ruptures (6). These merozoites invade other red cells and initiate another cycle of asexual reproduction in red cells → red cell rupture → merozoite release → re-invasion of red cells, etc (7). This cyclical asexual reproductive phase continues for months, even years, occurring every 48 or 72 hours (72 hours for *P. malariae*, 48 hours for the others). Some merozoites in red cells produce male and female gametocytes instead of entering the asexual reproductive cycle (8), and it is these that infect the next female mosquito to feed on the victim's blood (9). Some parasites (at stage 4) can remain sequestered and dormant in liver cells instead of maturing and dividing into merozoites; these dormant parasites are responsible for late relapses.

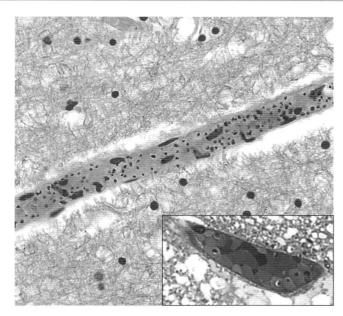

Fig. 8.36 Cerebral malaria. Main picture shows a tiny capillary with numerous black dots apparently within it. This is 'malarial' pigment, a fixation artifact occurring in association with red cells that contain malarial parasites. The inset is an epoxy resin thin section stained with Toluidine blue, showing the parasites within some of the tightly packed red cells.

widespread occlusion of capillaries in the brain, with secondary petechial hemorrhages. Similar capillary occlusion in the myocardium can produce acute cardiac failure.

Entameba histolytica is an important gastrointestinal parasite

This organism is confined to humans, and is transmitted by the orofecal route via the ingestion of food or water contaminated by amebic cysts passed in human feces. In brief, the lifecycle is:

* Ingestion of food or water containing encysted ameba from human feces.
* Cyst wall breaks down in small intestine to release ameba trophozoites.
* Ameba trophozoites penetrate mucosa of colon to produce shallow, flask-shaped ulcers.
* Ameba trophozoites may gain access to colonic submucosal blood vessels, with the potential for extracolonic spread (see below).
* Some trophozoites in the colon become encysted and are passed out in the feces.

Sometimes the ameba trophozoites feed harmlessly on colonic bacteria without significantly damaging the mucosal cells, and the infection is asymptomatic. When significant ulceration occurs (*Fig. 8.37*) amebic dysentery ensues, with abdominal pain and profuse diarrhea (which is often blood-

stained) during acute exacerbations, with intermittent cramping abdominal pain and mild diarrhea between major attacks. Without treatment the disease has a tendency to become chronic, and involvement of the appendix and cecal regions may lead to a large chronic inflammatory mass ('ameboma') in the right iliac fossa. Chronicity, with repeated acute exacerbations, over a period of months or years leads to chronic anemia (due to intermittent blood loss) and emaciation.

Extra-colonic amebiasis results from invasion of colonic submucosal vessels by amebic trophozoites in the ulcers. They pass in the portal venous system to the liver where amebic abscesses may form. Enlargement of a liver abscess may lead to local sub-diaphragmatic abscess and an abscess in adjacent lung tissue. Blood-borne spread from a lung or liver abscess, or from a large ameboma, may rarely produce a brain abscess.

Amebiasis is most common in tropical and subtropical countries, and cases in more temperate climes are usually acquired while living or working abroad. However, it can be a sexually transmitted disease in male homosexuals, due to anal sexual activity.

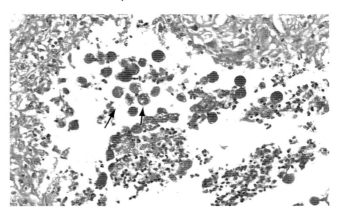

Fig. 8.37 Amebas in a colonic mucosal ulcer. In this photomicrograph the amebas are stained magenta by the PAS stain.

The Trypanosoma group of protozoa contains three distinct species which cause disease via insect vectors

Two of the species (*T. brucei gambiense* and *T. brucei rhodesiense*) are transmitted by tsetse flies and cause sleeping sickness in different parts of sub-Saharan central Africa ('African trypanosomiasis'). After inoculation by a tsetse fly bite, a small inflammatory skin nodule forms at the site but later heals. The parasites disseminate in lymphatics and bloodstream to produce fever, headaches and malaise, often with generalized lymphadenopathy. After a few months (in *T. brucei rhodesiense*) or months to years (in *T. brucei gambiense*), brain involvement becomes manifest as trypanosomes eventually reach the brain in significant numbers. Mixed cerebral symptoms include persistent headache, personality changes, lassitude and somnolence, tremor and ataxia, but progression is towards coma and death, within a year in *T. brucei rhodesiense* and within 3 years in *T. brucei gambiense*.

The third species is *Trypanosoma cruzi*, which is responsible for 'American trypanosomiasis' or **Chagas' disease**. It is largely confined to Central and South America but is seen in the USA in immigrants from these areas. Although most cases are transmitted to humans by an insect vector (reduviid bugs) from a large range of mammalian hosts (dogs, opossums, rats, etc), human-to-human transmission via blood transfusion is possible.

There is an **acute phase** during which organisms spread through the tissues via the bloodstream and lymphatics to infect many tissues, but particularly the nervous system, skeletal and myocardial muscle, and tissues and organs of the immune system. This phase may be asymptomatic, or marked by fever, malaise and lymphadenopathy. In a small percentage of patients there are severe symptoms with acute myocarditis or acute meningoencephalitis, often fatal ('acute Chagas' disease').

The patient enters a **chronic phase** lasting many years in which there may be very gradual tissue destruction, with immune damage playing an important part. The main features of this chronic Chagas' disease are:

- Slowly progressive cardiomyopathy (see page 178), leading to a dilated, chronically failing heart, ventricular aneurysms and dysrhythmias.
- Chronic dilatation of the esophagus and colon due to destruction of myenteric nerve plexuses, to produce changes similar to achalasia of the esophagus (see page 250) and Hirschsprung's disease (see pages 272–3).
- Potential for cross-placental transmission from infected mother, with high incidence of stillbirth or early abortion.
- Potential for reactivation to produce severe acute Chagas' disease if patient becomes severely immunosuppressed.

Leishmaniasis is transmitted by sandfly bites from a wide range of animal reservoirs, and produces three patterns of disease

The most common animal reservoirs in the west are dogs and rodents. The three patterns are cutaneous, mucocutaneous and systemic (visceral) leishmaniasis.

Cutaneous leishmaniasis is usually due to *Leishmania tropica* in Europe, and comprises a chronic ulcerating papule, usually in the skin of the face or arms following a sandfly bite, usually acquired in Southern Europe and the Mediterranean coastline or islands (see *Fig. 23.18*). The lesion is indolent and takes many months to heal, with scarring. The organisms are easily seen within dermal macrophages in early lesions (*Fig. 8.38*) but can be difficult to find in long-standing lesions. Different species in Asia,

Africa, and Central/South America cause similar skin lesions. One of the American species (*L. braziliensis*) occasionally produces:

Mucocutaneous leishmaniasis, in which a lesion of cutaneous leishmaniasis is followed, usually within months, by involvement of the nasal and nasopharyngeal mucosa, resulting in destructive chronic inflammatory masses.

Systemic (visceral) leishmaniasis is also known as kala-azar, and is due to *L. donovani*. It occurs in para-equatorial areas such as Central/South America, India and the Mediterranean coastline. Following a sandfly bite, the parasites

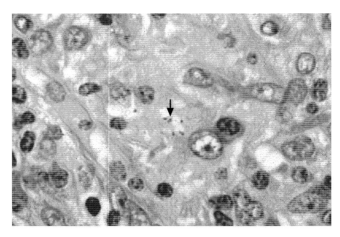

Fig. 8.38 Cutaneous leishmaniasis. Taken from a skin lesion which had been present for 14 days following a sandfly bite during a holiday in Cyprus. The organisms (arrowed) can be seen within the macrophages in the early dermal inflammatory infiltrate.

Fig. 8.39 Systemic leishmaniasis. From the bone marrow of a patient with systemic leishmaniasis. The parasites (*Leishmania donovani* – arrowed) are present in swollen macrophages in the hemopoietic bone marrow.

are distributed in the bloodstream, particularly to organs of the immune defense system such as the spleen, lymph nodes, bone marrow (*Fig. 8.39*) and liver. There is lymphadenopathy, hepatosplenomegaly, and evidence of marrow abnormality in the form of pancytopenia. Up to 80% of patients die if untreated.

Toxoplasmosis commonly produces benign reactive lymph node enlargement, but can be fatal in the immunosuppressed patient

The usual animal reservoir for *Toxoplasma gondii* is the domestic or feral cat, and most human disease is thought to be acquired by orofecal contact with *Toxoplasma* oocysts in cat feces, either directly or indirectly, via contaminated soil. In pregnant women the infection can be passed transplacentally to the fetus. There are the three main clinical patterns.

Acute lymphadenopathic toxoplasmosis is by far the most common. The main clinical feature is benign reactive enlargement of lymph nodes, particularly in the neck. This may be accompanied by an illness with many of the clinical features of infectious mononucleosis, including fever, malaise, sore throat and muscle discomfort. The blood picture shows similar features, with anemia and the presence of atypical lymphocytes in the blood smear. These symptoms may persist for weeks, and the lymphadenopathy may not return to normal for months.

Acute toxoplasma encephalitis is almost confined to immunosuppressed patients, and is now an important infective complication of AIDS. Most cases are probably the result of reactivation of quiescent or latent infection in patients who have previously had, and overcome, lymphadenopathic toxoplasmosis. The brain shows focal areas of necrosis and microvascular thrombosis associated with the presence of intact and ruptured toxoplasmal cysts, the ruptured cyst releasing large numbers of tachyzoites (*Fig. 8.40*). The CNS symptoms relate to the area of the brain involved, but in most cases there is raised intracranial pressure, altered mental state, fits and coma.

Congenital toxoplasmosis is due to transplacental spread from the infected mother. Severe infection early in pregnancy usually leads to spontaneous abortion or stillbirth. If the child survives in utero, it may be born with a structural brain disorder such as microcephaly or hydrocephaly, usually with foci of calcification in the brain, and choroidoretinitis. At birth, such neonates may have persisting jaundice, with a palpably enlarged liver. Less severe infections acquired when the mother contracts toxoplasmosis late in pregnancy may lead to an apparently normal infant, but symptoms due to toxoplasmosis may present later in childhood, particularly in the form of a choroidoretinitis (ocular toxoplasmosis).

Fig. 8.40 Acute encephalitis due to toxoplasmosis. In a portion of the brain alongside a small blood vessel a toxoplasma cyst has ruptured to release large numbers of minute organisms (arrow).

Trichomonas vaginalis most commonly causes vaginitis in women, and occasionally mild urethritis in men

This protozoan parasite is flagellated and highly motile, and can be easily identified under the microscope in a wet preparation of vaginal fluid in cases of infection. They are also frequently seen in cytological smear preparations taken for the diagnosis of cervical dysplasia (*Fig. 8.41*). The organism is transmitted by sexual intercourse, and in women produces a heavy vaginal discharge with an offensive smell, with secondary inflammation of the vaginal mucosa and often the vulval skin. Men are usually asymptomatic, or at the most have a mild urethritis. Because transmission is sexual, both partners should be treated whether symptomatic or not.

Fig. 8.41 *Trichomonas vaginalis* in a vaginal smear. Taken from a young woman with vaginal soreness and discharge, showing the greyish protozoan (arrows) and some darker-staining neutrophil polymorphs.

Giardia lamblia is a common intestinal parasite and may cause malabsorption syndrome

Giardia cysts occur in water, and infection is particularly likely to occur in areas of the world where sanitation is poor and water supplies are contaminated by human feces. The cysts are passed in the feces by infected humans and some other mammals, and there is potential for direct orofecal transmission. The organism is flagellated and attaches to the surface enterocytes of the duodenum and proximal jejunum (*Fig. 8.42*), and may interfere with the absorption of sugars and fats, leading to chronic malabsorption syndrome with the frequent passage of offensive soft or semi-liquid feces. Even without malabsorption the patient suffers from abdominal cramps and flatulence, although many remain asymptomatic carriers, passing both the sensitive trophozoites and the resistant cysts (which are the important source of reinfection and spread) in their feces.

Cryptosporidiosis is an important cause of infective diarrhea and is highly contagious

Infection can be spread from humans or animals by the orofecal route, but most outbreaks are the result of water supplies contaminated by human or animal feces.

The parasites live and replicate within the brush border of the absorptive enterocytes of the small intestine (*Fig. 8.43*), eventually producing oocysts which pass to the external environment in the feces. The infection produces profuse diarrhea and abdominal cramps, often lasting 2–3 weeks, being most severe and prolonged in patients with AIDS. Even after the patient has recovered from the acute illness, infective oocysts continue to be excreted in the feces.

Fig. 8.42 *Giardia lamblia* near duodenal mucosa. The ill-defined slightly purplish-stained organisms lie mainly free above the surface of the mucosa.

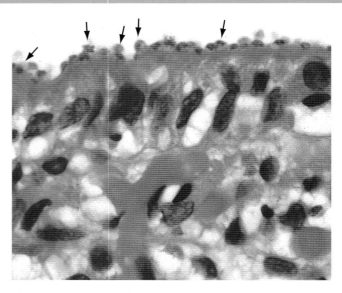

Fig. 8.43 Cryptosporidiosis in the small intestine. Showing the purple-staining Cryptosporidia (arrows) colonizing the surface of the enterocytes.

FLUKE (TREMATODE) INFECTIONS

There are many types of fluke infection worldwide, but the most important is schistosomiasis (bilharziasis), in which the water snail is the intermediate host. Different *Schistosoma* species affect different areas of the human body, and have different geographic distributions.

Schistosomiasis due to *Schistosoma haematobium* predominantly affects the human bladder

Schistosoma haematobium is widespread throughout Africa, including some tourist resorts on the North African coast. In simple terms, the organism's eggs pass in the urine of an infected human to contaminate fresh water, where they hatch and infect a freshwater snail, within the body of which they multiply to produce large numbers of infective cercariae which swim freely in the water. These can penetrate the skin of humans walking in the water and eventually migrate to the veins in the wall of the bladder, where they develop into sexually active adult worms which reproduce to form eggs. In the early stages there may be a localized itchy rash or lump at the site or sites of human skin (usually feet and lower legs) where the cercariae have penetrated. In the late stages (chronic schistosomiasis) the symptoms are due to the chronic inflammatory reaction in the bladder wall to the presence of schistosome eggs (*Fig. 8.44*). There is initially a florid chronic inflammatory and granulomatous reaction, followed by fibrosis. This leads to ulceration of the bladder mucosa which becomes chronic and is often attended by repeated attempts at re-epithelialization, which produces papillomatous masses of transitional epithelium, some of which may become malignant. The chronic

Fig. 8.44 Schistosoma in the bladder. There is a florid foreign body giant cell reaction and severe chronic inflammation in response to the presence of partly calcified schistosome eggs (arrows).

inflammation affecting the urothelium frequently leads to **squamous metaplasia**, and this may also be followed by the development of malignancy in the form of squamous carcinoma of the bladder.

Schistosomiasis due to *S. mansoni* and *S. japonicum* affects the alimentary tract and the liver

S. mansoni occurs in Africa and Central and South America, and *S. japonicum* occurs in the Far East. They gain access to humans in the same way as *S. haematobium*, but the organisms migrate not to the bladder but to the intestinal wall, where they produce ulceration, strictures and chronic fibrosis by chronic inflammatory, granulomatous and fibrous reaction to the presence of eggs. From the intestine some organisms migrate via the portal venous system to the liver, where they can produce a periportal fibrosis, sometimes leading to a pseudo-cirrhosis pattern. Because the damage is particularly marked in the portal triads, portal hypertension and hematemesis are important complications. Occasionally the eggs can be transferred to the lungs, where a foreign body granulomatous and fibrotic reaction can occur.

TAPEWORM (CESTODE) INFESTATIONS

Adult tapeworms are flat segmented worms (*Fig. 8.45*), each comprising:

* A head (or 'scolex'), which bears hooklets with which it attaches to the small intestinal mucosa of the host.
* Neck, from which the linked segments arise.
* Segments (proglottides), which are very small when they are formed in the neck region, but become larger

and more mature as they are pushed distally by new small segment formation.

The larger distal segments are sexually mature and contain a uterus within which eggs are formed (the worms are hermaphroditic). In most types (*Taenia saginata*, *Diphyllobothrium latum* and usually *Taenia solium*), the eggs pass out in the feces of the human host to be ingested by a variety of other animals (according to tapeworm species), within which the eggs hatch into 'oncospheres' which penetrate the blood vessels in the animal's intestinal wall and are carried around the body, often lodging in skeletal muscle where they become encysted and develop to contain a scolex or head.

Human infection is acquired by eating the affected animal's meat. In this pattern, the main effects on the human host are usually mild, often without significant symptoms. There may be mild abdominal pain and diarrhea, but sometimes large tapeworms may produce weight loss, malnutrition and vitamin deficiencies. This is because tapeworms have no alimentary tract, and nourish themselves by direct absorption of food and vitamins from the human small bowel lumen.

Important exceptions to this lifecycle pattern are hydatid disease and one variant of *Taenia solium* infestation (see below).

Fig. 8.45 A tapeworm (*Taenia saginata*). Mounted museum specimen of an almost entire tapeworm. From the scale it is easy to calculate its full length. At the top (the head) the worm is extremely small, with progressively enlarging segments distally.

Taenia saginata infestation is acquired by eating raw or undercooked infected beef

This disease has been largely eradicated in affluent nations owing to strict herd control, abattoir inspection, and examination of the butchered beast. It still occurs in poor countries, for example in parts of Africa, South America, Eastern Europe and the Middle East. In these areas, the use of human feces as a soil fertilizer, and inadequate treatment and disposal of sewage, play a part in the perpetuation of the cyclical infestation.

Taenia solium infestation is usually acquired by eating undercooked infected pork, but humans can also act as intermediate hosts by direct orofecal infection

Taenia solium can behave exactly like *T. saginata*, the ingestion of undercooked infected pork leading to the development of a mature worm in the small intestine. Like *T. saginata*, this infestation is usually asymptomatic or, at worst, responsible for mild abdominal discomfort and intermittent diarrhea. However, there is a much more serious pattern of illness when humans act as the intermediate host, in which the oncospheres hatch and spread. This may occur by direct human-to-human orofecal spread, the eggs hatching into oncospheres in the human stomach, then spreading in the bloodstream in the pattern normally seen in the cow (*T. saginata*) and pig. The oncospheres may spread to many sites (skin, muscle, internal organs, etc), where they encyst and form scolices, but the main target organs are the brain and spinal cord. The enlarging cysts may produce symptoms of a brain or spinal cord tumor. The symptoms are particularly severe when the cyst dies, as a vigorous inflammatory reaction results. Dead cysts are usually calcified and can be identified by brain imaging.

Echinococcus granulosus produces 'hydatid disease,' characterized by the formation of cysts, mainly in the liver

In this pattern, like the severe systemic variant of *T. solium* infection described above, humans act as the intermediate host, ingesting the eggs and developing migrating oncospheres, most of which pass to the liver (occasionally lungs) to produce slowly enlarging cysts containing daughter cysts within each of which is a scolex (*Fig. 8.46*). Rupture of a liver or lung cyst can lead to wide dissemination of scolices.

The main host is the dog, and the main alternative intermediate host is the sheep. Dogs acquire the infection by eating infected sheep, and humans become infected through contact with dog feces containing the eggs, probably by hand-to-mouth contamination. The disease is particularly

Fig. 8.46 Echinococcus granulosus. A collection of scolices of *Echinococcus granulosus* found on microscopy of the fluid contents of a hydatid cyst of the liver.

important in sheep farming areas such as Australia, New Zealand, the Mediterranean, South America, etc.

In the United Kingdom, Wales is the most common area for the disease to originate. The disease is also seen in some areas of North America, particularly Canada and Alaska; in these areas the moose is the main host rather than sheep.

Diphyllobothrium latum infestation is acquired by eating raw or undercooked infected freshwater fish

The worm gets into fish after a freshwater environment, particularly a lake, is contaminated by human feces due to inadequate sewage treatment and disposal. The eggs hatch into minute larvae in the water and are consumed by small crustaceans, which in turn are eaten by fish, some of which are caught and eaten by humans. It occurs worldwide, particularly in cold or temperate zones with abundant lakes. In the human small intestine the mature worms absorb food and vitamins, particularly Vitamin B_{12}, and may cause megaloblastic anemia (see pages 150 and 319–20).

ROUNDWORMS (NEMATODES)

Unlike tapeworms (cestodes) and flukes (trematodes), roundworms have a body cavity. They can affect humans in various ways, a few of which are briefly outlined below.

- Occupation of the human alimentary tract. Heavy infestations may produce abdominal pain and malnutrition, e.g. *Ascaris lumbricoides*, **trichuriasis**, or anemia due to the worm sucking blood from the intestinal mucosa, e.g. *Ancylostoma* **species**.
- Larval migration through the lungs may cause Löffler's syndrome (eosinophilic pneumonia), e.g. *Toxocara canis, Toxocara catis, Ascaris lumbricoides*.
- Multiple cysts containing larvae in tissues, particularly skeletal muscle, e.g. *Trichinella spiralis*.
- Obstruction of lymphatics, e.g. **filariasis**, often leading to marked lymphedema.
- Acute and chronic dermatitis, chronic skin ulcers and nodules, e.g. **Guinea worm**, **strongyloidiasis**, **Ancylostoma**, **Onchocerca**, **Loa-loa**.
- Eye lesions, e.g. **Toxocara** (ocular larva migrans), **Onchocerca** (river blindness), **Loa-loa** (migrating larva in conjunctiva).

The majority of the above are mainly tropical and subtropical diseases. Students are advised to read a microbiology or tropical medicine text for details of lifecycles and variety of clinical manifestations. A few of the more important are detailed below.

Ancylostoma species are hookworms which attach to the small intestinal mucosa and feed on the host's blood

Eggs in moist soil hatch into larvae which penetrate human skin and pass in the bloodstream to the lungs, from where they gain access to the small intestine in a similar manner to *Ascaris* larvae, as described below. On the way in, the penetrating larvae may cause a localized itchy rash, and blood eosinophilia and Löffler's syndrome may occur as the larvae pass through the bloodstream and lungs. When the worms are attached in the small intestine there may be only mild abdominal symptoms, but persistence leads to a chronic iron deficiency anemia due to the constant removal of blood from the small intestinal mucosa by the hookworm.

Ascaris lumbricoides eventually occupy the gut as mature roundworms, but the larval stage passes through the lungs

Ingested eggs hatch into larvae in the duodenum, the larvae passing into the bloodstream and reaching the lungs, where they may produce a transient Löffler's syndrome (eosinophilic pneumonitis). The larvae climb up the bronchi into the pharynx and are then swallowed to pass into the small intestine, where they develop into mature roundworms

Fig. 8.47 *Ascaris lumbricoides*. A freshly passed Ascaris roundworm in an enamel toilet bowl.

(*Fig. 8.47*). Unless there are large numbers of worms in the intestine the infestation may be asymptomatic, except in children, where there may be abdominal pain and failure to thrive. Heavy infestations in adults may produce similar symptoms. Mature worms produce eggs which are excreted in the feces. The disease is most common in tropical and subtropical areas, but may occur in rural areas in Europe and the USA, wherever sanitation facilities are poor.

Toxocariasis is a potentially important infection contractable by contact with dog and cat feces

This condition is particularly important in children who play in an environment where they may come into contact with dog and cat feces, and workers such as kennel maids. There are two main varieties, *Toxocara canis* and *Toxocara cati*, affecting dogs and cats, respectively. Eggs are passed from the animal's alimentary tract in the feces and may be ingested by humans by orofecal contamination. The eggs hatch in the human small intestine and penetrate into intestinal blood vessels, and are carried to the liver, brain, eyes, lungs and many other tissues, where they excite a florid chronic inflammatory granulomatous response, in which eosinophils are very numerous. There are two important clinical syndromes, one associated with the larvae locating in the eye ('ocular larva migrans' or 'ocular toxocariasis') and the other with widespread larval dissemination to other internal organs ('visceral larva migrans').

Ocular larva migrans is due to the florid granulomatous reaction in the eye, particularly in the retina, where it may lead to severe visual impairment. This pattern is mainly confined to children.

Visceral larva migrans is accompanied by severe systemic manifestations such as fever, raised white cell count with greatly increased numbers of eosinophils, with asthmatic symptoms and pneumonitis (if the larvae are numerous in the lungs) and hepatosplenomegaly (if the liver and spleen are involved). This mainly occurs in children under the age of 6. The larvae in the skin may produce an itchy rash, and severe cerebral symptoms may occur if the larvae reach the brain, although this is uncommon.

Pinworm infestation is very common in young children and usually presents clinically with perianal itching or soreness

The small pinworm (*Enterobius vermicularis*) is a very common parasite in children in temperate zones and of all social classes. The worm is small and difficult to see unless special methods are used to trap and identify it. The female worm is about 1 cm long, and is two to three times as big as the male. Infection is by direct or indirect orofecal transmission, directly from finger to mouth in young children who have scratched an itchy ova-laden perineum, or indirectly by contact with clothing or bedding in which the ova have come to rest. The ova hatch and mature into worms in the colon and rectum. The mature female migrates to the anus and perianal skin to deposit its ova, and the worms can sometimes be identified and trapped on the child's perianal skin at night, when the child is complaining particularly of itching. Sometimes placing a strip of transparent sticky tape over the anus may pick up eggs and even trap the female worms when they emerge to lay eggs at night. Once the eggs have been laid successfully, there is a very high chance of repeated reinfection by the orofecal route. However, the eggs can survive in clothing and bedding, etc., for days or even weeks.

Key Facts
Tissue reaction to protozoan and helminthic infection

The tissue response to protozoan and metazoan infections varies greatly between different organisms. Some common factors are evident:

- The immune response is operative in most infections with type I and type IV hypersensitivity responses. Immunosuppression is an important reason for fatal parasitic infection.
- Eosinophils play an important role in defense against parasitic infestation. Tissue and blood eosinophilia is frequently seen in such infections.
- Certain organisms induce tissue necrosis and acute inflammation, e.g. amebas.
- Certain organisms induce hypersensitivity responses and tissue damage is the result of the host immune response, e.g. fibrosis caused by *Schistosoma*.

CNS
Taenia solium (pork tapeworm), *Echinococcus granulosus* (hydatid cyst), *Trichinella spiralis*

EYE
Onchocerca volvulus, *Loa-loa*, *Toxocara catis/canis*

LUNG
Paragonimus westermani (liver fluke), *Strongyloides stercoralis*, *Wuchereria bancrofti* (filariasis), *Ascaris lumbricoides* (roundworm), *Echinococcus granulosus* (hydatid cyst)

LYMPHOID TISSUE
Wuchereria bancrofti (filariasis)

HEART
Trichinella spiralis

LIVER
Clonorchis sinensis, *Fasciola hepatica* (liver fluke), *Schistosoma mansoni/japonicum* *Echinococcus granulosus* (hydatid cyst)

LARGE INTESTINE
Enterobius vermicularis (pinworm), *Trichuris trichiura* (whipworm)

SMALL INTESTINE
Ascaris lumbricoides (roundworm), *Necator americanus* (hookworm), *Ancylostoma duodenale* (hookworm), *Taenia solium* (pork tapeworm), *Taenia saginata* (beef tapeworm)

BLADDER
Schistosoma haematobium

SKELETAL MUSCLE
Trichinella spiralis, *Taenia solium* (pork tapeworm)

SKIN
Onchocerca volvulus, *Loa-loa*, *Toxocara catis/canis*

Fig. 8.48 Metazoan infestations.

Environmental and nutritional factors in disease

9

ENVIRONMENTAL FACTORS IN DISEASE

Although an interplay between genetic and environmental factors often modifies the host response, many diseases are predominantly due to adverse environmental factors, the most important of which are mechanical trauma, extremes of temperature, exposure to radiation, electricity and chemicals, environmental pollution, and nutrition.

MECHANICAL TRAUMA

Mechanical trauma is responsible for a considerable proportion of emergency hospital admissions. The effects of the trauma will be dependent on:

- The nature of the trauma.
- The force of impact.
- The site or sites traumatized.

A special type of mechanical injury occurs with sudden changes in pressure, exemplified by blast injuries caused by proximity to explosions. In such cases, pressure waves may enter the body through air passages, causing traumatic rupture of lungs and intestines.

Skin and soft tissue injuries are common in trauma

The most frequent types of mechanical trauma are skin and soft tissue injuries. These may be divided into:

- **Abrasion** – removal of surface layers by friction.
- **Contusion** – rupture of small blood vessels, leading to extravasation of blood into tissues (bruising).
- **Laceration** – ragged tear in tissue.
- **Incision and puncture wounds** – caused by penetrating sharp objects, e.g. a knife, wooden stake, or broken glass.

Injuries to bone and tendon may be acute or chronic

Certain types of trauma lead to acute injuries. The most common type of acute bony injury after trauma is partial

Motor vehicle accidents

Trauma due to motor vehicle accidents is of major clinical and social importance. Damage inflicted is related to several factors, the most important of which are speed of travel, restraint, and protection from impact. There are three main types of injury:

1. **Injuries caused by sudden deceleration.** When a body is accelerated and then suddenly brought to a stop, the resulting internal stresses may cause severe damage.
   - The aorta may be transected, leading to severe internal bleeding.
   - The brain may sustain internal tearing of white matter tracts.
2. **Injuries caused by direct trauma.** These occur when a body impacts on parts of a vehicle or with road surfaces. There may be:
   - Lacerations to face and hands from windshield glass.
   - Fracture of sternum and ribs from impact with steering column.
   - Fracture of legs from collapse of car frame, or from impact of car on a pedestrian.
   - Contusional damage and laceration of liver, spleen and lungs.
   - Contusions of brain, and fracture of neck from impact damage to head.
3. **Injury secondary to impaired cardiorespiratory function.** Blood loss, unconsciousness, and interruption of the airway are common in victims of trauma and lead to secondary damage.
   - Brain is extremely vulnerable to hypoxia, developing neuronal death.
   - Kidneys may develop tubular necrosis.

or complete fracture of the bone. Fracture is associated with pain centered on the site of injury, and there is often considerable bleeding into the muscles and other tissues around the bone. Bone fracture is discussed in Chapter 24.

Acute musculotendinous injuries, such as torn muscle fibers, partially or completely ruptured tendons, and dislocated joints (particularly of the fingers and shoulder), are common sporting injuries.

More insidious is chronic trauma resulting in chronic musculoskeletal injuries, particularly osteoarthritis of joints (see pages 548–9). Thickening of tendon sheaths may result from repetitive minor trauma over a long period. It is particularly common in certain occupations, e.g. those that involve typing, and is a major contributor to so-called 'repetitive strain injury' (RSI).

Musculotendinous and joint injuries are discussed in Chapter 24.

DAMAGE FROM EXTREMES OF TEMPERATURE

Burns are caused by local heat injury

Direct exposure of the skin to severe heat produces burns, the severity of the burn being related to the degree of heat and the length of exposure.

The two factors that influence the outcome of burn injury are the depth of the burn (*Fig. 9.1*) and the surface area of skin affected.

Burns may be classified as major or minor, according to extent and depth. First-degree burns, although painful, are classed as minor and have little systemic impact. The immediate systemic consequence of a second-degree burn to more than 20% of the body is extravasation of fluid, including high-protein exudate, from the burn site. This loss causes hypovolemic shock, manifest by low blood pressure and failure of tissue perfusion. There is a hypermetabolic state, frequently requiring special nutritional support.

Victims involved in a fire frequently have other injuries that influence outcome, e.g. airways injury due to inhalation of hot air, carbon monoxide inhalation, and chemical inflammation of the lung caused by inhalation of toxic smoke.

In the period following a major burn, there are several further potential complications. There may be secondary infection of the burn, particularly by *Pseudomonas aeruginosa*, *Staphylococcus aureus*, streptococci and *Candida*, and lung damage due to shock (ARDS, see pages 206–7) can develop.

First-degree burns heal rapidly without scarring. Keratinocytes migrate from skin appendages such as hair follicles and eccrine ducts to form a new layer over the intact dermis and dermoepidermal basement membrane.

Full-thickness burns heal with dermal scarring. The only natural way to re-epithelialize is by migration of keratinocytes from the edges of the wound. This is assisted by skin grafting from an intact area of skin elsewhere. Despite graft-

Fig. 9.1 Depth of burns.

ing, excessive tissue scarring with contractures is a frequent complication.

Generalized heat injury can lead to death if untreated

Normally, heat gain by the body is counterbalanced by heat loss, mainly through the skin by radiation and evaporation; evaporation (of watery sweat from the skin surface) is the most important when ambient and internal body temperatures are high. The effectiveness of evaporation from the skin depends on ambient humidity, being minimal when the atmospheric humidity exceeds 70%. When body temperature rises above normal limits, the anterior hypothalamus initiates a number of physiological cooling responses, increasing blood flow to the skin to increase radiation and conduction loss, and stimulating increased sweat production by the eccrine glands in the skin. When these compensating heat loss mechanisms cannot lower the body temperature adequately, generalized heat injury (hyperthermia) may occur. It is most common in those exposed to a hot environment, particularly during strenuous physical exercise in high humidity. There are three patterns, of increasing severity:

Heat cramps are due to disturbances of electrolytes, which are lost in sweat. Treatment is by salt replacement.

Heat exhaustion is more severe. It occurs when fluid loss has been so severe that hemoconcentration occurs, and produces weakness, nausea, dizziness and headaches. Hypotension develops and the pulse is weak. Treatment involves oral rehydration and cooling.

Heat stroke is the most severe and only occurs when the body temperature rises above 41°C (106°F). In addition to the symptoms of heat exhaustion, the victim develops confusion, delirium with hallucinations, and loss of consciousness. Unless treatment is prompt there is a high risk of death from multiple organ failure or brain damage. Treatment is by fluid and electrolyte replacement and rapid lowering of body temperature.

Fig. 9.2 Frostbite of toes. Localized cold injury has caused necrosis of the toes in this person, exposed to the extreme cold while on a climbing expedition in the Himalayas. Similar changes may also occur in the fingers.

Localized cold injury leads to frostbite

The main syndrome caused by localized injury due to cold is frostbite, which occurs when part of the body is exposed to temperatures below freezing point. There is vasoconstriction and thrombosis in arteries, leading to tissue necrosis within a few hours (*Fig. 9.2*).

Hypothermia can cause death due to failure of cellular metabolism

Hypothermia is a generalized reduction in body temperature, usually due to prolonged exposure to low temperatures. It is most common in the elderly, in whom thermoregulatory mechanisms may be inefficient, and is particularly likely to occur if the person is immobile. It is not uncommon for hypothermia to complicate collapse from another disease process. For example, elderly patients are often found unconscious or semi-comatose in their poorly heated houses in winter. As well as an initial cause for collapse, such as a stroke, they are also found to have a low body temperature. Patients with hypothyroidism (myxedema) are particularly prone to developing hypothermia.

If the patient is warmed, recovery is possible. In severe cases patients die from cardiac failure or secondary bronchopneumonia. Acute pancreatitis is another complication.

DAMAGE FROM IRRADIATION

Ultraviolet radiation causes acute and chronic forms of skin damage

Melanin pigment in the keratinocyte cell layers of the skin has a protective function against the effects of ultraviolet (UV) radiation. As a result, Caucasians are particularly vulnerable to skin damage.

The most frequent type of damage is sunburn, in which dermal capillaries dilate and the epidermis undergoes necrosis, with blistering and eventual shedding. Healing occurs by re-formation of the epidermis from keratinocytes that migrate from undamaged basal cells.

Several skin rashes occur largely in areas exposed to light, and exposure to UV radiation is thought to be one of the factors involved in producing the skin damage (**photodermatitis**). However, there are other contributory factors, e.g. exposure to plant-derived allergens or an underlying intrinsic disease such as systemic lupus erythematosus. Testing may demonstrate skin sensitivity to UV radiation of a particularly narrow wavelength, and the application of a topical UV-blocking cream cures the rash.

UV radiation is a predisposing factor for development of neoplasia in skin

UV radiation is known to damage DNA in epidermal cells, and several malignant tumors of skin in Caucasians are believed to be caused by exposure to this type of radiation, particularly **malignant melanoma** and **basal cell carcinoma** (see Chapter 23).

In the rare autosomal recessive disease **xeroderma pigmentosum** there is an inherited deficiency of endonuclease, the enzyme partly responsible for the repair of DNA damaged, for example, by UV radiation. Children with this disorder develop severe abnormalities in the epidermis, followed by the development of multiple squamous cell carcinomas. Protection of the skin from sunlight prevents or greatly delays the development of malignant skin tumors in such cases.

Ionizing radiation causes damage to DNA

In terms of tissue damage, the main impact of ionizing radiation is on cell DNA. Ionizing radiation is normally present in the environment, and individuals may also be exposed to artificial sources, e.g. radiation used in diagnostic imaging. The ionizing radiations of medical importance are:

- X-rays and γ rays.
- α particles, β particles and neutrons.

To cause damage, ionizing radiation must be absorbed by tissues. It removes electrons from atoms of the tissue through which it passes, generating free radicals. These interact with DNA and cause strand breaks, base alterations and abnormal cross-linking. The DNA damage can either lead to immediate cell death or cell death at the next division, or may cause alterations in the genome, rendering a cell susceptible to neoplasia (see pages 30–1).

The extent and severity of radiation damage depends on the dose, duration of exposure, and sensitivity of individual cell types to the radiation.

The dose of radiation absorbed is expressed in grays (Gy; 1 Gy is equivalent to 100 rads, the previous dose unit). Because different types of ionizing radiation penetrate tissues to varying degrees, and different tissues vary in their sensitivity to radiation, doses are corrected mathematically as dose equivalents expressed in sieverts (Sv). (1 Sv is equivalent to 100 rems, the previous dose unit.)

In general, cell types with a high turnover (frequent mitoses) are the most sensitive; those with a low turnover are the least sensitive. This differential sensitivity of cells with a rapid mitotic and replication rate is the basis of the treatment of malignant tumors (composed of rapidly replicating cells) by ionizing radiation (radiotherapy).

There are three main types of exposure to ionizing radiation

The body is exposed to harmful amounts of ionizing radiation in three main ways:

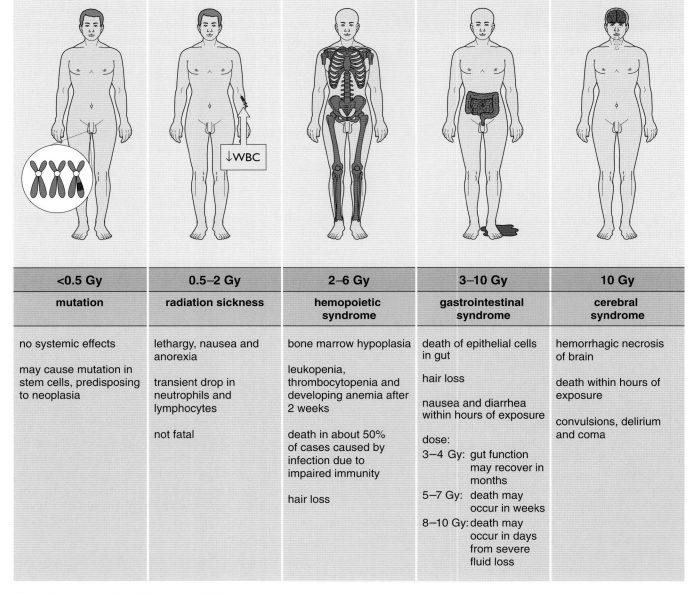

<0.5 Gy	0.5–2 Gy	2–6 Gy	3–10 Gy	10 Gy
mutation	**radiation sickness**	**hemopoietic syndrome**	**gastrointestinal syndrome**	**cerebral syndrome**
no systemic effects may cause mutation in stem cells, predisposing to neoplasia	lethargy, nausea and anorexia transient drop in neutrophils and lymphocytes not fatal	bone marrow hypoplasia leukopenia, thrombocytopenia and developing anemia after 2 weeks death in about 50% of cases caused by infection due to impaired immunity hair loss	death of epithelial cells in gut hair loss nausea and diarrhea within hours of exposure dose: 3–4 Gy: gut function may recover in months 5–7 Gy: death may occur in weeks 8–10 Gy: death may occur in days from severe fluid loss	hemorrhagic necrosis of brain death within hours of exposure convulsions, delirium and coma

Fig. 9.3 Responses to total body irradiation.

1. **Slow, cumulative, whole-body exposure.** This is usually due to natural or low-output industrial and medical sources. An important source of natural radiation is radon, a radioactive gas which naturally diffuses from hard rocks such as granite and may reach high concentrations in some buildings.
2. **Sudden, whole-body exposure.** This is usually due to industrial or military sources.
3. **High-dose, localized exposure.** This is mainly a result of therapeutic ionizing radiation used to treat tumors.

In the UK the annual average exposure to radiation is 2.5 mSv. Just over 10% of this is from medical usage. The clinical response to total body irradiation ranges from none to rapid death depending on the dose (*Fig. 9.3*).

Fig. 9.4 Photomicrograph of irradiation vascular damage.
After irradiation, vessels develop fibrinoid necrosis in walls (**F**) and hyalinization. Fibroblasts develop large hyperchromatic nuclei. The vascular changes lead to secondary ischemic damage to tissue.

Long-term effects of irradiation are related to chronic vascular damage

In addition to the acute effects of irradiation, tissues frequently show long-term or delayed effects of exposure. A common factor in such delayed effects is damage to blood vessels, which show intimal proliferation, hyalinization, and occasionally fibrinoid necrosis, long after exposure (*Fig. 9.4*). These changes cause secondary ischemic changes in tissue, with fibroblast proliferation and scarring. A summary of acute and delayed effects of radiation exposure is shown in *Fig. 9.5*.

Fig. 9.5 Summary of effects of irradiation on various tissues		
Tissue	**Acute effect**	**Chronic effect**
Skin	Desquamation and edema	Pigmentation and thinning Carcinoma
Bone		Bone necrosis Premature closure of epiphyses in children
Bone marrow	Marrow hypoplasia	Risk of leukemia
Ovary/testis	Destruction of germ cells	Atrophy and fibrosis
Lungs	Acute radiation pneumonitis	Alveolar wall fibrosis
Gut	Mucosal necrosis	Submucosal fibrosis and stricture
Kidney	Acute radiation nephritis with acute renal failure	Gradual loss of renal parenchyma, with chronic renal failure
Brain	Transient somnolence	Developmental delay in young children
Eye		Cataracts
Ear		Deafness
Thyroid		Hypothyroidism Risk of thyroid carcinoma

ELECTRICAL INJURY

Electrical injuries may be classified as:

- Lightning strikes.
- Low-voltage injury.
- High-voltage injury.

The severity of the injury depends on many factors, mainly the voltage and the resistance to current flow: the higher the voltage and the lower the resistance to current flow, the more severe the injury. Dry skin offers the greatest resistance to flow, and wet skin the least. There are two main effects of electrical injury:

- **Interference with normal body electrical activity**
The passage of current through the heart causes cardiac arrhythmia, particularly ventricular fibrillation. The passage of current through the brain, both low voltage and high voltage, produces unconsciousness because of depolarization of the neurons, and there may be cessation of activity in cardiorespiratory centers. Both may produce cardiorespiratory arrest. Spasm of skeletal muscles may cause bone fractures.
- **Generation of heat, causing burns** If there is prolonged contact with the electrical source (for some minutes), local generation of heat will cause burns. Prolonged exposure is particularly seen with alternating current sources as they cause tetanic spasms of muscles, preventing withdrawal from the electrical source. Even where there are not extensive burns, small localized skin burns may be apparent at the site of entry of the current in accidental or lightning strike electrocution, for example in the palm when a live electrical source has been grasped in the hand. Small localized burns may also be found at the exit point of the current. Identification of these sites, and histological confirmation of electric burn, are useful in forensic practice, aiding reconstruction of the event at the scene of a fatal electrocution. The histological appearances are characteristic, with extreme elongated spindling distortion of the cells and modification of their staining characteristics by heat coagulation of the protein. Similar changes are seen in tissues diathermied during surgery ('diathermy artefact').

CHEMICAL DAMAGE

Toxic chemicals can gain access to the body by many routes, including skin contact, inhalation, ingestion, and injection.

Exposure may be accidental (due to environmental or industrial exposure) or deliberate, the result of therapeutic, addictive or suicidal self-administration, or covert homicidal administration. Some chemicals have a direct toxic effect on cells, whereas others produce damage indirectly by acting as antigens and initiating a damaging immune response.

Ethyl alcohol is a potent toxin that affects many major organs

Ethyl alcohol consumption in alcoholic beverages is common in most societies. The pathopharmacology of ethanol and its psychological effects are important aspects of social medicine. In terms of structural pathology, ethanol has several main effects.

Acute intoxication. Ethanol is a depressant, leading to impaired consciousness and, ultimately, to respiratory depression at high levels. A frequent complication of excessive consumption is coma, during which aspiration of vomit into the lungs leads to death. Other acute effects of very high concentrations are acute gastritis (see pages 251–2) and acute alcoholic hepatitis (see pages 290–2).

Chronic ethanol abuse. This is frequently part of physical and psychological dependence on alcohol. The main pathological effects are:

- Chronic liver disease, leading to liver failure.
- Cardiomyopathy, leading to cardiac failure (see page 179).
- Pancreatitis, causing severe, intractable abdominal pain (see page 303).
- Peripheral neuropathy, often caused by associated vitamin deficiency.
- Brain damage, leading to cognitive decline and ataxia due to neuronal death.
- Fetal alcohol syndrome, seen in the offspring of mothers who are dependent on alcohol.

Substances of abuse cause disease by both direct and indirect effects

Substances of abuse taken for recreational purposes are a major social problem. Drugs abused are commonly stimulants, depressants, or hallucinogenics. They are taken by injection into the skin (skin popping), intravenously (mainlining), smoking, sniffing (snorting) or orally. Solvents are abused by inhalation (glue sniffing) and butane gas is inhaled. Associated pathology can be attributed to both direct and indirect effects.

Addiction to heroin and other opiates can lead to a wide range of pathologies

The pathological sequelae of opiate addiction can be divided into those due to the drug itself, those due to the presence of a contaminant in the injected drug (e.g. powdered talc, quinine, etc.), those due to unsterile administration, and those due to social pathology (risk of violence, etc.).

- **Direct opiate effect** – usually due to overdose, leading to depression of the cardiorespiratory center in the brain. Progressively slowing heart and breathing rates, with hypotension, eventually lead to coma, cardiorespiratory arrest and death due to acute pulmonary edema. Regurgitation of gastric contents while semi-comatose, with inhalation into the respiratory tract, is also a common cause of death.

- **Effects due to drug contaminants** – occur only with illegally purchased opiates which have been diluted ('cut') from the pure form with white powdery or crystalline substances such as talc or quinine. If talc has been used, there is a risk of multiple talc granulomas forming in the lung after intravenous drug injection, leading to progressive pulmonary fibrosis. Chronic quinine intoxication can lead to amblyopia. When the drugs are injected into the subcutaneous tissue (usually early in the addictive process), the contaminants may play a role in the frequent occurrence of skin ulcers.
- **Effects due to unsterile administration** – extremely important and common, and are due to a combination of injecting through dirty skin, use of dirty needles, and the sharing of needles and syringes between addicts. Bacterial infection (often staphylococcal) leads to bacteremia, septicemia and bacterial endocarditis, from which septic emboli can spread to anywhere in the body. Fungal infection (usually due to *Candida albicans*, another skin commensal; see page 122) has a similar pattern. Both candidal and staphylococcal endocarditis produce bulky vegetations on the heart valves (see *Fig. 10.47*). The most important viral infections, usually acquired through the sharing of needles and syringes with previously infected addicts, are hepatitis B and C (see pages 284 and 286) and HIV, leading to AIDS (see page 99).
- **Social pathology** is beyond the scope of this book, but it is worth noting that opiate addicts are very prone to accidental injury when under the influence of drugs and to criminal violence from fellow addicts and dealers. Addicts who turn to prostitution to fund their drug habit also have a high incidence of sexually transmitted disease.

Cocaine use produces both structural and social pathology

Although an overdose of cocaine can produce severe cerebral over-stimulation leading to fitting and death, this is rare. Probably the commonest cause of death in habitual cocaine users is involvement in road traffic and other accidents as a result of the inappropriate feelings of confidence and impregnability that the drug gives.

Persistent heavy nasal inhalation of cocaine can rarely lead to necrosis of the nasal septum due to intense persistent vasoconstriction of the small blood vessels in the septal mucosa and submucosa.

Cocaine is increasingly recognized as a reason for emergency admission with chest pain in young people. Sometimes the pain proves to be in the chest wall, but in a proportion there is true myocardial ischemia or infarction, the result of severe vasoconstriction in coronary arteries. Cocaine may also increase the production of clotting factors. The development of cardiac pathology is not related to dose or to frequency of cocaine use.

The social pathology of heavy cocaine abuse is immense, but beyond the scope of this book.

Crystal meth has dangerous physical and psychological effects

Crystal methamphetamine is an unpredictable and variable combination of amphetamine with various toxic volatile substances (such as methylamine); it exists in various forms (e.g. 'skank,' 'ice') which differ in purity, strength and toxicity. According to its form, the drug can be injected, snorted or smoked in a pipe, and produces a feeling of intense exhilaration lasting some hours. Unfortunately it also produces indiscriminate and uncontrolled, often aggressive, behaviour, hallucinations and paranoia, as well as rapid rises in blood pressure and heart rate which can occasionally be so severe as to produce cardiorespiratory failure, coma and death. These changes can occur with quite small doses.

Persistent smokers of crystal meth develop rapidly progressive rotting of the teeth and inflamed gums ('meth mouth').

The drug is highly addictive, the period of exhilaration being followed by profound depression and physical and intellectual lethargy which the user believes can only be overcome by taking more crystal meth. Addiction leads to abject poverty, poor self-care and low standards of hygiene, rendering the patient vulnerable to a wide range of infections, particularly sexually transmitted diseases.

MDMA (also known as Ecstasy or 'E') can lead to death by a combination of hyperpyrexia and dehydration or by disseminated intravascular coagulation

MDMA is 3.4 methylenedioxymethylamphetamine, and is now widely available on the illegal drugs market. It is commonly used by young people attending dance events. Under the influence of this stimulant and euphoriant drug, and the stimulating environment, they dance beyond exhaustion and may suffer severe dehydration and hyperpyrexia. A few individuals react inappropriately to the drug and develop a rapidly fatal disseminated intravascular coagulation state, with widespread rash, cerebral petechial hemorrhages, coma and death. The mechanism of this is not known.

Solvent abuse is an important drug-related cause of death in young teenagers

The most commonly used solvents currently inhaled by teenagers are those used in various glues ('glue sniffing'), and butane aerosols (e.g. cigarette lighter fuel). Inhalation leads to intoxication due to transient cerebral stimulation. Excessive dosage can lead to profound CNS depression and sudden death from cardiorespiratory arrest or inhalation of vomit.

Metals cause disease as a result of environmental, occupational and therapeutic exposure

Many metals have adverse effects if present in high levels. In most instances it is possible to distinguish acute toxic effects (often the result of suicidal or homicidal administration) from chronic toxic effects (usually environmental and occupational exposure). Complete lists of metals and their toxicity are presented in specialist texts. Some of the more common agents are listed in the blue box below.

Iron and copper accumulate in tissues as a result of inborn errors of metabolism

Iron can accumulate in tissues as a result of an inborn error of metabolism that leads to a disease termed **hemochro-**

matosis, in which cells contain vast excess of iron as ferritin. The defect causes excessive iron absorption from the gut, which comes to light because the accumulated iron causes cell death and dysfunction in several tissues. There may be:

- Cardiomyopathy leading to heart failure (see page 178–9).
- Diabetes because of iron in islet cells of pancreas (see page 569).
- Chronic liver disease due to cirrhosis (see page 294).
- Female infertility due to pituitary involvement.

Excessive iron can also accumulate in tissues in diseases associated with excessive breakdown of red cells, necessitating repeated blood transfusion. This is termed **secondary hemosiderosis** and mainly affects the liver (see page 293).

Copper toxicity is seen in an inborn error of metabolism termed **Wilson's disease**. Excessive copper is absorbed and accumulates in liver and brain owing to mutation in a gene coding for a copper transport protein. If untreated, there is death of neurons and hepatocytes, leading to permanent damage. The main effects are abnormal movement disorders, psychiatric disease and chronic liver disease.

Metals and toxicity

Lead toxicity

    Exposure: gasoline, earth, paints, water, car battery burning, foundries.

    At risk: workers in industry, children in poor socioeconomic circumstances.

    Effects: anemia with basophilic stippling of red cells (lead interferes with normal heme formation), motor neuropathy, contractions of intestinal smooth muscle and colic, deposition in growth lines in bones (visible in epiphyses on X-ray), encephalopathy in children.

Mercury toxicity

    Exposure: common industrial waste product.

    Acute toxicity: suicidal ingestion, gastrointestinal ulceration, and acute tubular necrosis.

    Chronic toxicity: (Minimata disease) cerebral and cerebellar atrophy with loss of neurons, dementia and ataxia; nephrotic syndrome.

Aluminium toxicity

    Exposure: ubiquitous in environment, but poorly absorbed.

    At risk: renal dialysis patients and some patients on total parenteral nutrition (TPN).

    Effects: osteomalacia-like syndrome, dementia with cerebral atrophy.

Arsenic toxicity

    Exposure: agricultural chemicals, particularly pesticides.

    Acute toxicity: suicidal or homicidal ingestion results in abdominal pain and collapse.

    Chronic toxicity: arsenical keratoses, skin cancer, peripheral neuropathy with myelin loss, angiosarcoma of liver.

Gold toxicity

    Exposure: therapeutic administration in arthritis.

    Effects: glomerulonephritis, skin rash.

Agrochemicals and disease

- **Organophosphates** are pesticides that work as acetylcholinesterase inhibitors. Chronic exposure causes muscle paralysis, autonomic dysfunction, and abdominal pain.
- **Paraquat** is a herbicide that causes massive free-radical generation. Accidental or suicidal ingestion leads to diffuse alveolar damage, renal necrosis, and hepatic necrosis.
- **Dioxin** causes chloracne in humans and has been shown to be embryotoxic in animals. It has been a contaminant in several processes producing other herbicides.

Fig. 9.6 Common chemical toxins available in domestic settings

Agent	Effects
Methyl alcohol	Metabolic acidosis, neurological damage
Ethylene glycol	Metabolic acidosis, oxalate deposition in kidneys, acute tubular necrosis
Carbon tetrachloride	Centrilobular necrosis in liver, tubular necrosis in kidneys
Carbon monoxide	Tissue hypoxia by forming carboxyhemoglobin
	Headache, dizziness and confusion (early features)
	Delayed damage to basal ganglia and white matter
	Coma and death with high saturation
Strong alkalis	Ulceration of oropharynx and esophagus.

Insecticides and herbicides are frequently implicated in disease

Environmental awareness has led to increasing scrutiny of the potential role of agrochemicals in disease. Several compounds have been found to accumulate in the food chain but, as yet, their significance in causing disease in humans is uncertain. For example, chlorinated hydrocarbons (DDT, dieldrin) are insecticides, chronic exposure leading to accumulation in the liver. Although toxicity to certain birds and carcinogenicity in rats is established, there is little evidence of toxicity in humans, despite extensive epidemiological surveys and evidence of massive exposure. However, recent concerns have been expressed that some compounds accumulating in the environment have estrogenic effects.

Importantly, the presence of agrochemicals must be weighed against the presence of highly toxic natural agents that are produced in plants as a result of infection by insects and fungi. Many of the toxins produced by nature are proven carcinogens, e.g. aflatoxins are highly carcinogenic substances produced by fungi in stored crops such as nuts.

Domestically available toxins are commonly used in suicides

There is ready access to chemicals in the domestic setting. Toxicity is mostly related to accidental or suicidal ingestion. The common agents are listed in *Fig. 9.6*.

Take a drug history: therapeutic agents are a frequent cause of disease

Therapeutic agents are a frequent cause of disease, and adverse drug reactions are responsible for many episodes requiring medical care, particularly skin rashes. Some reactions are dose related and may be attributable to pharmacokinetic variation between individuals. Others are idiosyncratic, often related to allergic and hypersensitive responses. Importantly, certain adverse reactions are delayed, e.g. drugs that are carcinogenic, impair fertility, or induce congenital malformations.

In addition to adverse effects of prescribed drugs taken in the correct dosage, therapeutic drugs are frequently used in suicide attempts.

NUTRITIONAL FACTORS IN DISEASE

Worldwide, nutritional factors are a very important cause of morbidity and mortality. In the developing world the major problem is under-nutrition; in the developed world, over-nutrition is a greater problem, in the form of obesity. A normal diet should provide energy, proteins, fatty acids, vitamins and minerals.

Under-nutrition can be caused by many factors, with a marked geographical variation

The causes of under-nutrition (starvation) in the developing world are usually:

- Insufficient food available.
- Severe infection, particularly gastroenteritis. Elsewhere, the main causes are:
- Malabsorption, due to intestinal disease.
- Anorexia nervosa and related psychological disorders.

In starvation there is inadequate intake of protein and carbohydrates. Hepatic stores of glycogen are rapidly depleted and the liver then breaks down amino acids and fatty acids to convert to glucose. The amino acids are derived from the breakdown of muscle protein, and the fatty acids from the breakdown of the fat stores, leading to loss of muscle bulk and subcutaneous fat. Lastly, serum proteins are catabolized to generate energy, resulting in

abnormally low levels of albumin. These metabolic disturbances can be reversed if a normal dietary intake of food can be resumed.

Many factors play a role in the etiology of obesity

Obesity can be regarded as a form of chronic calorie overdose, due to a combination of excessive calorie intake and inadequate calorie breakdown. The surplus calories are stored in the body's fat deposits as fat within adipocytes; the most obvious externally visible fat depot is the subcutaneous adipose tissue, leading to the appearance of obesity, but the surplus is also stored internally, for example in omental, mesenteric, perinephric and epicardial adipose tissue.

Briefly, the factors involved in obesity are:

- **Excessive food intake** (particularly of fats) – excessive or gluttonous eating habits are often imposed by parents in infancy and early childhood. Such strongly imprinted patterns are difficult to break. It is the calorie content, not the physical bulk, of the food that is important, though most obese persons consume large quantities of high-calorie food and drink.
- **Inadequate calorie breakdown** – due to insufficient physical activity. The largely sedentary, car-dependent lifestyle in the developed world is a particularly important factor.

Genetic factors have been claimed to play a role following the discovery of leptin, a protein made in the adipocytes which controls body fat levels, probably through an influence on those parts of the brain that regulate energy utilization. Mutations in the gene that codes for leptin may play a role in the predisposition to obesity.

Obesity predisposes to many diseases, serious and mild

Obesity has been linked to many diseases that are common in the developed world, the most serious and important of which are:

- Systemic hypertension.
- Type 2 diabetes mellitus.
- Hyperlipidemia and increased severity of atherosclerosis.
- Increased predisposition to heart disease.
- Osteoarthritis and other degenerative joint diseases.
- Gallstones and obstructive biliary disease.
- Increased predisposition to leg vein thrombosis and pulmonary embolus.

In addition, obese people frequently suffer from a wide range of mild disorders, including breathing disorders on exertion, fungal infections in skin creases, and the tendency to lower-leg ulcers which heal slowly and poorly.

Protein energy malnutrition

Protein energy malnutrition (PEM) is particularly seen in children in the developing world during periods of famine. When body weight falls to 60% of normal, a child is considered to have **marasmus** (*Fig. 9.7*). Metabolic changes of starvation lead to loss of subcutaneous adipose tissue and loss of skeletal muscle bulk. In addition, the hair is lost, the skin becomes thin and atrophic, and there is a predisposition to develop severe bacterial and viral infections, particularly TB and gastroenteritis, owing to the effects of malnutrition on the immune system. There is also vitamin deficiency.

When protein deprivation is greater than deprivation of energy (carbohydrates still being available in the diet), the condition of **kwashiorkor** develops, in which affected children are 60–80% of normal weight. However, the marked protein lack leads to severe hypoalbuminemia and generalized edema. A scaly skin rash develops and the liver is enlarged and shows fatty change because lipid carrier proteins cannot be made. As with marasmus, there is immune deficiency and vitamin deficiency.

Fig. 9.7 Marasmus. This emaciated infant died as a result of marasmus, complicated by gastroenteritis.

Vitamin deficiencies produce distinct clinical syndromes

In people with a well-balanced diet, vitamin deficiency is extremely rare. In most cases the manifestations of vitamin deficiencies are combined with some elements of protein–calorie malnutrition when the cause is starvation. However, individual vitamin deficiency syndromes can result from a number of factors, including impaired absorption due to bowel disease, impaired synthesis, and specific absence from the diet. The most important features of single vitamin deficiencies are given in *Fig. 9.8.*

Vitamin A deficiency can cause blindness

Vitamin A is a group of related natural retinoid substances: the storage and transport form is **retinol**, which is convertible to **retinal**, a visual pigment. A related oxidation product is **retinoic acid**, which influences the growth and differentiation of epithelial cells. The natural retinoids are derived in the body by conversion from the precursor, β-carotene (provitamin A), the dietary source of which is vegetables (particularly yellow vegetables such as carrots) and animal proteins (e.g. eggs, butter).

Vitamin A deficiency is largely confined to parts of the world where chronic malnutrition occurs, and manifests mainly as impaired night vision and dry eyes; severe and persistent deficiency causes corneal destruction, leading to blindness. Other effects are squamous metaplasia of the columnar epithelium of the respiratory tract, and some degree of immune deficiency.

Vitamin B₁ (thiamine) deficiency particularly affects chronic alcoholics

Although the deficiency may occur in the underdeveloped areas of the world, particularly where rice is the basis of the limited diet, in other parts of the world chronic alcoholism is the major cause. There are three manifestations of thiamine deficiency:

- A peripheral polyneuropathy initially producing foot drop and sensory loss, but later affecting the upper limbs ('dry beri beri').
- High-output cardiac failure, often associated with cardiac dilatation and severe leg edema ('wet beri beri').
- A brain disorder called Wernicke's encephalopathy, which is discussed in more detail on page 476.

All three conditions may occur together.

Vitamin B₂ (riboflavin) deficiency mainly affects the skin, eyes and tongue

Riboflavin is present in abundance in dairy products, meat and vegetables, and dietary deficiency is seen mainly in poor populations where chronic starvation is widespread, but also occurs in alcoholics and in some severe dietary faddists, particularly those who avoid meat and milk derivatives. A sore red tongue (glossitis) and angles of the mouth (cheilitis), often combined with a scaly desquamative skin rash, are common features. Superficial keratitis of the eye also occurs.

Fig. 9.8 Vitamin deficiency syndromes		
Vitamin	**Function**	**Consequences of deficiency**
A	Retinal function, epithelial growth control	Night blindness, keratomalacia, xerophthalmia
B₁ (thiamine)	Co-enzyme	Beri beri, Wernicke's encephalopathy
B₂ (riboflavin)	Co-enzyme	Dermatitis, glossitis, keratitis, neuropathy, confusion
B₆ (pyridoxine)	Co-enzyme	Neuropathy
B₁₂ (cobalamin)	Nucleic acid synthesis	Megaloblastic anemia. Subacute combined degeneration of spinal cord
Niacin	Co-enzyme NAD, NADP	Pellagra (diarrhea, dermatitis and dementia)
Folate	Co-enzyme in nucleic acid synthesis	Megaloblastic anemia, villous atrophy of gut
Vitamin C	Cofactor in hydroxylation	Scurvy
Vitamin D	Calcium and phosphate absorption	Rickets (childhood). Osteomalacia (adults)
Vitamin E	Antioxidant	Spinocerebellar degeneration
Vitamin K	Co-factor for coagulation factor synthesis	Bleeding due to coagulation defects

Vitamin B$_6$ (pyridoxine) deficiency is most commonly seen as a side-effect of long-term therapeutic drug administration

Some therapeutic drugs act as pyridoxine antagonists, and oral supplements of the vitamin must be given with the drug. Examples include penicillamine (given lifelong for Wilson's disease, see page 293) and for long periods for rheumatoid arthritis (see page 549), and isoniazid for the treatment of tuberculosis. The symptoms of pyridoxine deficiency are similar to those of riboflavine (see above).

Vitamin B$_{12}$ (cobalamin) deficiency is mainly caused by malabsorption

The main reasons for B$_{12}$ deficiency are outlined on page 149 in the discussion of the disease that results from the deficiency, megaloblastic anemia. With or without the anemia, the patient may suffer demyelination of the dorso-lateral columns of the spinal cord, producing the symptom complex called 'subacute combined degeneration of the cord.'

Folate deficiency also produces megaloblastic anemia

Folates are present in abundance in vegetables, fruit and meat, but cooking destroys much of them. Nevertheless, folate deficiency due to dietary inadequacy is rare except when the demand for folate is excessive, for example in pregnancy and infancy. Like vitamin B$_{12}$, folate is essential for nucleic acid synthesis, and requirements are greatly increased during periods of rapid growth. The bone marrow is particularly vulnerable, and megaloblastic anemia develops in folate deficiency, as it does in B$_{12}$ deficiency. Folate deficiency does not cause neurological disease, but severe maternal folate deficiency in the first trimester of pregnancy may lead to increased risk of neural tube defects in the fetus.

Niacin/nicotinamide deficiency produces the symptom complex called pellagra

Niacin/nicotinamide deficiency may be seen as a result of dietary inadequacy in poor populations whose staple is maize, but is most commonly seen in alcoholics. Pellagra syndrome comprises dermatitis (a typically symmetrical reddening, thickening and scaling of the skin), diarrhea, and dementia.

Vitamin C (ascorbic acid) deficiency leads to scurvy

Vitamin C is abundant in fruits and vegetables, with lesser amounts in meat and dairy products, and a balanced diet provides an adequate amount. People with an inadequate or alcohol-based diet may develop some of the features of scurvy, mainly hemorrhages due to weakness of capillary and venule walls in the skin and other organs; intracranial and intra-articular bleeds are particularly a problem in children, who may also manifest rickets-like bone changes (see page 538) owing to defects in the production of osteoid by osteoblasts during bone development. Vitamin C deficiency leads to interference with normal collagen synthesis, and this is the basis of the vascular and bone disorders.

Vitamin D deficiency produces rickets in children and osteomalacia in adults

The metabolism of vitamin D, causes of deficiency, and impact on the bone, are discussed in Chapter 24, page 538.

Vitamin E deficiency is rare, and causes neurological damage

Vitamin E is a collection of fat-soluble compounds, the most important of which is α-tocopherol. These compounds are abundant in a wide range of foods, and dietary inadequacy is rare. The commonest reason for deficiency is impaired fat absorptive capacity secondary to hepatobiliary, pancreatic or small intestinal disease. The clinical manifestations include ataxia, loss of joint position and vibration senses, and muscle weakness, particularly affecting the muscles of the eye. There is degeneration of axons in the dorsal columns of the spinal cord and spinocerebellar tracts particularly.

Vitamin K deficiency leads to abnormal bleeding

Vitamin K acts as a vital co-factor in the synthesis of many proteins, including the vital clotting factors produced in the liver. Deficiency can occur when there is malabsorption of fat (it is a fat-soluble vitamin) or when there is severe diffuse liver disease, and spontaneous bleeding may occur at many sites.

Blood circulatory system   10

GENERAL PATHOLOGY OF THE CIRCULATORY SYSTEM

Accumulation of excess fluid in tissues is termed 'edema'

An important consequence of disease of the blood circulatory system is the development of excess fluid in tissues, termed **edema**. Under normal circumstances only a little fluid leaks from vessels to form interstitial fluid, which is removed by lymphatic vessels. Excess fluid leaks from capillaries into tissues in three main circumstances:

1. More fluid leaves capillaries if the hydrostatic pressure in vessels is increased (interference with venous drainage, heart failure).
2. More fluid leaves capillaries with reduced plasma oncotic pressure (hypoproteinemia).
3. More fluid leaves capillaries if vascular permeability is altered (allergic responses liberating histamine, acute inflammation).

The two most important types of edema are seen as a consequence of cardiac failure:

Pulmonary edema is the accumulation of fluid in the alveoli of the lung. It is caused by increased hydrostatic pressure in the pulmonary vascular bed, resulting from failure of the left side of the heart (see page 172).

Subcutaneous edema is the accumulation of fluid in subcutaneous tissues. It is caused by increased hydrostatic pressure in the systemic venous system, resulting from failure of the right side of the heart (see page 172).

Hemorrhage is caused by rupture of blood vessels

Hemorrhage is caused by rupture of blood vessels. Massive exsanguination is usually caused by trauma to a major artery or vein, but may also result from bursting of a vessel weakened by disease.

Hematoma is an accumulation of blood within soft tissues. It is usually due to traumatic damage to vessels, but occasionally follows spontaneous rupture of diseased vessels.

Petechiae (1–2 mm diameter) and **purpura** (2–10 mm diameter) are small tissue hemorrrhages, often seen in the skin, due to either abnormal small vessel fragility, abnormal blood clotting or an abrupt increase in pressure within small venules and capillaries.

The accumulation of blood in an anatomic space is related to local bleeding. Examples include **hemopericardium:** usually due to rupture of the heart or the ascending aorta; **hemothorax:** blood in the pleural cavities due to trauma or rupture of the aorta; **hemoperitoneum:** usually due to rupture of an aortic aneurysm or traumatic damage to liver or spleen; **hemarthrosis:** a collection of blood in a joint space due either to direct trauma, or to a bleeding disorder such as hemophilia.

A clotted mass of blood forming in the circulation is called a 'thrombus'

A thrombus is a structured, solid mass composed of blood constituents that forms in the cardiovascular system (*Fig. 10.1*). This distinguishes it from a coagulum, which is

Fig. 10.1 Thrombus morphology. A thrombus is composed of elements derived from activation of the coagulation cascade, i.e. aggregated platelets, insoluble fibrin derived from soluble plasma fibrinogen, and entrapped red cells. These elements are usually arranged in a laminated pattern, layers of platelets alternating with layers of fibrin and entrapped red cells. This is shown in the photomicrograph of a thrombus, in which pale layers of platelets (**P**) are separated by pink-stained layers of fibrin and red cells (**F**).

unstructured and forms when blood clots outside the circulatory system.

The process of thrombus formation, termed **thrombosis**, is due to activation of the normal blood coagulation system. Aggregation of platelets, held together with a meshwork of fibrin, is a normal hemostatic mechanism, occurring constantly to plug small defects in blood vessel walls (*Fig. 10.3*). The result is the formation of a hemostatic plug composed of fibrin, platelets and entrapped red cells. The thrombus should be considered as a biologically active structure, rather than a passive physical plug. Peptide fragments derived from the coagulation cascade and factors released by platelets have effects on adjacent endothelium and the vessel wall, promoting repair.

Once the defect is plugged effectively and the vessel wall repaired, the small platelet/fibrin thrombus is normally removed by **fibrinolysis**, a multi-enzyme process that breaks down the supporting mesh of fibrin filaments, allowing dissolution of the thrombus (*Fig. 10.2*).

Fibrinolytic systems are activated to remove thrombus once formed

The products of the coagulation cascade are usually restricted to the immediate site of vessel wall damage.

Plasma inhibitors of coagulation act to limit the coagulation cascade. Loss of these inhibitors leads to an abnormal clotting state (thrombophilia). The most potent inhibitor of coagulation is antithrombin III, the action of which is potentiated by the action of heparin. Protein C is a vitamin K-dependent factor which is activated by thrombin in the presence of thrombomodulin and which, in concert with protein S, works by destroying activated cofactors V and VIII. Protein C also inactivates a circulating factor which normally prevents fibrinolysis (PAI-1).

Fig. 10.2 Fibrinolysis. The fibrinolytic system functions to degrade fibrin, thereby allowing lysis of formed thrombus. The enzyme that cleaves fibrin is termed plasmin, and this is formed from a precursor protein in plasma termed plasminogen. Plasminogen is converted to plasmin by the action of plasminogen activators. Other factors, grouped as plasminogen activator inhibitors, antagonize the process of forming plasmin, one such being PAI-1, which interacts with protein C. The end products of the fibrinolytic process are fibrin degradation products. These products also have anticoagulant activity. Plasminogen activators have been considered for therapeutic administration to promote the lysis of thrombus, for example in the immediate management of coronary artery thrombosis.

The endothelium normally prevents thrombosis in vessels

Normal endothelial cells act to prevent activation of the coagulation cascade, generating factors that bring about thrombolysis.

- Intact endothelium prevents platelets from coming into contact with collagen and von Willebrand factor (which cause platelet aggregation and degranulation).
- Prostacyclin (PGI₂) and nitric oxide prevent adhesion and aggregation of platelets to endothelium.
- Thrombomodulin on the endothelial surface binds to any locally formed thrombin generated as part of the activation of the coagulation cascade. The thrombomodulin–thrombin complex can then initiate

the anticoagulant effects of the vitamin K-dependent factor protein C and its cofactor protein S. Active protein C destroys factor V and factor VIII.
- Endothelium produces heparin-like molecules, which inhibit elements of the normal coagulation cascade.
- Endothelium synthesizes plasminogen activators, which produce plasmin, a proteolytic enzyme that lyses fibrin and inactivates parts of the coagulation cascade.
- Antithrombin III (AT-III) is a potent inhibitor of coagulation and works by inactivating proteases operating in the coagulation cascade. Heparin potentiates the activity of this system.

Events in thrombus formation

Endothelial damage results in exposure of collagen and von Willebrand factor, which mediate the adhesion of platelets. Platelets express surface glycoprotein receptor, which binds to these ligands.

- Glycoprotein Ia (GPIa) binds directly to collagen.
- Glycoprotein Ib (GPIb-IX) binds to von Willebrand factor (VIII:vWF), and this in turn binds to collagen. (Inherited deficiency of GPIb-IX results in a bleeding disorder termed Bernard-Soulier syndrome. Deficiency of VIII:vWF is termed von Willebrand's disease.)

Adherent platelets undergo a shape change and aggregate.

- ADP is released from granules, which stimulates further aggregation of platelets (as well as adhesion of further platelets), forming a platelet plug.
- Prostaglandin thromboxane A2 (TXA_2) is synthesized by platelets and causes platelet aggregation and vasoconstriction.
- Receptors are expressed on the platelet surface which interact with coagulation factors collectively referred to as platelet factor 3 (PF3). The coagulation system generates the insoluble protein fibrin.
- Platelets express glycoprotein complex IIb-IIIa on their surface (GPIIb-IIIa), which acts as a receptor for fibrinogen and vWF, helping form a firm hemostatic plug. (Inherited deficiency of GPIIb-IIIa results in a bleeding disorder termed Glanzmann's thrombasthenia.)
- GpIIb/IIIa inhibitor drugs are used to treat thrombotic diseases.

Fig. 10.3 Events in thrombus formation.

Fibrinolysis is brought about by formation of the protease plasmin (*Fig.10.2*). This is formed by the activation of its precursor, plasminogen, and acts to degrade fibrin into fibrinopeptides, collective termed fibrin degradation products (FDPs), together with fragments of cross-linked fibrin termed D-dimer. Plasminogen is converted into plasmin by the activity of plasminogen activators. The most important are tissue plasminogen activator, derived from endothelial cells (tPA) and urinary-type plasminogen activator (uPA). Under normal circumstances uPA and tPA are inhibited by plasminogen activator inhibitor 1 (PAI-1). However, activated protein C prevents this, thereby facilitating local fibrinolysis.

In normal vessels, excessive thrombosis is prevented by several physiological mechanisms (see pink box on page 152). In **pathological thrombosis** the process of thrombus formation proceeds beyond the capacity of the endogenous fibrinolysins to eradicate the thrombus. Thrombus continues to enlarge by the deposition of fresh layers of platelets and fibrin until a substantial mass is formed, which may reduce the lumen of the vessel.

Three main factors predispose to thrombus formation

Among the main predisposing factors to thrombus formation is **endothelial dysfunction**. Direct injury to endothelium, as seen in trauma and inflammation, may lead to thrombosis. Damage to endothelium occurs in association with atheroma (see page 158).

Change in the flow pattern of blood is a major factor in causing thrombus. Stasis allows platelets to come into contact with endothelium, and slow flow prevents blood diluting activated coagulation components. Turbulence of blood flow may cause physical trauma to endothelial cells and, with loss of laminar flow, bring platelets into contact with endothelium.

Changes in potential blood coagulability predispose to thrombus formation. This may be because of an increase in the concentration of fibrinogen in acute-phase responses. Increase in concentration of prothrombin and fibrinogen can also occur with estrogen-containing oral contraceptive therapy. Congenital lack of natural anticoagulant protein C, protein S or antithrombin III is a rare but important predisposing factor to thrombosis. Abnormal autoantibodies directed against platelet phospholipids (**antiphospholipid** antibodies) are an increasingly recognized cause of arterial and venous thrombosis.

A mutation in the coagulation factor V – so-called **Leiden mutation** – renders this factor resistant to inactivation and is a predisposing factor to abnormal arterial or venous thrombosis in 2–10% of the Caucasian population.

Thrombosis can occur at any place in the circulatory system

Thrombi that occur in different parts of the circulation have different causative factors and different macroscopic appearances. Those formed in fast-moving blood in arteries and cardiac chambers have a relatively high platelet/fibrin content and are very firm and pale, with prominent laminations. Thrombi that form in slow-moving blood, such as that in veins, have a high proportion of trapped red cells relative to fibrin/platelets, and are typically red, soft and gelatinous in texture, with poor laminations.

As most thrombi that form in small or medium-sized vessels occlude the lumen and prevent blood flow, they are termed **occlusive**. However, thrombi that form in the heart or aorta generally do not cause complete occlusion, appearing as raised plaques applied to the wall (**mural thrombi**).

Thrombi that occur on heart valves appear as polypoid masses and are termed **vegetations**. The main predisposing factors to thrombosis at different sites are shown in *Fig. 10.4*.

There are four main outcomes following vascular occlusion by a thrombus

Once a thrombus develops in a vessel there are several possible outcomes. The thrombus may enlarge along the vessel (a process termed **propagation**) or it may undergo lysis by the fibrinolytic system. The latter process may, in certain circumstances, be assisted by therapeutic administration of a fibrinolytic agent such as streptokinase.

There may be **organization** of the thrombus by ingrowth of granulation tissue from the vessel wall. Gradually the thrombus is replaced by granulation tissue, and new vascular channels develop, bridging the site of occlusion and re-establishing flow. This is termed **recanalization** (*Fig. 10.5*).

Alternatively, fragments may break off the thrombus and be carried by the circulation to impact in other vessels, a process termed **thromboembolism**.

EMBOLISM

Occlusion of a vessel by material travelling in the circulation is termed 'embolism'

Embolism can be defined as 'occlusion of a vessel by a mass of material that is transported in the bloodstream.' The mass of material is termed an **embolus**, and the most common type is due to fragments of circulating thrombus, termed **thromboemboli**.

Thromboembolism occurs when a mass of thrombus breaks off from its site of formation to enter the blood circulation, where it travels until it meets a blood vessel with a lumen too small to permit further passage. At this site it impacts, usually occluding the lumen of the vessel.

Fig. 10.4 Factors predisposing to thrombus at different sites

Site	Predisposition to thrombosis
Artery	Atheroma, aneurysms
Heart valve	Inflammation caused by infection
Ventricle	Inflammation following infarction Ventricular aneurysm
Atrium	Atrial fibrillation (→stasis) Mitral valve stenosis
Vein	Slow flow Changes in coagulability of blood
Cerebral venous sinus	Inflammation following infection Change in coagulability of blood

- Thromboemboli originating in systemic veins travel round to the heart to impact in the pulmonary arterial system, causing **pulmonary thromboembolism**.
- Thromboemboli originating in the heart (mural thrombus or vegetations) travel via the aorta to the systemic arterial circulation. There they commonly impact in arteries leading to the brain, kidneys, spleen, gut and lower limbs.
- Thromboemboli originating from mural thrombus in the common carotid arteries impact in the cerebral arterial system.
- Thromboemboli originating from mural thrombus in the abdominal aorta commonly impact in the renal arteries and arteries of the lower limbs.

**Fig. 10.5 Organization and recanalization of thrombus.
(a) Histology. (b) Macroscopic.** Granulation tissue containing many small blood vessels has completely replaced the thrombus that was occluding this vessel (a). Eventually, some of these vessels enlarge and flow is re-established. Such a recanalized artery is shown in (b), in which a coronary artery lumen has been replaced by three small lumina having been previously blocked by thrombus.

Pulmonary thromboembolism is an extremely common preventable condition

The most common preventable cause of death in hospital patients is pulmonary thromboembolism (*Fig. 10.6*). The vast majority of cases are caused by emboli arising from thrombosis of deep leg veins (calf, popliteal, femoral and iliac veins). Diagnosis of leg vein thrombosis is notoriously difficult, as symptoms and signs are non-specific; most cases are silent, resolving without detection.

The two main consequences of embolization to the pulmonary arterial tree are an increase in pulmonary arterial pressure (which puts a strain on the right side of the heart) and ischemia of the lung, with ventilated areas not being perfused by blood. The clinical consequences of pulmonary embolism depend on the extent of the pulmonary vasculature blockage and the timescale involved.

If 60% of the pulmonary vasculature is suddenly blocked, the heart cannot pump blood through the lungs. There is cardiovascular collapse, with electromechanical dissociation of the heart as it continues to beat but develops no output. This pattern of blockage is known as **massive pulmonary embolism**. Causing rapid death, it accounts for about 5% of all cases of pulmonary thromboembolism.

Accounting for about 10% of all cases of pulmonary thromboembolism, **major pulmonary embolism** occurs when there is blockage of middle-sized pulmonary arteries. Patients commonly experience breathlessness. Infarction of lung develops in only about 10% of such cases (see pages 190–1). It can lead to hemoptysis and, if adjacent to the pleura, pleuritic chest pain. It is not uncommon for patients to develop a subsequent massive thromboembolism if untreated.

In about 85% of all cases of pulmonary thromboembolism there is blockage of small peripheral vessels by small emboli (**minor pulmonary embolism**). Patients may be

Fig. 10.6 Pulmonary thromboembolism. The main pulmonary artery contains a mass of red thrombus (**T**), a thromboembolus. This originated by embolization from one of the femoral veins.

asymptomatic, or may experience breathlessness and pleuritic chest pain as a result of small infarcts. As with major pulmonary embolism, it is not uncommon for patients to develop a subsequent massive thromboembolism if untreated.

A very small number of patients develop **recurrent minor pulmonary embolism**. There is blockage of many small peripheral arteries over a period of many months by recurrent small emboli. This leads to obliteration of the vascular bed and right heart strain, causing pulmonary hypertension (see pages 190–1).

Embolism of material other than embolus is less common

The most common material to embolize in the bloodstream is thrombus, but other types of embolus can occur.

The most important and clinically significant is malignant tumor.

Tumor embolism is the way in which malignant tumors spread from the site of origin to distant metastatic sites using the bloodstream route. The malignant tumor infiltrates through the wall of a blood vessel (usually a venule or vein) at the primary site to occupy the lumen, and clumps of tumor cells of various sizes break off and are carried in the venous system until they reach a vessel too small to permit further passage, then impact there and often grow to produce a distant metastasis. For this reason, histological evidence of vascular invasion at the primary site at the time of tumor excision is regarded as a poor prognostic feature in tumor grading (see pages 79–81).

Fat and bone marrow embolus may occur following severe fracture trauma to bones. Fragments of fat released from traumatized adipocytes in the fatty bone marrow may enter the circulation through thin-walled veins torn by the fracture trauma. They pass through the venous system to the right side of the heart, and thence via pulmonary arteries to the lung capillaries, where some are trapped. However, some small lipid droplets can pass completely through the pulmonary capillary bed to enter the pulmonary veins and thereby gain access to the systemic circulation. They are then distributed to the small capillaries throughout the body; if many such fat droplets enter the cerebral circulation, they can occlude many brain capillaries, leading to coma and death. Larger fragments of bone marrow (including hemopoietic tissue) are too large to pass through the pulmonary capillaries, so are usually trapped in the lung.

Air embolism is usually due to accidental pumping of air into the venous circulation during intravenous injection or transfusion. If large quantities of air mixed with blood enter the right atrium, a bloody froth is formed and the patient may suffer cardiac arrest. In deep-sea divers, inhaled air may dissolve into the plasma due to the increased pressure at great depths, only to reform into bubbles of gas within the circulation if the diver comes to the surface too

Key Facts
Pulmonary embolus

- Usually follows thrombosis in leg veins, often deep veins in calf.
- Small pulmonary emboli impact in peripheral branches of pulmonary artery and cause **pulmonary infarcts** (often with clinical pleurisy).
- Large pulmonary emboli may impact in, and obstruct, a major pulmonary artery, causing sudden death (**massive pulmonary embolus**).
- A small pulmonary embolus (with infarction) may be followed by a much larger, fatal embolus ('**premonitary embolus**').
- Prevention of leg vein thrombosis is the best way of preventing pulmonary embolus.

Clinical conditions predisposing to leg vein thrombosis

Thrombosis arising in deep leg veins may be completely asymptomatic or may cause mild pain and tenderness in the muscles, sometimes with development of ankle edema.

Clinical situations predisposing to the development of deep leg vein thrombosis are:

- Immobility and bed rest.
- Postoperative period.
- Pregnancy and the postpartum period.
- Oral contraceptive therapy with high-estrogen preparations.

- Nephrotic syndrome.
- Severe burns.
- Trauma.
- Cardiac failure.
- Disseminated malignancy.

In many of these situations it is clinical practice to give prophylactic treatment with heparin to prevent the development of thrombosis, combined with physiotherapy to the legs.

quickly. This decompression sickness (known to divers as 'the bends') and the embolization of the bubbles of mainly nitrogen gas may occlude small vessels, leading to wide-spread anoxia of tissues, and even death.

Amniotic fluid embolism may occur rarely during childbirth; some of the amniotic fluid (containing fetal cells from the skin surface) may enter the maternal circulation through the exposed and bleeding placental bed in the uterus. The material passes in the venous circulation to the lung capillaries and may cause acute alveolar wall damage and disseminated intravascular coagulation (see pages 206 and 329).

Therapeutic embolization is being used increasingly to treat inoperable vascular malformations of the brain by interventional radiology. Wire, gelfoam, glue and balloons are all used to deliberately block vessels.

INFARCTION

Lack of perfusion of tissues by blood leads to infarction

Failure of adequate blood supply to a tissue causes cell damage through ischemia. Tissue necrosis due to interference with local blood flow is termed **infarction**. The vast majority of infarcts are due to obstruction of the arterial supply to a tissue, a minority being caused by interference to the venous drainage. The ischemic damage results in coagulative necrosis in tissues.

Infarction is a major cause of morbidity and mortality, the most important examples being myocardial infarction ('heart attack,' see page 174), cerebral infarction ('stroke,' see pages 458–9), pulmonary infarction (see page 156), gangrene of lower limb, and bowel infarction (see page 267).

Blockage of an artery generally causes coagulative necrosis in the target organ

Infarcts caused by blockage of an artery are shaped according to the territory of supply of the blocked vessel. Occlusion of small arteries in an organ such as the kidney or lung usually results in wedge-shaped infarcts, with the occluded vessel at the apex (*Fig. 10.7*).

Immediately following arterial occlusion, a damaged area is typically poorly defined, pale and swollen. Within about 48 hours the dead tissue becomes better demarcated and is pale and yellowed. As an acute inflammatory response develops in adjacent viable tissue, a red hyperemic border becomes visible, separating normal tissue from the area of infarction. After 10 days or so, ingrowth of granulation tissue and organization are advanced. The infarcted area is ultimately replaced by collagenous scarring.

Blockage of veins causes hemorrhagic necrosis (venous infarction)

Infarcts caused by blockage of venous drainage develop because tissue becomes massively suffused by blood. Blood

is unable to drain from the tissue via the veins, but arterial blood continues to pump in, causing congestion and a rapid rise in pressure in small blood vessels, which lead to vessel wall rupture. Eventually, when the pressure is so high that arterial blood cannot enter, the tissue is deprived of oxygenated blood and undergoes anoxic necrosis.

Affected areas are deeply congested by deoxygenated blood and may appear almost black (hemorrhagic infarction). The usual cause of venous infarction is torsion of the vascular pedicle of an organ. Examples include torsion of the testis, bowel volvulus, and strangulated hernia. Venous infarction is also seen in the brain with venous sinus occlusion by thrombosis.

Slow occlusion of a vessel may cause ischemia and not infarction

Infarction usually occurs when vascular occlusion is abrupt; when the blood flow is reduced over a period of time there are two possibilities. Alternative vascular channels can open up to compensate for the obstruction in the diseased vessel (collateral circulation). Development of collateral vessels is possible in many tissues, but not when an area is supplied by a single artery (end artery).

Alternatively, the tissue undergoes ischemic atrophy. Specialized cells shrink and eventually die over a long period of time, and tissue is converted into hyaline, pink-staining amorphous support tissue. Robust support cells such as fibroblasts may survive in the face of ischemia.

Fig. 10.7 Renal infarct. A recent infarct of the kidney shows a pale area of infarction (**I**), with an adjacent hyperemic border separating it from normal kidney.

SHOCK

Shock is a clinical state associated with generalized failure of tissue perfusion

In contrast to local failure of vascular flow, a systemic reduction in tissue blood flow, manifest by profound low blood pressure (hypotension), is clinically termed **shock**.

Among the many causes of shock are severe failure of the pumping mechanism of the heart (**cardiogenic shock**), blockage of major arteries (**obstructive shock**), and lack of blood to pump (**hypovolemic shock**) due to hemorrhage or severe fluid loss. Abnormal dilatation of peripheral vessels causing lack of venous return of blood may also be responsible, arising in cases of septicemic/endotoxic shock, anaphylactic shock and neurogenic shock.

Events in the early and later stages of shock are summarized in *Fig.10.8*. During the development of shock, protective mechanisms first operate to maintain perfusion of vital organs. The renin–angiotensin–aldosterone system causes retention of sodium and fluid, thereby expanding blood volume. There is increased catecholamine production by the adrenals, and increased sympathetic activity, causing tachycardia and vasoconstriction in certain vascular beds (the skin is cold and pale). ADH secretion is also increased, causing sodium and water retention.

With persistence of shock, systemic acidosis develops. This causes dilatation of previously constricted vessels, and blood pressure consequently falls. Blood is diverted from the gut and kidneys to maintain perfusion of the heart and brain. Output of urine falls and there is damage to renal epithelial cells. Gut stasis also develops, with necrosis of lining epithelial cells. In the late and irreversible stages of shock there is necrosis of cells in liver, heart and brain. Death is due to multiple organ failure.

Fig. 10.8 Early and late manifestations of shock

Tissue	Early shock	Late shock
Skin	Pale and cold	Cyanosed
Kidneys	Low urine production	Necrosis of tubular epithelium
Gut	Bowel stasis	Necrosis of lining epithelium
Lung	Tachypnea	Necrosis of alveolar epithelium
Liver	Fatty change	Necrosis of centrilobular cells
Brain	Reduced conscious level	Necrosis of neurons, coma
Heart	Tachycardia	Myocardial necrosis

ARTERIAL DISEASES

Arterial disease and its complications are an important cause of morbidity and mortality in most western societies, the main disease being atherosclerosis.

Thickening and hardening of arterial walls is termed 'arteriosclerosis'

Arteriosclerosis is the term used to describe thickening and hardening of the walls of arteries, without implying any particular cause. The effect of arteriosclerosis on the functions of the artery are twofold:

- The internal diameter of the arterial lumen is almost invariably reduced, with a consequent reduction in the amount of blood flowing through it.
- The thickened and rigid artery wall loses some of its ability to contract and relax, and also some of its elasticity.

Arteriolosclerosis is the term used to describe thickening and hardening of the walls of the arterioles. In most cases the structure of the wall of the affected arteriole is completely effaced, with destruction of the thin smooth muscle layer. Arteriolosclerosis is most frequently a consequence of systemic hypertension (see page 164) or diabetes mellitus (see page 382).

Atheroma is a specific degenerative disease affecting large and medium-sized arteries in the systemic circulation. Although it begins as a disease affecting the tunica intima, eventual involvement of the tunica media leads to thickening and hardening of the artery wall. At this stage the disease is called **atherosclerosis**, and is the most common cause of arteriosclerosis affecting large and medium-sized arteries.

Arteriosclerosis affecting small arteries is usually due to the affects of prolonged systemic hypertension (see page 460).

The main consequences of these structural abnormalities affecting arteries and arterioles are due to a combination of factors:

- The **reduction of the size of the lumen** leads to poor perfusion of blood to the tissues supplied by the affected vessels and consequent tissue hypoxia, which may be severe enough to cause cell death, particularly in cells that have a high oxygen requirement.
- The changes in the structure in the tunica intima, particularly the potential for damage to the lining endothelium, predisposes to **thrombus** formation (see pages 152–3).
- The changes in the structure of the media may result in loss of elasticity of the vessel wall. This is a major factor in the pathogenesis of **aneurysm** formation (see page 163), and occurs mainly in the large arteries affected by severe atherosclerosis, particularly the abdominal aorta below the origin of the renal arteries.

Atherosclerosis accounts for half of all deaths in the western world

Atheroma and its consequences constitute the most common and important cause of disease and death in the western world. Atheroma affects large and medium-sized arteries, rarely involving those under 2 mm in diameter, and is confined to arteries exposed to the high pressures in the systemic circulation. The pulmonary arteries normally show no evidence of atheroma except when heart or lung disease leads to pulmonary hypertension. Similarly, atheroma does not affect veins, although atheroma-like lesions can be seen in veins exposed to systemic arterial pressures, e.g. when lengths of vein are used to bypass blocked coronary arteries.

The arteries most severely affected by atheroma are the aorta, coronary, carotid, mesenteric, iliac and femoral arteries, and the cerebral arteries derived from both the vertebrobasilar and internal carotid arteries.

Atheroma is a disease of the intima of arteries

Atheroma is the accumulation of lipid-rich material in the intima of arteries associated with cellular reactions. The atheromatous lesions are termed **plaques** and are composed of a mixture of lipid, collagenous fibrosis, and inflammatory cellular responses. Although atheroma is essentially a disease of the tunica intima, it has an impact on the structure and function of the media.

The macroscopic appearance of atheroma varies according to the stage of evolution of a plaque (*Fig. 10.9*). Histologically, plaques show varying amounts of free lipid, collagen, and macrophages containing lipid (foam cells) (*Fig. 10.10*).

The sequence of changes that occurs in the development of a severe atheromatous lesion is summarized in *Fig. 10.11*.

The pathogenesis of atheroma

There have been many hypotheses as to the pathogenesis of atheroma, which must explain the origin of the lipid seen in plaques, the reason for development of the cellular elements of plaques, and the relation to known risk factors for atheroma development. Most opinions now favor a central role for endothelial dysfunction and injury in the development of atheroma.

The response to injury hypothesis (*Fig. 10.13*) proposes that the atheromatous plaque is a response to chronic low-grade injury to the endothelium. The known risk factors for atheroma can all cause endothelial dysfunction which, importantly, leads to defective production of nitric oxide (NO). NO secretion by endothelial cells normally prevents platelet aggregation, reduces macrophage migration, and limits smooth muscle cell activity. NO reduction in endothelial dysfunction allows platelet adhesion, migration of monocytes into the intima of arteries, and uptake of lipids into the media of vessels. Platelets release PDGF, and this stimulates the proliferation of intimal smooth-muscle cells (myointimal cells). These, in turn, synthesize excess collagen and elastin in the intima. Oxidization of LDL facilitates its uptake into monocytes by non-receptor-mediated pathways.

Remodeling of atheromatous plaques takes place and is mediated by extracellular proteases secreted from inflammatory cells. Local secretion of cytokines from inflammatory cells influences plaque composition. A high collagen component is believed to be important for stability of the plaque. Unstable plaques are characterized by loss of collagen, and the presence of free lipid in a large, soft core region.

Fig. 10.9 Atheroma in segments of aorta. The earliest changes are small fatty streaks (**F**), visible as pale areas beneath the endothelium in the aortic segment on the left. The central segment shows pearly white fibrolipid plaques (**P**), and the segment on the right shows ulcerated advanced plaques with adherent fibrin–platelet thrombus (**T**).

Fig. 10.10 Histology of atheroma. The plaque shows pale lipid-rich areas (**P**) and pink-stained fibrous areas (**F**). Late in the fibrolipid stage the media (**M**) beneath the plaque is thinned.

Fig. 10.11 Atheroma formation. (a) The pathogenesis of atheroma is believed to be damage to the endothelium associated with a variety of risk factors discussed later. This allows entry of cholesterol-rich low-density lipoproteins (LDLs) into the intima. (b) The lipid is taken up by macrophages in the intima. Normal receptor-mediated uptake of lipid can be bypassed by oxidization of LDL, which is taken up by a receptor-independent pathway. In this way, excessive lipid accumulates in intimal macrophages to form a visible pale bulge termed a **'fatty streak'**. (c) With the development and increased accumulation of lipid, macrophages release lipid into the intima. Cytokines secreted by macrophages stimulate proliferation of intimal cells with features of myofibroblasts. These cells secrete collagen and the plaque starts to become fibrotic. At this stage lesions are raised and yellow (lipid plaques). As the lesion develops, there is pressure atrophy of the media and the elastic lamina is disrupted. (d) Increased secretion of collagen forms a dense fibrous cap to the plaque, which is now hard and white (fibrolipid plaque). The advanced plaque shows free lipid as well as lipid in macrophages. Collagenization also affects the media, weakening the arterial wall. The endothelium is fragile and often ulcerates, allowing platelet aggregation and thrombosis. It is possible that platelet-derived growth factor causes further development of plaques by stimulating cell proliferation.

Clinicopathological consequences of atheroma

Atheroma produces disease in several ways:

- **Reduction of blood flow through arteries.** When atheroma affects small arteries, the enlargement of an intimal atheromatous plaque may severely reduce the size of the lumen (*Fig. 10.13a*). The main clinical implications are ischemic heart disease (pages 173–8),

peripheral vascular disease (page 162), and cerebrovascular disease (pages 457–9).

- **Predisposition to thrombosis.** If the fibrous cap and endothelium over an atheromatous plaque breaks down (termed plaque rupture or plaque fissure), collagen fibres in the abnormal intima are exposed to the circulating blood, and this initiates the formation of thrombus (*Fig. 10.13b*). In small-bore vessels such as the coronary or cerebral arteries, this thrombus may suddenly complete the occlusion of an already narrowed artery. In larger vessels, such as the aorta, a plaque of mural thrombus is formed, which may embolize to distal vessels. This complication is a manifestation of plaque instability, in which a plaque is undergoing remodelling.

- **Bleeding into a plaque.** If there is breakdown of the fibrous cap of a plaque due to instability, blood may dissect into the centre of the plaque, causing it to balloon into the vessel lumen and reducing blood flow (*Fig. 10.13c*). This is occasionally seen in coronary arteries, leading to myocardial infarction.

- **Weakening of vessel wall and aneurysm formation.** Severe atheroma in the intima eventually leads to thinning of the media, loss of smooth-muscle cells and elastic fibers, and progressive replacement by non-contractile inelastic collagen. The media becomes functionally incompetent, and this leads to generalized dilatation of the artery over a period of years to form an aneurysm (*Fig. 10.13d*). The abdominal aorta is the most common site for aneurysms secondary to atherosclerosis.

Key Facts
Atheroma

- A disease of the intima of systemic arteries.
- Plaques composed of macrophages, muscle cells, lipid (cholesterol rich), and collagen.
- Main risk factors are hypertension, smoking, high blood cholesterol, and diabetes.
- Complications are reduction of flow, initiating thrombosis, and aneurysm formation.

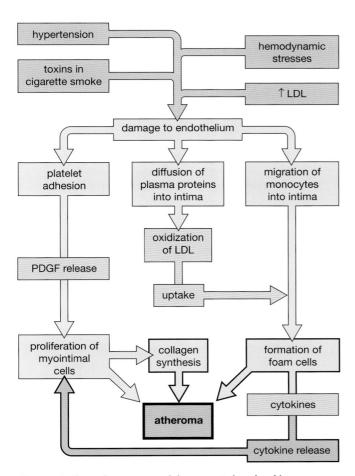

Fig.10.12 **Flow-chart summarizing events involved in pathogenesis of atheroma.**

Fig. 10.13 **Complications of arterial atheroma.** (a) Narrowing of artery by atheroma. (b) Thrombus on plaque. (c) Bleed into a plaque. (d) Aneurysm.

Atherosclerotic peripheral vascular disease causes gangrene

Atherosclerosis of arteries supplying the lower limbs is particularly common in diabetics, affecting them more than any other risk group. The iliofemoral and popliteal arteries are most commonly involved. Reduced flow leads to hypoxia of the calf muscles when their oxygen demands are high, e.g. during brisk walking or running. Patients complain of cramp-like pains in the calf muscles on exercise, which disappear after rest (**intermittent claudication**). More severe reduction in flow can produce similar changes at rest, and there are associated skin changes; there is hair loss, and the skin is smooth, shiny and slow to heal if traumatized.

Complete occlusion, usually by deposition of thrombus on the atheroma, produces **gangrene** (ischemic necrosis of all tissues), manifest as blue-purple, painful discoloration of the skin, followed by progressive blackening of the tissues. The toes are involved first, but the changes progress proximally until a line becomes demarcated where oxygenation is just adequate.

Understanding of risk factors for atheroma is largely based on epidemiological studies

Atheroma is almost ubiquitous in the western world, virtually all adults developing the disease to some degree. Fatty streaks can be seen in childhood, small fibrofatty atheromatous plaques in teenagers and young adults, and complicated atheroma lesions in early middle age; atheromatous lesions increase in number with age.

Epidemiological studies have identified risk factors associated with atheroma development. These can be grouped into constitutional, hard, and soft risk factors.

Constitutional risks for atheroma

- **Age** – The number and severity of atheromatous lesions increases with age.
- **Sex** – Clinically significant atheroma is considerably more common in men than in women up to the age of 55 years; thereafter, the incidence and severity increases rapidly in women, although men remain marginally more severely affected. It has been suggested that women are protected by estrogens before the menopause.
- **Familial traits** have an important bearing on atheroma in a small number of cases in which, independent of traits for hyperlipidemia, there is a familial increase in predisposition.

Hard risk factors for atheroma

- **Hyperlipidemia** – The severity of atherosclerosis has a direct correlation with serum levels of **cholesterol** or **LDL**. The risk increases in a linear fashion with serum cholesterol levels above 3.9 mmol/L (150 mg/dL). There is a less significant association with increased levels of triglyceride and elevated very low-density lipoprotein (VLDL). There is a *reduced* risk of atherosclerosis with high levels of high-density lipoproteins, and this is favoured by modest ethanol consumption (less than 30 mg/day).

Atherosclerosis is much more common in patients with some forms of familial hyperlipidemia (types II and III).

- **Hypertension** – There is a link between persistent high blood pressure and the severity of atheroma, most evident for raised diastolic blood pressure.
- **Diabetes mellitus** is a major risk factor for the development of atheroma, and has been related to induced hypercholesterolemia in this disease.
- **Cigarette smoking** – There is a link between cigarette smoking and death from coronary artery disease, the most important clinical consequence of severe atheroma.

Soft risk factors for atherosclerosis

- **Exercise** reduces the incidence of sudden death from ischemic heart disease, one of the main effects of atherosclerosis, but it is uncertain whether it has an effect on the development of atheroma.
- **Overweight** individuals have an increased risk of death from ischemic heart disease, but this may be a reflection of diet and resultant hyperlipidemia.
- **Stress and personality** traits have been linked to death from ischemic heart disease in some studies.

ANEURYSMS

Diseases that damage the arterial media predispose to aneurysm formation

An aneurysm is an abnormal focal dilatation of an artery. Aneurysms can cause signs or symptoms from a local mass effect, for example by pressing on an adjacent structure. However, the main complications are due to rupture, causing local bleeding, and predisposition to thrombosis. Although it is the most frequent cause, atherosclerosis is not the only disease that produces aneurysms: any abnormality that weakens the media may produce an aneurysm. Other types and causes of aneurysm are given in *Fig. 10.14*. Apart from developmental causes, a common factor in this type of pathology is loss of elastin and muscle in the arterial wall mediated by a local inflammatory response.

AORTIC DISSECTION

In aortic dissection, a tear in the intima leads to tracking of blood into the arterial media, which splits. The most common site for this is the aorta, where the split forms a false channel, usually between the inner two-thirds and the outer third of the medial thickness. The possible outcomes are summarized in *Fig. 10.15*.

Among the predisposing factors are hypertension, present in 70% of cases, and degenerative changes in the aortic media (medial mucoid degeneration), which sometimes arise as part of a hereditary disorder, e.g. Marfan's syndrome due to defective fibrillin, and Ehlers–Danlos syndrome.

Atheroma is also a predisposing factor, the original intimal tear occasionally occurring at the edge of an atheromatous plaque. This pattern is particularly important in the distal aorta.

Fig. 10.14 Types of aneurysm

Type	Site	Cause	Incidence
Atherosclerotic	Abdominal aorta	Thinning and fibrous replacement of media	Common
Syphilitic	Ascending aorta and arch	Inflammatory destruction of media and fibrous replacement	Now rare
Berry	Cerebral arteries	Congenital defect(s) in elastic lamina/media	Common
Infective (mycotic)	Any	Destruction of wall by bacteria in infected thrombus	Rare

Fig. 10.15 Outcome following aortic dissection. (a) External rupture, usually lower down the thoracic aorta, with massive fatal hemorrhage into the thoracic cavity. (b) Retrograde spread (back towards the heart) with rupture into the pericardial cavity and fatal hemopericardium. (c) Internal rupture, with blood tracking back into the lumen by rupturing through the inner media and intima, to produce a double-channeled aorta. This is rare.

HYPERTENSION

Hypertension may be classed as primary or may be secondary to a known cause

Elevated blood pressure (hypertension) is an important and treatable cause of disease, and is divided into primary or secondary groups. In the population, blood pressure is a continuous variable, with increasing risk of disease associated with increasing blood pressure. Hypertension can be arbitrarily defined as sustained diastolic pressure greater than 90 mmHg. However, there is no threshold below which a person has no risk of developing diseases in which blood pressure is a pathogenic factor.

Primary (essential) hypertension is elevation of blood pressure with age, but with no apparent cause. It accounts for over 90% of all cases and is usually seen after the age of 40 years. The phenotype of high blood pressure in essential hypertension is the result of interactions between genetic predisposition, obesity, alcohol consumption, physical activity and other, as yet unidentified, factors.

Accounting for about 10% of all cases, **secondary hypertension** is due to an identifiable cause, the most common of which is renovascular disease that elevates blood pressure by activation of the renin–angiotensin–aldosterone system.

Depending on the clinical course of the disease, both primary and secondary hypertension can be classified into two types. With **benign hypertension** there is gradual elevation of blood pressure over many years, and with **accelerated hypertension** (malignant hypertension) blood pressure elevation is severe and becomes worse over a short period. The pathological changes seen in blood vessels differ between benign and accelerated hypertension.

Arterial wall thickening and hyaline arteriolosclerosis are features of benign hypertension

In benign hypertension, vessel changes develop gradually in response to a persistent stable elevated blood pressure. The changes in small arteries are shown in *Fig. 10.16*, and those in arterioles in *Fig. 10.17*.

These degenerative changes in the walls of small vessels such as arterioles lead to a reduction in effective lumen, with consequent tissue ischemia, and to increased fragility of vessels in the brain, predisposing to hemorrhage.

Destruction of small vessel walls is seen in malignant hypertension

When the blood pressure rises suddenly and markedly, acute destructive changes occur in the walls of small blood vessels, together with proliferative reparative responses in the walls of small arteries (*Figs 10.19* and *10.20*).

These changes lead to cessation of blood flow through the small vessels, with multiple foci of tissue necrosis, e.g. in the glomeruli in the kidney.

Hypertension mainly affects the heart, brain, kidneys and aorta

The pathological consequences of hypertension are seen in four main tissues:

- **Heart.** With increasing pressure, the left ventricular myocardium undergoes hypertrophy. Continued remodeling of the heart leads to dilatation and left ventricular failure.
- **Brain.** Hypertensive patients are prone to develop **intracerebral hemorrhage** due to rupture of

Fig. 10.16 Small arterial changes in benign hypertension. There is hypertrophy and thickening of muscular media (**M**), thickening of the elastic lamina (**E**), fibroelastic thickening of the intima (**I**), and reduction in the size of the vessel lumen (**L**).

Fig. 10.17 Arteriolar changes in benign hypertension. There is hyaline wall thickening (hyaline arteriolosclerosis) (**H**), increased rigidity (with limited capacity for expansion and constriction), and reduction of luminal size.

Factors that regulate blood pressure

Blood pressure can be elevated by increasing cardiac output or by increasing peripheral vascular resistance. The former is raised by increasing the blood volume or by increasing cardiac contractility and rate, and the latter may be increased by humoral, neural and autoregulatory factors. These regulatory processes are summarized in *Fig. 10.18*.

There is great interest in understanding genetic predispositions to hypertension. Very rare single-gene disorders have been identified that can cause hypertension:

- Mutations in genes coding for proteins involved in aldosterone metabolism.
- Mutations in genes coding for sodium ion handling.

The search is on to identify common polymorphisms in genes that will explain both population and individual predispositions to hypertension.

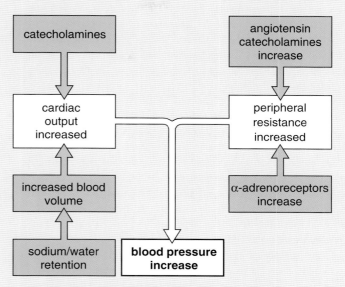

Fig. 10.18 Regulation of blood pressure.

intracerebral blood vessels (see page 460). Small vessel damage produces microinfarcts in the form of small areas of brain destruction filled with fluid (**hypertensive lacunae**).

- **Kidney.** Arteriolosclerosis leads to progressive ischemia of the nephron, with eventual destruction of glomeruli. This disease is slowly progressive, as individual nephrons are picked off one at a time. When sufficient nephrons have been damaged, progressive **chronic renal failure** occurs. When hypertension has produced renal failure the kidney is said to show **hypertensive nephrosclerosis**. It is a common and important cause of chronic renal failure in the middle-aged and elderly.
- **Aorta.** Hypertension predisposes to the development of severe atheroma, abdominal aortic aneurysms, and dissections (page 163).

Fig. 10.19 Accelerated hypertension change in small arteries.
Loose myxomatous fibrous intimal proliferation (**I**) can be seen, together with reduction of luminal size (**L**) and normal media (**M**).

Fig. 10.20 Accelerated hypertension change in arterioles.
Fibrinoid necrosis, visible as replacement of the wall by material stained bright red (**F**), is seen in the wall of a renal arteriole in malignant hypertension.

Secondary hypertension accounts for less than 10% of cases

In a minority of cases some structural abnormality is considered to be responsible for the development of systemic hypertension. For example, **stenosis of one renal artery** (usually at its origin) by atherosclerosis can produce hypertension, treatable by surgery. Associated with a rise in renin and angiotensin II levels in the circulation from the ischemic kidney, the hypertension can be cured in the early stages by removing the affected kidney.

Hypertension is also a feature of **diffuse renal disease,** such as glomerulonephritis and pyelonephritis. The hypertension is transient in the initial acute phase of glomerular diseases (e.g. acute nephritic syndrome), but is permanent in chronic diffuse renal disease.

Pheochromocytoma, an adrenaline/noradrenaline (epinephrine/norepinephrine)-secreting tumor, usually of the adrenal medulla, produces hypertension that is initially paroxysmal (see page 348).

Coarctation of the aorta is a congenital malformation in which there is increased peripheral resistance due to a structural narrowing of the aorta. In such cases the hypertension is not truly systemic, as it affects only the arterial system proximal to the coarctation and, thus, mainly the arms, head and neck (see page 186).

Hypertension is a feature of **adrenal cortical diseases**, conditions associated with excess production of glucocorticoids and mineralocorticoids by the adrenal cortex (Cushing's syndrome and Conn's syndrome, see page 346). It is also a feature of **pre-eclampsia** (see page 436), may be seen in association with endocrine disorders such as thyrotoxicosis, acromegaly and, occasionally, hypothyroidism, or there may be a **neurogenic cause** such as raised intracranial pressure.

Pulmonary arterial hypertension is usually due to disease in the lung or the left side of the heart

Most pulmonary hypertension is 'secondary' in that it develops as a consequence of one of two types of raised pressure in the pulmonary capillary bed (*Fig. 10.21*).

Pulmonary capillary pressure may be raised due to raised pressure in the left atrium and left ventricle. This back pressure is the result of inadequate emptying of the left heart chambers (left heart failure), the increased pressure in these chambers being reflected along the pulmonary veins and into the pulmonary capillary beds (pulmonary congestion). Important causes are left ventricular failure due to hypertensive or ischemic heart disease, aortic valve stenosis, and mitral valve stenosis (leading to left atrial failure).

Alternatively, pulmonary capillary pressure may be raised because of destruction of the pulmonary capillary bed as a result of primary lung disease.

VASCULITIS

Vasculitis syndromes are a mixed group of diseases, affecting blood vessels of all types

Vasculitis implies inflammation and damage to the vessel wall. It can affect capillaries, venules, arterioles, arteries and, occasionally, large veins. A pathological classification divides vasculitis into three groups depending on the size of vessel predominantly involved (see *Fig. 10.22*). Some patterns of vasculitis are associated with antineutrophil autoantobodies (ANCA), discussed in the blue box. Clinically, patients usually present with constitutional symptoms of fever and malaise. Arthralgia and myalgia are common. Organ- and tissue-specific manifestations are also present, and depend on the type of vasculitis and how it affects different sites (*Fig. 10.23*).

The different vasculitis syndromes are associated with different types of inflammation involving the walls of affected blood vessels.

Neurophilic vasculitis (necrotizing vasculitis) is associated with necrosis of the wall of the affected vessel, with

Fig. 10.21 Causes of pulmonary hypertension
SECONDARY
Increased pulmonary blood flow
Cardiac shunts (ASD, VSD) (see page 185)
Destruction of lung capillary bed
Emphysema Interstitial fibrosis of lungs
Mechanical arterial occlusion
Multiple pulmonary thromboemboli (see page 155) Foreign body emboli (drug addicts)
Alveolar hypoxia causing pulmonary vasoconstriction
High altitude Obesity Chronic obstructive airways disease
Pulmonary venous congestion
Mitral valve disease especially stenosis (see page 182) Chronic left ventricular failure (see page 172)
PRIMARY
Idiopathic
Primary pulmonary hypertension: a rare disease of young women caused by increased tone in pulmonary vessels, leading to progressive vascular changes and death. Pulmonary veno-occlusive disease: a rare disease causing fibrous obliteration of pulmonary vessels. Some cases thought to be due to vascular thrombosis.

Laboratory medicine

In some types of vasculitis it is possible to detect autoantibodies that react against granules of neutrophils; one type has a cytoplasmic pattern on immunofluorescence (c-ANCA) and is directed to proteinase-3 (PRC-ANCA); the other shows a pattern of perinuclear staining (p-ANCA) and is directed against myeloperoxidase (MPO-ANCA).

In the absence of p-ANCA, c-ANCA is present in the serum of 90% of patients with Wegener's granulomatosis and, rarely, in other types of vasculitis. p-ANCA is present in polyarteritis nodosa and other types of necrotizing vasculitis.

Identification of these antibodies in serum is used in the diagnostic evaluation of patients with possible vasculitis.

Fig. 10.23 Clinical syndromes and likely vasculitis

Organ	Likely vasculitis
Lung and kidney	Wegener's granulomatosis Microscopic polyangiitis
Upper respiratory tract	Wegener's granulomatosis
Lung and skin	Henoch–Schönlein purpura Cryoglobulinemic vasculitis
Associated with asthma and eosinophilia	Churg–Strauss syndrome
Kidney	Microscopic polyangiitis Wegener's granulomatosis
Peripheral nerve	Polyarteritis nodosa
Heart	Kawasaki disease Polyarteritis nodosa
Skin only	Drug-related

deposition of fibrin (fibrinoid necrosis) and infiltration by neutrophils.

Giant cell vasculitis is associated with histiocytic infiltration of the vessels wall and the formation of multinucleate giant cells.

Granulomatous vasculitis is associated with the formation of histiocytic granulomata in relation to damaged vessels.

Lymphocytic vasculitis shows infiltration of vessel wall by lymphoid cells.

Fig. 10.22 Vasculitis syndrome

Immune complex (hypersensitivity) vasculitis is the commonest form of vasculitis

Immune complex vasculitis (hypersensitivity vasculitis) is the most common of all the vasculitides. It affects capillaries and venules, and usually presents as a skin rash (*Fig. 10.24*). It is often a manifestation of allergy to a drug ('drug-induced vasculitis'), occasionally arising as an allergic rash in viremia or bacteremia. It also occurs in Henoch–Schönlein purpura (the commonest type seen in children) and cryoglobulinemia. This is a form of neutrophilic vasculitis that involves the postcapillary venules, with some capillary involvement (*Fig. 10.25*). The extravasation of red cells in the dermis is manifest as a transient palpable purpuric skin rash.

Patients are typically ANCA-negative, and the pathogenesis is due to immune complexes between an antigen and antibody becoming trapped in the walls of venules. These activate complement, setting off a local acute inflammatory response, with neutrophil chemotaxis.

Fig. 10.24 Purpuric skin rash in immune complex (hypersensitivity) vasculitis.

Microscopic polyangiitis is the commonest form of ANCA-positive vasculitis

Microscopic polyangiitis is the commonest form of ANCA-positive small-vessel vasculitis and usually affects adults, leading to renal problems, skin rashes and, less frequently, involvement of the respiratory tract and bowel.

Polyarteritis nodosa (PAN) is a systemic disease that affects small and medium-sized arteries

Polyarteritis nodosa is a systemic disease characterized by inflammatory necrosis of the walls of medium-sized arteries, but can also affect small vessels. The clinical effects of the disease are the result of vessel occlusion leading to small areas of infarction, and the tissues most seriously affected are the kidneys, heart, alimentary tract, liver, central nervous system, peripheral nerves, skeletal muscle, and skin (*Fig. 10.26*). Although the disease is systemic, it is patchy and focal, only parts of some arteries being involved. Affected vessels show necrotizing vasculitis (*Fig. 10.27*).

The cause of the disease is unknown, but it is likely to be immune-complex mediated. There is an association with chronic hepatitis B virus antigenemia.

Fig. 10.25 Immune complex (hypersensitivity) vasculitis.
Histologically the capillaries and venules in the upper dermis show destruction of small vessel walls by neutrophils, with adjacent dark-stained particles of neutrophil nuclear debris (neutrophilic vasculitis), and extravasated red cells in the area around the vessel. Occasionally the vessel walls show fibrinoid necrosis. This pattern of vasculitis mainly affects skin, but occasionally a similar small-vessel vasculitis occurs in the kidney, the lining of the joints and the alimentary tract mucosa in Henoch–Schönlein syndrome.

Fig. 10.26 Pathological effects of polyarteritis nodosa		
Organ	**Effects**	**Clinical features**
Kidney	Microinfarcts	Acute renal failure
Gastrointestinal tract	Microinfarcts	Mucosal ulceration
Central nervous system	Infarction	Focal neurology
Nerves	Necrosis	Mononeuritis multiplex
Skeletal muscle	Fiber necrosis	Myalgia and weakness
Heart	Infarction	Cardiac failure

Giant cell arteritis is common in the elderly

Giant cell arteritis is a systemic disease that mainly involves large arteries in the head and neck region. It particularly affects the temporal arteries, hence the alternative term, **temporal arteritis**. Increasing in incidence with age, it is rare under the age of 50 and is more common in females.

Patients have ill-defined symptoms of malaise and tiredness, with headaches. In many cases there is an associated disease of muscle, polymyalgia rheumatica. Investigations characteristically reveal a very high ESR. Diagnosis is by biopsy of the temporal artery, and histological findings are shown in *Fig. 10.28*.

A frequent complication is sudden blindness due to involvement of the ophthalmic artery; treatment with steroids is urgently indicated in this condition.

Buerger's disease is an inflammatory disease of vessels that is related to smoking

Buerger's disease causes inflammatory occlusion of peripheral arteries in the upper and lower limbs. It is related to heavy cigarette smoking and is seen mainly in males. Pathologically there is segmental chronic inflammatory infiltration of the walls of arteries and veins, with secondary thrombosis. Small foci of neutrophils may also be seen.

Patients develop peripheral vascular insufficiency, and eventually gangrene.

STRUCTURAL ABNORMALITIES OF VEINS

Dilatation and congestion of veins is common in many sites

The most common abnormality of veins is dilatation and congestion with blood. Such abnormal veins are given different names in different sites.

Varicose veins are persistently distended superficial veins in the lower limbs (long and short saphenous veins). They are the result of incompetence of the valves, which allows the veins to become engorged with blood under the influence of gravity. A saphenovarix is a localized distension of the superficial saphenous veins in the groin, producing a smooth, rounded mass.

Hemorrhoids (or 'piles') are greatly distended veins of the internal hemorrhoidal plexus of submucosal veins in the anal canal and at the anorectal junction. They present as prolapsed mucosa-covered masses, which often protrude through the anal orifice. Bleeding may follow trauma, and pain may follow from gross protrusion and anal sphincter spasm.

Varicocele is persistent distension of the veins of the pampiniform plexus of veins in the spermatic cord within the scrotum.

All of these conditions in the pelvis and lower limbs can be aggravated by any pelvic or abdominal condition that causes pressure on the veins, preventing adequate venous return. For example, pregnancy is an important and common precipitating factor in the development of varicose veins and hemorrhoids.

Esophageal varices and prominent periumbilical veins are distended venous channels that develop in portal hypertension secondary to cirrhosis of the liver (see page 251).

Fig. 10.27 Polyarteritis nodosa. The artery wall shows infiltration by mixed inflammatory cells, in which neutrophils and eosinophils are most numerous. Fibrinoid necrosis (**F**) of the artery wall is common. The inflammatory destruction leads to necrosis of muscle cells and destruction of the elastic lamina; healing is followed by fibrous replacement of these specialized structures. During the acute inflammatory phase the extensive damage to the intima predisposes to thrombosis, which is often followed by vessel occlusion and infarction of the target tissue.

Fig. 10.28 Giant cell arteritis. In giant cell arteritis the vessel wall is thickened and infiltrated by a mixture of inflammatory cells. This is largely composed of T lymphocytes, but has foci of histiocytes and giant cells (**G**). The histiocytic giant cells are mainly related to fragments of the disrupted elastic lamina (**E**). Complication by thrombosis is common.

TUMORS AND MALFORMATIONS OF VESSELS

Angiomas are developmental malformations derived from blood vessels

Developmental malformations derived from blood vessels are very common and are termed **angiomas** or **hemangiomas**.

- Hemangiomas are composed of dilated vascular spaces.
- Capillary angiomas are composed of small capillary-like vessels.
- Cavernous angiomas are composed of wide, vein-like vessels (*Fig. 10.29*).
- Angiomas with mixed patterns are common.

Vascular tissues (usually abnormal) are an important, often predominant, component of mixed connective tissue hamartomatous malformations in the subcutaneous tissue of the neck and upper trunk in young people. In some cases lymphatic vessels are the predominant feature, and in children such malformations may consist almost entirely of enormously dilated lymphatic vessels (**cystic hygroma**). Other connective tissues present include adipose tissue, abnormal nerves, and some smooth muscle.

Large vascular malformations are an important cause of intracerebral hemorrhage

The brain is an important site for vascular malformations. They are usually large and consist of both arterial and venous-type vessels. These often communicate directly and are termed **arteriovenous malformations** (AVM). They may produce symptoms by local brain compression, resulting in focal neurological signs. The most serious complication is spontaneous bleeding leading to intracranial hemorrhage.

True vascular tumors are rare

True tumors of blood vessels are rare, but include Kaposi's sarcoma, which is becoming a more important and common tumor.

Numerically the most common tumor is the so-called **glomus tumor (glomangioma)**, which presents as a tender, painful nodule on the finger, often close to the nail. The tumor contains vascular channels surrounded by glomus cells.

Angiosarcoma (*Fig. 10.30*), a malignant tumor of blood vessel endothelium, most commonly occurs as a raised bluish-red patch on the face or scalp of elderly people. It enlarges progressively, often ulcerating, and later metastasizes to regional lymph nodes. This tumor may also occur in limbs that have very long-standing chronic lymphedema, but this is now very rare, and was most commonly seen in the arms of women who had had a total axillary clearance as part of radical surgery for breast cancer. Angiosarcomas

Fig. 10.29 Cavernous angioma. Cavernous angioma is composed of vein-like vascular spaces filled with blood. In this example the lesion has arisen in the liver.

in the liver have been associated with industrial exposure to vinyl chloride, which is used in various chemical industries (particularly plastic manufacturing).

Hemangioendotheliomas behave as low-grade malignant tumors and are derived from endothelial cells. **Hemangiopericytomas**, also of low-grade malignant potential, are derived from the pericytes surrounding blood vessels. Occurring mainly in the subcutaneous tissues of the limbs, they occasionally develop in other sites.

One form of Kaposi's sarcoma is seen with AIDS

Kaposi's sarcoma is believed to be derived from endothelial cells. However, this is still debated. There is a strong and possible causative association with human herpes virus-8 (HHV8). There are four patterns of disease, the natural histories of which seem to be related to the clinical setting in which the tumor develops. Only one form is seen in AIDS.

Endemic Kaposi's sarcoma is seen in Africa. In children it is a highly malignant condition based in lymph nodes, but in adults it runs a more indolent course, with hematogenous spread.

Classic Kaposi's sarcoma is a rare tumor that develops in the lower limbs of elderly men. It behaves as a low-grade malignant skin neoplasm, with hematogenous and lymph node metastasis.

Kaposi's sarcoma in therapeutic immunosuppression resembles classic Kaposi's sarcoma, behaving as a low-grade malignant neoplasm in the skin.

Epidemic Kaposi's sarcoma is seen in patients with AIDS. It is a highly malignant tumor of skin, with spread to lymph nodes and visceral organs.

Kaposi's sarcoma progresses through three phases, which are summarized in *Fig. 10.31*. The nodular phase is shown in *Fig. 10.32*.

Fig. 10.30 Angiosarcoma. An angiosarcoma is composed of neoplastic endothelial cells, which form vascular-like channels in tissues. This is a highly malignant tumor.

Fig. 10.31 Stages of Kaposi's sarcoma	
Phase	**Macroscopic appearance (skin and oral mucosa)**
Patch phase	Flat, bruise-like, purple lesions
Plaque phase	Slightly raised, firm, purple lesions
Nodular phase	Dome-shaped, firm, purple lesions

Fig. 10.32 Nodular phase of Kaposi's sarcoma. Histology shows plump spindle cells with compressed, slit-shaped vascular channels containing red cells.

DISEASES OF THE HEART

HEART FAILURE

Cardiac failure develops when the heart cannot maintain the circulation

When the pumping effort of the heart falls short of sustaining a circulation sufficient for metabolic needs, **cardiac failure** is said to have occurred. Conditions in which the circulation fails because of a low blood volume, e.g. bleeding or fluid loss, are excluded from this definition. The main broad groups of conditions causing cardiac failure are those demanding extra work of the heart (e.g. hypertension, valve diseases) and those that damage heart muscle (e.g. ischemia).

Cardiac failure can be either acute or chronic

Acute cardiac failure takes place when there is a sudden onset of pathology. There is abrupt failure of chamber emptying, the failing chambers dilate, and compensatory mechanisms cannot be brought into operation. Circulatory collapse with low blood pressure is termed 'cardiogenic shock' (see page 158).

Chronic cardiac failure occurs when there is a gradual increase in the severity of a disease. It has a major impact on organ systems other than the heart, and is manifest by tiredness, breathlessness, and the development of edema. In the face of inadequate circulation, several compensatory responses take place:

- The ventricles of the heart enlarge, and contract more effectively.
- Constriction of arterioles causes redistribution of blood flow.
- Activation of the sympathetic and renin–angiotensin systems causes retention of salt and water, and changes in vascular tone.
- There is desensitization of cardiac muscle to sympathetic stimulation.

Acute or chronic cardiac failure may develop when compensatory mechanisms break down.

Failure of the left side of the heart leads to poor systemic arterial perfusion and increased pressure in the pulmonary venous and capillary systems

When the left heart fails to pump efficiently, the chambers fail to empty completely at systole and become dilated. A dilated chamber is a failing chamber. Incomplete emptying leads to a progressive rise in pressure in one chamber, which is reflected back into the chamber or vessels that precede it in the circulation. In the left heart this leads to dilatation of the left atrium, dilatation and increased pressure in the pulmonary veins and, eventually, increased pressure in the

Fig. 10.33 Pulmonary edema – left heart failure. This histological section shows lung alveoli filled with pink-stained edema fluid (**F**).

Fig. 10.34 Congested liver – right heart failure. Chronic passive venous congestion of the liver causes dark areas where centrilobular zones are congested by blood, contrasting with pale periportal areas. This appearance is similar to that of the cut surface of a nutmeg, hence the term 'nutmeg liver.'

pulmonary capillaries. The high pressure in the pulmonary capillary system forces the fluid component of blood out into the alveolar air sacs, which become filled with low-protein fluid. This is manifest clinically as **pulmonary edema**, and presents with acute breathlessness due to fluid in the air sacs (*Fig. 10.33*).

Another consequence of left heart failure is that insufficient blood is pumped out into the aorta and arterial system, which leads to hypotension, poor perfusion of tissues, and poor tissue oxygenation.

Failure of the right side of the heart leads to poor perfusion of the lungs and increased pressure in the systemic venous system

As the right side of the heart fails, the chambers dilate and there is increased intrachamber pressure, preventing adequate emptying of the systemic venous blood from the venae cavae into the right atrium. This rise in systemic venous pressure has a number of clinical manifestations:

- The raised pressure in the superior vena cava can be observed in the neck in the form of jugular vein engorgement (**raised jugular venous pressure**).
- The raised pressure in the inferior vena cava is reflected back into the venous system of the liver and other organs, and may manifest as a **tender, palpably enlarged, congested liver** (*Fig. 10.34*),
- The raised pressure in the small venules and capillaries of the lower limb, supplemented by the effect of gravity, leads to increased pressure in the lumina of these small vessels, with transudation of fluid into the interstitial tissues producing **subcutaneous edema**, particularly around the ankles.

Congestive cardiac failure is failure of both the right and the left sides of the heart

Failure of both sides of the heart is termed 'congestive cardiac failure.' Biventricular failure most commonly arises when there is right heart failure secondary to pulmonary capillary congestion as a result of primary left heart failure.

When left heart failure is long-standing and severe, the back-pressure effects cause permanent congestion and increased pressure in the pulmonary capillary system. This gives rise to increased back pressure in the pulmonary arterial system, which leads to right heart failure as a result of the right heart having to pump against an increased peripheral resistance.

Congestive cardiac failure may also be caused by unusual diseases that simultaneously affect the muscle of both ventricles.

Key Facts
Heart failure

- Left-sided failure causes pulmonary edema.
- Main causes of left-sided failure are myocardial infarction, hypertension, and valve disease.
- Right-sided failure causes venous congestion and peripheral edema.
- Main causes of right-sided failure are chronic lung disease and chronic left-sided failure.
- Congestive cardiac failure is failure of both sides of the heart.

Molecular changes in the myocardium are important in the pathophysiology of cardiac failure

Increasing interest is being shown in the phenotype of cardiac myocytes in the failing heart.

In heart failure, compensatory mechanisms are brought into play at the level of changes in signaling pathways aimed at improving cardiac reserve and function. Albeit beneficial, these augmentations have cumulative damaging effects.

- Cardiac muscle is extensively remodeled in the failing heart, both in terms of contractile proteins and in the extracellular matrix.
- In the failing heart expression of the myosin isoforms involved in contraction are reduced, correlating with impaired systolic function.
- Uncoupling of adrenergic receptors to the G-protein cAMP pathway is seen in failing hearts owing to abnormal receptor phosphorylation.

Signal	Benefit	Adverse effects
Adrenergic	Contractility Myocardial hypertrophy	Myocyte toxic effects Myocyte apoptosis
Angiotensin II	Myocardial hypertrophy	Change in gene expression of contractile proteins
Cytokine (TNFα)	Myocardial hypertrophy	Remodeling of extracellular matrix with dilatation

These insights into the molecular pathophysiology of cardiac failure are directing the search for new therapeutic agents.

ISCHAEMIC HEART DISEASE

The most common disease of the heart is caused by myocardial ischemia

Ischemic heart disease is the most common type of cardiac disease and the leading cause of death in the western world, accounting for about 30% of all male deaths and 23% of all female deaths.

The main cause of ischemic heart disease, also called **coronary heart disease**, is atheroma of coronary arteries. The risk factors predisposing to the development of ischemic heart disease are similar to those predisposing to the development of atheroma (see page 160).

Because of its greater bulk and work requirement, the myocardium of the left ventricle has the higher oxygen demand and is more prone to ischemia. Coronary heart disease can be divided into chronic and acute presentations, the acute forms being termed the acute coronary syndromes.

Stable angina is caused by low flow in atherosclerotic coronary arteries

Angina is episodic chest pain that takes place when there is a demand for increased myocardial work, usually through exercise, in the presence of impaired perfusion by blood. Pathological studies of patients with angina show that they have at least one stenosis of over 50% of the lumen in a main coronary artery. High-grade stenosis limits flow, but this may be modifiable by drugs, depending on the nature of the plaque. Atheromatous plaques in coronary arteries may be one of two types, eccentric or concentric (*Fig. 10.35*).

Over a long period, repeated episodes of impaired flow may lead to the development of fine fibrosis in the myocardium, with death of individual cardiac muscle fibers. Anastomotic vessels frequently develop to compensate for areas of vascular stenosis.

Acute coronary syndromes are largely caused by complicated atheroma

Thrombus formation, stimulated by instability in an atheromatous plaque, is the main cause of acute episodes of ischemic heart disease, termed **acute coronary syndromes**. Thrombosis at this location is caused by two main processes:

Main syndromes caused by disease of coronary arteries

Atherosclerosis of coronary arteries causes:

Chronic manifestation	Acute manifestations
Stable angina	Unstable angina
Cardiac failure	Non-ST-elevation myocardial infarction
	ST-elevation myocardial infarction
	Sudden cardiac death

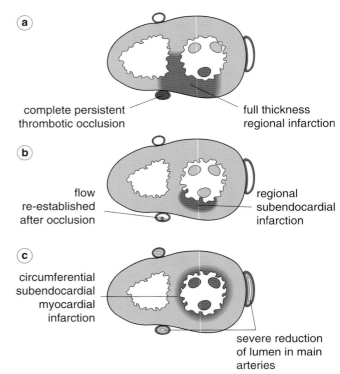

Fig. 10.35 Plaques in coronary arteries. Eccentric plaques, often rich in lipid, affect only one segment of the wall of a coronary artery. Improvement of flow at the site of such plaques may be achieved by vasodilator drugs, which can cause relaxation of the normal (unaffected) part of the vessel wall. **Concentric plaques**, usually mostly collagenous, affect the whole of the arterial wall and, as the whole wall is abnormal, drug therapy cannot improve flow over a narrowed segment.

Fig. 10.36 Patterns of myocardial infarction. The three main patterns of myocardial infarction are regional full thickness (a), regional subendocardial (b), and circumferential subendocardial (c).

- 25% of cases are due to superficial ulceration of endothelium over a plaque.
- 75% of cases are due to plaque fissuring, resulting in a deep cleft in a lipid-rich plaque that either precipitates thrombus development in the lumen or causes bleeding into the body of the plaque, with resultant ballooning into the lumen.

Importantly, such complications may be in low-grade stenoses, areas that will not have caused previous angina on exertion. The initial manifestation of coronary artery atherosclerosis may therefore be an acute coronary syndrome, with no history of previous chest pain on exertion.

Unstable angina is caused by fissuring of atherosclerotic plaques

Fissuring of plaques may cause a syndrome of sudden-onset angina that increases in frequency and severity, termed **crescendo angina** or **unstable angina**. On initial presentation it is clinically difficult to discriminate between unstable angina and early forms of myocardial infarction. A definition is that there is no elevation of serum cardiac troponin, which would indicate death of cardiac muscle.

As there is a plaque fissure and thrombosis has been initiated, there is a risk of subsequent total thrombotic occlusion of the vessel. A proportion of patients with unstable angina will progress to myocardial infarction or may die from secondary development of a ventricular arrhythmia. It is estimated that between 5% and 8% of patients who present with unstable angina will die within 6 months.

Acute myocardial infarction may be full or partial thickness

Death of cardiac muscle following arterial occlusion occurs in two main patterns, either full thickness or partial thickness (subendocardial) (*Fig. 10.36*). The difference in these two patterns is generally related to the severity and duration of coronary arterial occlusion following plaque instability and arterial thrombosis.

Regional myocardial infarction (90% of cases) involves one segment of the ventricular wall. The cause of this pattern is nearly always thrombus formation on a complicated atheromatous plaque. If there is complete persistent occlusion of the arterial branch supplying that area, the infarct is full thickness (*Fig. 10.37*). If there is lysis of the thrombus or a collateral supply to the myocardium, the infarct will be limited to the subendocardial zone (**regional subendocardial infarction**).

A third pattern, termed **circumferential subendocardial infarction** (10% of cases), is caused by a general hypoperfusion of the main coronary arteries. This is usually due to an episode of modest hypotension critically reducing flow in arteries already affected by high-grade atherosclerotic stenosis. Circumferential subendocardial infarction involves the subendocardial zone of the ventricle, the region at the end of the arterial perfusion zone, which fails to be perfused and undergoes necrosis (*Fig. 10.38*).

Clinical patterns of infarction correlate generally with pathology

The clinical definition of myocardial infarction requires that there be a demonstrated elevation of serum cardiac troponin levels. Additional categorization is based on the presence or absence of changes in the ST segment on ECG.

- ST-elevation myocardial infarction (STEMI), with evolution of the ECG to develop Q waves, usually correlates with a full-thickness regional myocardial infarct.

Fig. 10.37 Regional full-thickness myocardial infarction. The full thickness of the lateral wall of the left ventricle is infarcted (**I**).

Fig. 10.38 Circumferential subendocardial infarction. The subendocardial zone around the whole circumference of the left ventricle is infarcted and dark in color.

- Non-ST-elevation myocardial infarction (NSTEMI) usually correlates with a partial-thickness lesion and no subsequent development of Q waves on the ECG.
- Circumferential subendocardial infarction is generally not associated with the development of Q waves.

The site of regional myocardial infarction depends on which vessel is involved

The extent and distribution of the area of myocardial infarction depends upon which coronary artery branch is occluded (*Fig. 10.39*). The vast majority of infarcts affect the left ventricle and the septal region. Infarction of the right ventricle can occur, but is very rare by comparison.

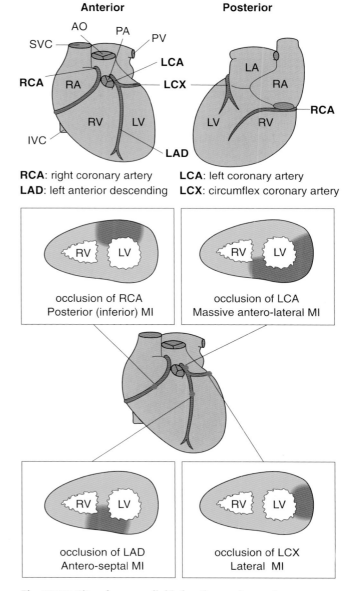

Fig. 10.39 Site of myocardial infarction and vessel involvement.

Myocardial infarction induces acute inflammation, followed by organization and scarring

The end result of myocardial infarction is replacement of the necrotic area by collagenous scar. The entire process, from fiber necrosis to scar formation, takes 6–8 weeks, the macroscopic and histological appearances of the infarct changing with time (*Fig. 10.42*).

Sudden cardiac death is due to either infarction or arrhythmias

Most deaths caused by ischemic heart disease do not occur in hospital. Patients either have no warning symptoms or die shortly after their onset. Death is usually due to ventricular fibrillation.

Patients who have had symptoms of previous ischemic heart disease, e.g. angina or previous infarction, tend to develop cardiac arrhythmias arising from muscle adjacent to an area of old scarring, and have not had a new thrombotic episode.

Those with no previous cardiac history have usually had a new thrombotic event arising from a complicated atheromatous plaque. This has given rise to acute myocardial ischemia, which precipitates the arrhythmia.

Sudden cardiac death is the most important immediate consequence of myocardial ischemia.

Many complications of myocardial infarction occur in the first 2 weeks

If the patient survives the immediate impact of acute myocardial infarction, or is successfully resuscitated from cardiac arrest or acute pulmonary edema, the next hurdle is the short-term complications. These include:

- **Further episodes of cardiac dysrhythmia**, particularly ventricular fibrillation. Bradyarrhythmias are particularly seen with posterior (inferior) infarcts, as the AV node is often involved.
- The **development of left ventricular failure** is most common with very large areas of infarction, which cause cardiac dilatation as the necrotic wall softens in organization.
- **Rupture of the ventricular wall** at any time, usually 2–10 days after the infarct, particularly during early organization and softening (*Fig. 10.40*). Blood bursts through the wall, instantly filling the pericardial cavity (hemopericardium). The sudden rise in intrapericardial cavity pressure prevents cardiac filling (**cardiac tamponade**), leading to rapid death. Rarely, intracardiac rupture may occur through the septum, causing a left-to-right shunt and the development of severe left ventricular failure if large.
- **Papillary muscle dysfunction or infarction** leads to mitral valve incompetence, as one valve leaflet is no longer able to close during systole.
- **Mural thrombus formation** on the inflamed endocardium over the area of infarction (*Fig. 10.41*). Fragments can break off and embolize to various organs (particularly the brain, spleen, kidney, gut and lower limbs), producing infarction.
- **Acute pericarditis** may occur due to inflammation over the infarct surface.

Fig. 10.40 Rupture of myocardial infarct. The area of infarction (**I**) has ruptured and a track of blood runs from the ventricular chamber (**V**) to the epicardial surface. In this instance death was rapid after the development of hemopericardium.

Fig. 10.41 Mural thrombus over myocardial infarct. A plaque of mural thrombus (**T**) lies over an area of infarction at the apex of the left ventricle.

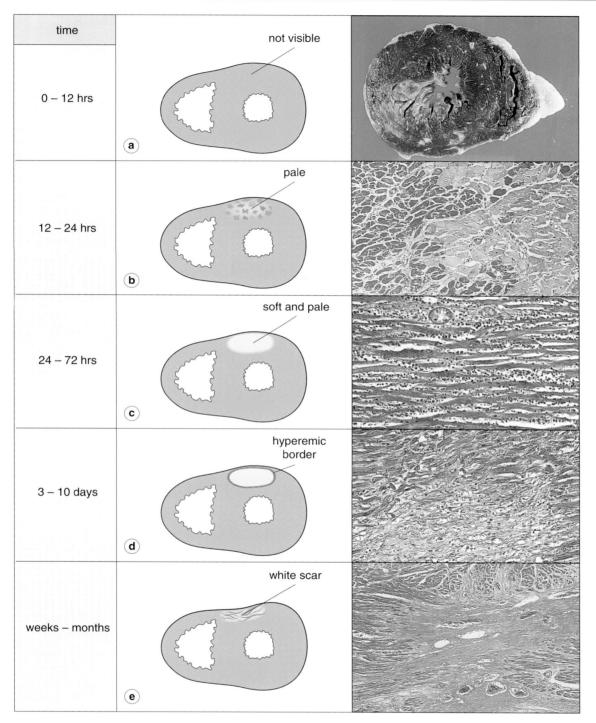

Fig. 10.42 Appearances of myocardial infarct. Myocardial infarcts go through a series of changes with time. Between 0 and 12 hours an infarct is not macroscopically visible; however, the ischemic muscle can be detected by showing loss of oxidative enzymes with nitroblue-tetrazolium (NBT) when the infarcted area appears uncolored (a). Between 12 and 24 hours the infarcted area is macroscopically pale with blotchy discoloration. Histologically (b) infarcted muscle is brightly eosinophilic with intercellular edema. Between 24 and 72 hours the infarcted area excites an acute inflammatory response. Macroscopically the dead area appears soft and pale with a slight yellow color. Histologically neutrophils infiltrate between dead cardiac muscle fibers (c). Organization of the infarcted area occurs between 3 and 10 days. Macroscopically a hyperemic border develops around the yellow dead muscle. Histologically there is replacement of the area by vascular granulation tissue (d). With time, progressive collagen deposition occurs and over a period of weeks to months the infarct is replaced by collagenous scar (e).

Long-term complications of myocardial infarction

If patients survive the immediate and short-term effects of myocardial infarction, long-term complications may arise, among which is **chronic intractable left-heart failure** due to inadequate left ventricular pumping action. This is particularly common when the infarct has been extensive and full thickness.

There may be **ventricular aneurysm formation** due to gradual distension of that part of the left ventricular wall where the muscle has been replaced by rigid but inelastic fibrous scar. Ventricular aneurysms frequently become filled with laminated thrombus, but embolic complications are uncommon (*Fig. 10.43*). This occurs in around 10% of long-term survivors.

Recurrent myocardial infarction is a risk because of the underlying coronary artery insufficiency; a patient who has had a myocardial infarct is always prone to develop a further episode.

Dressler's syndrome is a form of immune-mediated pericarditis associated with a high ESR. It develops in a very small number of cases after infarction (2–10 months after the acute event).

Fig. 10.43 Left ventricular aneurysm. After an infarct, stretching of collagenous scar causes aneurysmal bulging of the ventricular wall (**V**).

CARDIOMYOPATHY AND MYOCARDITIS

Cardiomyopathies are diseases primarily affecting heart muscle

Once cases of ischemic heart disease, valvular heart disease, and hypertensive heart disease have been excluded, there remains a group of patients who have presented with abnormal cardiac function due to primary disease of the myocardium, termed **cardiomyopathies**. There are three main etiological groups:

- **Inherited cardiomyopathy:** caused by mutation in a gene coding for a product important in myocardial function.
- **Idiopathic primary cardiomyopathies** – no known cause and not inherited.
- **Secondary cardiomyopathies** – a defined cause that directly affects cardiac muscle function is identified (*Fig. 10.44*).

The cardiomyopathies usually cause progressive development of cardiac failure. The timescale varies according to the cause of disease; development may occur over weeks or years. In some instances sudden cardiac death is the first manifestation of disease.

Diagnosis is based on clinical features supplemented by imaging (radiology and echocardiography) and cardiac catheter studies. These investigations allow cardiomyopathies to be grouped according to functional abnormalities of the myocardium, and structural changes to the heart. To obtain a histological diagnosis of disease, **endomyocardial biopsy** may be performed at the same time as cardiac catheterization.

Primary cardiomyopathies are classified according to myocardial dysfunction

Primary cardiomyopathies follow two main patterns according to the dysfunction of the myocardium.

In **hypertrophic cardiomyopathy** the heart walls (especially the left ventricle) are enormously thickened and hypertrophied, often in an asymmetrical pattern, particularly affecting the interventricular septum (*Fig. 10.45*). Catheter studies show an abnormal pressure gradient along the left ventricular cavity. Histologically there is disorganized branching of hypertrophied muscle fibers, which show loss of the normal parallel orientation. In about 50% of cases hypertrophic cardiomyopathy is inherited as an autosomal dominant disorder; it presents most often in young adults and juveniles, and may cause sudden death on exertion. Less dramatic presentations include angina and breathlessness on exertion in a young person, or repeated fainting attacks. There have been developments in the genetic understanding of this group of disorders (see pink box on page 179).

In **dilated (congestive) cardiomyopathy** the ventricles are dilated, the chamber walls stretched thin, and the muscle is poorly contractile (*Fig. 10.46*). Typically, there is an elevated ventricular end-diastolic pressure. The cause is not known, but some cases may follow viral myocarditis.

The least common form of cardiomyopathy is when there is abnormal rigidity of the myocardium (**restrictive cardiomyopathy**). This may be seen in association with subendocardial fibroelastosis in rare childhood conditions.

Sudden arrhythmic death syndrome (SADS) may run in families

Several cardiac conditions can cause the development of a fatal ventricular dysrhythmia presenting as sudden unexpected death. In some instances this is the result of a defined cardiomyopathy, for example hypertrophic cardiomyopathy. Arrhythmogenic right ventricular cardiomyopathy (ARVC) is a condition in which the wall of the right ventricle is extensively replaced by adipose tissue. In 50% of cases this is inherited and can cause sudden cardiac death. Patients known to have this condition have an annual death rate of 2.5% per year. Several genes have been identified.

In other cases the cause is related to conduction disturbances in the heart. Some of these conditions can be identified by noting prolonged QT interval on ECG. Several heritable causes have been defined due to mutations in genes coding for ion channels.

Myocarditis is an uncommon disease in which there is diffuse inflammation of the myocardium

Inflammation of the myocardium, termed **myocarditis**, is generally uncommon. Although it is considered by many to be a cardiomyopathy (inflammatory cardiomyopathy), others categorize this pattern of disease separately. The myocardium shows interstitial edema and infiltration with lymphocytes and macrophages.

The disease can be caused by **direct infection**, e.g. *Trypanosoma cruzi* (Chagas' disease), Coxsackie A and B viruses, HIV, influenza, Epstein–Barr virus, and fungi; **toxin-mediated damage**, e.g. diphtheria, typhoid and septicemic states; and **immune hypersensitivity**, e.g. acute rheumatic fever (see page 187). There are also idiopathic causes, such as giant-cell myocarditis. Diagnosis can be helped by endomyocardial biopsy.

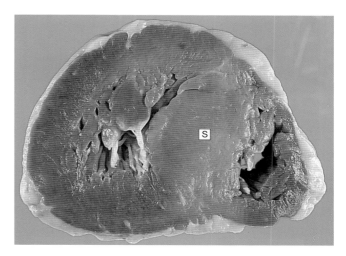

Fig. 10.45 Hypertrophic cardiomyopathy. In hypertrophic cardiomyopathy there is marked left ventricular hypertrophy. This often preferentially affects the septum (**S**).

Fig. 10.44 Causes of secondary cardiomyopathies
Multisystem diseases
Diabetes
Amyloid
Thyroid disease
Hemochromatosis
Inflammatory and infective diseases
Myocarditis
Chagas' disease
Toxic and metabolic disturbances
Alcohol
Drugs (e.g. daunorubicin)
Primary muscle disorders
Muscular dystrophy
Mitochondrial cytopathy

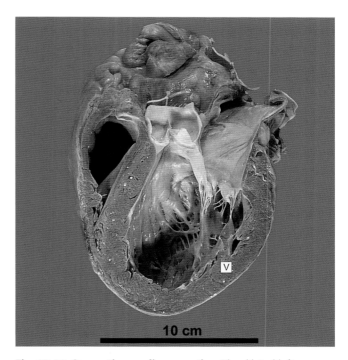

Fig. 10.46 Congestive cardiomyopathy. The dilated left ventricle (**V**) has a thin wall.

Genetic basis of cardiomyopathy

A genetic basis has now been identified in 90% of all cases of hypertrophic cardiomyopathy and in about 30% of congestive cardiomyopathies.

- In hypertrophic cardiomyopathy mutations in two genes cover over 80% of cases. These are cardiac myosin-binding protein C (MYBPC3) and β-myosin heavy chain (MYH7), which each account for about 40% of all disease.

- Some individuals have more than one mutation, suggesting a gene dose effect in these compound-heterozygous or double-heterozygous cases.
- Mutations in genes coding for proteins of the contractile cytoskeleton are noted in a small proportion of cases. The Online Mendelian Inheritance in Man database lists over 12 genetic variants of hypertrophic cardiomyopathy.

Type OMIM into the Google search engine to review genes associated with cardiomyopathy.

CARDIAC TUMORS

Neoplasia affecting the heart is uncommon

The pericardium and heart may be involved by metastatic disease, the most common cause being local extension of a carcinoma of the lung.

Atrial myxoma is a tumor composed of stellate cells in a myxoid matrix, which arises from the atrial lining and may cause symptoms similar to infective endocarditis.

Cardiac rhabdomyomas are tumors of muscle seen in association with tuberous sclerosis.

DISEASES OF THE PERICARDIUM

The main disorder of the pericardium is pericarditis

The main disorder of the pericardium, pericarditis, is often complicated by the development of a pericardial effusion.

In acute pericarditis there is acute inflammation of the pericardium, in which both pericardial surfaces are coated with a fibrin-rich acute inflammatory exudate (*Fig. 10.47*). Loss of smoothness leads to the clinical sign of a friction rub.

The most common cause of acute pericarditis is myocardial infarction (see page 176). The next most common cause encountered in community practice is the transient pericarditis that can occur in some **viral disorders.** Other causes of clinically significant pericarditis are:

- **Postoperative,** following open heart surgery. The pericarditis is diffuse, and heals by fibrosis.
- **Bacterial pericarditis,** usually associated with severe bacterial infection of the lungs. An important cause in the past was pulmonary TB, producing tuberculous pericarditis.

- **Malignant pericarditis,** usually due to infiltration of the pericardium by local spread from a primary bronchial tumor.
- **Uremic pericarditis,** rarely seen now that chronic renal failure can be treated by dialysis.
- **Immune pericarditis,** formerly an important component of the pancarditis associated with rheumatic fever, is now rare. Occasionally seen in patients with autoimmune disease, such as SLE and rheumatoid disease.

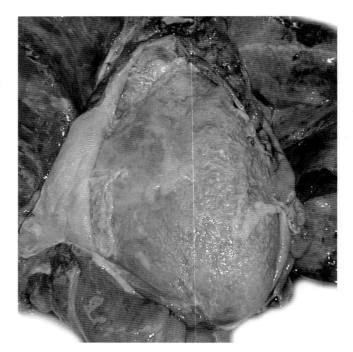

Fig. 10.47 Fibrinous pericarditis. The epicardial surface is covered by a shaggy fibrous inflammatory exudate.

DISEASES OF ENDOCARDIUM AND VALVES

Primary diseases of the non-valvular endocardium are rare

As a long-term result of myocardial infarction that involves the endocardial surface, the endocardium is damaged and thickened, and may be a predisposing site for mural thrombosis, although this complication is more frequent in the immediate post-infarct period.

Similar patchy areas of endocardial thickening can be seen (particularly in the left atrium) where the flow through the mitral valve has been modified by valve disease. A jet of blood squirting through the incompetent mitral valve during systole can produce a patch of endocardial thickening (jet lesion) where the jet hits the atrial wall.

Endocardial thickening in the right side of the heart is rare, but may occur in the carcinoid syndrome or in some congenital heart diseases, where there is a left-to-right shunt.

Diffuse endocardial thickening in the left heart is seen in two uncommon diseases. In **endocardial fibroelastosis** the endocardium becomes greatly thickened and replaced by fibroelastic tissue, mainly in the left heart, often extending over the papillary muscles. This disease occurs in babies and young children, presenting with unexplained heart failure. Its cause is not known. In **endomyocardial fibrosis** there is fibrous thickening of the endocardium and the inner myocardium, leading to limitation of cardiac contraction. Occurring particularly in Central Africa, this condition is often associated with peripheral blood eosinophilia; its cause is not known.

Both of the above conditions lead to cardiac failure by restricting contraction of the cardiac chambers during systole; they are sometimes classified as a form of cardiomyopathy (**restrictive cardiomyopathy**) by clinicians, despite the fact that the primary structural abnormality is endocardial.

Mechanical disturbance of heart valves results in cardiac disease

Mechanical disturbances of heart valves are an important cause of cardiac disease. The two main types of mechanical defect are narrowing or abnormal rigidity of a valve, resulting in **stenosis**, and failure of the valve to close fully, resulting in **incompetence**.

The principal causes of valve disease are congenital abnormality, post-inflammatory scarring, degeneration with aging, dilatation of the valve ring, degeneration of collagenous support tissue of the valve, and acute destruction by necrotizing inflammation.

Any structurally abnormal valve is more liable than usual to develop colonization by microorganisms (infective valvulitis).

Inflammatory disorders of heart valves cause vegetations and late scarring

Inflammation of the endocardium of heart valves (valvulitis) is an important cause of valve disease, which results either from **immune-mediated damage** initiating inflammation in the valve cusps (seen in acute rheumatic fever, see page 187), or from **damage due to infection**, e.g. in bacterial and fungal endocarditis.

Inflammatory damage to heart valves has two important consequences:

- Valve collagen is exposed, causing **thrombus deposition**. The thrombus develops as exophytic nodules or irregular warty growths on the valve leaflets, called **vegetations** (*Fig. 10.48*).
- Inflammation and thrombus formation on the valve causes organization with collagenous scarring. This causes physical distortion to the valve cusps and renders them mechanically and functionally abnormal.

The valves on the left side of the heart (mitral and aortic) are much more frequently the site of endocarditis and thrombotic vegetation formation than those of the right side of the heart (tricuspid and pulmonary); thus, embolic material from valve thrombosis passes into the systemic circulation and produces infarcts in the systemic organs.

Some vegetations form on valves as a consequence of hypercoagulability of blood

In patients who are severely debilitated, for example with widespread metastatic carcinoma or severe chronic infections, small, non-infective, firm, platelet-rich vegetations (**marantic vegetations**) may form on the valves of the left side of the heart. The reason for this is hypercoagulability of the blood caused by an acute-phase response, manifest by a very high ESR.

Fig. 10.48 Heart valve vegetations. A thrombotic vegetation (**V**) on the mitral valve caused by inflammation of the valve.

Vegetations may form on the heart valves in SLE (Libman–Sacks endocarditis). This is related to the presence of high titers of anticardiolipin antibodies, which cause platelet aggregation.

Rheumatic fever is a major cause of chronic scarring of heart valves

The main cause of chronic scarring of valves is rheumatic fever, the incidence of which has decreased in many countries in recent years. Acute rheumatic fever is a disease of children, and is discussed on page 187.

The rheumatic pericarditis and myocarditis that arise in the acute phase usually resolve without long-term ill-effects. However, the damage to the valves heals by progressive fibrosis, with fibrous thickening of the valve leaflets and associated chordae tendineae. The valve leaflets become thickened, fibrotic and shrunken, often with fusion to their partners, and there is frequent secondary deposition of calcium.

Many patients with chronic scarring of valves give no history of having had rheumatic fever; the non-committal term 'post-inflammatory scarring' is used in such cases.

Mitral stenosis causes left-sided heart failure and predisposes to atrial thrombosis

Mitral stenosis is caused by post-inflammatory scarring of the valve cusps. A history of rheumatic fever is obtained in only about half of cases, and a chronic rheumatic etiology cannot be assumed in all instances.

Valve cusps are thickened and there is fusion of commissures. Chordae tendineae are thickened and fused, resulting in a funnel-shaped, narrowed valve orifice with a slit-like opening (*Fig. 10.49*).

Failure of the left atrium to empty through the stenosed valve leads to left atrial hypertrophy and dilatation. Back pressure causes pulmonary hypertension and pulmonary vascular congestion, which commonly causes hemoptysis. Left-sided cardiac failure develops. Atrial fibrillation is a common complication, with resultant development of left atrial thrombosis. (*Fig. 10.50*).

Mitral incompetence leads to left-sided heart failure and has many causes

Regurgitation from the left ventricle back into the atrium is the result of mitral valve incompetence, the main causes of which are post-inflammatory scarring (commonly rheumatic), papillary muscle dysfunction after infarct, left ventricular dilatation, cusp destruction by infection (infective endocarditis), and floppy mitral valve syndrome.

If the valve is suddenly rendered incompetent (papillary muscle rupture or infective perforation), severe acute pulmonary edema develops.

In most cases regurgitation develops slowly and results in left ventricular enlargement and a giant left atrium (caused by its filling with blood in systole). Progressive left-sided cardiac failure develops with time.

Mitral valve prolapse (floppy valve syndrome) is now much more common than rheumatic mitral valve disease. The valve leaflet becomes degenerate, with myxoid degeneration of the central zona fibrosa. The valve leaflet is soft and bulges upwards into the atrium during systole

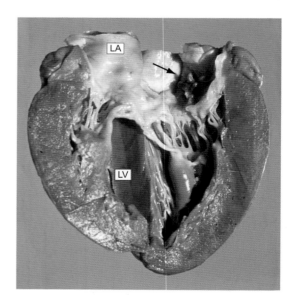

Fig. 10.50 Mitral stenosis with left atrial thrombosis. This heart has been opened to show the left atrium (**LA**) and left ventricle (**LV**), with the mitral valve between them. The valve and its chordae tendineae have been damaged by rheumatic endocarditis, leading to thickening and fusion of both, with functional stenosis. The combination of stasis in the dilated left atrium and coexisting atrial fibrillation has led to thrombus formation (arrow).

Fig. 10.49 Mitral stenosis. Looking down onto the valve from above, the mitral valve orifice is reduced to a narrow slit (**S**). This is caused by chronic rheumatic heart disease.

(*Fig. 10.51*). The posterior mitral leaflet is most commonly involved, and mild valve incompetence is the result of the hypermobility of the leaflet. However, there is a danger of rupture of one of the chordae, leading to severe valve incompetence. It is most common in women and usually presents in young adulthood. In some cases there is a family history.

Aortic valve disease is a cause of sudden cardiac death

The aortic valve is frequently affected by disease, resulting in either stenosis or incompetence.

Fig. 10.51 Mitral valve prolapse. Looking down on the mitral valve, the ballooning of the leaflets due to mitral valve prolapse is seen.

Fig. 10.52 Calcific aortic valve disease. The valves become thick and fibrotic, with fusion of the commissures and heavy calcification. The thickening and fusion lead to reduction of the valve lumen, so that flow out of the valve is greatly reduced during systole (aortic stenosis). Furthermore, because the valve leaflets are rigid and fused, they are unable to close completely and there is flow of blood back into the left ventricle during diastole (aortic regurgitation).

Aortic stenosis is most commonly due to calcification of a congenital bicuspid aortic valve (*Fig. 10.52*), post-inflammatory scarring after rheumatic fever, or senile calcific degeneration. Isolated fibrosis and calcification of the aortic valve, with no evidence of mitral valve involvement or evidence of previous rheumatic fever, is the most common valve disease, although its cause is unknown. The disease is most commonly seen in bicuspid aortic valves, a common congenital malformation, but can also been seen in originally normal valves with three cusps.

Aortic regurgitation has four main causes:

• Retraction of cusps due to post-inflammatory scarring.
• Erosion of cusps by inflammation in infective endocarditis.
• Retraction of cusps due to age-related calcification.
• Dilatation of the aortic wall and valve ring caused by inflammatory diseases (e.g. syphilis, ankylosing spondylitis).

Mixed stenosis and regurgitation is common.

Progressive obstruction of the outflow of the left ventricle causes the development of left ventricular hypertrophy. When stenosis is severe, patients may develop angina due to low flow in coronary arteries. They may also have episodes of syncope and are at risk of sudden cardiac death because of cardiac arrhythmias.

With aortic regurgitation, patients usually remain asymptomatic until the left ventricle, having undergone hypertrophy, fails acutely. Because of the serious nature of aortic valve disease surgical intervention is offered early in the disease course.

Disease of the pulmonary and tricuspid valves is uncommon

The valves of the right side of the heart are infrequently involved in disease, but in rheumatic heart disease may be damaged by post-inflammatory scarring. Endocarditis of the right side of the heart is seen in association with intravenous drug abuse.

For reasons that are as yet unclear, the carcinoid syndrome, caused by excess secretion of 5-hydroxytryptamine by tumor, can result in endocardial fibrosis of the right side of the heart and pulmonary stenosis.

Infective endocarditis is caused by infection of heart valves or other areas of endocardium

Infection of the endocardium, whether on heart valves or elsewhere, is termed 'infective endocarditis'. There are two broad groups of cases.

In one group, patients are predisposed to infection by a **structural abnormality of heart valves** or by congenital cardiac defects. The incidence of this pattern has increased in western countries in recent years, mainly as a result of patients surviving with structurally abnormal hearts and heart valves. The infective organisms responsible are of low pathogenicity and are derived from normal commensal organisms of skin, mouth, urinary tract and gut. Organisms that enter the blood in trivial episodes of bacteremia become enmeshed in platelet aggregates on the surface of abnormal endocardium, growing to cause persistent infection. The main underlying abnormalities in this group are congenital bicuspid aortic valves, post-inflammatory scarring, mitral valve prolapse syndrome, and prosthetic valves.

Infection of **normal valves** accounts for the remaining cases of infective endocarditis. In contrast to the first group, infection is with pathogenic organisms that directly invade the valve and cause rapid destruction. This pattern of disease is predisposed by conditions that promote the entry of pathogenic organisms into the blood. It is seen in intravenous drug addicts, after open-heart surgery, and following septicemia from other causes.

Infective endocarditis occurs as two main clinical syndromes

Following on from the two main groups of cases of infective endocarditis described earlier, there are two main clinical disease patterns.

Acute infective endocarditis is usually due to a virulent organism, e.g. *Staphylococcus aureus*, and can occur on a previously normal heart valve. The bacteria proliferate in the valve and cause necrosis, with the generation of thrombotic vegetations. The pathogenic bacteria lead to destruction of the valve leaflets, with perforation and acute disturbance of valve function leading to acute cardiac failure. The disease is rapidly progressive and often fatal.

Diagnosis of infective endocarditis

The diagnosis of infective endocarditis is based on clinical suspicion, knowing the risk factors for development of disease. It should also be considered in patients with unexplained fever, septicemia, heart failure, or embolic infarct.

Investigations commonly reveal a raised ESR, raised white cell count, and a normochromic normocytic anemia.

The most important diagnostic procedure is **blood culture** to isolate an organism. A negative blood culture may be caused by prior administration of an antibiotic (which will not have cured the infection), or may be due to a special organism such as a fungus, *Coxiella* or *Chlamydia*.

Echocardiograms can be used for detection, if vegetations on valves are large.

Subacute bacterial endocarditis generally occurs on structurally abnormal valves. The causative organisms are generally poorly virulent (e.g. *Streptococcus viridans*) and proliferate slowly in thrombotic vegetations on the damaged valve surface. In most cases they cause very gradual valve destruction, stimulating the formation of thrombus with potential for systemic embolization. Many of the effects of this pattern of infection are through immunological phenomena and the generation of cytokines from persisting low-grade inflammation.

The main clinical effects of subacute infective endocarditis are:

- Small emboli of infected thrombotic material enter the systemic circulation, producing infarcts in many organs, particularly the brain, spleen, and kidneys. These necrotic areas may, in turn, become infected by organisms in the occluding thrombus.
- Gradual destruction of valve cusps leads to features of valve incompetence with cardiac failure.
- Immune complexes against antigens in the infecting organism are trapped in small vessels. They cause skin

Cardiac transplantation is increasingly being performed for severe disease

Cardiac transplantation is now a technically straightforward surgical operation, and many of the problems of transplant rejection are being overcome; immunosuppression with cyclosporine has greatly improved the management of the almost inevitable rejection episodes.

Transplantation of the heart is mainly undertaken for advanced irreversible myocardial disease, particularly cardiomyopathy and severe ischemic disease, and particularly in young people. Where the severe heart disease is associated with poor lung function, combined heart–lung transplants can be carried out. Because donor hearts are difficult to obtain, poor HLA matching is not usually a contraindication, although poor matches are usually associated with more severe rejection reactions.

Two patterns of rejection are seen:

- Acute cellular rejection, in which there is myocardial fiber necrosis, interstitial edema with lymphocytic infiltrate, and inflammation of the endocardial lining.
- Chronic vascular rejection associated with thickening of the intima in the coronary arteries leads to ischemic damage in the myocardium, with interstitial fibrosis.

petechiae and microhemorrhages in the retina and skin, particularly around the finger nails. They also cause a form of glomerulonephritis.

- Cytokine generation from low-grade infection leads to systemic features of fever, weight loss and malaise.
- There may be anemia and splenomegaly.

HEART DISEASE IN CHILDREN

The most important heart diseases in children are congenital cardiac malformations

Most cardiac malformations are manifest at or shortly after birth, usually by some sign of cardiac failure such as cyanosis, breathlessness, feeding difficulties, and failure to thrive. Certain maternal factors are known to increase the incidence of congenital cardiac malformations, particularly maternal rubella infections and chronic alcohol abuse, but in the majority of cases no teratogenic factors can be identified.

Congenital cardiac defects may be divided into two main groups: lesions that cause **obstruction to blood flow**, and those that cause **abnormal shunting** of blood between the two sides of the heart.

The latter group normally cause a left-to-right shunt because of the higher pressure in the left side of the heart. This is not associated with clinical cyanosis.

If there is an increase in resistance to blood moving on from the right side of the heart (either from obstruction of the right ventricular outflow or from pulmonary hypertension), there is a right-to-left shunt; with blood bypassing the lungs to enter the systemic circulation, cyanosis develops.

The most common congenital heart defects cause left-to-right shunts

The most common group of malformations result in a shunt of blood from the left side of the heart to the right.

Atrial septal defects (ASDs) are due to a defect in the interatrial septum. The lesion is usually located at the level of the fossa ovalis, which is incompletely closed (ostium secundum defect) (*Fig. 10.53*).

Ventricular septal defects (VSDs) are due to a defect in the interventricular septum. The larger defects involve the muscular wall of the septum, but small defects are often confined to the tiny membranous area (*maladie de Roger*) (*Fig. 10.54*).

Patent ductus arteriosus is due to persistent patency in the ductus arteriosus, an embryological connection between the aorta and the pulmonary trunk or left main pulmonary artery. In intrauterine life the ductus is an important channel, allowing blood oxygenated in the placenta to bypass the lungs, but it closes at or shortly after birth, when the lungs become aerated and expand. Persistence of the duct is most common in females (*Fig. 10.55*).

The severity of the symptoms depends on the size of the shunt. In the case of small ASDs or VSDs the flow can be minor and largely asymptomatic, sometimes presenting in mid-adult life with unexplained right heart failure. Patent ductus usually requires treatment in childhood.

Defects leading to permanent right-to-left shunts are less common

The most important and common congenital abnormality of the heart to cause right-to-left shunting is **Fallot's tetralogy** (*Fig. 10.56*), which consists of:

Fig. 10.53 Atrial septal defect.

Fig. 10.54 Ventricular septal defect.

Fig. 10.55 Patent ductus arteriosus.

- **VSD**.
- **An overriding aorta**, which sits astride the VSD, so that it receives blood from both right and left ventricles.
- **Pulmonary stenosis**, usually due to thickening of the subvalvular muscle in the pulmonary outflow tract, but sometimes associated with fused stenotic valve cusps.
- **Right ventricular hypertrophy**.

Because the abnormal aorta receives blood from the right ventricle as well as the left, the systemic circulation contains deoxygenated blood and the patient has clinical **cyanosis**. The pulmonary stenosis leads to inadequate perfusion of the lungs. Affected individuals develop a right-to-left shunt and have cyanosis. With growth, the pulmonary stenosis remains fixed and eventually there is severe right ventricular outflow obstruction. Most cases are surgically corrected.

Surgical correction of this complex disorder is usually aimed at closing the VSD, rechanneling the flow into the aorta from the left ventricle only, and relieving the pulmonary stenosis. This technique has greatly increased survival. Complications include bacterial endocarditis (see page 112), and consequent cerebral infarction or brain abscess.

Some congenital malformations are not associated with significant shunting of blood

Of those congenital malformations not associated with significant shunting, the most common are aortic stenosis, coarctation of the aorta, and transposition of the great vessels.

With **aortic stenosis** there is stenosis of the valve, which is usually bicuspid. Symptoms tend to appear later in life, when fibrosis and calcification of the abnormal valve lead to functional stenosis and incompetence (see *Fig. 10.52*). Less commonly the stenosis occurs in the muscular tissue below the aortic valve (**subvalvar stenosis**), or in the aortic wall above the valve (**supravalvar stenosis**). These two variants are present in infancy and may be associated with coarctation of the aorta.

In cases of **coarctation of the aorta** there is a stenotic narrowing of the aorta, usually located at or just beyond the site of the ductus arteriosus, which appears closed (*Fig. 10.57*). The stricture produces hypertension proximal to the stenosis, and hypotension distal to it. The proximal hypertension can produce symptoms such as headache and dizziness, whereas the distal hypotension produces generalized weakness and poor peripheral circulation. Further symptoms may be due to the associated stenotic aortic valve that is present in about half of cases.

Transposition of the great vessels is a complex malformation in which the connections between the right and left ventricle and aorta and pulmonary artery are disordered, the aorta emanating from the right ventricle and the pulmonary artery from the left. Survival is possible only if other shunts are present at either atrial (a), ventricular (b) or ductus (c) level (*Fig. 10.58*).

Cardiac disease is uncommon in children, with the exception of congenital malformations and rheumatic heart disease

Cardiomyopathy may occur in young children, but it is more common in juveniles. Some cardiomyopathies in young children are associated with abnormal storage in some of the autosomal recessive storage disorders, e.g. glycogen storage disease.

Fig. 10.56 Fallot's tetralogy.

Fig. 10.57 Coarctation of the aorta.

Fig. 10.58 Transposition.

The myocardium can be involved in some muscular dystrophies, but presentation in childhood is rare.

Acute rheumatic fever is still an important disease of children in certain developing countries

Rheumatic fever is an immune disorder that follows an infection in children, usually a streptococcal tonsillitis or pharyngitis. Certain strains of streptococci, especially group A β-hemolytic streptococci, produce particular antigens to which antibodies are developed by certain susceptible individuals; these antibodies may cross-react with host cardiac antigens.

The disease occurs mainly in children between the ages of 5 and 15 years, and was once prevalent in the UK, Europe and USA. It is now rare outside certain developing countries with low socioeconomic standards. The disease is a systemic disorder which, in the acute phase, presents with fever, malaise and, sometimes, synovitis and polyserositis. However, the most important target organ is the heart. Patients develop characteristic lesions (**Aschoff's nodules**) in various parts of the heart (*Fig. 10.59*). Diagnostic criteria have been established (*Fig. 10.60*).

Rheumatic fever causes a pancarditis in the acute phase

The components of the pancarditis are:

- **Rheumatic pericarditis**. Aschoff's nodules form in the pericardium, associated with an acute pericarditis. The exudate can produce a pericardial effusion, which may distend the pericardial cavity.
- **Rheumatic myocarditis**. Aschoff's nodules developing in the myocardium are associated with interstitial edema and mild inflammation, sometimes with muscle-fiber necrosis. The myocarditis is usually clinically mild, but may produce left ventricular failure.
- **Rheumatic endocarditis**. Aschoff's nodules may form anywhere in the endocardium, producing slight irregularity of the endocardial surface. However, Aschoff's nodules in the valves lead to greater irregularity, and there may be erosion of the overlying endocardium, particularly at the points at which the valves contact each other at the line of closure. In these sites, small aggregations of fibrin and platelets accumulate to form small vegetations. The aortic and mitral valves are most prone to develop severe lesions, probably because of the higher pressures to which they are exposed and the more vigorous and traumatic valve closure.

In the acute phase of rheumatic fever the greatest dangers to the patient are the pericarditis and myocarditis; however, the main morbidity of rheumatic fever is the long-term effects of the immune damage causing chronic scarring of valves (page 182).

Fig. 10.59 Histology of the Aschoff's nodule. The Aschoff's nodule is composed of an area of degenerate collagen, surrounded by activated histiocytic cells and lymphoid cells. These lesions stimulate fibroblast proliferation and lead to scarring.

Clinical and laboratory diagnosis of acute rheumatic fever

Fig. 10.60 Jones' criteria for the diagnosis of rheumatic fever

Major manifestations

Carditis
Polyarthritis
Skin rashes (erythema marginatum and erythema nodosum)
Neurological symptoms (Sydenham's chorea)

Minor manifestations

Fever
Polysynovitis (flitting arthropathy)
Arthralgia
Raised ESR or raised C-reactive protein
Prolonged PR-interval on ECG

Diagnosis requires two major features **or** one major and two minor features **plus** raised anti-streptococcal antibody levels (anti-streptolysin O titre) **or** positive throat culture for group A β-hemolytic streptococcus.

Case-based questions

Case 1 A pulseless, cold, painful foot

A 69-year-old man is admitted to hospital, having been referred urgently by his own doctor. His right foot had become acutely painful and was described by his doctor as cold, blue and pulseless. His medical records indicate that he has been a lifelong cigarette smoker, and has been treated medically for hypertension in the past 5 years. A clinical diagnosis of critical ischemia of the right lower limb is made.

Based on your understanding of the pathology of the cardiovascular system, what investigations are suggested in this patient to establish the cause of his critical lower limb ischemia?

Case 2 Cardiac arrest

You are sitting talking to the nursing staff on the Coronary Care Unit, where you have several patients. Hearing a shout from behind you, you turn and see a nurse calling for help with one of your patients who had been on the unit for 3 days. The patient is a 55-year-old man who you admitted with a classic history, confirmed by investigation, of a large lateral Q-wave myocardial infarct. He had been treated with thrombolytic therapy following admission. He has been given oxygen and has also required a small dose of a diuretic and ACE inhibitor because of mild features of left ventricular failure.

As you cross to attend the patient and help in the cardiac arrest, **which pathological complications of myocardial infarction are you considering, and how might this determine your approach to assessment of the patient?**

Case 3 Abdominal pain

A 60-year-old warehouse supervisor, visits his local family practitioner because he has become concerened about vague abdominal pain and backache that he has been experiencing for about six months. His friend has recently been told he has cancer, and this was what made him go to see a doctor. He smokes 20 cigarettes a day, and has done so since he started work at the age of 14, but is otherwise well. On examination, his doctor notes a large pulsatile abdominal mass. An abdominal aortic aneurysm is diagnosed and he referred to hospital for consideration of surgical intervention.

1. **What is the most likely cause of this patient's aneurysm?**
2. **Describe the histological changes occurring in the wall of the aorta in this condition?**
3. **What complications may occur?**
4. **What are the other main types of aneurysm and their causes?**

Brief answers to these case-based questions are given on pages 585–6. More detailed answers and other study resources are available online at www.studentconsult.com.

Respiratory system 11

THE RESPIRATORY SYSTEM COMPRISES THE UPPER RESPIRATORY TRACT, THE AIRWAYS AND THE LUNGS

The respiratory system consists of the upper respiratory tract, the airways and the lungs. Diseases of the nose and larynx are considered along with those of the ear in Chapter 12, as these conditions are clinically seen together.

The main diseases of the airways and lung are caused by infection and inflammation. Exposure to environmental agents has an important role in causing disease, especially smoking and occupational exposure to dusts. Carcinoma of the lung is particularly feared because of its aggressive nature. Another important category of disease is vascular disease of the lung, with pulmonary thromboembolism being the most common.

One consequence of severe disease of the respiratory system is impairment of oxygenation of blood, resulting in respiratory failure.

RESPIRATORY FAILURE IS DEFINED BY THE PRESENCE OF A LOW LEVEL OF BLOOD OXYGEN

Normal respiratory function maintains blood gases within physiological limits. The normal PaO_2 varies between 10.7 kPa and 13.3 kPa (80–100 mmHg), and the normal $PaCO_2$ varies between 4.7 kPa and 6.0 kPa (35–45 mmHg). Respiratory failure is defined as when the PaO_2 falls below 8 kPa (60 mmHg).

There are two types of respiratory failure, which are defined according to whether blood carbon dioxide is also abnormal:

- **Type I:** PaO_2 is low, but $PaCO_2$ is within the normal range.
- **Type II:** PaO_2 is low and $PaCO_2$ is raised (>6.7 kPa/50 mmHg).

Respiratory failure can be caused by a wide range of conditions affecting ventilation, gas exchange, or perfusion of the lung. Failure of ventilatory drive may be caused by depression of respiratory centers, for example following neurological damage. Mechanical failure of ventilation may result from massive rib fracture, diseases of muscle or diseases of peripheral nerves.

Blood gas analysis

Analysis of arterial blood gases is vital in distinguishing the severity and different types of respiratory failure. The only direct clinical sign of respiratory failure is central cyanosis, detected reliably when the PaO_2 is <6.7 kPa (50 mmHg) in a person with a normal hemoglobin levels. Loss of consciousness occurs when the PaO_2 is <4.0 kPa (30 mmHg).

Disorders of conduction of air and ventilation cause both hypoxia and CO_2 retention.

A low PaO_2 alone (breathing normal air) usually means that there is mismatch between ventilation and perfusion of lungs, but that alveolar ventilation is normal.

Hypoxia due to an increase in the proportion of blood passing through the lung without being oxygenated (increased shunt fraction) is seen in pulmonary collapse, and in situations in which the lung becomes consolidated.

Failure of diffusion of gas because of abnormal thickening in alveolar septa leads to hypoxemia, but hypercapnia does not develop.

Chronic respiratory failure has major effects on the cardiovascular system

Chronic hypoxemia has two main consequences:

- **Pulmonary hypertension** due to pulmonary vasoconstriction leads to increased pulmonary artery pressure. In time, pulmonary arteries develop intimal proliferation and narrowing. Pulmonary hypertension leads to right ventricular hypertrophy.
- **Polycythemia** is due to stimulation of erythropoietin release from the kidney. This can lead to increased blood viscosity and predisposes to increased risk of thrombosis.

Hypercapnia, when severe, causes tremor of the outstretched hands, a bounding pulse, vasodilatation and increased cardiac output, and confusion leading to coma.

COLLAPSE OF THE LUNG IS TERMED 'ATELECTASIS'

Several conditions lead to atelectasis, which has important clinical consequences of disturbing respiratory function:

- Obstruction of an airway leads to resorption of air from the lung distal to the obstruction.
- Compression of the lung is most commonly seen when fluid or air accumulates in the pleural cavity (see page 218).
- Scarring in the lung may cause contraction of parenchyma and collapse.
- Loss of normal surfactant (developmental or acquired) from terminal air spaces leads to generalized failure of lung expansion, termed **microatelectasis**.

VASCULAR AND HEMODYNAMIC DISEASE OF THE LUNGS

The main cause of pulmonary edema is pulmonary capillary congestion due to left ventricular failure

Pulmonary edema is caused by an increase of fluid in alveolar wall (pulmonary interstitium) which, if severe, subsequently affects alveolar spaces. The main cause of pulmonary edema is failure of the left ventricle, causing increased pressure in the alveolar capillaries.

Fluid leaks from capillaries into the pulmonary interstitium, and there is an increase in the flow of fluid into pulmonary lymphatics. This increases the stiffness of the lungs,

Fig. 11.1 Heart-failure cells. The alveolar spaces contain macrophages which show brownish discoloration of their cytoplasm owing to the hemosiderin content (arrows).

giving rise to a subjective sensation of dyspnea. Such a condition may remain stable for a long time.

In severe left ventricular failure, fluid also leaks into alveolar spaces, resulting in severe acute impairment of respiratory function.

Capillary rupture leads to leakage of red cells into the interstitium, as well as into alveoli. Hemoglobin is phagocytosed by macrophages, which accumulate iron pigment and lie in alveoli and the interstitium. They are often termed 'heart-failure cells' (*Fig. 11.1*).

Pulmonary hypertension results in structural damage to pulmonary vessels

Increased pulmonary arterial pressure in pulmonary hypertension causes irreversible structural changes in pulmonary arteries, leads to increased demand for work on the right side of the heart, right ventricular hypertrophy and right heart failure (**cor pulmonale**). The main causes of pulmonary hypertension are listed in *Fig. 10.22*, the most important being:

- Chronic obstructive pulmonary disease.
- Fibrosis of the lungs.
- Chronic pulmonary venous congestion.

In long-standing pulmonary hypertension structural changes develop in the lung, including medial hypertrophy in muscular arteries (with increase in amount of smooth muscle) and pulmonary veins (arterialization). There is narrowing or occlusion of the lumina of pulmonary arteries by intimal proliferation. Alveolar macrophages containing hemosiderin are prominent (*Fig. 11.1*). Fibrosis in the interstitium of the lung develops in long-standing cases.

The clinical effects of pulmonary hypertension are breathlessness and the development of right-sided cardiac failure.

Pulmonary emboli cause infarction of lung in a minority of cases

Occlusion of the pulmonary arteries by thromboemboli was introduced on pages 155–6 in the chapter on the cardiovascular system. This is a very common condition. Most emboli arise in the deep leg veins and pass in the venous circulation, through the right side of the heart, to lodge in the pulmonary arteries. The outcome of pulmonary thromboem-bolism depends on the size of the thrombus and local hemodynamics.

Occlusion of large pulmonary arteries by large masses of thrombus leads to collapse, with no structural changes seen in the lungs themselves. The pattern of cardiac arrest is often a pulseless-with-electrical activity (PEA) arrest, also termed electromechanical dissociation (EMD) arrest.

Pulmonary infarction (*Fig. 11.2*) occurs in only about 10% of emboli because the normal dual circulation to the lung, from both pulmonary arteries and bronchial arteries, protects against ischemic necrosis. Infarcts are typically hemorrhagic and appear as wedge-shaped peripheral lesions

Fig. 11.2 Pulmonary infarction. Macroscopically, pulmonary infarcts are typically hemorrhagic because of blood entering from the bronchial circulation. (a, b) Pulmonary infarcts (**P**) appear as wedge-shaped subpleural red areas. There is often an overlying area of fibrinous inflammatory exudate which gives rise to pleuritic chest pain as well as a pleural rub that may be found on examination. On cut surface, areas of infarction are hemorrhagic and airless, as seen in (c). Note the peripheral pulmonary artery branch occluded by pale thromboembolus (E). Blood in the alveolar spaces in areas of infarction is responsible for the clinical sign of hemoptysis. With time, infarcts become organized to form a fibrous scar.

in the lung. Healing of areas of infarction is through organization and fibrosis, leaving a residual peripheral scar. In patients who have pulmonary infarcts as well as a chest infection the necrotic tissue can become colonized with bacteria, leading to a so-called septic pulmonary infarct, which can develop into a lung abscess.

In other instances of pulmonary thromboembolism, local hemodynamics do not lead to an infarct. Perfusion is reduced to a lung area which remains ventilated. Patients experience dyspnea and there may be tachycardia and hypotension. This pattern of thromboembolism may be detected by imaging studies that match ventilation (V) against perfusion (Q). A V/Q mismatch may indicate a pulmonary thromboembolus.

Recurrent small thromboemboli do not lead to pulmonary infarction. Organization of such thrombi in the small peripheral pulmonary arteries causes permanent occlusion, which over months and years leads to progressive obliteration of the pulmonary vasculature. Over time this loss of the pulmonary vascular bed can cause pulmonary hypertension.

Pulmonary vasculitis (angiitis) is caused by several disease processes

Several uncommon diseases are characterized by inflammatory cellular infiltration of pulmonary blood vessels (**angiitis**), resulting in necrosis of pulmonary parenchyma.

The main forms of this process are caused by inflammatory destruction of vessels as part of a necrotizing vasculitis (see pages 166–7).

In Wegener's granulomatosis, mainly the nose, lung and kidneys are affected: Churg–Strauss syndrome is caused by infiltration of the lung by eosinophils.

Diagnosis is made on the basis of clinical features, in conjunction with lung biopsy.

Key Facts
Vascular and hemodynamic disease of the lungs

- Pulmonary arteries undergo vasoconstriction in response to hypoxia. Poor lung ventilation may therefore exacerbate pulmonary hypertension.
- Pulmonary edema is most commonly caused by left ventricular failure.
- The common causes of chronic pulmonary hypertension are chronic left-sided heart failure (causes chronic pulmonary venous congestion), COPD and fibrosing lung disease.
- Pulmonary hypertension causes right-sided cardiac failure.
- Pulmonary thromboembolism is most commonly from deep leg vein thrombosis.
- Large pulmonary emboli cause acute right heart failure and death.
- Pulmonary infarcts are typically hemorrhagic, but only happen in about 10% of emboli.
- Pulmonary embolism may be detected by detecting a ventilation/perfusion mismatch on imaging studies.
- Rare cases of pulmonary hypertension are caused by syndromes of recurrent small pulmonary emboli.
- Rare vasculitis syndrome can also lead to pulmonary infarcts.

INFECTIVE DISEASE OF THE RESPIRATORY SYSTEM

Infective diseases of the upper respiratory tract (nose, pharynx, larynx, trachea and bronchi) are frequent in western countries, but most are minor and transient. Infections of the lower respiratory tract (bronchus to alveoli) are a serious cause of morbidity and mortality.

Infection of bronchi and bronchioles is most commonly due to viruses

Inflammation of bronchi and bronchioles is extremely common (*Fig. 11.3*). Most cases are due to self-limiting viral diseases. For example, influenza causes tracheobronchitis with necrosis of the lining epithelium, and respiratory syncytial virus causes epidemics of bronchiolitis in very young children. In rare cases destruction and scarring of airways can occur.

Adenovirus and measles viruses can cause severe inflammation of bronchioles, which heals by fibrosis leading to permanent damage to lungs (obliterative bronchiolitis).

Bacterial infection of airways is common and precedes the development of bronchopneumonia. *Bordetella pertussis* causes whooping cough and, in fatal cases, is associated with bronchial and bronchiolar inflammation.

Infective inflammation and consolidation of the lung is termed 'pneumonia'

Pneumonia is one of the most common infective conditions and is the fifth most common cause of death in the USA. There are three ways of classifying pneumonias, as shown in *Fig. 11.4.*

A pathological classification of pneumonia is based on the main location of inflammatory responses within the lung parenchyma. The vast majority of bacterial infections cause inflammatory exudation and infective spread within the air spaces of the lung. There are two main patterns of bacterial pneumonia, termed **bronchopneumonia** and **lobar pneumonia**. A characteristic of both of these patterns is filling of the alveolar spaces by an inflammatory exudate which renders the affected areas of lung macroscopically solid and airless (**consolidation**). Viral infections and certain other organisms tend to cause inflammatory changes within the interstitium of the lung but little involvement of the air spaces, being termed interstitial pneumonia.

A clinical classification of pneumonia is best suited for planning investigation and initiating therapy. This is because knowledge of the circumstances in which a person develops a pneumonia is a strong clue as to the likely causative organism, allowing antimicrobial therapy to be started while awaiting definitive conformation of the cause by microbiological investigation.

Pneumonitis also refers to interstitial lung inflammation

The term pneumonitis is used to refer to inflammatory disease dominated by interstitial inflammation. Therefore, interstitial pneumonia is also a form of pneumonitis. However, there are other causes of pneumonitis, including the effect of inhaled toxins and allergens, certain drug reactions, and the response to irradiation. Certain multisystem autoimmune diseases also cause pneumonitis, for example the so-called connective tissue diseases. Non-infective

Fig. 11.3 Acute bronchitis. In acute bronchitis the airway mucosa is red and edematous. There is often an overlying mucoid purulent exudate.

Fig. 11.4 Classifications of pneumonia
Pathological classification
How infection spreads within the lung
Air space spread (typically bacterial)
•   Bronchopneumonia (via bronchi to alveoli)
•   Lobar pneumonia (alveoli to alveoli)
Interstitial spread (typically viral)
•   Interstitial pneumonia
Microbiological classification
Causative organism determined by microbiology
Clinical classification
Circumstances surrounding development of disease
Community-acquired disease
Hospital-acquired disease (nosocomial)
Disease acquired in special environments
Disease in immunosuppressed patients
Aspiration pneumonia

Fig. 11.5 Bronchopneumonia. The cut surface of the lung shows pale areas in the lower lobe (**P**), which are areas of consolidation.

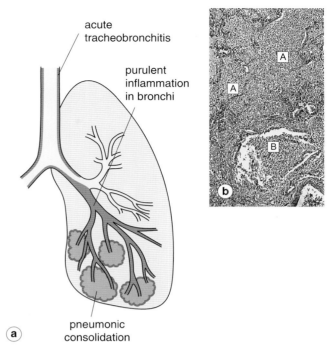

Fig. 11.6 Bronchopneumonia. In bronchopneumonia, inflammation centered on bronchi (**B**) spreads out to cause inflammation in the alveoli (**A**), which contain acute inflammatory infiltrate. Consolidation is in the dependent parts of the lung.

causes of pneumonitis are discussed in the section on restrictive lung diseases (see page 205).

Bronchopneumonia occurs when organisms colonize bronchi and extend into alveoli

In bronchopneumonia, primary infection centered on bronchi spreads to involve adjacent alveoli, which become filled with an acute inflammatory exudate, and affected areas of lung become consolidated. Initially, consolidation is patchy within the lung (involves lobules), but if untreated it becomes confluent (involving lobes).

This pattern of disease, which is most common in infancy and old age, is predisposed to by the presence of debility and immobility. Patients who are immobile develop retention of secretions; these gravitate to the dependent parts of the lungs and become infected, hence bronchopneumonia most commonly involves the lower lobes.

Macroscopically, affected areas of lung are firm, airless, and have a dark red or gray appearance (*Fig. 11.5*). Pus may be present in the peripheral bronchi. Histologically, there is acute inflammation of bronchi, and alveoli contain acute inflammatory exudate (*Fig. 11.6*). Involvement of the pleura is common and leads to pleurisy.

If treated, recovery usually involves focal organization of lung by fibrosis. Common complications include lung abscess, pleural infection (pleurisy, see pages 218–9), and septicemia. The causative organisms for this pattern of pneumonia depend on the circumstances predisposing to infection.

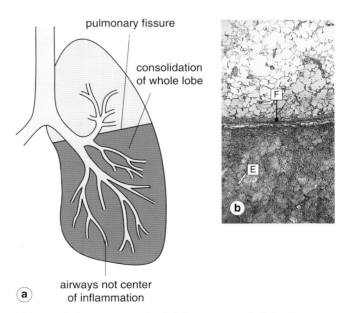

Fig. 11.7 Lobar pneumonia. In lobar pneumonia, infection spreads rapidly through air spaces to consolidate a whole lobe (a). Histologically (b), alveoli are filled with acute inflammatory exudate (**E**), which is limited by the pulmonary fissures (**F**).

Fig. 11.8 Lobar pneumonia. The upper (**U**) and lower (**L**) lobes are consolidated compared to the congested but uninvolved middle lobe (**M**).

Fig. 11.9 Acute pleurisy in lobar pneumonia. The pleural surfaces over consolidated lobes (**L**) are covered by a patchy, white, fibrinous exudate, causing acute pleurisy.

Lobar pneumonia occurs when organisms widely colonize alveolar spaces

In lobar pneumonia, organisms gain entry to distal air spaces rather than colonizing bronchi (*Fig. 11.7*). Rapid spread through alveolar spaces and bronchioles causes acute inflammatory exudation into air spaces. Macroscopically, the whole of a lobe becomes consolidated and airless (*Fig. 11.8*).

This pattern of disease is seen in adults. Vagrants and alcoholics who have poor social and medical care are particularly prone to this pattern of pneumonia, which is often caused by *Streptococcus pneumoniae* or *Klebsiella* spp.

Patients with lobar pneumonia are usually severely ill, and there is usually associated bacteremia. If treated promptly, many patients recover and the lungs return to normal structure and function by resolution. In other cases the exudate in alveoli is organized, leading to lung scarring and permanent lung dysfunction. Common complications are the development of pleurisy (*Fig. 11.9*), lung abscess, and septicemia.

Community-acquired pneumonia is usually caused by Gram-positive bacteria

No cause is identified by microbiology in about 30% of cases of community-acquired pneumonia, usually because of the administration of antibiotics. The most common cause of community-acquired pneumonia is *S. pneumoniae*, accounting for about a third of all cases. In cases associated with bacteremia there is a mortality rate of about 25%. In children, patients over the age of 60 and those with chronic obstructive airways disease, *Hemophilus influenzae* infection is common. *Legionella* causes disease particularly in mid-adult life, accounting for under 5% of cases (with a 10% mortality rate).

Atypical pneumonia caused by *Mycoplasma pneumoniae* accounts for about 10% of cases of community-acquired infection between the ages of 20 and 60 years. Increasingly, infection with *Chlamydia pneumoniae* is responsible for many cases of pneumonia in neonates and working adults.

Pneumonia due to *Mycobacterium tuberculosis* is particularly seen in socially deprived patients with poor medical care. It is common in developing countries, and is once more an increasing cause of disease in developed countries.

Viral pneumonia probably accounts for 10–20% of cases, often complicated by the development of superadded bacterial infection. *Staphylococcus aureus* may cause a very severe pneumonia following viral infection (especially influenza), and particularly causes the development of lung abscesses (see *Fig. 11.18*).

In dramatic contrast to pneumonias acquired in hospital, Gram-negative bacteria account for less than 1% of community-acquired pneumonias. The organism most commonly responsible is *Klebsiella pneumoniae*, which causes a lobar pattern of pneumonia in debilitated and poorly nourished patients, such as alcoholics.

Hospital-acquired pneumonias are mainly due to Gram-negative bacteria

Hospital-acquired (nosocomial) infection is defined as 'that which occurs 2 days or more after admission to hospital.'

This happens in up to 5% of all patients admitted to hospital and is predisposed to by old age, serious illness, cigarette smoking, reduced lung defenses (anesthetics, reduced consciousness), and mechanical ventilation in critical-care units.

Gram-negative bacteria (e.g. *Klebsiella, Escherichia coli, Pseudomonas, Proteus, Serratia* spp.) cause 60% of cases, and organisms responsible for community-acquired pneumonia also cause nosocomial disease, but with much reduced frequency. For example, *Pneumococcus* accounts for infection in about 5% of nosocomial cases. Importantly, certain institutions harbor *Legionella* (see pink box on page 120), which can be a cause of nosocomial pneumonia.

Microbiological diagnosis of nosocomial infection may be difficult because Gram-negative organisms frequently colonize the oropharynx following hospital admission, contaminating expectorated sputum. Specimens obtained by bronchial lavage are often more useful in establishing the cause of infection and the antimicrobial sensitivity.

The pattern of lung involvement in tuberculosis depends on host immune response

Pulmonary tuberculosis is an example of a granulomatous disease. The histopathological characteristics of granulomatous inflammation are described in Chapter 4. A characteristic feature of the granulomata that develop in tuberculosis is the presence of necrosis, termed caseation.

There are different tissue patterns according to the level of host immunity.

- If there has been no previous exposure to the organism, a pattern of disease termed primary tuberculosis develops.
- If a person has previously been exposed and is sensitized to the organism, a pattern called secondary tuberculosis develops.
- If exposure has occurred, but immune responses become abnormal (e.g. by immunosuppression), the pattern of primary TB develops.

In primary TB the initial lung lesion remains small, but infection spreads to peribronchial lymph nodes

When infection with TB first occurs (e.g. in childhood), the organisms are inhaled and cause an area of infection and necrosis at the periphery of the lung, often just beneath the pleura (a **Ghon focus**). Bacteria are then conveyed to local nodes at the lung hilum which enlarge through granulomatous inflammation and caseation (*Fig. 11.10*). These early changes may produce no significant symptoms, and the outcome of the infection will depend on the balance between the host response to disease and the virulence and number of organisms.

In the vast majority of cases the Ghon focus and caseating granulomas in the lymph nodes heal leaving a zone of caseation surrounded by a wall of collagen (see *Fig. 11.11*). Once the immune system has been exposed to *M. tuberculosis* the patient is sensitized to the organism. The disease does not progress, and organisms are confined within the shell of collagen. Importantly, viable bacteria may remain walled off within the healed primary complex (latent tuberculosis).

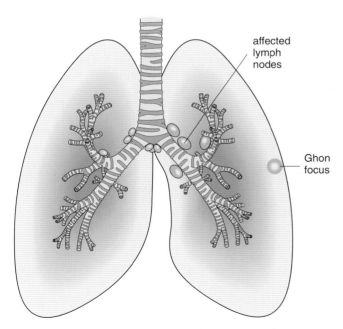

Fig. 11.10 The primary pattern in pulmonary TB. The peripheral Ghon focus and enlarged peribronchial lymph nodes constitute the **primary complex**. The usual outcome is healing by progressive fibrosis surrounding the caseous necrosis.

affected lymph nodes

Ghon focus

Fig. 11.11 Healed Ghon focus in an elderly man. This close-up photograph shows an old, healed Ghon focus at the periphery of the lung. An incidental finding at autopsy, the lesion is a mass of yellowish caseous necrosis surrounded, in this case, by only a thin fibrous capsule.

Fig. 11.12 Caseating TB in peribronchial lymph node. This photomicrograph shows part of a lymph node which has been virtually replaced by pink-staining caseating tuberculous necrosis; only a thin rim of the original lymph node remains. Nodes such as this can rupture into the airways or bloodstream to initiate the spread of tuberculosis.

Rarely, the primary complex will progress in patients with poor natural immunity

In patients who are unable to mount a vigorous immune and reparative response, further spread of mycobacteria occurs, with continuing enlargement of the caseating granulomas in the lymph nodes (*Fig. 11.12*). Known as progressive primary tuberculosis, spread occurs by the enlarging nodes eroding either through the wall of a bronchus or into a thin-walled blood vessel.

The Ghon focus usually remains small, although rarely it may rupture through the visceral pleura, discharging organisms into the pleural cavity to produce tuberculous pleurisy.

Bronchial spread of organisms produces tuberculous bronchopneumonia

If an infected lymph node erodes into a bronchus, tuberculous caseous material containing living tubercle bacilli passes down bronchi and bronchioles under the influence of gravity, spreading the infection to the furthest reaches of the lungs (*Fig. 11.13*), where extensive, confluent caseating granulomatous lesions develop. This pattern of disease used to be termed 'galloping consumption,' and historically was usually rapidly fatal.

Bloodstream spread of organisms produces miliary TB

If the enlarging caseating infected lymph node erodes a vessel wall, tubercle bacilli are carried in the bloodstream to many parts of the body, including the remainder of the lung, causing miliary tuberculosis (*Fig. 11.14*). Patients are generally extremely ill, and this pattern carries a high mortality.

Fig. 11.13 Tuberculous bronchopneumonia. As shown in the diagram (a), if the enlarged caseous nodes erode the bronchial wall, tubercle bacilli can enter into the lower portions of both the same and the opposite lung. New enlarging caseating granulomas form, often in the lower lobes. This is shown in the photomicrograph (b), where a caseating tubercle (**T**) is situated close to an infected bronchiole (**B**), down which the tubercle bacilli have passed.

In secondary TB initial infection is at the apex of the upper lobe of a lung, with little lymph node involvement

In secondary TB, organisms may be acquired exogenously or from a healed primary complex.

In this pattern an apical lesion (often called an **Assmann focus**) begins as a central area of caseous necrosis surrounded by a granulomatous inflammatory response. In most cases destruction of the lung leads to cavitation. There is little involvement of lymph nodes, as spread of organisms to regional nodes is prevented by the immune response.

Fig. 11.15 Healed fibrocaseous TB. This photomicrograph shows the histology of a small nodule from the apex of an adult who had no history of TB. There is a central area of pink-staining caseous material surrounded by a thick, pale-pink collagenous shell, representing healing of a small Assmann focus.

Fig. 11.14 Miliary tuberculosis of lung. If an enlarged caseous node drains into a pulmonary vein (a), there is systemic dissemination of organisms (kidneys, liver, spleen). If drainage is into a pulmonary artery, miliary dissemination into the lung occurs (b). This slice of the lung of a child shows numerous tiny yellow-white dots. Each of these is a small caseating tuberculous granuloma caused by bloodstream spread. In (c) the photomicrograph shows the histological appearances of miliary TB in the lung; there are many small early tubercles, most of which have giant cells at their centre. There is, as yet, little caseation.

In adults secondary TB heals by fibrosis around the caseating mass

In adults with vigorous immune responses, healing of the apical lesion occurs, leaving a central area of caseous necrotic material containing bacteria surrounded by a thick, dense

collagenous wall, which may also be calcified (*Fig. 11.15*). If the patient's immune response becomes weakened later in life this latent tuberculosis can lead to spreading infection (reactivated fibrocaseous tuberculosis).

In adults with poor immune responses, secondary TB progresses locally

In adults with poor immune responses, progressive enlargement of the apical lesion occurs, with caseous necrosis destroying lung tissue. A large caseous mass is formed as a result, which is surrounded by a thin cellular reaction, inducing little collagen to wall off the lesion (progressive pulmonary tuberculosis). As the lesion grows, so too does the risk of erosion into blood vessels or airways.

The release of tubercle bacilli into the main bronchi allows them to be coughed into the atmosphere in droplets, transmitting the infection to other people (so-called open tuberculosis), as well as producing TB bronchopneumonia by passage down bronchi to the lower lobes.

Bloodstream spread of organisms can lead to single-organ infections

Sometimes only small numbers of tubercle bacilli escape into the blood and, if host defenses are effective, most of the organisms die. However, for reasons that are not yet certain, some bacilli settle in specific organs and may remain dormant for many years, only proliferating and producing overt disease at a later date, often after the initial lung and lymph node lesions have healed. Known as metastatic tuberculosis or isolated organ tuberculosis, the organs particularly involved in this pattern of disease include the adrenal glands (see page 197), kidney (see page 383), fallopian tube (see page 428), epididymis (see page 398), brain and meninges (see page 469), and bones and joints.

Aspiration pneumonia is caused by chemical and infective damage to lungs

Aspiration into the airway is usually associated with regurgitation during episodes of unconsciousness, but is also seen in patients who have impaired swallowing due to neuromuscular disease, e.g. after a stroke, or with motor neuron disease.

Gastric acid causes chemical pneumonitis, which can lead to adult respiratory distress syndrome (see page 206). Patients develop increasing respiratory dysfunction, and chest radiography shows opacification of lungs. Food material excites a foreign body histiocytic response in the lung, and organisms from the oropharynx cause infection.

Organisms causing infection are usually mixed, but include anaerobes, e.g. *Fusobacterium* and *Bacteroides*. In cases of aspiration pneumonia in hospital patients, *Staphylococcus aureus* and oropharyngeal Gram-negative bacteria are common.

The development of lung abscess (see page 200) is a frequent complication of aspiration pneumonia.

Atypical pneumonia is characterized by inflammation in alveolar septa

In contrast to lobar pneumonia and bronchopneumonia, in which there is inflammatory exudation into air spaces, certain forms of infection of the lung are characterized by inflammation of the alveolar septa by chronic inflammatory cells. This pattern of inflammation (acute interstitial pneumonitis), may be caused by several factors, including infection by *Mycoplasma*, some viruses, *Chlamydia* and *Rickettsia*.

Patients with this pattern of infection develop fever, a dry cough and dyspnea, with little to find on clinical examination of the chest, e.g. absence of consolidation. This pattern of infection is therefore termed **atypical pneumonia**.

Pneumonia acquired in special environments

- *Legionella* pneumonia is acquired from exposure to buildings with contaminated air-conditioning or water supplies.
- Psittacosis is caused by *Chlamydia psittaci*, usually acquired from avian excreta. It is therefore seen after exposure to pet birds, especially parrots.
- Histoplasmosis is a disease with a similar clinical pattern to that seen in TB. It is seen in the midwest and the southeastern regions of the USA, and is acquired by inhaling fungal spores in dust. Pathology shows granulomatous inflammation and fibrosis.

Virus infections of the lung cause inflammation of lung interstitium

Most viral infections of the lung cause an interstitial inflammatory response by lymphoid cells (interstitial pneumonitis), which in most cases is self-limiting. In severe cases, damage to alveolar lining cells leads to alveolar exudation of fibrin similar to that seen in adult respiratory distress syndrome (see pages 206–7).

Influenza causes rhinitis, pharyngitis, tracheobronchitis and interstitial pneumonitis. Some patients develop a superinfection with bacteria, especially *Staphylococcus aureus*. Certain strains of influenza virus have been associated with particularly severe forms of influenza pneumonia. In such examples infection, mainly in younger adults, causes severe pneumonitis associated with necrosis of the alveolar lining cells, hemorrhagic exudation into the lungs, and the development of adult respiratory distress syndrome. This is associated with a high case fatality rate. Human transmission of the H5N1 strain of avian influenza has been linked to a high case fatality rate. Pandemics of influenza of high virulence are an established historic fact, and it is likely that a pandemic of a virulent strain will affect the population within the next decade.

SARS coronavirus causes severe acute respiratory syndrome (SARS), and has caused epidemic forms of pneumonitis with a high case fatality rate.

Cytomegalovirus causes a self-limiting interstitial pneumonitis, commonly seen in small children. Severe infection may be seen in immunocompromised adults.

Measles may cause an interstitial pneumonitis characterized by the formation of multinucleate giant cells. Inflammation of bronchioles with scarring can be a complication. In poorly nourished or immunocompromised individuals, measles infection of the lung can be fatal (see *Fig. 8.31*).

Varicella infection may cause an interstitial pneumonitis (chickenpox lung) and can lead to miliary small scars in the lung parenchyma, visible on chest radiography. In immunocompromised individuals it may be fatal.

Fungal infections of lung cause destructive inflammation

Fungal infections of the lung are mostly seen in immunosuppressed patients, but rare cases occur in normal patients by exposure to an agent indigenous to a geographic area.

Aspergillus infection of the lung can cause several patterns of disease, including a pneumonia that leads to extensive necrosis and infarction of the affected lung because of vessel wall invasion (*Fig. 11.16*) by the fungus.

Histoplasmosis, coccidioidomycosis and sporotrichosis all cause chronic granulomatous inflammation of the lung, with fibrosis in a pattern resembling TB (see page 308).

Cryptococcal pneumonia is mainly seen in immunocompromised patients.

Candida pneumonia is seen in severely debilitated patients and causes severe acute inflammation, leading to a bronchopneumonic pattern of disease.

Immunosuppressed patients develop opportunistic pneumonias

The diagnosis and treatment of pneumonia in immunosuppressed patients is becoming increasingly important, particularly with the growing incidence of AIDS (see page 471). Infection may be with several types of organism, many being opportunistic infections.

- Routine bacterial pathogens responsible for community pneumonias are generally more severe in immunosuppressed patients.
- Mycobacterial infection can be with *M. tuberculosis* or with atypical mycobacteria.
- Viruses, e.g. cytomegalovirus (CMV) and herpes simplex.
- Fungi, e.g. *Candida*, *Aspergillus* and *Pneumocystis carinii* (see *Fig. 11.16*).

Bronchiectasis stems from abnormal dilatation of the bronchial tree and predisposes to infection

Abnormal dilatation of main bronchi is termed **bronchiectasis** (*Fig. 11.17*). Patients have recurrent cough and hemoptysis, and expectorate copious quantities of infected sputum. Recurrent episodes of chest infection are common, with a mixed flora of organisms including anaerobes.

Although any bronchi may be involved, the most common site is at the base of the lungs. Airways are dilated, may contain purulent secretions, and show chronic inflammation in the wall with replacement of the epithelium by inflammatory granulation tissue; it is this that bleeds, giving rise to the frequent clinical sign of hemoptysis. With repeated episodes of infection extending into the adjacent lung there may be fibrous scarring leading to respiratory failure.

The pathogenesis of this condition is shown in the pink box. Complications of bronchiectasis include chronic suppuration, the formation of a lung abscess, hematogenous spread of infection (particularly predisposing to brain abscess), and the development of serum amyloid A-derived systemic amyloidosis (see page 575).

Pathogenesis of bronchiectasis

Bronchiectasis is predisposed by two main factors:

Interference with drainage of bronchial secretions

- Obstruction of proximal airway, e.g. tumor, foreign body.
- Abnormality in the viscosity of bronchial mucus, e.g. cystic fibrosis (see page 221).
- Immotile cilia syndrome, in which cilia are abnormal, leading to stagnation of secretions (see page 220).

Recurrent and persistent infection weakening bronchial walls

- Predisposed to by retention of secretions (as above).
- Immunodeficiency states, particularly hypogammaglobulinemia.
  In many cases in adults, no cause can be found (**idiopathic bronchiectasis**).

Fig. 11.17 Bronchiectasis.
This is a lower lobe of lung surgically resected for bronchiectasis. Large dilated air passages (P) extend out to the lung periphery.

Fig. 11.16
***Aspergillus* pneumonia.**
Aspergillus invades widely in lung, frequently involving vessel walls. In (a) the section has been stained to show *Aspergillus* hyphae invading lung as well as vessel wall. This causes infarction of lung, seen on the cut surface (b) as large areas of organizing infarction (I).

Bacterial lung abscess is predisposed to by several diseases

A bacterial lung abscess appears as a cavity, typically 1–3 cm in diameter, containing pus and surrounded by fibrosis and organizing inflammation (*Fig. 11.18*). There are many diseases that cause or predispose to the development of a lung abscess, including infection in a pulmonary infarct, unresolved acute pneumonia (particularly due to staphylococci), aspiration of gastric contents (see page 198), and bronchiectasis.

The main complications of an abscess are rupture into pleura, causing empyema and pneumothorax; hemorrhage from erosion into a pulmonary vessel; and bacteremia causing cerebral abscess.

Fig. 11.18 Lung abscess. (a) A lung abscess is seen as a cavity filled with green purulent material (**A**). The histological section (b) shows the cavity of a peripheral lung abscess (**A**) containing pus, with a wall (**W**) composed of acute inflammatory granulation tissue. This was derived from an infected area of infarction.

ASTHMA

Asthma is characterized by reversible airways obstruction in small airways

Asthma is a syndrome of reversible airways obstruction that presents clinically as recurrent breathlessness, cough and wheeze. It is characterized by functional obstruction of small airways by a combination of bronchospasm and mucous plugging, which fluctuates with time and is frequently reversible with bronchodilator drugs. It is a common disorder, affecting around 10% of children and 5% of adults.

- **Atopy** is the commonest cause of asthma in patients under the age of 30 and is caused by IgE production following exposure to environmental allergens such as are in house dust. Th2 lymphocytes mediate some of this process.
- **Intrinsic asthma** shares pathological features with atopic asthma, except that an external allergen trigger is not found. Cold exposure and exertion may trigger attacks.
- **Childhood asthma** is often stimulated by viral infections and may be related to the small size of airways in children, as it frequently abates with age.
- **Occupational asthma** is triggered by factors in the work environment, including the direct actions of chemical irritant gases or dusts that modify local immune networks.
- **Aspirin-induced asthma** is triggered by exposure to aspirin or non-steroidal anti-inflammatory drugs. This develops in patients with pathological susceptibilities involving arachidonic acid-mediated inflammatory responses.

Tissue diagnosis does not form part of the routine diagnostic assessment of a patient with asthma. Occasionally, patients die following an acute episode of asthma. **Status asthmaticus** refers to severe, acute disease that does not respond to drug therapy and may cause death from acute respiratory insufficiency. At postmortem the lungs are typically hyperinflated and histological features typical of asthma are seen in the airways (*Fig. 11.19*). Patients with asthma are also predisposed to develop pneumothorax, which may cause a severe decline in respiratory function and may be fatal if not recognized and treated.

Asthma is due to a complex chronic inflammatory response in bronchial mucosa

The main changes that take place in asthma are shown in *Fig. 11.19* and biological mechanisms are discussed on page 202.

A complex inflammatory response involving eosinophils, mast cells and lymphoid cells is seen in asthma, whatever the underlying cause. The prevailing view is that asthma is an inflammatory condition with both acute and chronic components affecting different structural elements in the

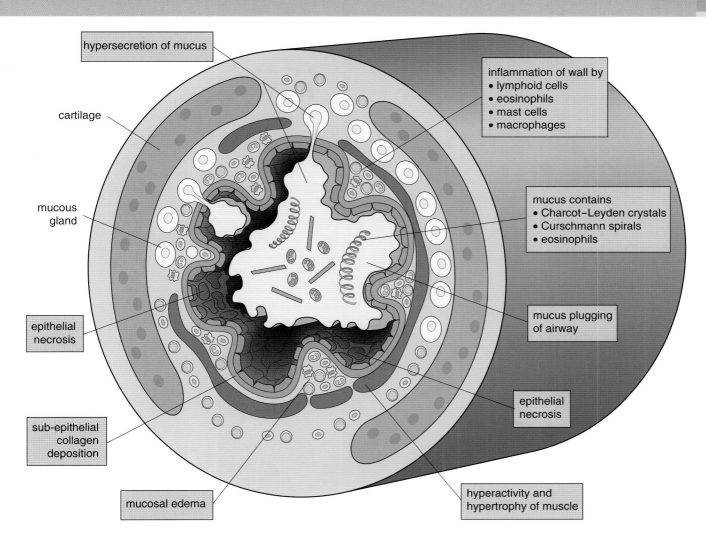

hypersecretion of mucus

inflammation of wall by
• lymphoid cells
• eosinophils
• mast cells
• macrophages

cartilage

mucous gland

mucus contains
• Charcot–Leyden crystals
• Curschmann spirals
• eosinophils

epithelial necrosis

mucus plugging of airway

epithelial necrosis

sub-epithelial collagen deposition

mucosal edema

hyperactivity and hypertrophy of muscle

airways. It is believed that a variety of triggers may stimulate acute exacerbations. Some of the proposed mediators and mechanisms in the pathogenesis of asthma are described in the pink box on page 202.

Most people with asthma have mild disease with acute episodes of bronchospasm that are triggered by well-recognized causes. In the majority of patients symptoms are controlled by drug therapy with inhaled β_2-adrenoceptor agonists and corticosteroids.

A minority of patients have severe disease in which airway obstruction persists and there are frequent relapses despite drug therapy. Chronic disease leads to permanent structural changes in the airways and pulmonary vessels. Chronic alveolar hypoventilation may cause pulmonary vasoconstriction and pulmonary hypertension. The condition can then move on to a state that becomes indistinguishable from chronic obstructive pulmonary disease (COPD) (see pages 202–9), sometimes termed 'chronic asthma.'

Patients with COPD from a variety of causes may also have a reversible airways obstruction component to their disease, but otherwise these patients do not have typical 'asthma.'

Fig. 11.19 Structural changes in asthma.
The main events that take place in the airways in asthma are shown diagrammatically. There is:

• Bronchoconstriction due to increased responsiveness of bronchial smooth muscle.

• Hypersecretion of mucus leading to plugging of airways.

• Mucosal edema leading to narrowing of airway lumen.

• Extravasation of plasma in submucosal tissues due to leakage from vessels contributes to mucosal edema.

• Infiltration of bronchial mucosa by eosinophils, mast cells, lymphoid cells and macrophages.

• Focal necrosis of airway epithelium.

• Deposition of collagen beneath bronchial epithelium in long-standing cases.

• Sputum contains Charcot–Leyden crystals (derived from eosinophil granules) and Curschmann spirals (composed of mucus plugs from small airways).

Notes on cellular mechanisms of asthma

Immune mechanisms are dominant in many cases of asthma (type I hypersensitivity response); 80% of asthmatics show an atopic tendency.

Although **mast cells** are thought to be important in asthma, and although they release histamine, antihistamines are not clinically useful in therapy. Mast cells may be activated in asthma by stimuli other than aggregation of IgE receptors.

T cells, particularly Th2 cells are prominent in the mucosal cellular infiltrate. They can release a variety of cytokines such as IL-4 and IL-13, and are under intense study in pathogenesis.

A variety of **cytokines** orchestrate and amplify the inflammatory response in asthma. Anti-cytokine therapies are undergoing clinical trials.

Eosinophils are thought to be important in the pathogenesis of asthma. They migrate into the mucosa in response to chemotactic factors, releasing many mediators of inflammation:

- Leukotrienes LTC$_4$ and LTD$_4$ can constrict airways.
- Factors derived from eosinophils are likely to be responsible for the structural remodeling seen in bronchi.

Stimulation of afferent nerves by inflammatory mediators can release local neuropeptides that may mediate edema and the hypersecretion of mucus. Such neural mechanisms are believed to play an important role in pathogenesis and are beginning to be targeted by new therapies.

Inflammation of bronchial walls can give rise to airflow restriction by causing depletion of surfactant in small airways, making them open with difficulty. In long-standing cases collagen is deposited beneath bronchial epithelium, and this may predispose to increased susceptibility to epithelial necrosis.

CHRONIC OBSTRUCTIVE PULMONARY DISEASE

Chronic obstructive pulmonary disease (COPD) is defined as 'a disease state characterized by airflow limitations that is not fully reversible. The airflow limitation is usually both progressive and associated with an abnormal inflammatory response of the lungs to noxious particles or gases' (Global Initiative for Obstructive Lung Disease: GOLD). Airflow is limited for one of two main reasons: either because **airways resistance is increased** (normally due to narrowing) or because the **outflow pressure is reduced** (elastic recoil of lungs is lost). The three main pathologies contributing to COPD are **emphysema** (destruction of air spaces and loss of elastic recoil), **chronic bronchitis** (mucus hypersecretion and luminal narrowing of airways) and **bronchiolitis** (narrowing of small airways by inflammation and scarring).

Generalized emphysema is characterized by dilatation of air spaces

Emphysema can be defined as 'a permanent dilatation of any part of the respiratory acinus (air spaces distal to the terminal bronchiole), with destruction of tissue in the absence of scarring.' One component of pathogenesis is thought to be parenchymal destruction by extracellular

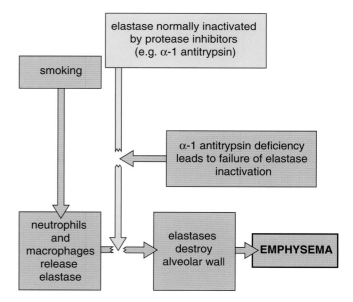

Fig. 11.20 Pathogenesis of emphysema. Normally, proteases secreted by inflammatory cells are inactivated by extracellular proteases, one example being α_1-antitrypsin. If proteases are not inactivated they can destroy lung tissue. Emphysema is caused by an imbalance in the activity of proteases and protease inhibitors. Smoking increases local release of proteases. Congenital lack of protease inhibitors may allow protease activity to persist and contribute to disease. Polymorphisms may cause inefficient protease inhibitors.

Fig. 11.21 Generalized emphysema. (a) Normal distal lung acinus. (b) Centriacinar emphysema. (c) Centriacinar emphysema. (d) Panacinar emphysema. (e) Panacinar emphysema (Gough–Wentworth section). The normal lung acinus distal to the terminal bronchiole consists of respiratory bronchioles, alveolar ducts and terminal acini. In centriacinar emphysema there is dilatation of the respiratory bronchioles at the center of the acinus (b). This is seen in a very high-power macroscopic photograph (c) of a portion of affected lung, in which the dilated air spaces (**D**) are surrounded by normal-sized alveoli. In panacinar emphysema (d), there is dilatation of the terminal alveoli and alveolar ducts, which later affects respiratory bronchioles, thereby affecting the whole acinus. The extent of this process in a whole lung can be seen in (e), which is a Gough–Wentworth preparation made by taking a slice, 1 mm thick, through a whole lung and mounting it on paper. The dilated air spaces (**D**) caused by emphysema are evident in all lobes.

proteases, normal defensive protease inhibitors being reduced (*Fig. 11.20*). There are two main forms of generalized emphysema, defined by the location of damage in the respiratory acinus (*Fig. 11.21*).

In practical terms, there is loss of elastic recoil in lungs as connective tissue in the alveolar walls is destroyed. The area available for gas exchange is also reduced. Individuals with severe emphysema have reduced oxygen uptake despite increased ventilation. Although they manage to maintain blood oxygenation by a rapid respiratory rate, they feel breathless on the slightest exertion and become hypoxic (type I respiratory failure). In pure emphysema, cyanosis, hypercapnia and cor pulmonale develop only late in the disease, after a progressive decline in respiratory function.

Macroscopically the lungs are voluminous and, on cut surface, show large dilated air spaces. More than one pattern of emphysema may exist in the same lung.

Centriacinar emphysema (centrilobular emphysema) is the most common form and most cases are associated with cigarette smoking (*Fig. 11.21b* and *c*). It is most often seen in the upper lobes, with sparing of lower lobes.

It is likely that the pathogenesis of this type of emphysema is related to the secretion of extracellular proteases by local inflammatory cells. Cigarette smoke may also inhibit the effect of protease inhibitor α_1-antitrypsin, thereby potentiating tissue destruction.

Panacinar emphysema involves the whole respiratory acinus and is also commonly associated with smoking (*Fig. 11.21 d* and *e*). As with centriacinar emphysema, its pathogenesis is probably related to excessive activity of extracellular proteases. In contrast to centriacinar disease, this form affects both upper and lower lobes. Individuals with congenital deficiency of α_1-antitrypsin also develop this pattern of emphysema at an early age.

Chronic bronchitis causes increased airflow resistance in large airways

Chronic bronchitis is a functional disorder, defined clinically as 'cough productive of sputum on most days for 3 months of the year for at least 2 successive years.' The structural changes are shown in *Fig. 11.22*. The main problem relates to hypersecretion of mucus associated with hyperplasia of mucous glands.

Not everyone with mucous hypersecretion will have COPD, but smokers with this feature commonly go on to develop airways obstruction. Airways obstruction in chronic bronchitis is related to luminal narrowing and mucous plugging. This leads to alveolar hypoventilation, hypoxemia and hypercapnia (type II respiratory failure). Individuals with chronic bronchitis and type II respiratory failure are typically cyanosed, but do not usually have distressing dyspnea. Hypoxic pulmonary vasoconstriction may cause secondary pulmonary hypertension and, with time, lead to right-heart failure (cor pulmonale).

Fig. 11.22 Chronic bronchitis. In chronic bronchitis the main abnormality is secretion of abnormal amounts of mucus, causing plugging of the airway lumen (**P**). Hypersecretion is associated with hypertrophy and hyperplasia of bronchial mucus-secreting glands (**M**). This can be appreciated by the **Reid index**, the ratio of gland:wall thickness in the bronchus, which is increased in cases of chronic bronchitis. Inflammation in chronic bronchitis is typically not present, although individuals with excessive mucus production frequently develop coincidental respiratory tract infections, leading to secondary inflammation. Squamous metaplasia (**S**) is common in patients who have persistent or recurrent superimposed infections.

Bronchiolitis is an early smoking-related lesion

Cigarette smokers develop inflammation of airways <2 mm in diameter, at a level which is distal to the cartilage-walled larger bronchi. Macrophages and lymphoid cells infiltrate the airway wall, causing bronchiolitis. This may progress and lead to scarring and narrowing of these airways. Bronchiolitis is believed to contribute to functional airways obstruction.

Chronic obstructive pulmonary disease is associated with several causes

The main risk factors that have been suggested for COPD are lifetime smoking exposure, recurrent chest infections in childhood, atopy and asthma, occupational exposure to dusts (especially mining), low socioeconomic status, and a series of incompletely understood genetic factors.

Exacerbations of COPD are usually infective

COPD is a slowly progressive condition but can be subject to acute exacerbations in which patients experience dyspnea and wheeze, often associated with the production of purulent sputum. Such acute deterioration can be caused by viral and bacterial infections or short-term exposure to air pollution. This leads to narrowing of peripheral airways and may also precipitate acute deterioration of chronic cor

Key Facts
Chronic obstructive pulmonary disease

- Definition: a disease state characterized by airflow limitations that are not fully reversible. The airflow limitation is usually both progressive and associated with an abnormal inflammatory response of the lungs to noxious particles or gases.
- Cigarette smoking remains the most important cause of COPD. Other risks are recurrent chest infections in childhood, atopy, asthma, and occupational exposure to dusts (especially mining).
- Respiratory bronchiolitis is one of the earliest lesions seen in smokers.
- Chronic bronchitic airways show mucous hypersecretion with mucous gland hyperplasia.
- Chronic bronchitis and bronchiolitis cause airway narrowing.
- Emphysema causes loss of elastic recoil in lungs and contributes to functional airways obstruction.
- Generalized emphysema is defined as permanent dilatation of any part of the respiratory acinus, with destruction of tissue in the absence of scarring.
- There are two patterns of generalized emphysema: centrilobular and panacinar.
- Many patients with COPD have a reversible component to functional airways obstruction.
- Pulmonary hypertension and right-sided heart failure are common in long-standing chronic obstructive pulmonary disease.
- Acute deterioration in COPD is usually caused by viral or bacterial infection.

pulmonale, with cyanosis, peripheral edema and deterioration of conscious level due to hypoxia. Treatment relates to underlying pathology and is aimed mainly at increasing alveolar oxygen saturation. Controlled oxygen is administered and may alleviate hypoxia-mediated pulmonary vasoconstriction (cor pulmonale). Bronchodilator drugs facilitate alveolar ventilation by opening up airways. Corticosteroids may serve to minimize any inflammatory response and reduce mucosal edema, thereby also opening up peripheral airways. Bacterial infection which may be causing inflammation may be treated with appropriate therapy. Physiotherapy to encourage expectoration of secretions can be the most important factor in opening peripheral airway in the subgroup of patients with mucus hypersecretion who have mucus plugging.

DIFFUSE PARENCHYMAL LUNG DISEASES

A group of lung diseases is characterized by widespread inflammatory pathology in the interstitium and alveolar spaces. Patients present with dyspnea, and onset varies from acute to chronic. Imaging typically reveals diffuse shadowing in both lungs. Once infective causes have been eliminated by investigation (see pneumonias, page 192, et seq) a set of parenchymal inflammatory diseases remains and must be distinguished by further investigation.

Two main clinical patterns of diffuse parenchymal lung disease are recognized.

- **Acute parenchymal lung disease** is characterized by exudation and edema affecting most air spaces in both lungs. This clinical syndrome is associated with severe acute life-threatening disease requiring treatment in an intensive care facility. The main disease encountered in clinical practice presenting as an acute diffuse parenchymal lung disease is the adult respiratory distress syndrome (ARDS).
- **Chronic parenchymal lung disease** is usually characterized by focal involvement of the alveoli in both lungs over a period of months to years. Individual alveoli go through phases of exudation, inflammation, chronic inflammation with subsequent cell proliferation and fibrosis. It is this latter pattern of disease that leads to a group of diseases characterized by **chronic pulmonary fibrosis.** In clinical practice, patients with chronic disease patterns present with cough, dyspnea, and systemic features. The main diseases in this category are the group of idiopathic interstitial pneumonias, which includes cryptogenic fibrosing alveolitis (idiopathic pulmonary fibrosis), and extrinsic allergic alveolitis.

Alveolar wall damage followed by fibrosis leads to restrictive lung disease

Both acute and chronic forms of parenchymal lung disease lead to reduced compliance of the lungs, i.e. they are difficult to expand with respiration. The main reason for this pattern of respiratory dysfunction is an abnormality of the alveolar walls that renders them rigid, usually due to edema or fibrosis. Those affected complain of breathlessness (dyspnea), as they feel the greater effort needed to inflate the lungs. Fibrosis and edema of alveolar walls causes them to thicken, such that a diffusional defect develops, with consequent hypoxia.

Damage to alveolar walls can vary from an acute exudative reaction into alveolar spaces, through to a smoldering chronic inflammatory response limited to the interstitium. As with other chronic inflammatory processes, fibrosis is a common outcome. These parenchymal inflammatory diseases are therefore associated with four main histological patterns of reaction in lung:

- Hemorrhage and fibrin exudation into alveoli (so-called **hyaline membranes**).
- Edema and inflammation of the interstitium.
- Macrophage accumulation in alveolar spaces.
- Fibrosis in the interstitium or the alveolar spaces.

In the various types of diffuse parenchymal lung disease, these differing tissue responses are present to differing degrees. In acute syndromes the majority of alveoli become involved, with dominant exudative and inflammatory responses, giving rise to widespread and symptomatic disease. In the chronic syndromes either the pattern of involvement is focal, or the type of response is dominated by low-grade chronic inflammation and fibrosis.

Adult respiratory distress syndrome (ARDS) is an acute restrictive lung disease caused by diffuse alveolar damage

The adult respiratory distress syndrome is an acute form of diffuse parenchymal lung disease. It is the result of diffuse alveolar damage leading to exudative and inflammatory responses in the lung and consequent widespread systemic metabolic derangements. Many conditions predispose to this condition, most commonly systemic sepsis and severe trauma (*Fig. 11.23*). Systemic liberation of chemical mediators of inflammation, particularly cytokines, is important in the progression of disease. The pathophysiology of this condition is presented in the pink box (*Fig. 11.25*). *Fig. 11.24* summarizes the main features and outcomes in ARDS.

Fig. 11.23 Conditions causing ARDS

ARDS follows a wide variety of direct or indirect insults to the pulmonary vascular endothelium or the alveolar epithelium:

- Major trauma, especially associated with raised intracranial pressure
- Septicemia
- Pulmonary aspiration of gastric contents
- Inhalation of toxic fumes or smoke
- Major burns
- Near-drowning
- Pneumonia from many causes, requiring ventilation
- Disseminated intravascular coagulation
- Massive blood transfusion
- Amniotic fluid embolism
- Acute pancreatitis
- Cardiac surgery with bypass
- Radiation injury
- Certain types of anti-tumor chemotherapy
- Paraquat poisoning

Pathophysiology of ARDS

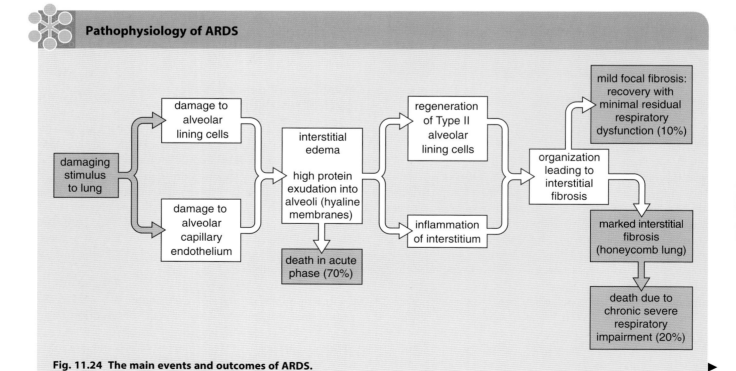

Fig. 11.24 The main events and outcomes of ARDS.

red cell

alveolar capillary

a

Type I
pneumocyte

interalveolar septum
containing elastic and
collagen fibers

damage to vessel
wall and extravasation
of red cells

hyaline membrane

fibrin
exudation

neutrophil adherence
and degranulation

b

activation of
macrophages

necrosis of
Type I alveolar
lining cells

collagenous
scarring

c

fibrosis organizing
alveolar exudate

proliferation of
fibroblasts

hyperplasia of
Type II
pneumocytes

The normal alveolar wall is shown diagrammatically in *Fig. 11.25a*. The alveolar wall showing pathological charges centered on the same group of vessels can be seen in *Figs 11.25b* and *c*.

The events that take place in the lung in ARDS are termed **diffuse alveolar damage** (DAD) and occur in two phases:

1. Acute exudative phase, with destruction of alveolar lining cells.
2. Late organization phase, with cell proliferation and fibrosis.

Following the damaging stimulus there is a latent period of 4–24 hours before symptoms develop. Dyspnea develops before changes are visible on chest radiographs. ARDS develops progressively over a period of 24–48 hours.

In the **acute phase** (*Fig. 11.25b*) there is:

- Necrosis of alveolar epithelium.
- Exudation of fibrin and fluid into alveolar spaces, forming hyaline membranes.
- Microthrombosis in alveolar capillaries.
- Adherence and activation of neutrophils, with release of neutrophil enzymes.
- Hemorrhage into alveoli.

In the **organization phase** the lungs are congested and ventilation is impaired by disturbance of alveolar walls, with exudation into alveolar spaces (*Fig. 11.25c*). There is regeneration of type II alveolar lining cells and organization of hyaline membranes with pulmonary fibrosis. Organization may result in interstitial fibrosis with thickening of alveolar walls, or may cause fibrous obliteration of alveolar spaces.

If ARDS has been caused by septicemia, endotoxin causes endothelial and neutrophil activation, with activation of complement. Treatment with high concentrations of oxygen may, paradoxically, increase damage by generation of oxygen-derived free radicals. ARDS is often complicated by secondary infection in the lungs.

In severe cases of ARDS from any cause, cytokines liberated from the lung vascular bed can enter the systemic circulation and may cause systemic endothelial activation, with systemic neutrophil activation leading to multiorgan failure (**systemic inflammatory response syndrome**).

Fig. 11.25 Adult respiratory distress syndrome. (a) Normal alveolar wall. (b) Acute phase of ARDS. (c) Organization phase of ARDS.

Diffuse parenchymal lung diseases has several causes, but may be idiopathic

Several conditions are grouped together on the basis of a common process of progressive inflammatory infiltration or fibrosis in the lungs. The conditions represent a group of acute and chronic lung disorders collectively referred to as **interstitial lung diseases** or **diffuse parenchymal lung diseases**. A proportion of these diffuse parenchymal diseases have a defined cause. The same tissue responses can be initiated by a wide range of extrinsic factors, both inhaled (e.g. industrial dust disease) and non-inhaled (drugs, radiation), as well as intrinsic disease such as scleroderma and rheumatoid disease (*Fig. 11.26*). Many of these diseases are of unknown cause and are grouped as the **idiopathic interstitial pneumonias**.

The end-stage of chronic pulmonary fibrosis is termed 'honeycomb lung'

The end result of long-standing pulmonary fibrosis, from whatever cause, is conversion of the lung into a mass of cystic air spaces separated by areas of dense collagenous scarring. This is termed 'honeycomb lung,' as the cut surface has been thought to resemble a honeycomb (*Fig. 11.27*).

This is an end-stage process resulting from any of the causes of chronic parenchymal lung disease given in *Fig. 11.26*, and is the result of the sequence of damaging stimuli and reparative changes. Honeycomb lung leads to chronic respiratory impairment (restrictive lung disease), with reduced diffusion capacity.

The alveolar wall fibrosis greatly reduces the pulmonary capillary network, leading to right ventricular hypertrophy and the development of pulmonary hypertension, with eventual right heart failure (cor pulmonale). Death results from a combination of respiratory and cardiac failure.

Fig. 11.26 Causes of diffuse parenchymal lung disease
Atypical pneumonias (*Chlamydia*, *Mycoplasma*, some viruses)
Connective tissue diseases (rheumatoid disease and scleroderma; see Chapter 25)
Sarcoidosis (see Chapter 25)
Drug-induced damage (particularly anti-tumor chemotherapeutic agents)
Radiation damage (see page 142)
Idiopathic interstitial pneumonia (several histological subtypes) *(see Fig. 11.28)*
Pneumoconiosis (diseases caused by inhaling inorganic dusts)
Extrinsic allergic alveolitis (disease caused by immune reactions to inhaled organic dusts)

Fig. 11.27 Honeycomb lung. Macroscopically (a) honeycomb lung appears as large, cystically dilated air spaces surrounded by fibrosis. The pleural surface has a bosselated, leathery appearance. In a Gough–Wentworth preparation (b) the extent of abnormality and interstitial fibrosis can be better appreciated. Histology (c) shows coalescence of air spaces, both alveoli and bronchioles, to form cysts lined with cuboidal epithelium. Focal squamous metaplasia is frequently seen, as well as proliferation of smooth muscle around terminal bronchioles.

Interstitial pneumonia can lead to pulmonary fibrosis

There are at least seven different histological patterns of interstitial pneumonia (*Fig. 11.28*). Once all grouped as an entity termed fibrosing alveolitis, recent studies have shown that the different patterns have clinical prognostic importance. Different types tend to have an association with certain causative factors. Certain patterns of disease have the potential to develop progressive pulmonary fibrosis. High-resolution CT scanning of the lungs is able to distinguish between the different patterns of disease with reasonable certainty. In cases of diagnostic difficulty a lung biopsy may be performed to determine the pattern of disease more precisely.

Cryptogenic fibrosing alveolitis (idiopathic pulmonary fibrosis) is characterized by UIP in the lungs

Cryptogenic fibrosing alveolitis, also termed idiopathic pulmonary fibrosis, is the result of usual interstitial pneumonia

---

Fig. 11.28 Histological types of interstitial pneumonia

Usual interstitial pneumonia (UIP): commonest pattern – focal alveolar involvement with inflammation, fibroblastic foci, and interstitial fibrosis. Typical pattern found in cryptogenic pulmonary fibrosis

Non-specific interstitial pneumonia (NSIP). Uniform widespread involvement of alveoli by inflammation. Often seen in connective tissue disease or drug-related disease

Cryptogenic organising pneumonia (COP) (also termed bronchiolitis obliterans organizing pneumonitis BOOP) characterized by macrophages and granulation tissue buds in alveolar spaces. Steroid-responsive disease

Acute interstitial pneumonia (AIP) dominated by exudative pathology and hyaline membranes as seen in ARDS

Respiratory bronchiolitis-associated interstitial lung disease seen in smokers. Characterized by inflammation of the respiratory bronchioles, filling of bronchiolar lumen and alveoli with pigmented macrophages. Response to corticosteroids

Desquamative interstitial pneumonia (DIP) seen in smokers. Characterized by 'ground glass' imaging appearance, numerous macrophages in the alveoli and a response to corticosteroids

Lymphocytic interstitial pneumonia (LIP) characterized by interstitial lymphoid infiltrates and mainly seen in association with connective tissue diseases

---

(UIP). Investigations reveal no obvious cause, hence the designations cryptogenic and idiopathic. There is an association with smoking and exposure to wood or metal dusts in an occupational setting. The condition typically presents with insidious onset of dyspnea and tachycardia, developing over about 18 months, most commonly in the sixth decade. A restrictive pattern of respiratory disturbance develops, with impaired diffusion of gas across alveolar walls. High-resolution CT scans reveal a mixture of reticular densities and diffuse patchy shadowing in basal parts and subpleural zones of the lower lobes which becomes more extensive as the disease progresses. In patients whose disease progresses, honeycomb lung develops.

Extrinsic allergic alveolitis is caused by immune reaction to inhaled allergens

Extrinsic allergic pneumonitis, also called **hypersensitivity pneumonitis**, is caused by immune reaction in the lung to inhaled antigens. There are two main groups of allergen: **animal proteins**, e.g. proteins in bird droppings, and **microbial agents** that contaminate vegetable-derived material. The latter are thermophilic actinomycetes and fungi that colonize rotting crops (e.g. hay, compost, sugar cane, maple bark).

Many clinical syndromes result from this process, their names reflecting the circumstances of allergen exposure, e.g. farmer's lung (*Actinomyces* in moldy hay), bird fancier's lung (budgerigar and pigeon feces), bagassosis (*Actinomyces* in moldy sugar cane, called 'bagasse').

There are two types of clinical problem caused by inhalation of allergens:

- Symptoms resulting from acute exposure to antigen. After inhalation, there is a type III hypersensitivity response. Immune complexes generated at the site of allergen entry in the lung activate complement and there is inflammation. Those affected have dyspnea, fever and cough 4–8 hours after exposure to antigen which resolves after 12–24 hours.
- Symptoms resulting from chronic pulmonary fibrosis. Repeated exposure to antigen results in a type IV cell-mediated hypersensitivity reaction, with small granulomas visible histologically. This causes interstitial fibrosis and insidious onset of cough and dyspnea, eventually leading to honeycomb lung in about 5% of cases.

Goodpasture's syndrome is immune mediated

Diffuse damage to the interstitium of the lung is seen in Goodpasture's syndrome, which is caused by autoantibodies reactive to type IV collagen in basement membrane in the lung and in renal glomeruli. Patients develop hemoptysis and renal failure.

PNEUMOCONIOSIS

Pneumoconiosis is a respiratory disease caused by inhalation of dusts

Disease of the lungs caused by inhalation of dusts is termed 'pneumoconiosis,' the majority of cases being caused by non-fibrous mineral dusts. Lung damage occurs when the dust interacts with defense mechanisms in the lung. The normal fate of inhaled dust is for it to be coughed out of the lung or ingested by macrophages. If a dust is toxic to macrophages, there is local inflammation, secretion of cyto-kines and stimulation of fibrosis. Fibrosis in the lung causes a restrictive pattern of respiratory dysfunction. The main dusts causing industrial pulmonary fibrosis are various forms of silicates, often mixed with other materials such as iron oxide or coal.

There are two types of coalworker's pneumoconiosis: one mild, one severe

The risk of developing coalworker's pneumoconiosis is related to the degree of exposure to dust. There are two types of pathology.

Simple coalworker's pneumoconiosis (*Fig. 11.29*) is diagnosed by the presence of small nodules, 2–5 mm in diameter, in the lung fields on chest radiography. This pattern of disease is not associated with any clinically significant impairment of respiratory function.

Progressive massive fibrosis (PMF) is characterized by large nodules in the lungs, more than 10 mm in diameter (*Fig. 11.30*). The disease progresses relentlessly and may present long after active exposure to coal dust. Patients have severe respiratory impairment, with a mixed restrictive and obstructive pattern.

Silicosis is caused by inhalation of quartz-containing dust

Silicosis is caused by inhalation of silicon dioxide (quartz). The main occupational exposure is from slate mining, metal foundries, stone masonry, tunneling, granite quarrying, and coal mining through granitic rocks. Changes are seen on chest radiographs as small nodules, 3–5 mm in diameter. There may also be calcification of the periphery of hilar

Fig. 11.29 Simple coalworker's pneumoconiosis. Histologically there is accumulation of anthrosilicotic dust in macrophages at the center of the acinus, with associated emphysema of focal dust type.

Fig. 11.30 Coalworker's pneumoconiosis: progressive massive fibrosis. (a) Cut surface (b) thin section of whole lung. The nodules in progressive massive fibrosis (N) are most common in the upper lobes; they become so extensive as to occupy up to 30% of the lung fields. There is usually surrounding irregular emphysema. There are three main pathological types of nodule in PMF:

- Amorphous collection of acellular proteinaceous material containing little collagen and abundant carbon pigment, which frequently cavitates and liquefies. This type is seen in response to coal with a low silica content (a).
- Dense collagenous tissue and macrophages, heavily pigmented by carbon dust, seen in response to coal with high silica content (b).
- Caplan's syndrome occurs in miners with rheumatoid disease. The nodules have the appearance of large, carbon-pigmented rheumatoid nodules (see page 567).

lymph nodes. Disease may progress even after cessation of exposure.

Short heavy doses produce acute silicosis with pulmonary edema and alveolar exudation.

Prolonged exposure leads to the formation of multiple fibrous nodules composed of collagen in the lungs (*Fig. 11.31*). These expand and cause extensive destruction of lung tissue. PMF may also develop. Histologically, silica particles can be seen in nodules under polarized light.

The development of tuberculosis is a common complication of silicosis (silicotuberculosis). It is presumed to be due to impaired local defenses consequent upon the accumulation of silica in macrophages.

The pathogenesis of silicosis is thought to be a toxic effect on macrophages, which stimulates cytokine generation, precipitating fibrogenesis.

Asbestos causes several major diseases of the lung and pleura

Now that its harmful effects have been realized, asbestos exposure has declined rapidly in most parts of the world. Patients who present with asbestos-related diseases are generally over the age of 40 and suffered exposure before legislation became effective in the late 1960s. An insidious feature of asbestos-related disease is that there is often a long latent period of up to 50 years between exposure and clinical onset of disease.

The diseases produced by asbestos are:

- **Pleural plaques.** Benign plaques of collagenous fibrosis in the pleural surfaces.
- **Pleural effusions** and pleural thickening. Spontaneous effusions in the absence of obvious other cause, and dense pleural thickening, which may compress the lungs.
- **Asbestosis.** Progressive chronic fibrosis of lungs.
- **Malignant mesothelioma.** A highly malignant tumor of the mesothelium (see pages 220 and 271).
- **Carcinoma of the lung** (see pages 212–7).

Occupational asbestos exposure has been extensive

Asbestos is a fibrous silicate mineral that was widely used between 1890 and 1970 as a building, insulating and fire-resistant material. As well as the hazards of mining and refining asbestos, exposure of individuals has occurred in the building industry, and in industries using asbestos for its insulating properties, e.g. dockyard workers and spray-lagging operatives.

There are two main forms:

- Serpentine asbestos (including white asbestos) is the most common form, and fibers persist in the lung for a limited time.
- Amphibole asbestos (including blue and brown asbestos), the fibers of which persist in the lung for many years. This form is the main cause of malignant mesothelioma.

The risk of disease is proportional to the duration and intensity of exposure.

Asbestosis causes pulmonary fibrosis, and fibers can be seen in the lung

Pathological findings are of interstitial fibrosis of the lungs which, in the early stages, is maximal at the lung bases. Asbestos bodies may be seen histologically (*Fig. 11.32*).

Fig. 11.31 Silicosis of lung. In silicosis, nodules of collagen (**C**) contain silica particles. In this case, as is common when coal-mining exposure has occurred, there is additional carbon pigmentation, resulting in black peripheral staining.

Fig. 11.32 Asbestos bodies. Asbestos bodies are long, thin asbestos fibers coated with hemosiderin and protein to form brown filaments with a beaded or drumstick pattern.

Asbestosis is caused by heavy exposure to asbestos, usually with a latent period of 25 years before clinical symptoms become evident.

Diagnosis is made on the basis of occupational exposure, changes on chest radiographs (linear shadows in lung bases), and a pattern of restrictive defects on lung-function testing.

The disease progresses with increasing restrictive defect, which is associated with interstitial fibrosis. Pulmonary hypertension and cor pulmonale develop in the late stages.

GRANULOMATOUS DISEASE IN LUNGS

Some progressive lung diseases are characterized by the presence of histiocytic and giant-cell granulomatous inflammatory responses. The most important are TB (caused by *M. tuberculosis*), sarcoidosis, granulomatous vasculitis, and fungal infections, e.g. histoplasmosis.

Granulomas also develop as a response to some foreign bodies in the lung, e.g. in some pneumoconioses such as chronic berylliosis, and in response to some inhaled allergens.

Sarcoidosis causes granulomatous inflammation of the lung with interstitial fibrosis

A multisystem disease of unknown cause, sarcoidosis is characterized by the presence of non-caseating granulomas in tissues. From the histology it is evident that a type IV immune response takes place, yet no allergen or infective organism has been conclusively demonstrated. In 90% of cases the main tissues involved are those of the lungs and draining hilar lymph nodes. Sarcoidosis is also discussed in Chapter 25.

Patients with lung involvement present with slowly progressive dyspnea and cough, and are found to have lung shadowing on chest radiographs, with enlargement of hilar lymph nodes. Histology shows non-caseating histiocytic granulomas in the lung interstitium. Around 75% of patients recover with steroid therapy; 25% show progression to interstitial fibrosis and the development of honeycomb lung.

Pulmonary eosinophilia is caused by several diseases

Infiltration of the interstitium of the lungs with eosinophils is a feature of several diseases, and is often also associated with blood eosinophilia and elevated serum IgE. The clinical features of asthma with reversible airways obstruction are often present.

The main causes are:

- Allergic bronchopulmonary aspergillosis.
- Drug reactions (penicillin, nitrofurantoin, aspirin).
- Helminth infections (microfilariasis, schistosomiasis).
- Idiopathic (Loeffler's syndrome, Churg–Strauss syndrome).

NEOPLASTIC DISEASE OF THE LUNGS

Carcinoma of the lung is the most common cause of death from neoplasia in industrialized nations. Once mainly a disease of males, it is now increasingly common in females. The peak incidence is between the ages of 40 and 70 years, reflecting cumulative exposure to several potential causative carcinogens.

The incidence of lung cancer is related to the main causative factors of cigarette smoking and industrial carcinogens.

Cigarette smoking increases the risk of developing lung cancer, with precursor lesions of metaplasia and dysplasia occurring in the respiratory tract after exposure to cigarette smoke. The risk of cancer increases with the number of cigarettes smoked and the age at which smoking was started.

Occupational and environmental factors are known to predispose to development of lung cancer, especially exposure to radioactive material, asbestos, nickel, chromium, iron oxides, and coal gas plants. Radon, the natural radioactive gas, is thought to contribute significantly to respiratory exposure to radiation in certain geographic areas.

There are two main clinical groups of lung cancer

The four main histological types of carcinoma of the lung are squamous cell carcinoma (50%), small-cell anaplastic carcinoma (oat-cell carcinoma) (20%), adenocarcinoma (including bronchoalveolar carcinoma) (20%), and large-cell anaplastic carcinoma (10%).

Because of differences in natural history and response to treatment, many clinicians group tumors into either small-cell lung carcinoma (SCLC) or non-small-cell lung cancers (NSCLC). A small proportion of tumors may show a mixed pattern of differentiation, particularly mixed adenocarcinoma/squamous carcinoma; 70% of all tumors arise in relation to the main bronchi (central or hilar tumors, see *Fig. 11.33*). 30% of lung cancers arise from peripheral airways or alveoli (peripheral tumors, see *Fig. 11.34*).

Lung cancers spread by four main routes

All types of carcinoma of the lung spread by the common routes of metastasis.

Local spread: tumors spread locally into surrounding lung. Peribronchial spread to distant parts of the lung is common. Direct extension into pleura and adjacent mediastinal structures is a feature of advanced disease.

Lymphatic spread: ipsilateral and contralateral spread into the peribronchial and hilar lymph nodes may cause symptoms by compressing adjacent structures.

Transcelomic spread: tumor cells may seed within the pleural cavity, causing a malignant pleural effusion.

Hematogenous spread: the main sites of bloodborne spread are to the brain, bone, liver and adrenal glands.

Fig. 11.33 Central carcinoma of the bronchus. Central carcinomas of the lung (**L**) appear as friable white masses of tissue that extend into the lumen of bronchi and invade into the adjacent lung.

Fig. 11.34 Peripheral carcinoma of the lung. Peripheral carcinomas of the lung (**C**) appear as ill-defined masses, often occurring in relation to scars, and frequently extend to the pleural surface.

Fig. 11.35 Squamous cell carcinoma of the lung. Squamous cell carcinoma of the lung shows a range of differentiation, from well-differentiated lesions producing lots of keratin (**K**), through to lesions with only a few keratin-producing cells.

Fig. 11.36 Adenocarcinoma of the lung. This micrograph shows an acinar pattern of adenocarcinoma of the lung, with prominent gland-like spaces (**S**) lined by a columnar epithelium.

Squamous cell carcinoma is the most common type of cancer of the bronchus

Squamous cell carcinomas are believed to be derived from metaplastic squamous epithelium, which develops to line the main bronchi as the result of exposure to agents such as cigarette smoke (*Fig. 11.35*).

Tumors, which are most common in males, are usually central and close to the carina, frequently presenting with features related to bronchial obstruction. Compared with other types, they are relatively slow-growing and may be resectable.

Adenocarcinoma of the lung is usually a peripheral tumor

Adenocarcinomas (*Fig. 11.36*) have an equal gender incidence and are not as closely linked with cigarette smoking as other types. They characteristically develop as a peripheral tumor, although they may also occur as a central lesion arising from a main bronchus. A proportion of adenocarcinomas are thought to originate in areas of existing lung scarring **(scar cancers)** (see *Fig. 11.34*).

Bronchoalveolar carcinoma is a special type of adenocarcinoma

Bronchoalveolar carcinoma of the lung is a special type of adenocarcinoma, accounting for about 5% of all cases and derived from alveolar or bronchial epithelial cells (Clara cells and type II pneumocytes). A distinct histological feature is spread through the lung along alveolar septa. In the absence of metastasis, this subtype has a better prognosis than other forms of lung cancer.

Small-cell anaplastic carcinoma is the most highly malignant of lung cancers

Small-cell anaplastic lung cancer (also called **oat-cell carcinoma** because the cell nuclei histologically resemble oat grains) is a highly malignant condition (*Fig. 11.37*). Tumors arise from bronchial epithelium, but exhibit differentiation into neuroendocrine cells containing neurosecretory granules.

Tumors are usually centrally located and are associated with a rapid rate of growth, relative to other forms of lung cancer. It is usual for metastases to be present at the time of diagnosis. Because of the neuroendocrine type, this form of cancer is often associated with ectopic hormone production.

Large-cell anaplastic carcinoma lacks features of differentiation by light microscopy

Large-cell anaplastic carcinomas are insufficiently differentiated to permit further classification by light microscopy (*Fig. 11.38*). However, if electron microscopy is used, features that favor either a squamous or an adenocarcinomatous origin can be often seen. This is therefore a diagnostic grouping of convenience, as further histogenetic subdivision is of no clinical or biological importance. They have a poor prognosis and are frequently widely disseminated at diagnosis.

The natural history of lung cancer allows no opportunity for screening

There are no early symptoms of lung cancer and it is probable that a lesion may have been growing for many years before presenting clinically. Symptoms at presentation are usually a manifestation of locally advanced disease.

- Cough (80% cases): infection distal to airway blocked by tumor.
- Hemoptysis (70% cases): ulceration of tumor in bronchus.
- Dyspnea (60% cases): local extension of tumor.
- Chest pain (40% cases): involvement of pleura and chest wall.
- Wheeze (15% cases): narrowing of airway.

Systemic features of malignancy, such as weight loss, anorexia and malaise, are also common at presentation.

Fig. 11.37 Small-cell anaplastic carcinoma of the lung. This type of carcinoma shows neuroendocrine differentiation. Cells are round to oval and have little cytoplasm.

Fig. 11.38 Large-cell anaplastic carcinoma of the lung. These tumors are composed of pleomorphic large cells with no distinguishing differentiation features by light microscopy.

Smoking and lung cancer

- If smokers who smoke fewer than 20 cigarettes a day stop, the increased risk of lung cancer decreases, reaching that of a non-smoker after 13 years.
- If smokers who smoke more than 20 cigarettes a day stop, they retain a small increased risk over non-smokers for life.
- For passive smokers the risk of developing lung cancer is twice as great as that for those not exposed to smoke.

Tissue diagnosis of lung cancer

Diagnosis is made on the basis of clinical features, imaging and obtaining histological confirmation of the nature of the disease.

- Sputum cytology: examination of expectorated sputum by cytology.
- Cytology of pleural effusion: examination of pleural fluid by cytology.
- Percutaneous needle aspiration under image guidance: cytological preparation obtained.
- Bronchoscopy and biopsy: small tumor biopsy obtained.

Molecular pathology of lung cancer

Lung cancer is characterized by multiple genetic alterations. Loss of part of chromosome 3p is common, but the gene(s) important in development are not yet determined. Rb and P53 are often inactivated.

Dominant oncogenes are activated in particular; *ras* proteins are mutated in about 20% of NSCLC, but not in SCLC, and seem to be associated with a poorer prognosis.

Overexpression of epidermal growth factor receptor is commonly seen.

At present, such molecular information is used as a research tool. The expectation is that a temporal sequence of mutational events may be uncovered that gives insight into the behavior of these tumors.

Several initiatives to detect lung cancer by mass screening using chest radiography revealed that over half of the asymptomatic tumors detected at screening were inoperable, with no improvement in overall survival.

Metastatic spread is a frequent presenting feature of lung cancer

Metastatic spread is present in 70% of patients at presentation, 30% of patients presenting with symptoms caused by metastatic disease.

Bloodstream spread may present with pathological fracture (bone metastasis), leukoerythroblastic anemia (extensive marrow replacement), CNS symptoms (brain metastasis), or hepatomegaly and jaundice (liver metastasis).

Local spread and spread to intrathoracic nodes causes several important clinical syndromes. For example, Horner's syndrome (ptosis, enophthalmos, small pupils, lack of sweating on the ipsilateral side of the face) is caused by invasion of the cervical sympathetic chain, and superior vena caval obstruction is caused by enlarged right paratracheal nodes compressing veins. Recurrent laryngeal nerve palsy results from spread to the left hilar region, and brachial neuritis is due to direct invasion of the plexus by apical tumors, leading to pain in the T1 dermatome and wasting of intrinsic hand muscles. Pericarditis is due to direct tumor invasion.

Lung cancer frequently causes non-metastatic syndromes

Systemic syndromes associated with non-metastatic effects are common in lung cancer and may be a presenting feature of disease.

Endocrine disturbances, seen in 12% of patients with lung cancer, are nearly all associated with small-cell lung cancer because it has a neuroendocrine phenotype with neurosecretory granules. Common syndromes include inappropriate ADH secretion (low sodium and plasma osmolality and high urine osmolality) and ectopic ACTH secretion associated with a Cushing's syndrome (see page 346). Hypercalcemia is most common with squamous cell carcinomas, in contrast to other endocrinopathies, and is due to the secretion of parathormone-related protein.

Several neurological syndromes can be caused by lung cancer, including peripheral sensory/motor neuropathy, cerebellar degeneration causing ataxia, proximal myopathy, dermatomyositis, and Lambert–Eaton myasthenic syndrome, which is associated with small-cell tumors and may precede the clinical detection of tumor.

Hypertrophic pulmonary osteoarthropathy (finger clubbing, swelling of wrists and ankles with periosteal new bone formation) is seen in 2–3% of squamous cell carcinomas and adenocarcinomas.

Staging and histological type determine outcome in lung cancer

The factors that determine the outcome of lung cancer, and its likely response to treatment, are histological type and stage. For example, squamous cell carcinomas grow slowly and carry a better prognosis if detected at an early stage and are operable; some forms of bronchoalveolar cell carcinoma have a better prognosis than other forms of lung cancer (see page 214); and small-cell tumors metastasize widely and have the poorest prognosis.

Survival is better for early-stage disease, except for small-cell carcinoma. The TNM system and staging used for carcinoma of the lung is discussed in *Fig. 11.39.*

215

Most lung cancers are inoperable

NSCLC: 75% of all cases are inoperable owing to age, poor lung function, or advanced stage on careful assessment (CT and MRI scanning or mediastinoscopy). The best survival is seen in bronchoalveolar-cell carcinomas, with 20–50% 5-year survival rates. Overall, others show 5–30% of cases surviving for 5 years. Inoperable cases may be treated with radiotherapy, depending on the clinical circumstances. The role of chemotherapy is limited.

SCLC: limited disease, in which tumor is confined to one side of the chest, is seen in only 30% of cases, the rest having extensive disease. SCLC is sensitive to radiotherapy and chemotherapy, but the extent of disease means that survival is still poor despite local control of tumor. Treatment offers good palliation of pain, cough and dyspnea. Radiotherapy and combination chemotherapy cause a complete local response in 30% of cases, with an overall median survival of 11 months and a 1-year survival of 45%.

Carcinoid tumors of the lung have variable malignant potential

Carcinoid tumors of the lung are neuroendocrine tumors, representing about 5% of all pulmonary neoplasms. They grow either as bronchial lesions that protrude into the lumen or as locally infiltrative lesions extending from the bronchus into the adjacent lung.

Histological examination shows that lesions having no atypical cytological features behave in a benign fashion. Others, particularly the infiltrative group, show mitoses and nuclear atypia. This group has the potential for local recurrence or metastasis in a small proportion of cases, being termed **atypical pulmonary neuroendocrine tumors**. The term 'pulmonary carcinoid' is perhaps inappropriate for such lesions, as a clinical carcinoid syndrome is unusual in most cases, and most lesions do not secrete 5-hydroxytryptamine.

Staging of carcinoma of the lung

Non-small cell lung cancer

For non-small cell lung cancer, tumor stage has an important bearing on prognosis. Tumors are evaluated using a lung cancer-specific TNM system, and on this basis can be divided into stages I–IV.

For stages I and II the main form of therapy that will be considered is surgery. The key features offering a reasonable prospect for surgery are listed in *Fig. 11.39*. For stages III–IV combinations of chemotherapy and radiation therapy offer the best option, mainly with an expectation for palliation of symptoms rather than cure.

Small cell lung cancer

For small cell lung cancer the detailed TNM staging system is not commonly used in clinical practice because metastatic disease is commonly present at diagnosis and survival is generally not affected by the local and regional extent of tumor. A two-stage system has been devised which is of much more clinical relevance and is widely used in practice.

- **Limited stage**. Limited-stage small cell lung cancer refers to tumor confined to one hemithorax, the mediastinum and the supraclavicular nodes, and which can be encompassed within a clinically acceptable therapeutic irradiation field.
- **Extensive stage**. Extensive-stage small cell lung cancer refers to any tumor that extends beyond the definition of limited-stage disease.

Fig. 11.39 Features that go with a reasonable prospect for surgery in non-small cell lung cancer

- Tumors <3 cm.
- Tumors are in a lobar bronchus or at least 2 cm distal to the carina.
- No involvement of the chest wall, diaphragm, pericardium, trachea, great vessels, esophagus or vertebrae.
- No contralateral lymph node involvement.
- No distant metastases (including separate tumor nodules in same lobe).
- Absence of a malignant pleural effusion.
- Absence of associated atelectasis or obstructive pneumonitis in the adjacent lung.

For limited-stage disease most patients will be offered treatment with combination chemotherapy and radiotherapy to the affected side of the chest. Those who respond may be offered prophylactic cranial irradiation in an attempt to minimize the development of cerebral metastases.

For extensive-stage disease most patients will be offered treatment with combination chemotherapy. Radiotherapy is generally used to treat sites of metastatic disease, especially in the brain, bone, and for the relief of vena-caval obstruction.

There is about 80% 10-year survival for resected cases showing no atypical features, whereas atypical forms have about 50% 5-year survival.

Tumor permeation of pulmonary lymphatics leads to severe breathlessness

Metastatic tumor, whether from lung or extrapulmonary sites, may diffusely infiltrate pulmonary lymphatic vessels, producing the syndrome of **lymphangitis carcinomatosa** (*Fig. 11.40*).

This presents as severe breathlessness, as blockage of lymphatics causes failure of removal of interstitial fluid, which accumulates in lung parenchyma in much the same way as in early cardiogenic pulmonary edema. The chest radiograph shows diffuse shadowing, and dilated intrapulmonary lymphatic vessels may be visible as linear streaks. This is a dire condition which is rapidly fatal.

Metastases and hamartomas are common pulmonary mass lesions

After primary cancers, the two most common mass lesions in the lung are metastases and hamartomas.

Metastatic tumors are common by bloodborne spread, particularly from the kidney, breast, testis, and gastrointestinal tract.

Bronchial hamartomas are common benign lesions composed of tissue normally encountered in the lung. Most are 1–3 cm in diameter and consist largely of cartilage, being firm and glistening white in appearance. Other elements are bronchial epithelium, fat, and muscle. They are asymptomatic and are mainly discovered at postmortem examination.

Fig. 11.40 Lymphangitis carcinomatosa. Diffuse permeation of pulmonary lymphatics by malignancy may occur with lung tumors or from metastases. Macroscopically, surface lymphatics packed with tumor may be visible on the pleural surface. Histologically, tumor cell clumps (**T**) are evident in lymphatics throughout the lung.

Coin lesions on chest radiographs

A rounded solitary lesion on a chest radiograph is termed a 'coin lesion.' This appearance has several main causes.

If all age groups are considered, one-third of cases are caused by a carcinoma of the lung, increasing to a half of all cases in patients over the age of 50.

The common lesions are:

- Primary bronchial or lung carcinoma.
- Metastatic tumor (especially of the kidney).
- Bronchial hamartoma.
- Carcinoid tumor.
- Granulomatous inflammation (e.g. TB).
- Lung abscess.

The uncommon lesions are pulmonary cysts, pulmonary angiitis, fungal mycetoma, and vascular malformations.

Key Facts
Lung cancer

- Caused by inhaled environmental agents, particularly smoking and radon.
- Peak incidence 40–70 years, most common form of cancer.
- Four main types: squamous cell, small-cell anaplastic, adenocarcinoma and large-cell anaplastic.
- Bronchoalveolar carcinoma is a special form of adenocarcinoma with a better prognosis than other types.
- Clinical division is into small-cell and non-small cell types (all others).
- Tumors may be central (all types) or peripheral (mainly adenocarcinomas).
- Small-cell carcinoma is neuroendocrine, highly malignant, and may be associated with ectopic endocrine syndromes.
- Only a small proportion of carcinomas are operable because of high stage at presentation.
- TNM staging used for NSCLC.
- Simple staging used for SCLC–Limited and Extensive.
- Overall survival 5–30% at 5 years, highly dependent on type and stage of disease.

Mass lesions in the mediastinum can be caused by many different lesions arising from structures in its anterior, middle, posterior, inferior and superior parts (*Fig. 11.41*).

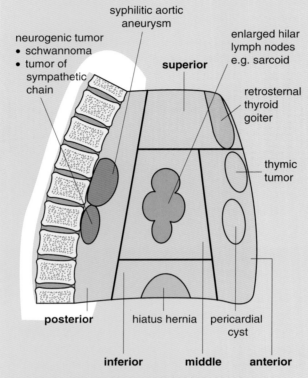

Fig. 11.41 Mass lesions in the mediastinum.

PATHOLOGY OF THE PLEURA

The pleura is lined by a sheet of mesothelial cells. There is constant generation of fluid from the parietal pleura and resorption of pleural fluid by the visceral pleural surface. The formation of fluid is influenced by hydrostatic and osmotic gradients, as well as by changes in the permeability of local vessels.

Several types of fluid may accumulate in the pleural space. If the accumulation is large, there may be compression of the lung.

- **Pus**: empyema due to infection.
- **Blood**: hemothorax due to trauma or surgery.
- **Chyle**: chylothorax due to leakage from the thoracic duct.
- **Fluid effusion** (either transudate or exudate): can be caused by several main diseases (see *Fig. 11.42*).

Bronchoalveolar lavage (saline injected into a lung segment down a bronchoscope. Saline is aspirated and examined for cells and organisms):

- Atypical infections, e.g. pneumocystis.
- Interstitial lung diseases.

Bronchial biopsy (biopsy down bronchoscope):
- Neoplasia.
- Sarcoid.
- Allergic aspergillosis.

Transbronchial biopsy (forceps advanced to lung periphery down bronchoscope and samples parenchyma):
- Diffuse lung disease.
- Transplant monitoring.
- Infection diagnosis.

Percutaneous lung biopsy by needle:
- Localized mass lesions.
- Atypical infections.
- **Open lung biopsy**:
- Chronic diffuse lung shadowing of uncertain cause.

- **Transudate**: low-protein fluid due to movement of excess fluid through normal vessel walls. Commonly due to high hydrostatic pressure in cardiac failure.
- **Exudate**: high-protein fluid (containing fibrinogen/fibrin) due to movement of fluid through damaged vessel walls. Commonly due to infection, infarction or tumor (see *Fig. 11.42*).
- **Air**: 'pneumothorax'.

Pneumothorax may be spontaneous, traumatic or iatrogenic

The presence of air in the pleural space is termed 'pneumothorax.' Spontaneous pneumothoraces can be divided into those that occur secondary to disease in the lungs, and those that occur in otherwise healthy individuals. Traumatic pneumothorax may be due to chest injury, or may be iatrogenic. The causes are summarized in *Fig. 11.43*.

Infection of the pleura is the most common cause of pleurisy

Acute inflammation of the pleura is termed **pleurisy**, the most common cause of which is infection. Macroscopically, fibrinous exudate is seen over the pleural surfaces, and there is variable exudation of fluid. Certain infections result in accumulation of pus in the pleural cavity (**empyema**). Aspiration of an infected pleural effusion reveals a high-protein

Fig. 11.42 Pleural effusion

Type of effusion	Pathogenesis	Causes
Transudate Less than 30 g protein/L	Increased hydrostatic pressure	Cardiac failure
	Decreased oncotic pressure	Vena caval obstruction Hypoalbuminemia
Exudate More than 30 g protein/L	Infections	Bacterial, including TB Other organisms
	Neoplasm	Metastatic carcinoma Primary carcinoma of lung Mesothelioma of pleura
	Pulmonary infarction	Thromboembolic disease
	Autoimmune disease	Rheumatoid disease Systemic lupus erythematosus
	Abdominal disease	Pancreatitis Subphrenic abscess

Investigation of pleural effusion

The investigation of a pleural effusion involves aspirating a sample for laboratory investigation. It is also common for a biopsy sample of pleura to be taken, using a specialized needle.

- **Cytology**: this will detect neoplastic cells, and distinguish acute and chronic inflammatory conditions on the basis of the presence of appropriate inflammatory cells.
- **Biochemistry**: analysis of protein concentration helps in deciding whether an effusion is a transudate or an exudate.
- **Microbiology**: if the aspirate is turbid, it is important to search for infective causes. TB is best cultured from a pleural biopsy rather than from fluid.
- **Histology**: biopsy of the pleura will assist in histological identification of neoplastic conditions and TB.

Fig. 11.43 Causes of pneumothorax

Spontaneous pneumothorax

Primary

- Thin young men
- Rupture of congenital subpleural apical bleb

Secondary

- Rupture of emphysematous bulla
- Asthmatics
- Rupture of congenital cyst
- Pleural malignancy
- Cystic fibrosis
- Pneumonia
- Sarcoidosis
- Whooping cough

Traumatic pneumothorax

- Penetrating chest wounds
- Rib fractures
- Esophageal rupture

Iatrogenic pneumothorax

- Subclavian cannulation
- Positive pressure artificial ventilation
- Pleural aspiration
- Esophageal perforation during endoscopy
- Lung biopsy

exudate. Neutrophils predominate in acute infections, whereas lymphoid cells predominate in TB. There is a wide range of causative organisms, mostly spreading from initial lung infection, including *Streptococcus pneumoniae*, *Hemophilus*, *Klebsiella*, *Pseudomonas* and *Bacteroides* spp.

Viral infections of the pleura are most commonly due to Coxsackie viruses, echoviruses and adenoviruses.

The fibrinous exudate of acute pleurisy may become organized to form fibrous pleural adhesions and can lead to fibrous pleural thickening. Calcification may also be seen in the pleura as a result of old tuberculous pleurisy.

The most common tumor of the pleura is metastatic carcinoma

Metastatic tumors are the most common cause of neoplasm in the pleura. The most frequent primary sites are the lung and breast, causing pleural effusion.

Metastasis to the pleura is usually associated with a high-protein exudate. Diagnosis can be made by cytology of aspirated fluid or by needle biopsy of the pleura.

Malignant mesothelioma is caused by exposure to asbestos

Primary neoplasms of the pleura are rare except after exposure to asbestos, when tumors termed malignant mesotheliomas develop. After exposure, there may be a latent period of up to 50 years before development of the tumor.

Patients have chest pain and breathlessness, and there is commonly a pleural effusion. Diagnosis is made on pleural biopsy. Histologically, mesotheliomas have spindle cells and glandular patterns.

These are highly malignant tumors that spread around the pleural cavity and pericardium, encasing the lung and mediastinal structures (*Fig. 11.44*). Death is usual within 10 months of diagnosis, and metastasis is rare.

Exposure to asbestos also causes development of benign collagenous thickenings of the pleura, termed **pleural plaques**.

LUNG DISEASE IN CHILDREN

Common developmental abnormalities of the lung

Bronchial atresia leads to severe narrowing of a bronchus supplying an area of lung. Overexpansion of the lung segment may occur as a result of air trapping.

Pulmonary hypoplasia reflects incomplete development of the lung, which is smaller than normal. This is often seen with other congenital abnormalities and is associated with lung compression by other abnormal masses and oligohydramnios.

Bronchogenic cysts are usually attached to the trachea and represent accessory bronchial buds, which become sealed off from the rest of the main airways. They are lined by a respiratory epithelium and contain mucinous fluid.

Bronchopulmonary sequestration is due to the development of a portion of lung that does not communicate with the normal bronchial tree. Patients develop an abnormal lung mass and the abnormal areas develop dilated airways. There are recurrent infections, with frequent development of an abscess.

Fig. 11.44 Malignant mesothelioma. Mesothelioma is seen as a thick sheet of white tumor that encases the whole of the lung.

Neonatal respiratory distress syndrome is also called hyaline membrane disease

The neonatal respiratory distress syndrome (NRDS) is due to a deficiency of surfactant in the lungs. It is primarily a disease affecting premature infants, but is also seen in infants born to diabetic mothers, as excess production of insulin by the fetus suppresses surfactant production.

A very common condition, the incidence of NRDS increases with increasing prematurity (20% incidence at 32–36 weeks' gestation; 60% incidence at <28 weeks' gestation).

The pathogenesis of the disease is illustrated in *Fig. 11.45*. With the development of disease, the chest radiograph shows a 'ground glass' opacity in the lung fields. The mortality from NRDS is 50% in infants weighing under 1000 g. The lungs of infants who die from the condition appear airless, dark red and dense. Depending on the stage of disease, atelectasis, epithelial necrosis, hyaline membranes, and organization may be seen histologically.

There are four main extrapulmonary complications of NRDS: hypoxic-related intracerebral hemorrhage; failure of closure of ductus arteriosus (normal closure stimulated by oxygenation); necrotizing enterocolitis caused by hypoxic/ischemic damage to gut; and bronchopulmonary dysplasia, which is caused by high-pressure ventilation and oxygen toxicity to alveolar lining cells. Lungs show fibrous obliteration of bronchioles, peribronchial fibrosis, and overdistended alveoli.

Administration of synthetic surfactant and respiratory support allows recovery in the majority of cases. Prevention can be assisted by administering corticosteroids to mothers about to deliver prematurely, as this stimulates surfactant production in the fetus.

Immotile cilia syndrome leads to recurrent chest infections

Recurrent chest infections in childhood may be due to defective cilial function – the **immotile cilia syndrome**.

Pathogenesis of NRDS

There are five main risk factors for the development of NRDS. The immature or damaged lung is unable to make enough surfactant, the lecithin-rich surface-active lipid secreted by type II pneumocytes. Normally this reduces surface tension in alveoli and keeps them open. In NRDS, lack of surfactant means that alveoli collapse with microatelectasis.

Hypoxia leads to damage of alveolar lining cells, and pulmonary arterial constriction. Endothelial damage causes plasma to leak into alveoli, being deposited as fibrin. The fibrin appears as bright, pink-stained membranes lining air spaces, hence the name **hyaline membrane disease**. The presence of fibrin further impairs gas exchange and makes hypoxia worse. The process is similar to that in diffuse alveolar damage, illustrated in *Fig. 11.25*.

Later, regenerative changes in the lung lead to organization of hyaline membranes and fibrosis.

Fig. 11.45 Pathogenesis of NRDS.

Key Facts
Neonatal respiratory distress syndrome

- Caused by a deficiency of surfactant.
- Risk factors: prematurity, diabetic mother, neonatal aspiration, multiple birth, caesarean section.
- Alveolar collapse causes hypoxia, damage to endothelial and alveolar lining cells, and fibrin exudation.
- 50% mortality if weight <1000 g.
- Complications: intracerebral bleed, patent ductus arteriosus, necrotizing enterocolitis, bronchopulmonary dysplasia.

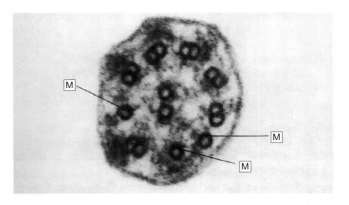

Fig. 11.46 Cilial dysmotility syndrome. Electron micrograph of cilia from a person with recurrent chest infections since childhood. The outer dynein arms are absent and there are abnormal single microtubules (**M**), which prevent normal motility.

Imaging studies show reduced clearance of tracer substances inhaled into the lungs, and biopsy of cilia-bearing nasal mucosa shows uncoordinated beating using time-lapse photography. In some individuals cilia are seen to have an abnormal structure, with absence of structural components such as the dynein arms (*Fig. 11.46*).

A syndrome of absent frontal sinuses, bronchiectasis and situs inversus (organs on the wrong side), termed **Kartagener's syndrome**, is due to defective cilial motility.

Cystic fibrosis is characterized by abnormally thick mucus

Cystic fibrosis is the most common autosomal recessive disorder in the Caucasian population, with an incidence of 1:2500 newborns, 1:25 adults being a heterozygous carrier of the CF gene. It is a multisystem disease and, most importantly, causes recurrent chest infections in childhood, associated with pancreatic exocrine dysfunction. The disease is caused by the production of an abnormally viscid mucus that cannot be cleared from the lungs and causes blockage of the main pancreatic ducts.

- 40% of cases present with respiratory disease.
- 30% present as failure to thrive and malabsorption.
- 20% present at birth with meconium ileus (due to abnormally viscid intestinal mucus).
- 10% present with liver disease, recurrent nasal polyps or sinusitis.

Diseases of other organs are discussed in relevant chapters.

The molecular pathogenesis of the disorder is defective function in a membrane chloride channel of epithelial cells, which causes reduced release of sodium and water to liquefy mucus. This is shown in the pink box (*Fig. 11.47*). In the respiratory tract, bronchi and bronchioles become obstructed by abnormally viscid mucus, which leads to four main problems:

- The obstruction and stagnation of secretions leads to repeated bouts of infection, particularly with *Staphylococcus aureus* and the mucoid form of *Pseudomonas*.
- Bronchiectasis is a frequent complication leading to hemoptysis (see page 199).
- Hyperinflation of lungs due to air trapping behind mucin plugs increases the risk of developing pneumothorax.
- Hypoxia, scarring and destruction of the pulmonary vascular bed lead to pulmonary hypertension and cor pulmonale (see page 190).

The median age of survival is just over 30 years.

Molecular pathogenesis of cystic fibrosis

The gene for cystic fibrosis (CF gene) is on the long arm of chromosome 7. It encodes a protein termed the **cystic fibrosis transmembrane conductance regulator** (CFTR).

In normal mucus-secreting epithelia (a) chloride channels open in response to increased concentration of cAMP (generated by stimulation of cell surface receptors), which activates a protein kinase (PKA). Phosphorylation of the CFTR protein opens the channels, and secretion of chloride, water and sodium is facilitated.

In the main mutation causing CF (b) (70% of cases), the protein is not present in the cell surface, stimulated chloride secretion cannot occur, cells do not secrete water and sodium, and mucus is extremely viscid. Such cases have severe clinical disease.

Over 100 other different mutations of the CF gene lead to expression of an abnormal CFTR in the cell membrane, with only partial activity in response to cAMP (c). Such cases have moderately viscid mucus and milder clinical disease.

The detection of the CF gene now allows for fetal diagnosis and carrier detection. Gene therapy to place a normal CF gene in respiratory tract epithelial cells is a real possibility, using an inhaled viral vector.

Fig. 11.47 Molecular pathogenesis of cystic fibrosis.

Case-based questions

Case 1 Chest infection

A 70-year-old retired postman is admitted to hospital for transurethral resection of the prostate under general anaesthesia. He has no significant past medical history and is on no medication. However, he has smoked 10 cigarettes a day for 40 years (20 pack-years). He undergoes an uneventful operation but is slow to mobilize postoperatively, and on the third day of his admission complains of cough productive of yellow-green sputum. On examination, he is pyrexial (temperature: 38.5°C) and has bilateral, coarse, expiratory crepitations. He was started on amoxycillin pending the results of microbiology. However, his symptoms worsened, with the production of increasing quantities of foul-smelling sputum, a swinging pyrexia and confusional state. Following further investigation, *Klebsiella pneumoniae* was cultured; his antibiotic treatment was altered and he made a slow recovery.

1. **What is the most likely diagnosis for his initial symptoms?**
2. **What predisposing factors for the development of a chest infection did this man have?**
3. **What would be the pathological changes in the lungs?**
4. **What are the possible causes for the progression of his illness?**

Case 2 Lung fibrosis

A 55-year-old man is admitted to hospital for investigation of respiratory problems. He has retired early and has sold his business to concentrate on breeding racing pigeons, a consuming passion since the death of his son several years earlier in a road traffic accident. He tells you that he has experienced recurrent episodes of feeling unwell, accompanied by a cough and severe shortness of breath lasting between 12 and 24 hours. Although he has a cough, he says that he does not bring anything up. In addition, over the previous year or so he has noticed a gradual loss of weight with episodic fevers, and he reckons that he is not so fit, being unable to climb the stairs to his pigeon loft because of shortness of breath. He is a non-smoker and has been otherwise well on no medication. There is no family history of disease.

He has come during one of his attacks and on examination he is noted to have clubbing of the fingers,

is pyrexial, centrally cyanosed and tachypneic. There are coarse expiratory crepitations throughout the lung fields.

A chest X-ray has been reported as showing interstitial pulmonary fibrosis. His lung function tests show a pattern of restrictive ventilatory deficit.

1. **What is your differential diagnosis?**
2. **What else do you want to know from his medical history, and what other investigations would you perform?**
3. **What pathological process is going on in the lung?**
4. **What are its long-term complications?**

Case 3 Chronic lung disease

A 58-year-old man who runs a shop selling spare parts for motor cycles is admitted to hospital because he can barely speak as he is short of breath. He tells you that he has always had a bad chest, coughing every day and producing copious green sputum. He also gets breathlessness on exertion. Over the past 3 days his chest has become so much worse that he can barely move. He has smoked 30 cigarettes a day for over 40 years (60 pack-years), and also said that he occasionally developed chest pain on exertion which, to you, sounds like angina. He has only recently been prescribed a course of antibiotics, but has been on no other medication. He has no significant family history of disease.

On examination, he is centrally cyanosed and pyrexial. He has a bounding pulse and shows peripheral vasodilatation. His jugular venous pressure is elevated, and he has pitting ankle edema and mild hepatomegaly. Examination of his chest reveals a right parasternal heave, coarse expiratory crepitations at the left base, and expiratory wheeze.

Treatment with β-agonists results in an immediate slight improvement in PEFR and, with appropriate antibiotics and physiotherapy, he gradually improves but remains breathless on exertion and continues to produce sputum on most days.

1. **What is the most likely diagnosis?**
2. **What is the pathogenesis of his chest problem and what is the pathology in the bronchi?**
3. **What are the main risk factors for developing this disease?**

Brief answers to these case-based questions are given on page 586. More detailed answers and other study resources are available online at www.studentconsult.com.

Oral and ENT pathology 12

MOUTH AND OROPHARYNX

The mouth is lined largely by non-keratinizing squamous epithelium, but there is abundant scattered salivary tissue located in the submucosa, with ducts opening onto the surface. The mouth comprises the lips, the buccal cavity, the palate, the tongue, the alveolar ridges of the mandible and maxilla (in which the teeth are embedded), the teeth, and **Waldeyer's ring**, which is formed by the lymphoid tissue of the posterior tongue, the palatine tonsils, and the oropharynx.

Cleft palate and cleft lip are the most common major congenital malformations of the mouth

Cleft palate and cleft lip frequently occur together, as they arise as a result of the same process, i.e. a failure of fusion of embryological midline structures (see page 70) at about 8 weeks' gestation. A few cases are associated with a chromosomal abnormality (e.g. trisomies 13 and 18), but the teratogenic factors cannot usually be identified in individual cases. In minor degrees of cleft palate only the soft palate is cleft, the most obvious feature on examination being a bifid uvula. Severe degrees also affect the bone of the hard palate, and the cleft may involve the alveolar ridge, in which case there is coexistent cleft lip.

A high, arched palate is a very frequent minor congenital abnormality. It is usually asymptomatic, although there may be a predisposition to middle ear infections and sinusitis.

Most infections of the lips and buccal cavity (infective stomatitis) are due to either viruses or fungi

Herpes simplex virus (HSV) type 1 produces herpetic stomatitis. In the early stages blisters develop on the gingiva and palate, leaving shallow ulcers after rupture. Severe herpetic stomatitis is important in immunosuppressed patients, particularly AIDS patients. Herpes labialis (cold sore) is the result of viral latency, with reactivation of previous virus infection, usually as a consequence of sun or cold exposure, fever, upper respiratory tract infection or trauma.

Virulent disseminated eruption can occur in immunosuppressed patients and infection may seed to the brain to produce HSV encephalitis. The eye can also be infected, resulting in a keratoconjunctivitis.

Herpes zoster may affect the mouth when the disease involves the trigeminal nerve ('trigeminal shingles'), producing clusters of vesicles in the mouth, invariably unilaterally.

In infectious mononucleosis, the **Epstein–Barr virus** (glandular fever) most commonly produces symptoms at the back of the mouth, particularly in the tonsils and pharynx. However, the anterior part of the oral cavity may show small petechial hemorrhages, usually on the palatal mucosa.

Coxsackie A virus produces tiny vesicles in the mouth, with small vesicles in the skin of the hands and, occasionally, that of the feet (hand, foot and mouth disease). This transient, mild infection is mainly seen in children, often in school-based epidemics.

Fungal infection of the mouth with *Candida albicans* is common

Candida albicans infection of the mouth is most frequently seen in infants in the form of 'thrush.' It is manifest as white patches on the palatal (*Fig. 12.1a*), buccal, and tongue surfaces; the white patches are composed of tangled fungal hyphae (*Fig. 12.1b*) mixed with acute inflammatory cells and some desquamated epithelium. The underlying epithelium is acutely inflamed and red, a feature that becomes apparent when the white patch is scraped away.

In adults, acute candidal infection of the mouth is less common unless there are predisposing factors such as diabetes mellitus, immunosuppressive therapy, or a natural immunosuppressed state, for example in advanced malignancy or with HIV infection. However, infection is not uncommon in apparently normal women who are taking oral contraceptives or who are pregnant. **Denture stomatitis**, due to *Candida* lodging under the denture plate, is also seen in adults with no other predisposing factors.

Infective stomatitis due to bacteria is now rare

Bacterial infections are common and important at the back of the mouth and oropharynx. However, although dental caries and periodontal disease are a consequence of bacteria on and around the teeth, bacterial infections of the front of the mouth are now uncommon.

Acute necrotizing ulcerative gingivitis occurs mainly in young males with poor dental hygiene (*Fig. 12.2*). There is acute sloughing ulceration of the interdental papillae, which rapidly spreads along the gingival margins, producing an expanding area of yellow slough surrounded by a narrow zone of hyperemic mucosa, which often bleeds heavily. The gingiva are very painful, and the breath smells

Fig. 12.1 *Candida albicans* infection of the palate. In (a) the white sheets are fungal mycelia in a thickened horny layer. The underlying mucosa is red and inflamed. Palatal mucosa stained with PAS (b) shows masses of superficial fungal hyphae.

foul. Extension of the necrosis and inflammation leads to destruction of the periodontal tissues. The necrotic areas are heavily populated by a mixture of fusiform and spirochetal organisms (*Fusobacterium* and *Borrelia* species), which are probably the causative organisms.

In the developing world, overwhelming bacterial cellulitis of the mouth and the destructive bacterial gingivitis known as **cancrum oris** are still occasionally seen.

Not all types of stomatitis are infective

The most common type of inflammation of the lips, tongue and buccal mucosa is associated with **aphthous ulceration**. Tiny, often extremely painful, shallow ulcers form against a background of red mucosa (*Fig. 12.3*). The ulcer crater is covered by a creamy exudate composed of fibrin and inflammatory cells, mainly neutrophils. The ulcers are recurrent but of short duration. Large ulcers (up to 3 cm across) occasionally occur, sometimes persisting for several weeks before healing with fibrosis. This is, however, a much less common variant.

Oral ulcers that are clinically and histologically identical to aphthous ulcers are a feature of **Behçet's syndrome**.

Fig. 12.2 Acute necrotizing ulcerative gingivitis.

Fig. 12.3 Aphthous ulcer on lower lip. This example is unusually large.

There is associated ulceration of the genital mucosa, which is usually extensive and painful. In this syndrome the ulcers do not resolve quickly without treatment, and are often refractory to the treatments that normally improve ordinary aphthous ulcers. The cause of aphthous ulcers is not known.

Many common skin diseases can affect the oral mucosa

The skin diseases that most frequently involve the oral mucosa are lichen planus, erythema multiforme, discoid lupus erythematosus (DLE) and systemic lupus erythematosus (SLE), pemphigus vulgaris, and pemphigoid.

Of these, **oral lichen planus** is the most common, presenting with white lines against a background of a red buccal mucosa (*Fig. 12.4*). The disease may also affect the tongue and gingiva. Unlike lichen planus in the skin, erosion (due to separation of the epidermis) is common in the mouth. The disease may be particularly chronic, with older lesions producing patchy areas of white thickening. The histological appearances are similar to those seen in the skin (see pages 510–1). There is a dense lichenoid inflammatory infiltrate associated with degeneration of the basal layer of the epithelium, and occasional apoptotic keratinocytes termed Civatte bodies are also seen. In buccal and gingival lesions the overlying epidermis is frequently very thin.

Erythema multiforme in the mouth is probably most often seen as an adverse drug reaction. However, spontaneous episodes without a drug history are seen, particularly in children and juveniles in whom no obvious causative factor can be identified, although some follow a viral illness. The lesions range from small, red mucosal areas with central blisters, to very extensive erosive blistering lesions (*Fig. 12.5*). The latter pattern is sometimes called Stevens–Johnson syndrome. Unlike the skin lesions, erythema multiforme in the mouth nearly always blisters.

Oral involvement in **SLE** and **DLE** produces ulcerated and erosive lesions that can be clinically and histologically difficult to distinguish from lichen planus (see page 508).

The histological appearances of **pemphigus vulgaris** and **pemphigoid** are typical: both produce blisters and mucosal erosions (see page 111).

Pigmentation of the lips and buccal mucosa is usually non-neoplastic

Most pigmented patches in the mucosa of the mouth are due to increased melanin production in dark-skinned races. Melanocytic neoplasms such as nevi and malignant melanoma are rare in the mouth.

Amalgam tattoo is a specific type of pigmentation that is seen only in the mouth. It is due to the deposition of metal oxides in the buccal mucosa as a result of entry of dental amalgam into the submucosa during dental procedures. The histology is characteristic, with black material being deposited on collagen fibers, in the basement membranes around vessels and nerves, and in the perimysium of any skeletal muscle.

Patches of pigmentation around the lips are a characteristic feature of the **Peutz–Jeghers syndrome** (see page 263), and pigmentation within the mouth is a now-rare manifestation of **Addison's disease** (see page 345).

Polypoid nodules of the mouth and gingiva are common

The most common type of polypoid nodule is the so-called **fibrous** or **fibroepithelial polyp**, which can form anywhere on the cheek or tongue. Those associated with the gingival margins are sometimes called **fibrous epulis**. The etiology is not known, but some may be related to chronic trauma from teeth or dentures. Macroscopically they are usually smooth-surfaced and pale pink.

Each nodule is composed of a densely compacted fibrocollagenous core covered by slightly thickened squamous epithelium. Although clinically similar to fibrous epulis, **giant-cell epulis** is often darker red and occurs in the gingiva, being attached to the periodontal ligament. It is

Fig. 12.4 Oral lichen planus. The buccal mucosa shows the characteristic feature of reticulate white lines on a red background.

Fig. 12.5 Oral erythema multiforme. Large, confluent, blistering lesions over the entire surface of the lower lip.

composed of large multinucleate giant cells in a fibrous stroma and is covered by squamous epithelium.

Pyogenic granulomas, which are histologically and macroscopically similar to those seen in the skin, are sometimes seen in the mouth, particularly in pregnancy (sometimes called 'pregnancy epulis') (*Fig. 12.6*).

Fig. 12.6 Pyogenic granuloma.

White patches in the mouth are an important physical sign

Many conditions produce white thickening of the mucosa in the mouth, including lichen planus, *Candida* infection, and chronic friction from teeth or dentures (**frictional keratosis**) (*Fig. 12.7*). In most cases the cause is not apparent, but it is seen mainly in smokers, particularly pipe smokers. It is important as a physical sign as this is one way in which premalignant epithelial dysplasia may present.

The most frequent tumors in the mouth are squamous cell carcinomas derived from the lining epithelium

True benign squamous tumors of the mouth are very rare; most of the lesions that have the appearance of benign squamous 'papilloma' are either viral warts or localized areas of thickened hyperkeratotic squamous epithelium secondary to chronic trauma. Invasive squamous carcinoma is the most important and common lesion.

Established invasive squamous carcinomas present as raised, nodular lesions that develop central ulceration with a hard, raised edge. Tumors on the lip (*Fig. 12.8*) and tongue are usually recognized at an early stage and are amenable to surgery.

Squamous carcinomas in the floor of the mouth (*Fig. 12.9*) may be asymptomatic, remaining so until local invasion is extensive and surgical removal difficult. Lesions in the cheek may also present late, mainly because patients ignore them, ascribing their development to denture trauma.

Squamous carcinomas of the oral cavity are strongly associated with tobacco use, particularly pipe smoking. Molecular analysis has revealed that approximately 50% of cases also contain human papilloma virus sequences, particularly types 16, 18 and 33.

Fig. 12.8 Oral squamous carcinoma. Squamous carcinoma of the lip, showing typical raised edges and central ulceration.

Fig. 12.7 Frictional keratosis. The squamous epithelium is thickened and irregular, and there is an overlying thick horny layer of keratin.

Fig. 12.9 Squamous carcinoma of floor of mouth. The irregular tumor with raised edges is arrowed.

Squamous carcinomas of the mouth may arise in areas of epithelial dysplasia

Non-invasive epithelial dysplasia may precede the development of invasive squamous carcinoma. Clinically, such areas may present as thick, white patches raised above the level of surrounding mucosa, or as areas of red, velvety epithelium level with the surrounding mucosa. Such areas require biopsy to establish the presence of epithelial atypia and to exclude the development of early invasive tumor. The characteristics of dysplastic epithelium and carcinoma in situ are discussed and illustrated in Chapter 6, page 94.

Key Facts
Squamous cell carcinomas of the mouth

- Male preponderance – most associated with smoking.
- Affect the elderly (65+).
- Lips are the most common site (particularly lower lip).
- Actinic damage is a possible etiological factor.
- Tongue is the second most common site, usually occurring in the anterior two-thirds, on the lateral border. May present with thick white patch, eventually ulcerating.
- Floor of mouth and cheek are less common sites in UK and USA, but common in Indian subcontinent.
- Palate is the least common site.
- Most are well differentiated and keratinizing.
- May arise in pre-existing dysplasia.
- Infiltrate locally and metastasize to regional lymph nodes in the neck.

Abnormalities of the salivary gland, including tumors, may present in the mouth

As the mouth is lined by stratified squamous epithelium, with salivary gland tissue in the submucosa, abnormalities of the salivary gland may present in the mouth.

The most frequent abnormality is a **mucocele** (or **mucous retention cyst**). These small cystic nodules on the lower lip (mucosal aspect) are the result of obstruction of the minor labial salivary gland ducts, with cystic dilatation and retention of secretions. They are frequently traumatized, with escape of mucoid secretion into the surrounding tissues. A variant of salivary mucocele occurs beneath the tongue, in association with the ducts of the sublingual and submandibular salivary glands, forming a large, thin-walled, bluish cyst commonly called a **ranula**.

Salivary calculi from the submandibular or parotid glands may produce a swelling in the region of the sites of emergence of their respective ducts into the mouth, i.e. sublingual and buccal regions. The swelling may be due to retained secretion or to the calculus (**sialolith**) itself.

Salivary gland tumors may occur anywhere in the mouth, but are less common than tumors in the major salivary glands

Although salivary gland tumors that occur in the mouth are less common than those in the major salivary glands, they are more likely to be malignant.

Any of the tumors that occur in the major salivary glands, such as parotid and submandibular glands (see below), can also occur in the minor salivary gland tissue of the mouth. As with the major salivary glands, **pleomorphic salivary adenoma** is the most common type of tumor, and the palate is the most common intraoral site. The one salivary tumor that almost never involves the mouth is **adenolymphoma of the parotid**. Malignant salivary tumors may also occur in the minor intraoral salivary tissue.

Salivary gland tumors are mainly benign, and most commonly affect the parotid gland

The parotid gland is the most common site for salivary gland tumors, less than 25% occurring in the other large salivary glands (submandibular and sublingual) and the minor salivary tissues of the mouth. The most common tumor (90%) is the benign **pleomorphic adenoma** (formerly called 'mixed salivary tumor'), the histological features of which are illustrated in *Fig. 12.10b*. The peak incidence is in late middle-age and beyond, the tumor presenting as a slow-growing, smooth, painless swelling. Despite its apparent encapsulation, there may be small nodules attached to the main tumor which can be left behind at surgery if the main tumor is shelled out without a surrounding zone of normal salivary gland. This can lead to apparent recurrence of this benign tumor. Adequate surgical excision in the parotid may be difficult because of the need to spare the facial nerve, which runs between the deep and superficial parts of the parotid.

Key Facts
Salivary gland tumors

- Most common in major salivary glands: parotid > submandibular > sublingual.
- Most commonly benign: pleomorphic salivary adenoma > Warthin's tumor.
- Salivary adenoma can occur anywhere, including the minor salivary glands in the mouth.
- Warthin's tumor is almost always in the parotid.
- Adenoid cystic carcinoma is the most common malignant tumor.
- Adenoid cystic carcinoma is slow-growing but very locally invasive, spreading particularly in perineural spaces.

Fig. 12.10 Pleomorphic salivary adenoma. (a) Clinical picture of an unusually large tumor in the parotid. (b) Histology showing a mixture of adenomatous epithelial tissue and a pale myxoid stroma. The tumor is well circumscribed and is compressing adjacent normal parotid.

Fig. 12.11 Warthin's tumor of parotid. Histology showing a combination of glandular and lymphoid tissue.

Fig. 12.12 Adenoid cystic carcinoma. This micrograph shows the typical histological appearance, the so-called cribriform pattern.

The second most common tumor is the **monomorphic adenoma**. This is behaviorally identical to the pleomorphic adenoma, but has histological differences.

Warthin's tumor (adenolymphoma) is almost entirely confined to the parotid gland, usually occurring in the lower border near the angle of the mandible. It is most common in middle-aged men and presents as a painless, spherical, smooth-surfaced tumor, which may fluctuate in size. Larger tumors may be fluctuant because of central necrosis or due to the presence of mucin. Histologically the tumor is unusual, with an epithelial component of tall eosinophilic columnar cells forming clefts and cystic spaces within lymphoid tissue containing germinal centers (*Fig. 12.11*).

Malignant tumors of salivary tissue are rare and are particularly important in the intraoral minor salivary tissue

The most common malignant salivary tumor is the **adenoid cystic carcinoma** (*Fig. 12.12*). It can occur in the major salivary glands, such as the parotid and submandibular glands, but is proportionally more common in the intraoral salivary tissue, e.g. the palate. A slow-growing but locally invasive tumor, it frequently ulcerates in its intraoral location. Although it metastasizes late, the tumor has a poor prognosis because of its very extensive local invasion, with a particular tendency to grow in the perineural spaces. The tumor often extends considerably further than is apparent to the naked eye, and primary surgical excision is often unsuccessful in eradicating it completely, so further recurrence is very frequent. This, combined with poor radiosensitivity, makes management of this tumor difficult. The second operation for recurrence frequently requires radical and disfiguring orofacial surgery.

Two less common malignant tumors of salivary tissue are:

- **Mucoepidermoid carcinoma**, which arises mainly in the parotid in elderly people, occasionally developing in the palate. These lesions are of variable malignancy: some behave like pleomorphic adenoma, others are more aggressive from the outset.
- **Acinic cell carcinoma** occurs mainly in the parotid in the middle-aged and elderly, and is more common in

women than in men. It is sometimes called 'acinic cell tumor' because the majority behave in a benign fashion like pleomorphic adenoma, only rarely showing extensive local infiltration and lymph node metastasis.

Calculus formation in the ducts of the major salivary glands leads to chronic sialadenitis

Calculi or inspissated secretions that form in the major salivary ducts lead to obstruction in the flow of salivary secretions. The back-pressure effects lead to dilatation of the ducts and atrophy of the salivary acini, associated with increased interstitial fibrosis and lymphocytic infiltrate. This is called chronic sialadenitis. This condition can also occur as a result of viral infection, particularly paramyxovirus (mumps), and in autoimmune conditions such as Sjögren's syndrome.

COMMON DISORDERS OF THE TEETH AND RELATED STRUCTURES

The most common disorder of teeth is dental caries

Dental caries is the result of damage to the enamel and dentine by acid formed within bacterial plaque (*Fig. 12.13*). Bacterially generated acid in the mouth is usually neutralized by the alkaline secretions of the salivary tissue. However, when the acid is made by bacteria in plaque, the physical density of the plaque prevents saliva from reaching the enamel surface of the tooth. The acid dissolves the calcium hydroxyapatite of the enamel and progressively penetrates the full thickness of the enamel, decalcifying it as it goes. This produces a visible cavity in the tooth. As the cavity forms, bacteria can penetrate deeper into the

Fig. 12.14 Dental caries. Note the disruption of the dentinal structure, with large numbers of darkly stained bacteria penetrating towards the pulp cavity down the linear dentinal tubules.

tooth until the dentine is reached, and then penetrate the dentine layer through the hollow dentinal tubules (*Fig. 12.14*), which become distended with bacteria and tissue debris. This, combined with the continuing demineralizing effect of the acid, leads to liquefaction of the dentine. Eventually the dentine layer may be fully penetrated, and both bacteria and acid reach the soft central dental pulp.

Along the line of attack, the enamel and dentine are destroyed and the odontoblasts die. Although there is limited capacity for tissue reaction because the tissues are poorly cellular, in chronic lesions the odontoblasts may produce secondary dentine in an attempt at repair and restitution.

The consequences of carious attack are a pit or crater in the enamel, a penetrating destruction of the dentine and, when the dentine is fully penetrated, acute pulpitis due to bacterial and acid damage to the soft tissues of the pulp.

  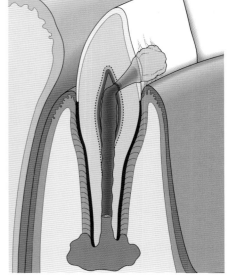

Fig. 12.13 The development of dental caries and its sequelae. (a) Acid destruction of enamel beneath plaque. (b) Dentinal caries (see *Fig. 12.14*), with acute pulpitis and pulp abscess. (c) Apical periodontal infection and abscess.

The most important complications of dental caries are pulpitis and periapical inflammation or abscess

Spread of bacteria and acid into the soft pulp space through carious penetration leads to necrosis of some of the pulp tissues, with an associated acute inflammatory reaction (mainly vessel dilatation, edema, and neutrophil infiltration). When there is extensive tissue necrosis a **pulp abscess** may form (*Fig. 12.15*). The combination of bacterial and acid necrosis with increased intrapulp pressure due to inflammatory edema leads to extensive necrosis of all the pulp tissues. Inflammatory stimulation of the nerve twigs in the pulp produces severe pain, localized or diffuse toothache being the main symptom of **acute pulpitis**.

Where the penetration of the enamel and dentine has been through a narrow carious channel, the pulp cavity remains largely isolated from the mouth cavity (**closed pulpitis**). However, where there has been extensive destruction of the enamel and dentine, the pulp cavity may be exposed to the oral cavity (**open pulpitis**). In these cases the pulp cavity is often completely replaced by inflammatory granulation tissue, which progresses through the phases of vascular granulation tissue, fibrous granulation tissue, and fibrous scar. The scarred pulp forms a polypoid protrusion into the oral cavity, and may become re-epithelialized.

Inflammation and death of the pulp is often followed by **apical periodontal infection**, the inflammation initially being confined to the small space beneath the tooth apex, between the apex and the surrounding bone. At first the infection is acute, with a predominantly acute inflammatory reaction that is rich in neutrophils, and there is often abscess formation (periapical abscess). The inflammation eventually becomes chronic, with a heavy infiltrate of lymphocytes and plasma cells, and granulation tissue formation (**chronic periapical periodontitis**). The enlarging inflammatory mass often erodes the bone around the apex of the tooth, producing an osteolytic, rounded lesion composed of chronic inflammatory granulation tissue, which may contain small neutrophil accumulations. This is sometimes called a **periapical granuloma** and is the most common cause of tooth-related cystic lesions in the bone.

Expansion of acute or chronic inflammatory lesions at the apex of abnormal teeth may produce inflammation in surrounding tissues with, for example, abscesses in the mandible pointing through the skin of the neck or producing sublingual cellulitis. Similar lesions in the upper jaw can break through the floor of the maxillary sinus to produce chronic sinus inflammation.

Periodontal disease, not associated with apical abnormality, is usually a consequence of gingivitis

Some form of gingivitis (inflammation of the gums) is present in almost every mouth, and is usually the result of neglected oral and dental hygiene. **Acute gingivitis** particularly affects young men, manifesting as swelling and soreness of the gums, often with bleeding and ulceration. Large numbers of bacteria are present in the ulcerated areas, and are probably causative.

Chronic gingivitis (*Fig. 12.16a*) occurs as a result of accumulation of bacterial plaque. It usually begins in childhood, when it is asymptomatic. Regular brushing of teeth, beginning in childhood, minimizes the accumulation of bacterial plaque and reduces the likelihood of significant gingivitis in later life. In adults bacterial plaque becomes calcified, separating the gingiva from the tooth. There is chronic inflammation in the gingival epithelium and submucosa, with large numbers of lymphocytes and plasma cells.

Chronic periodontitis results from the consequences of chronic gingival inflammation in relation to the presence of calculous plaque between the gingiva and the tooth. These are:

- **Destruction of the periodontal ligament,** leading to loosening of the tooth in its socket (*Fig. 12.16b*).
- **Progressive deepening of the pocket between tooth and gingiva,** which contains ever-increasing amounts of subgingival plaque (*Fig. 12.16b*).
- **Progressive inflammatory destruction of the alveolar bone,** leading to severe gingival recession (*Fig. 12.17*).
- **Periodontal abscess formation** (*Fig. 12.16c*) if the chronic inflammatory process becomes accelerated by acute bacterial infection. This accelerates destruction of the alveolar bone, and pus may extrude into the alveolar cavity or alongside the tooth in the subgingival pocket.

Fig. 12.15 Acute pulpitis. The pulp cavity contains an acute abscess.

Fig. 12.16 Chronic periodontal disease and its complications. (a) Chronic gingivitis. (b) Destruction of periodontal ligament. (c) Periodontal abscess.

Cysts related to the teeth can produce osteolytic lesions in the bones of the jaw

Dental cysts can be simply classified into those due to a developmental abnormality, and those that are secondary to inflammatory disease associated with the teeth.

Among the most important **developmental cysts** are **odontogenic keratocysts**, which usually occur in young males and are related to the mandibular molar region. They may be asymptomatic or may present with an intraoral swelling. Treatment is difficult, and they tend to recur after incomplete removal.

Dentigerous cysts mostly involve the third molars or the canine teeth. A typical cyst envelops the crown of an unerupted or displaced tooth and is attached to its neck.

The most important **inflammatory cyst** is the **radicular cyst**. It is far more common than the developmental cysts, and usually occurs in adults in association with caries of the permanent dentition. Most commonly involving the upper

Fig. 12.17 Chronic periodontal disease. Clinical picture showing severe gingival recession.

lateral incisors, it follows the development of a periapical granuloma resulting from caries.

Tumors derived from dental precursor tissues are rare

The most common tumor derived from odontogenic epithelium is the **ameloblastoma**. It is benign and does not metastasize. Tumors are mainly seen in the mandible of middle-aged adults, the vast majority developing at the angle of the mandible. They are slow-growing lesions that locally invade the bone, tumor expansion often leading to separation of the teeth and, occasionally, to loosening. They are composed of islands of odontogenic epithelium, often with a mixed fibrous stroma. The odontogenic epithelium forms islands with peripheral, tall ameloblastic epithelial cells surrounding loose epithelium, resembling the stellate reticulum of the developing tooth. Squamous metaplasia may occur, which is a source of potential confusion with invasive squamous carcinoma. Radiologically the tumor may resemble a unilocular or multilocular cyst.

The oropharynx is a common site of viral and bacterial infections (sore throat)

A red, inflamed, sore oropharynx is a symptom commonly encountered in family practice, and is usually due to a viral infection which also involves the nasopharynx and larynx. It is a common component of the common cold, influenza, and other viral upper respiratory tract infections, and is often severe in glandular fever (infectious mononucleosis).

Bacterial pharyngitis is much less common, and is usually due to infection by β-hemolytic streptococci; it is an important precursor of **acute post-streptococcal glomerulonephritis** and **acute rheumatic fever**.

Enlargement of the palatine tonsils as a result of inflammation is common

The mucosa-associated lymphoid tissue around the pharynx (Waldeyer's ring) comprises the palatine tonsils (tonsils), the nasopharyngeal tonsil (adenoids), and the lymphoid tissue in the submucosal region of the posterior third of the tongue (lingual tonsil). As part of the immune system, the lymphoid tissue in these areas reacts to inflammation or infection in the region by undergoing lymphoid hyperplasia. The changes are most easily seen in the prominent palatine tonsils; **reactive lymphoid hyperplasia** is the most common cause of tonsillar enlargement, particularly in children and juveniles, often occurring as a response to a viral or bacterial pharyngitis.

Acute tonsillitis usually occurs as a component of a widespread acute bacterial pharyngitis, usually due to β-hemolytic streptococci. The tonsils are swollen (*Fig. 12.18*), red owing to mucosal hyperemia, and partly covered by a creamy acute inflammatory exudate (**acute parenchymatous tonsillitis**). Sometimes there are scattered, creamy yellow spots on the surface (**acute follicular tonsillitis**) due to beads of pus extruding from the mouths of the infected epithelium-lined crypts. Acute streptococcal pharyngitis and tonsillitis may be complicated by the development of a peritonsillar abscess (**quinsy**) or, rarely, by spreading cellulitis in the neck (**Ludwig's angina**) or retropharyngeal abscess formation. Acute tonsillitis may also be a component of a severe viral pharyngitis, e.g. in glandular fever and some adenovirus infections.

In adults the tonsils usually become progressively smaller as the lymphoid component atrophies. However, in some cases the lymphoid element remains prominent, in association with enlarged crypts distended by keratin, in which numerous bacterial colonies (particularly *Actinomyces* species) are seen. This is sometimes called **chronic tonsillitis**, although the organisms are considered to be commensals.

Diphtheritic pharyngotonsillitis (due to infection by *Corynebacterium diphtheriae*) is now very rare because of widespread immunization.

Tumors of the tonsil are usually squamous cell carcinoma or malignant lymphoma

Benign tumors of the tonsil are very rare, and most are malignant. Squamous papillomas of the tonsillar region are mainly benign viral overgrowths, and occur on the faucial pillars rather than on the tonsil.

Squamous cell carcinoma presents as a mass or an ulcer with raised edges, usually in elderly men. The tumor invades the tongue and fauces, and lymphatic spread to neck nodes occurs early. Often, late presentation means that local and lymph node spread is advanced, and complete surgical removal is impossible.

Lymphomas of the tonsil are nearly always non-Hodgkin's lymphomas. Most are high-grade lesions and can

Fig. 12.18 Acute tonsillitis. The tonsils are swollen and acutely inflamed, almost meeting in the midline.

occur in children and young adults; a smaller number are low-grade lesions, which tend to occur in elderly patients. Sometimes there is associated lymphoma in the rest of Waldeyer's ring or in the gastrointestinal tract (lymphoma of mucosa-associated lymphoid tissue – MALT; see Chapter 15). Lymphoma of the tonsil has a better prognosis than squamous carcinoma because of the good response to chemotherapy.

PATHOLOGY OF THE NOSE AND NASOPHARYNX

The nose is lined by tall columnar ciliated respiratory-type epithelium, bathed in mucus produced by numerous mucus-secreting glands. The surface area is greatly increased by projections of bone (turbinates) and by the presence of communicating sinuses (maxillary, ethmoid, etc.) lined by identical epithelium. In the roof of the nasal cavity is a patch of specialized olfactory epithelium which is responsible for the sense of smell. The nasopharynx communicates with the middle ear via the eustachian tube.

The skin of the nose is susceptible to a large number of dermatological disorders

Skin disorders associated with exposure to sunlight are common on the nose, including basal cell carcinoma and solar keratoses (see pages 141 and 524).

Common inflammatory diseases include **rosacea** and **discoid lupus erythematosus** (see page 533). Rosacea affecting the nose may lead to the bulbous disfigurement called **rhinophyma**, particularly in elderly men.

Pale, firm nodules in the skin of the nose are a frequent presenting symptom. The most common causes are:

- **Nodular sebaceous hyperplasia** or **sebaceous adenoma** – the nose is very rich in sebaceous glands.
- **Basal cell carcinoma** – these enlarge and eventually develop central ulceration (*Fig. 12.19*).

Fig. 12.19 **Basal cell carcinoma of the nose.** A characteristic lesion with raised pearly edges and central ulceration.

The only certain way to distinguish a basal cell carcinoma from the other, less aggressive, lesions is to use excision biopsy.

Acquired structural deformity of the nose is almost invariably the result of trauma

Most nasal fractures will heal without therapeutic interference, but certain complications require surgical management. The complications of nasal fracture include:

- **Hematoma formation**, leading to nasal obstruction and risk of infection, with possible subsequent collapse of the cartilaginous nasal pyramid (**saddle nose**).
- **Deviation of the septum** due to dislocation of the septal cartilage. This may lead to marked nasal obstruction.
- **Deviation of the nose**, which is cosmetically unpleasing.

The most common nasal symptom seen in family practice is rhinitis

Rhinitis (a runny, blocked and perhaps sore nose) is usually due either to infection or to allergy.

Infective rhinitis is usually viral in origin, e.g. the common cold, influenza. Viral necrosis of surface epithelial cells is followed by exudation of fluid and mucus from the damaged surface (runny nose). Later submucosal edema produces swelling, which may lead to partial blockage of the narrow nasal airways.

In **allergic rhinitis** a type I hypersensitivity reaction to inhaled materials such as grass and flower pollens produces a mixed serous–mucous exudate, and submucosal edema leads to nasal blockage. In allergic rhinitis, where the antigenic stimulus may persist for many weeks, the submucosal edema may persist and worsen. An irregular, swollen, polypoid mucosa can develop, in which one or more **nasal polyps** may develop (*Fig. 12.20*), usually bilaterally.

Fig. 12.20 **Nasal polyp after excision.**

Typical nasal polyps are smooth-surfaced, creamy, semi-translucent, ovoid masses. Histologically they are characterized by immense edema and a scattered infiltrate of chronic inflammatory cells (including plasma cells); eosinophils are often very numerous in allergic polyps.

In acute rhinitis there is usually associated inflammation of the sinus linings

Acute maxillary sinusitis is the most important type of sinus inflammation, ethmoidal and frontal sinusitis being less significant. Swelling of the mucosa around the drainage foramen of the maxillary sinus may prevent drainage of maxillary sinus secretions into the nasal cavity, causing stasis. Stasis of maxillary secretions predisposes to secondary bacterial infection, with alteration of the retained maxillary fluid from seromucous to frankly purulent. In severe cases the infection may spread into the ethmoids and frontal sinuses, with the risk of spread to the meninges.

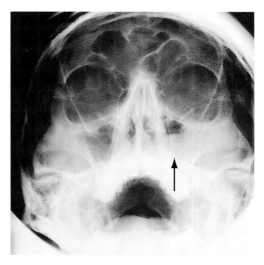

Fig. 12.21 **Maxillary sinusitis.** This X-ray, taken to show the maxillary sinuses, shows a fluid level in the left sinus (arrow) due to retention of secretions.

Chronic maxillary sinusitis may follow acute sinusitis, chronic inhalational insult, or nasal obstruction

Failure of an acutely inflamed sinus to drain, even after the resolution of the acute rhinitis that initiated it, leads to chronic maxillary sinusitis, with a chronically thickened and inflamed mucosa and persistent fluid accumulation (*Fig. 12.21*).

Chronic inhalation of irritant material is sometimes the result of industrial exposure, but most commonly involves cigarette smoke. Chronic rhinitis and maxillary sinusitis develop, initially as a toxic allergic reaction, but such cases are always liable to secondary bacterial infection or exacerbation during a viral infection.

Obstruction to maxillary sinus drainage may result from a severely deviated nasal septum, or from the presence of nasal polyps.

Nosebleeds (epistaxis) and loss of smell sense (anosmia) are common complaints

The nasal submucosa is highly vascular, and bleeding from the nose (**epistaxis**) is common. In most cases the cause is readily apparent, e.g. trauma, especially a blow to the nose or vigorous nose-picking, or acute rhinitis (*Fig. 12.22*). The most common site for bleeding is a small patch on the anterior septum. This area is particularly prone, being the site of numerous submucosal anastomoses (Little's area). However, persistent nosebleeds may be an indication of significant underlying disease.

Granulomatous inflammation in the nose is an important disorder worldwide; most cases are due to leprosy, TB or fungal infections, and are largely confined to the developing world. However, **sarcoidosis** may involve the nose (see page 570), and a specific form of granulomatous vasculitis, **Wegener's granulomatosis**, frequently presents with nasal lesions; Wegener's granulomatosis is considered in more detail in Chapter 10.

Fig. 12.22 Causes of epistaxis

Local disease	Little's area (particularly in acute rhinitis)
	Trauma
	Nasal tumors
Systemic disease	Hereditary telangiectasia
	Hypertension/mitral stenosis
	Bleeding diathesis, particularly thrombocytopenia
	Anticoagulant therapy
	Hemophilia and other clotting disorders
	Fevers

Fig. 12.23 Causes of anosmia (loss of sense of smell)

Obstructive	Acute and chronic rhinitis (allergic and infective)
	Acute and chronic sinusitis
	Nasal polyps
	Intranasal tumors, benign and malignant
Sensorineural	Fracture of cribriform plate
	Frontal lobe trauma
	Frontal lobe tumors
	Pituitary tumors

True benign tumors of the nose and paranasal sinuses are uncommon

The lesion most commonly mistaken for a benign tumor clinically is most often seen in the nasal vestibule (see *Fig. 12.23*), just inside the nostril, arising from the squamous epithelium of the vestibule. Although clinically it is labeled a 'squamous papilloma', histological examination shows that the vast majority of these lesions are viral warts identical to those seen on the skin.

Among the most frequently occurring benign tumors are **hemangiomas** (so-called 'bleeding polyps'). Usually located on the septum, they are responsible for repeated nosebleeds. Some are vascular chronic inflammatory lesions, resembling the pyogenic granulomas seen on the skin.

Juvenile angiofibroma is a rare tumor that occurs in male children and juveniles. It is mainly located in the nasopharynx rather than the nose. During puberty these lesions can grow quickly, mimicking a malignant tumor in their rapid growth and tendency to erode bone. They frequently ulcerate, and present with bleeding.

Transitional cell papilloma and **inverted papilloma** occur in adults. Although benign, they tend to recur or to be difficult to eradicate. Malignant change can supervene, but is rare.

The most frequent malignant tumors of the nose and sinuses are squamous and transitional cell carcinomas

The most common site for malignant tumor in the nasal cavity is in the anterior region near the nostrils; the tumor is usually squamous carcinoma. Further back in the nose there is an increasing proportion of transitional cell carcinomas (*Fig. 12.24*).

Malignant tumors of the sinuses are most common in the maxillary sinus, but some originate in the ethmoid sinus.

The major effects of tumors in the nose and nasal sinuses result from local invasion, often with destruction of the cheek, the palate and, most dangerously, the orbit.

Fig. 12.24 Transitional cell carcinoma of the nose. The tumor is composed of transitional respiratory epithelium, producing deeply invading masses.

obstruction to Eustachian tube;
secretory otitis media → hearing
loss and tinnitus

diplopia due to invasion of the VI cranial nerve | nasal obstruction, epistaxis, serous nasal discharge | metastases in cervical lymph nodes

Fig. 12.25 Clinical manifestations and complications of carcinoma of the nasopharynx.

Malignant melanomas can also occur, mostly affecting the middle-aged and elderly; in the nose they are often highly pigmented.

The nasopharynx is an important site of malignant tumors

The nasopharynx is that part of the pharynx lying immediately behind the nasal cavities. It is lined by respiratory-type columnar epithelium, and there is a considerable amount of lymphoid tissue in the submucosa, which is part of the mucosa-associated lymphoid tissue (MALT). Squamous metaplasia is frequent in adults, and much of the lining epithelium eventually becomes squamous lined. Carcinoma of the nasopharynx is particularly common in China, and is usually a squamous carcinoma or an undifferentiated carcinoma. Because the nasopharynx is an inaccessible site, these tumors may remain small and undetected until after they have spread to the lymph nodes in the neck (*Fig. 12.25*). The vast majority of patients with nasopharyngeal carcinoma have lymph node metastases when they first present. One of the histological characteristics of both squamous and anaplastic carcinomas is the presence of abundant lymphoid tissue in the stroma.

Malignant lymphoma also occurs in the nasopharynx, presumably arising from the submucosal lymphoid tissue forming part of Waldeyer's ring.

PATHOLOGY OF THE EAR

Congenital malformations of the pinna are very common

The most common congenital malformations related to the pinna are discussed in the section concerning ear disease in children (see page 242).

Acquired diseases of the pinna are frequently seen in community practice

Among the most commonly seen pinnal lesions are **keloids:** firm, dermal nodules that develop in the dermis, usually following trauma. The most common site is the earlobe following ear-piercing, particularly in girls of Afro-Caribbean origin. Attempts at surgical excision of these unsightly nodules are usually followed by the development of even larger keloids.

Trauma to the pinna is usually the result of a violent blow, sustained during criminal assault, or to contact sports such as boxing and rugby. The most common lesion is a tense, tender hematoma, incomplete resolution of which leads to physical distortion of the pinna (**cauliflower ear**).

Inflammatory skin disease particularly affects the back of the pinna and the groove behind the ear. **Atopic eczema** is the most common disease, particularly in children with the atopic tendency. Inflammation of the skin around the meatus is usually part of an **otitis externa** involving the full length of the meatus (see page 238).

Chondrodermatitis nodularis helicis presents as a small intractable and often tender ulcer, usually on the helix (*Fig. 12.26*). It is most common in the elderly and there may be degeneration of the pinnal cartilage beneath the ulcerated area. The cause is unknown, but may be ischemic.

Fig. 12.26 Chondrodermatitis nodularis of the pinna.

Fig. 12.27 Early squamous cell carcinoma of the pinna. In the early stage these lesions are clinically very similar to those of chondrodermatitis nodularis, and biopsy may be necessary to separate them.

Tumors and **pre-tumorous conditions** occur mainly in the elderly. They are usually squamous cell carcinomas (*Fig. 12.27*) or basal cell carcinomas (both of which tend to be single lesions), or solar or actinic keratoses (which may be multiple). These conditions are discussed in Chapter 23.

The most common abnormalities of the external auditory meatus are wax retention and inflammation

Wax retention leading to conductive deafness (see page 241) is a frequent complaint encountered by the family practitioner. The situation is often made worse by inept attempts to remove wax, using penetrating foreign bodies such as cotton wool buds.

There are two patterns of inflammation of the external auditory meatus (**otitis externa**). Inflammation may be **localized**, due to a boil (furuncle) in the ear canal, or **diffuse**, usually due to either bacterial or fungal infection (*Fig. 12.28*). A common fungus is *Aspergillus niger*, black threads of which can be identified in the inflammatory exudate and may even be visible in the ear canal. **Allergic otitis externa** is usually a response to topical ear drops.

Viral warts, basal cell carcinomas and squamous cell carcinomas can occur in the external auditory meatus, but all are rare.

Perforation of the tympanic membrane usually results from middle ear infection, but may occasionally follow trauma

The tympanic membrane (eardrum) is a three-layered structure. There is a central sheet of fibrocollagenous support tissue containing numerous elastic fibers, covered on the external surface by stratified squamous epithelium continuous with that of the external auditory meatus, and on the

Fig. 12.28 Otitis externa. The external auditory meatus is inflamed and covered by a scaling exudate, which spreads onto the pinna. Some of the pinnal changes are due to superimposed allergic otitis, a response to antibiotic eardrops given for the original infection.

inner surface by low cuboidal epithelium continuous with that lining the middle ear.

Infection (usually **acute otitis media**) is the most important cause of perforation, particularly in children. Less commonly, trauma, e.g. sustained during attempted removal of foreign bodies, may result in perforation. Most central perforations of the drum (*Fig. 12.29*) heal spontaneously.

The most important complications of a central perforation are predisposition to recurrent middle ear infection (otitis media), with impaired hearing, and failure to heal.

Fig. 12.29 Auroscopic view of a central perforation of the eardrum.

After perforation most eardrums heal by fibrosis

Although small central perforations heal spontaneously by fibrosis within a few days, larger perforations sometimes fail to heal and may require surgical closure using a fascial graft. A healed perforation is sometimes visible as a white scar or thinned area on the eardrum.

Acute otitis media is an important cause of earache and temporary hearing loss in children

Upper respiratory tract viral infections in children are frequently accompanied by the changes of acute inflammation in the lining of the middle ear, and in the inner lining of the tympanic membrane. Secondary bacterial infection may supervene, increasing the risk of a central perforation of the tympanic membrane. Children are particularly prone, probably because the narrow eustachian tube can become obstructed by the hyperplastic submucosal lymphoid tissue at its lower end (**adenoids**).

The main complications of acute otitis media include persistent perforation of the eardrum, tubotympanic chronic suppurative otitis media, otitis media with effusion (OME or 'glue ear'), and acute mastoiditis.

Acute otitis media often presents as a gastrointestinal upset in children.

Acute mastoiditis is now rare

In the pre-antibiotic era, secondary bacterial infection of a viral otitis media was common, leading to acute suppurative otitis media and the risk of bacterial infection spreading to the mastoid air cells. From the mastoid air cells, suppuration could extend into the brain to cause meningitis and brain abscess. This is now rare.

Chronic suppurative otitis media usually follows permanent perforation of the eardrum

Recurrent chronic inflammation in the middle ear is an important cause of chronic earache, deafness, and persistent discharge from the external auditory meatus. It usually occurs in people with a persistent, non-healing perforation of the eardrum. Chronic suppurative otitis media (CSOM) is usually subdivided into two broad groups:

- **Tubotympanic disease**, in which the perforation is in the pars tensa of the eardrum, and the discharge is typically copious and mucopurulent. The mucosal lining of the middle ear becomes chronically inflamed with a heavy infiltrate of lymphocytes and plasma cells, leading to thickening and the formation of inflammatory granulation tissue, often in the form of **chronic inflammatory granulation polyps**. These inflammatory masses can protrude through the perforated tympanic membrane, and large polyps may even present at the external auditory meatus. Some chronic inflammatory polyps contain large numbers of cleft-like crystals of cholesterol esters, often surrounded by a foreign body giant cell reaction; this is called **cholesterol granuloma**. The source of the cholesterol is not known, but it may be derived from red blood cells, as cholesterol granuloma is particularly important in otitis media in which there has been hemorrhage.
- **Atticoantral disease**, in which the perforation is located in the eardrum at the attic region, and is typically associated with the development of **cholesteatoma**. Atticoantral disease is also associated with a higher risk of major complications, e.g. brain abscess and other intracranial infection.

Key Facts
Complications of middle ear infection

COMMON

- Chronic inflammatory polyps
- Cholesterol granuloma
- Cholesteatoma

LESS COMMON

- Acute mastoiditis.
- Extradural abscess.
- Subdural abscess.
- Meningitis.
- Brain abscess.
- Lateral sinus thrombosis.
- Facial paralysis.
- Labyrinthitis.
- Petrositis.

Cholesteatoma is an important middle ear disease

Cholesteatoma is a form of epidermoid cyst. Most commonly located in the epitympanic recess (attic) and mastoid antrum, it often extends into the mastoid process. Its precise pathogenesis is disputed, but it is frequently associated with an atticoantral perforation of the eardrum. It is a cystic structure lined by squamous epithelium (*Fig. 12.30*), which constantly produces keratin. This leads to expansion of the lesion, damaging the small structures in the cavity. The area may become colonized by Gram-negative saprophytic bacteria, which probably stimulate continuing keratin formation. The enlarging keratinous mass, lined by stratified squamous epithelium, can eventually erode bone and may destroy the labyrinth, mastoid air cells, and facial nerve. It may even erode through the skull forming the base of the middle cranial fossa. Although they are non-neoplastic, cholesteatomas have the same effects as a slow-growing benign tumor.

Fig. 12.30 Cholesteatoma. In the auroscopic view of a cholesteatoma (a), the lesion is manifest as an irregular white mass. Histology (b) shows a cystic mass of keratin, which is lined by keratinizing squamous epithelium.

OME (glue ear) in children is commonly associated with upper respiratory tract infections

In otitis media with effusion (OME), mucoid fluid accumulates in the middle ear cavity because it is unable to drain through the child's narrow eustachian tube. This is possibly associated with lower tube blockage due to reactive hyperplasia of the adenoid lymphoid tissue.

The fluid is sterile, and is often thick and tenacious, resembling grayish-brown liquid glue, hence the common term 'glue ear.' It is associated with conductive deafness and intermittent earache. Because of the stasis of the fluid within the middle ear, there is a predisposition to acute suppurative otitis media due to secondary bacterial infection.

Tympanosclerosis is a hyaline degeneration of the eardrum submucosa. Appearing either as a crescentic white area or as chalky-looking patches, it may occur in the tympanic membrane in association with OME. It is most commonly seen after the insertion of a grommet.

The most important primary disease of the small bones of the middle ear is otosclerosis

In otosclerosis the normal bone of the auditory ossicles is replaced and thickened by newly deposited woven bone (see page 536). The disease, which is usually bilateral and eventually produces deafness, may be hereditary. There is an adult female preponderance. The disease usually starts at the otic capsule between the cochlea and vestibule, and may spread to involve the footplate and limbs of the stapes. It is the involvement of the stapes and of the cochlea that leads to deafness.

The two most important diseases affecting the inner ear are Ménière's disease and sensorineural deafness

Ménière's disease has three components:

* **Tinnitus** (ringing or buzzing).
* **Paroxysmal vertigo**.
* **Unilateral deafness**.

Although it is usually initially unilateral, up to 50% of patients may eventually develop disease in the other ear, sometimes many years later. Its cause is unknown, but the most important abnormality is marked distension of the cochlear duct by excess fluid, such that the vestibular membrane of Reissner, which separates two fluids of different compositions, bulges into the scala vestibuli (*Fig. 12.31*). This membrane may rupture, allowing the two fluids to mix. Histological study of the disease is hampered by the difficulty of obtaining untraumatized cochlea at postmortem examination.

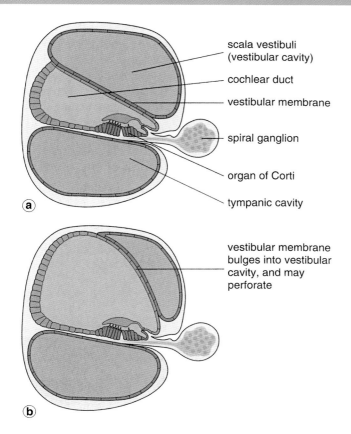

scala vestibuli
(vestibular cavity)

cochlear duct

vestibular membrane

spiral ganglion

organ of Corti

tympanic cavity

(a)

vestibular membrane
bulges into vestibular
cavity, and may
perforate

(b)

Fig. 12.31 Changes in Menière's disease. Cross-section of cochlea. (a) Normal cochlea. (b) Affected cochlea.

Many diseases of the ear are associated with temporary or permanent hearing loss

Hearing loss can be classified as **conductive** (usually due to some abnormality in the external or middle ear), **sensorineural** (usually due to some abnormality in the inner ear, auditory nerve or brain), or **mixed** (i.e. with features of both conductive and sensorineural hearing loss).

Conductive hearing loss occurs when sound waves cannot be transmitted to the inner ear

Conductive hearing loss is the most common type of temporary hearing loss encountered in family practice. In most cases it is due to occlusion of the external auditory canal by **wax**, and the hearing improves when the wax is carefully removed. Other common causes of conductive deafness are:

- **Acute otitis externa**, particularly if accompanied by marked swelling and exudate in the external auditory meatus and canal.
- **Acute and chronic otitis media and its complications**. Fluid accumulation in the middle ear in acute infection, and chronic inflammation and granulation tissue formation in chronic otitis media, are important

causes of conductive hearing loss. Also responsible for partial hearing loss are erosion by cholesteatoma complicating otitis media, and the accumulation of mucoid glue in otitis media with effusion.
- **Barotrauma**, e.g. after blast injuries, may lead to temporary hearing loss, which may be permanent if there is damage to the auditory ossicles. Perforation of the tympanic membrane in blast injuries is potentially recoverable.
- **Perforation of tympanic membrane by trauma or infection**.
- **Otosclerosis**.

Less common causes of conductive deafness include severe congenital malformations of the pinna and external auditory meatus, e.g. anotia.

Sensorineural deafness is due to damage to the inner ear, or to the nerve tracts transmitting messages to the brain

The most common type of permanent hearing loss is **presbyacusis**, a pattern of sensorineural hearing impairment in the elderly. There is decrease in hair cells (associated with atrophy of the epithelial tissue in the basal turn of the cochlea), atrophy of the stria vascularis, and neuronal loss in the spiral ganglia, all of which lead to a progressive sensorineural hearing loss. This type of deafness is characterized by loss of high tones combined with distortion.

The other important causes of acquired sensorineural deafness are:

- **Excessive noise**. Formerly, this was often the result of industrial exposure. However, it is now becoming an important cause in juveniles and young adults because of the use of personal stereo systems at loud volumes.
- **Ototoxic drugs**, particularly aminoglycosides, e.g. gentamicin.
- **Post-infective**, e.g. non-inherited congenital deafness following maternal rubella (now rare), cytomegalovirus, and toxoplasmosis. Non-congenital post-infective deafness can follow meningitis, and this is the most common cause in children.
- **Acoustic neuroma** and **head injury** are important causes of acquired sensorineural deafness in adults.

There are many causes of sensorineural hearing loss, some of which are rare congenital syndromes beyond the scope of this book.

Tumors of the ear are not common, and occur mainly in the external ear

Tumors affecting the pinna have already been discussed (see page 238). Both **basal cell carcinoma** and **squamous cell carcinoma** can originate in the epithelium of the external auditory meatus, and may spread to involve the middle ear.

The most important primary tumor presenting in the middle ear is a **paraganglioma**. Derived from the glomus jugulare, it is a neuroendocrine tumor. There is a female preponderance and most patients are between 40 and 60 years old. The tumors are slow growing and may present late, causing damage by destruction of the ossicles and perforation of the eardrum.

In children, **rhabdomyosarcoma** is an important tumor of the ear (see next section).

Schwannoma of the vestibulocochlear nerve is an important cause of unilateral hearing loss. As with paraganglioma, it is more common in women than in men, usually presenting between the ages of 30 and 50 years.

EAR DISEASE IN CHILDREN

There are many minor congenital malformations of the ear

There are many minor variations in the structure of the pinna, such as the presence of a small spur (**Darwin's tubercle**) on the helix, or prominent forward-facing ears owing to a poorly formed antihelix (**bat ears**); such conditions may require surgical treatment for cosmetic reasons, but they are not associated with significant morbidity.

In the skin immediately in front of the ear a small, raised nodule or polyp may arise, situated in front of the tragus. This common malformation, which is termed an **accessory lobule**, often contains a small island of cartilage.

Preauricular sinus is a persistent minute pit, usually situated in the skin immediately in front of the top of the helix. It sometimes contains a small plug of keratin, causing symptoms particularly when infected, with swelling and tenderness, often associated with a persistent watery or bloodstained discharge. The pit may be the only visible surface feature of a fairly extensive branched system, and surgical eradication may be difficult.

Severe pinnal malformations (e.g. congenital absence, or the presence of only rudimentary structures) are usually associated with abnormalities of the external auditory meatus and structures within the middle ear, as a result of maldevelopment of the first and second branchial arches. The inner ear is usually normal.

Middle ear disease is common in children

Acute otitis media and otitis media with effusion (glue ear) are particularly common in children, partly as a result of the narrow eustachian tube and the prominent adenoid lymphoid tissue at its lower end.

Infection of the external ear in children is frequently the result of the presence of an unsuspected foreign body.

Deafness in children

Temporary hearing loss is typically the result of acute otitis media or glue ear.

Permanent hearing loss, which is usually of the sensorineural type, may be congenital, due either to maternal infection or to a rare inherited disorder (see above). Acquired permanent hearing loss in children is an important complication of acute bacterial meningitis.

Rhabdomyosarcoma is the most important malignant tumor of the ear in children

Rhabdomyosarcoma is a highly malignant pleomorphic tumor composed of striated rhabdomyoblasts. It may present as a mass in the ear, but there is often a history of symptoms that have been misinterpreted as otitis media. The tumor grows rapidly and may infiltrate the parapharyngeal tissues and the mastoid air cells, sometimes extending upwards to invade the skull and brain.

THE LARYNX AND RELATED STRUCTURES

The larynx and related structures are illustrated in *Figs 12.32* and *12.33*.

The supraglottic and glottic regions are frequently inflamed in acute pharyngitis

Viral and bacterial infections of the pharynx frequently involve the supraglottic and glottic regions, producing hoarseness and temporary voice loss. Infection usually extends into the subglottic and tracheal regions, and perhaps down into bronchi, producing cough and tracheal soreness. This symptom complex, which is known as **upper respiratory tract infection** (**URTI**), is very common but

Fig. 12.32 Larynx viewed from above. E = epiglottis; **F** = false cord; **T** = true cord; **V** = ventricles.

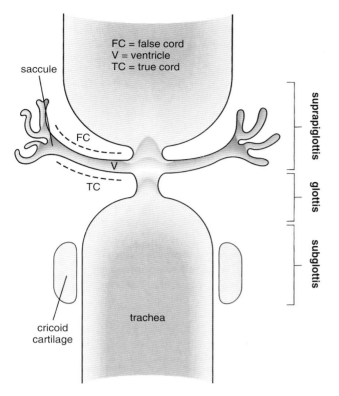

saccule

FC = false cord
V = ventricle
TC = true cord

FC

V

TC

supraglottis

glottis

subglottis

cricoid
cartilage

trachea

Fig. 12.33 Diagram of larynx showing supraglottic, glottic and subglottic regions. The supraglottis includes the epiglottis, false cords, ventricles and saccules. The glottis comprises the true vocal cords, anterior and posterior commissures and vocal processes of the arytenoids. The subglottis is the area below the true vocal cords, as far as the level of the lower border of the cricoid cartilage.

usually transient and trivial. It can have serious consequences in young children and in the elderly or debilitated.

In young children the small airway can become obstructed by mucosal and submucosal swelling (croup). Acute epiglottitis, usually due to *Haemophilus influenzae* infection, can produce fatal obstruction.

In the elderly and debilitated the cough reflex is poor, and infected material cannot be cleared from the tracheo-bronchial tree. It may pass into small peripheral bronchi and bronchioles under the influence of gravity, producing **bronchopneumonia** (see Chapter 11, page 193).

Inflammatory changes in the larynx may also result from allergic and toxic damage

Allergic pharyngolaryngeal edema can arise as a life-threatening type I hypersensitivity reaction, which is usually associated with swelling of the face (**angioneurotic edema**). Bronchospasm may also occur as part of the same reaction, increasing the severity of the asphyxia.

Acute toxic laryngitis is rare, but is occasionally seen following the inhalation of toxic fumes during exposure in a fire (inhalation of fumes from polystyrene material being particularly important), although the direct physical effect

of heat may also be responsible. Industrial exposure to toxic fumes is also an important cause.

Chronic laryngitis is most commonly seen in heavy cigarette smokers. Chronic inflammatory infiltrates are present in the larynx, and there may be thinning or keratotic thickening of the overlying epidermis. In the latter pattern, dysplastic change may occur in the basal layer. This is considered to be a predisposing factor in the eventual development of squamous carcinoma.

Benign thickenings, nodules and polyps of the larynx are a common cause of hoarseness

Chronic laryngitis may lead to permanent thickening of the laryngeal mucosa and submucosa, particularly where there is associated excess production of keratin (smoker's keratosis).

Singer's nodes are minute smooth, round nodules located at the nodal point at the junction between the anterior third and the posterior two-thirds of the vocal cords (*Fig. 12.34*). Particularly seen in singers and professional voice users, they are covered by smooth epithelium, and the submucosa shows fibrosis.

Fig. 12.34 Singer's nodules. The nodules (arrow) occur at the points of contact of the true cords.

Diffuse inflammatory edema (sometimes polypoid) is the result of an unusual pattern of edema (**Reinke's edema**) with hyaline change and occasional stromal hemorrhage (*Fig. 12.35*). Histologically there is marked fibrinoid degeneration of the stroma. Excessive bleeding may lead to hematoma formation, particularly after strenuous vocal activity.

Fig. 12.35 Reinke's edema. Diffuse swelling of the cords due to Reinke's edema.

Laryngeal cysts occur most commonly in the aryepiglottic folds, rather than on the true vocal cords. These translucent structures, which are filled with thick mucus, are retention cysts resulting from blockage of the ducts of mucus glands.

Warty papillomas on the larynx are usually due to infection by the human papilloma virus (HPV 11 and 16)

In adults warty papilloma is usually solitary and confined to the vocal cords; its viral nature is less obvious than those in children. Clinically it may be difficult to distinguish from an early verrucous carcinoma (see page 245), and there are also histological similarities.

As the name suggests, **juvenile laryngeal papillomatosis** is largely confined to children. It consists of multiple soft, pink papillomas on the vocal cord, also extending into other parts of the larynx and sometimes even down the trachea. These lesions have the histological features of a florid viral wart (*Fig. 12.36*). They are difficult to eradicate, often requiring repeat multiple excisions, as they are typically both persistent and recurrent.

Carcinoma of the larynx is an important malignancy in cigarette smokers

Carcinoma of the larynx is most common in male cigarette smokers over the age of 40 years, but is becoming increasingly common in women smokers. It is a squamous carcinoma and can occur in the **supraglottic region**, e.g. the aryepiglottic folds, false cords and ventricles; the **glottic region**, in the true vocal cords and anterior and posterior commissures; or the **subglottic region**, arising below the true vocal cords and above the first tracheal ring.

Tumors of the true vocal cords (**glottic**) are most common. They have the best prognosis if detected early (an early symptom being hoarseness), because the true vocal cords have a poor lymphatic drainage except at the commissures. The tumor remains localized to the larynx for a long time and, except in neglected tumors that have invaded local tissues widely, metastasis to lymph nodes is rare.

Supraglottic tumors can be resected with sparing of the true vocal cords. However, as these areas are better supplied with lymphatics, lymph node metastasis is more common than in glottic tumors, and may be the presenting symptom.

Subglottic tumors are the rarest type, and have a poor prognosis because of late presentation; symptoms are often manifest only when extensive growth and local spread lead to stridor and voice loss due to vocal cord involvement.

Some invasive squamous carcinomas of the larynx arise in areas of severe dysplasia and carcinoma in situ

Mild dysplasia of the laryngeal epithelium is a common feature of smoker's keratosis, the chronic hyperkeratotic

Fig. 12.36 Juvenile laryngeal papillomatosis. Histology showing warty thickening of the epithelium due to HPV virus.

laryngeal thickening that occurs in heavy smokers. More extensive and severe dysplasia merges with **carcinoma in situ** (*Fig. 12.37*), and there may be small foci suggesting microinvasion. There is some dispute as to the proportion of invasive squamous carcinomas that arise in pre-existing areas of carcinoma in situ, but common sense seems to suggest that, as in the colon and other sites, there is a sequence in the larynx of mild dysplasia, through moderate dysplasia, severe dysplasia and carcinoma in situ, culminating in invasive carcinoma (*Fig. 12.38*). The histological appearances of these pre-invasive states are illustrated in *Fig. 12.39*.

Most invasive squamous carcinomas are well-differentiated keratinizing squamous carcinomas, but occasionally

Fig. 12.37 Carcinoma in situ of the larynx. The mucosa of the true cords is thickened, irregular and granular, with a small polyp. Histological examination reveals severe dysplasia of the covering epithelium. To the naked eye there is no evidence of invasion.

poorly differentiated forms occur, which are sometimes spindle celled. An important variant is **verrucous carcinoma**, which usually affects one or both of the true vocal cords. Clinically it presents as an often large, warty papillary tumor, with all the clinical features of malignancy. However, histologically it appears very bland, being composed of benign-looking squamous epithelium with hyperkeratosis. Despite the innocent histology, these tumors are locally destructive and require surgical removal to prevent fatal obstruction or laryngeal destruction. Metastasis is virtually unknown, but occasionally follows attempts at radiotherapy treatment.

Fig. 12.38 Invasive squamous carcinoma of the larynx. In this resected specimen of the larynx, there is extensive replacement of the left vocal cord by tumor (**T**).

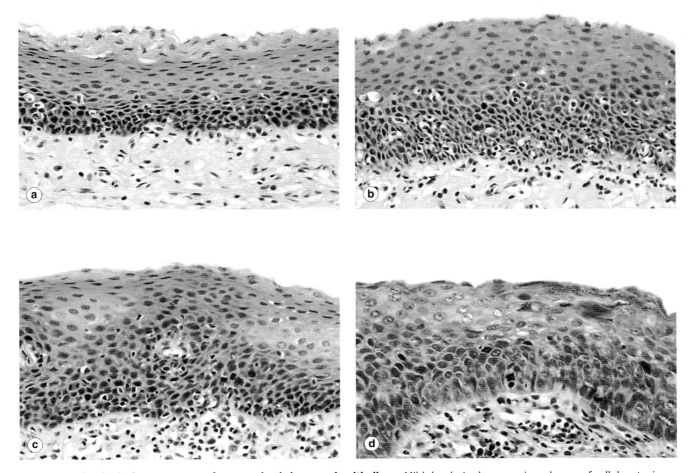

Fig. 12.39 Histological appearances of preneoplastic laryngeal epithelium. Mild dysplasia shows a minor degree of cellular atypia confined to the basal third of the epithelium (a). Dysplastic changes in the middle third are indicative of moderate dysplasia (b), and extension into the upper third indicates severe dysplasia (c). Severe dysplasia can be present both with and without surface keratosis. Full-thickness dysplasia indicates carcinoma in situ (d), and occasionally these lesions exhibit microinvasion.

PRIMARY TUMORS   **SECONDARY TUMORS**

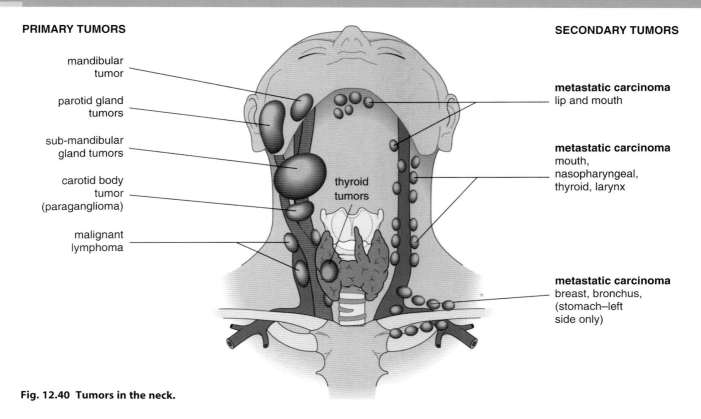

mandibular tumor

parotid gland tumors

sub-mandibular gland tumors

carotid body tumor (paraganglioma)

malignant lymphoma

thyroid tumors

metastatic carcinoma
lip and mouth

metastatic carcinoma
mouth, nasopharyngeal, thyroid, larynx

metastatic carcinoma
breast, bronchus, (stomach–left side only)

Fig. 12.40 Tumors in the neck.

It is important that students know the differential diagnosis of lumps in the neck

A simple approach is based on the precise location of the lump in the neck *Fig. 12.40*), together with its texture (solid or cystic).

The location of solid lumps can be divided into those:

- **Related to the thyroid gland**, e.g. multinodular goiter, solitary thyroid nodule, thyroid carcinoma, etc.
- **Related to the submandibular salivary gland**, e.g. pleomorphic salivary adenoma, chronic sialadenitis.
- **Related to the cervical lymph node groups**. These occur mainly in the jugular chain and in the supraclavicular region.
- **Related to the mandible**, e.g. mandibular cysts, abscesses and tumors of both dental and bony origin.
- **Related to the carotid bifurcation**. These are almost always neuroendocrine tumors derived from the carotid body, the chemodectoma.

Tumors or lumps associated with the thyroid gland are discussed in Chapter 16, those related to the mandible on page 233, and those related to the salivary glands earlier in this chapter.

The lymph nodes in the neck frequently enlarge by benign hyperplasia in response to infection and inflammation

The lymph nodes in the neck, particularly those in the jugular region, respond to local inflammation and infection by reactive hyperplasia, which is either follicular or parafollicular in pattern (see Chapter 15, page 307). Common sources of primary infection include the tonsils, teeth, pharynx, sinuses and, occasionally, the ear. Reactive lymph node enlargement may also occur when there has been localized skin inflammation, e.g. in the scalp or behind the ear. Three important diseases may present with benign lymph node enlargement in the neck.

Infectious mononucleosis (glandular fever) is often associated with severe inflammation of the tonsils. The diagnosis can be confirmed by examination of the peripheral blood film for atypical mononuclear cells, and by the Paul–Bunnell test, although the diagnosis can be made on histological examination of the node if it is foolishly removed surgically.

In cases of **cervical tuberculosis** the lymph nodes are often matted and inflamed. They may be slightly fluctuant, and in neglected cases they even point and discharge onto the surface ('scrofula'). Histological appearances are characteristic, with extensive caseating necrosis. It is always advisable to send part of an excised tuberculous node for culture in case the organism is an atypical or resistant mycobacterium.

Toxoplasmosis usually develops in a juvenile or a young adult. Toxoplasmic lymphadenitis is discussed and illustrated in Chapter 15 (pages 307–8). Patients with toxoplasmosis may have circulating atypical lymphocytes, rather like patients with infectious mononucleosis. In a fully developed case, lymph node histology is characteristic.

The lymph nodes in the neck are a common site for metastatic tumor deposition

The jugular nodes are the eventual drainage site for many of the mucosal structures in the head and neck, as well as the skin of the head and scalp. Consequently they are a common site for metastatic carcinoma deposits from sites such as the lip, tongue, mouth, nasopharynx, oropharynx, larynx, salivary glands, and thyroid. Attempts at complete surgical removal of tumors in these sites often include a block dissection of the lymph nodes of the neck on the affected side; where the primary tumor has crossed the midline, the nodes of the other side are also dissected.

The supraclavicular lymph nodes are important sites for metastatic tumor deposits in the bronchus, breast and (on the left side) stomach (Troisier's node).

Enlargement of one or more lymph nodes in the neck may be a presenting symptom of some types of malignant lymphoma

Malignant lymphoma, a primary malignant tumor of cells of the lymphoid system, is discussed in Chapter 15 and will not be considered in detail here. One form of Hodgkin's disease commonly presents with cervical lymphadenopathy.

Cystic or fluctuant lumps in the neck are usually either midline or lateral

The most common and important midline cystic lesion is the **thyroglossal duct cyst** (*Fig. 12.41*). This is a remnant left from the migration of the thyroid gland from the posterior part of the tongue to the neck during embryological development. It presents in young children, sometimes in the form of a cyst, or occasionally as a persistent sinus; it may present in young adult life, when the lesions may be quite large.

Occasionally a nodule in the thyroid is fluctuant and is diagnosed as a '**thyroid cyst.**' These 'cysts' are almost always benign adenomas showing central degenerative changes.

The most common and important lateral cystic lesion is the **branchial cyst** (*Fig. 12.42*). Derived from cystic remnants of the branchial arches, it produces diffuse fluctuant swelling in the lateral aspect of the neck, often beneath the angle of the mandible.

Fig. 12.41 Thyroglossal duct cyst. Note the midline location.

Fig. 12.42 Branchial cyst. Note the lateral location.

Case-based questions

Case 1 – A young vagrant with foul gums

A 19-year old male, a homeless vagrant, is seen in the Emergency Department in a drunken state. He is bleeding from the mouth but has no history of trauma. On examination there is acute, sloughing ulceration of the gums surrounded by inflamed red mucosa, with many areas of bleeding. The breath is foul and the teeth are dirty, with a large build-up of plaque and calculus. A smear from the ulcerated areas shows numerous fusiform and spirochaetal organisms.

1. **What is the diagnosis?**
2. **What are the predisposing factors?**
3. **What are the organisms?**
4. **What are the long-term complications?** ▶

▶ ### Case 2 – An old man with a white patch inside his cheek

A 72-year-old retired bookbinder is referred by his dentist because of an area of white thickening of the buccal mucosa. On examination there is an ill-defined thick white patch on the buccal mucosa on the left. The lesion is biopsied.

1. What are the most likely causes?
2. Why was it considered important to biopsy the lesion?

Case 3 – An old man with a white ulcerated patch on his tongue

A retired docker from the port of Hull, aged 74, is seen because of an area of white thickening on the lateral border of the anterior third of his tongue. He had smoked for many years and, while working, had developed a taste for Russian vodka. He describes the lesion as a slowly enlarging thick white patch present for many months. It was causing him no concern until a small, slightly painful ulcer developed in the centre of the patch. The lesion is biopsied to confirm the clinical diagnosis before curative treatment is initiated.

1. What is the most likely clinical diagnosis?
2. If the biopsy confirms the clinical diagnosis, what is the most frequent and effective treatment?
3. What is the commonest site for the spread of the lesion?

Case 4 – A woman with an unsightly swelling on her jaw

A 57-year-old woman has come somewhat unwillingly to hospital because of a smooth, enlarging mass at the angle of her jaw on the left side. She says it has been present for some years, had given her no trouble, but had slowly enlarged and was now becoming disfiguring. Her anxious daughter obviously fears cancer, and the lump can no longer be disguised by cosmetics. On examination the mass appears to be in the parotid gland, is firm and rubbery, with a smooth, well-circumscribed outline, and is non-tender.

1. What is the differential diagnosis?
2. What precautions must be taken during surgery, and why?
3. Are you able to reassure the daughter?

Case 5 – A child with acute earache and hearing loss

A 5-year old girl is referred by her GP to the ENT clinic with a 'glue ear' on the right side following a recent upper respiratory tract infection. The child is in pain and has a degree of hearing loss. On examination, the ear is tender and the drum appears dull, with radial vessels clearly visible. The drum is bulging and immobile on testing with a pneumatic speculum. The child has a pyrexia of 38°C. The left ear is full of debris, but the visible part of the drum appears normal.

1. What is the most likely explanation for her earache, deafness and pyrexia?
2. What are the major complications of this condition?
3. What is the underlying pathology in this condition?
4. What is the likely organism in this age group?
5. What are the treatment options?

Case 6 – A singer with a hoarse voice

A 42-year-old nightclub singer is unable to fulfill her demanding schedule of bookings because of increasing hoarseness of voice, which has been present for many months. Initially, the symptom gave her voice a smoky, throaty timbre that was much appreciated by her audience, but the symptoms have worsened so that she is scarcely capable of singing at all. She had reduced her smoking from 30 per day to fewer than five, but there has been little or no improvement.

1. What is the diagnosis?
2. What would her larynx look like on direct laryngoscopy, and what is the nature of the lesions?

Case 7 – An old man with loss of voice

A 68-year-old retired pig farmer, who still lives on the farm which is now run by his son, has been a heavy smoker of hand-rolled cigarettes for over 50 years. He has had a hoarse voice for as long as he can remember. He attends hospital complaining of complete loss of voice for about 1 month. On laryngoscopy, the left vocal cord is completely replaced by a large white friable mass which extends to the anterior commissure. The right vocal cord is thickened and irregular.

1. What is wrong with his left vocal cord?
2. What is wrong with his right vocal cord?
3. What is the most likely sequence of events?
4. What will happen in the future if the lesion is not successfully treated?

Brief answers to these case-based questions are given on pages 586–7. More detailed answers and other study resources are available online at www.studentconsult.com.

Alimentary tract **13**

DISEASE OF THE ALIMENTARY TRACT

The alimentary tract extends from the lips to the anus, and the diseases that occur in each component of the tract vary from site to site. Diseases of the various components of the mouth as far as the oropharynx are dealt with in Chapter 12. In this chapter we deal with the esophagus, stomach, small intestine, large intestine, rectum and anus.

DISEASE OF THE ESOPHAGUS AND ESOPHAGOGASTRIC JUNCTION

From its origin at the cricoid cartilage to its termination at the esophagogastric junction, the esophagus is normally lined by stratified non-keratinizing squamous epithelium.

The esophageal wall contains both striated muscle (in its upper portion) and smooth muscle (in the lower portion). A competent lower esophageal sphincter is essential to prevent the reflux of gastric contents back into the esophagus.

Reflux esophagitis (gastroesophageal reflux disease – GERD) is the most common abnormality of the esophagus encountered by the family practitioner

Reflux of gastric acid into the lower esophagus produces a burning pain in the centre of the lower chest or hypochondrium, commonly known as heartburn. Factors predisposing to acid reflux include those that increase intra-abdominal pressure, e.g. over-eating, pregnancy, and poor posture; and those that render the lower esophageal sphincter lax or incompetent, e.g. hiatus hernia (see page 251), smoking, and alcohol ingestion.

The normal squamous epithelium of the lower esophagus is sensitive to the effects of gastric acid and is frequently damaged. Several complications may arise:

- **Reflux esophagitis**. The esophageal mucosa becomes acutely inflamed.
- **Peptic ulceration of lower esophagus**. Small ulcers usually develop, which become chronic, with fibrosis.
- **Lower esophageal stricture**. Chronic peptic ulceration causes progressive fibrous thickening of the lower

esophagus wall. The resultant narrowing causes difficulty in swallowing.
- **Barrett's esophagus**. Persistent esophageal reflux causes metaplasia of the lower esophageal mucosa, the squamous epithelium being replaced by glandular epithelium containing goblet cells (*Fig. 13.1*). This is also termed **columnar epithelial-lined esophagus** (CELO).

Barrett's esophagus predisposes to the development of adenocarcinoma

Barrett's esophagus can progress from metaplastic glandular epithelium to epithelial dysplasia, and then to frank adenocarcinoma. The columnar epithelium may show features of intestinal metaplasia, in which the epithelium resembles that of the small intestine, or may resemble that of the cardiac region of the proximal stomach.

Fig. 13.1 Barrett's esophagus. The lower esophageal mucosa (**E**) is replaced by darker columnar epithelium, with an area of ulceration (**U**) at the esophagogastric junction (**EGJ**). The arrow marks the abnormally high squamocolumnar junction.

Patients with Barrett's esophagus are kept under surveillance through repeated endoscopy and biopsy to detect early neoplastic changes. Treatment by esophageal surgery is then possible before the development of invasion.

Esophagitis is rarely caused by agents other than reflux

Acute esophagitis may be caused by infective or physical agents. Bacterial infection is very rare, but fungal infection (mainly by *Candida albicans*) is an important cause of severe erosive esophagitis, particularly in immunosuppressed patients.

Viral infections of the esophagus (particularly by herpes simplex and cytomegalovirus) are increasingly being seen in AIDS patients and those receiving immunosuppressive therapy.

Acute esophagitis is also produced by irradiation and by ingestion of caustic agents. Certain skin diseases, such as pemphigus, epidermolysis bullosa and Behçet's syndrome, may cause esophageal ulceration, with extensive separation of the epithelium from the submucosa producing blistering, followed by erosion.

Any esophageal obstruction causes difficulty in swallowing, known as 'dysphagia'

Four main types of lesion cause obstruction:

- **Lesions in the lumen**. Swallowed foreign bodies, especially in children.
- **Lesions in the wall**. Benign neoplasm or carcinoma of the esophagus, fibrosis caused by chronic inflammation.
- **Lesions outside the wall**. Esophageal diverticulum, tumors in the mediastinum (e.g. invasion by carcinoma of the lung).
- **Lesions affecting function**. Achalasia (see below), Chagas' disease, motor neuron disease (see page 471).

Esophageal obstruction may be complicated by reflux of food into the airways, resulting in aspiration pneumonia (see page 198), and by malnutrition due to the inability to maintain adequate intake.

Achalasia of the esophagus is due to abnormal innervation

In achalasia, lack of coordinated muscle contraction and relaxation at the lower end of the esophagus leads to retention of the food bolus, the result of peristaltic spasms combined with sluggish relaxation at the esophagogastric sphincter. The condition is mainly seen in middle age. Over a period of time the esophagus becomes markedly dilated (megaesophagus). Its cause is unknown, but in long-standing cases reduced numbers of ganglion cells in the muscle plexus have been noted. This condition also predisposes to the development of carcinoma of the esophagus.

In South America, infection with *Trypanosoma cruzi* causes a very similar condition, with destruction of the myenteric plexus, termed **Chagas' disease**.

Dysphagia is commonly seen in family practice

Although esophageal stricture, achalasia and malignant tumors are the most important causes of dysphagia, they are not the most common.

In family practice, complaints of difficulty in swallowing, and the feeling of a lump in the throat, are common among young and middle-aged women. The patient describes an apparent obstruction in the cricoid region of the upper esophagus, and the swallowing problem is not directly related to food ingestion, but difficulty is particularly experienced in swallowing saliva and drinks. Called **globus pharyngeus**, the condition is associated with spasm of the cricopharyngeus muscle, identifiable on barium swallow. Although probably psychosomatic in most cases, it may be a manifestation of hiatus hernia, reflux esophagitis or peptic ulceration.

Esophageal perforation is most often caused by medical procedures

Perforation of the esophageal wall is extremely serious as it liberates secretions (including gastric juices) into the mediastinum, causing **mediastinitis**. Patients have chest pain and develop clinical shock. A chest radiograph may show air in the mediastinum.

Perforation most commonly occurs after instrumentation of the esophagus, e.g. after dilatation of strictures or endoscopy. Tearing of the lower esophagus may occur after severe vomiting with a full stomach, leading to perforation and hemorrhage from local vessels (**Mallory–Weiss tear**).

The most common malignant tumors of the esophagus are squamous carcinomas and adenocarcinomas

There is great geographical variation in the incidence of esophageal carcinoma, which is particularly common in the Far East, especially in China and Japan. Tumors are most common in males after the fifth decade, and can be divided into two main histological types.

Squamous carcinomas are most common in the middle and lower esophagus. They mostly develop in men who are heavy alcohol drinkers or heavy smokers, and may be preceded by epithelial dysplastic change. The disease usually presents late, when the tumor has become large enough to compromise the esophageal lumen and cause dysphagia. Regional lymph node spread is early and common.

Adenocarcinomas mostly affect the lower esophagus, arising in areas of epithelial metaplasia (**Barrett's esophagus**). Some adenocarcinomas may represent a primary carcinoma of the stomach that has infiltrated into the lower esophagus. These tumors tend to metastasize via lymphatics at an earlier stage than squamous carcinomas.

The prognosis for both types of carcinoma is poor, that for squamous carcinoma being slightly better than adenocarcinoma because it is more responsive to radiotherapy. Fewer than 10% of patients survive for 5 years.

Squamous carcinomas of the upper esophagus, located in the post-cricoid region, are very rare and are usually linked to the Plummer–Vinson syndrome, most common in middle-aged and elderly women.

Rare malignant primary tumors of the esophagus include malignant melanomas, small cell neuroendocrine carcinomas, and sarcomas.

Benign tumors of the esophagus are uncommon

Most of the rare benign esophageal tumors are leiomyomas derived from the smooth muscle of the muscularis propria. Less common are tumors derived from nerves, i.e. schwannomas and neurofibromas. They produce smooth spherical nodules projecting into the lumen, and are usually covered by intact mucosa unless they become large, at which stage ulceration of the stretched overlying mucosa can occur.

In hiatus hernia the stomach moves into the thorax

Hiatus hernia, in which the upper part of the stomach moves through the diaphragmatic esophageal hiatus into the thoracic cavity, is a common and important condition.

Patients often complain of symptoms of reflux esophagitis, and there may be peptic ulceration in the intrathoracic part of the stomach and lower esophagus. In **sliding hiatus hernia** (95% of cases), the stomach herniates through the diaphragmatic hiatus through which the lower esophagus normally passes. In **paraesophageal hiatus hernia**, the stomach protrudes through a separate defect alongside the esophagus (*Fig. 13.2*); these rarely induce reflux, but can become strangulated or obstructed.

Esophageal varices are an important cause of vomiting blood

At the lower end of the esophagus the submucosal venous plexus drains into both the systemic venous system and the portal venous system. When the pressure in the portal venous system is high, e.g. as a result of severe diffuse long-standing liver disease, the esophageal submucosal venous channels become enormously dilated to form esophageal varices, which may protrude slightly into the lumen. Rupture of the varices, or ulceration of the overlying mucosa, can produce torrential hemorrhage into the esophagus and stomach, often precipitating vomiting of blood (**hematemesis**).

The most common cause of esophageal varices is portal hypertension associated with cirrhosis of the liver (see Chapter 14).

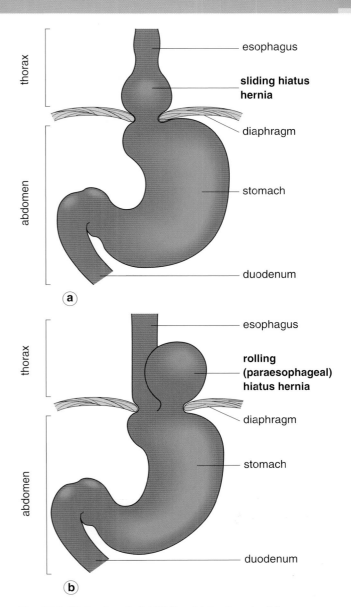

Fig. 13.2 Hiatus hernia (a) Sliding hiatus hernia. (b) Paraesophageal hiatus hernia.

DISEASE OF THE STOMACH

The stomach has three mucosal zones: the **cardia**, which is immediately adjacent to the esophageal junction; the **body** (fundus), which contains long tubular glands secreting acid and intrinsic factor; and the **pylorus** (antrum), which contains the majority of gastrin-secreting cells. Each zone is affected by different types of pathology.

Gastritis is characterized by inflammation of the gastric mucosa

Inflammatory changes in the mucosa and submucosa of the stomach are known as **gastritis**, and may be either **acute** or **chronic**. This may be assessed by endoscopic examination of the mucosa and confirmed by biopsy.

Acute (erosive) gastritis is characterized by focal loss of the superficial gastric epithelium (*Fig. 13.3*). Patients develop dyspepsia with vomiting and, occasionally, if the erosions are numerous, hematemesis may occur. This pattern of acute gastritis is caused by shock, stress associated with severe burns or raised intracranial pressure, nonsteroidal anti-inflammatory drugs, and very heavy acute alcohol ingestion.

Severe **necrotizing ulcerative gastritis** follows suicidal ingestion of strong alkalis and acids.

Chronic gastritis has been revealed by endoscopic examination to be more common than formerly thought, and carries a recognized risk of development of malignancy (see page 253). Chronic gastritis leads to mucosal atrophy and intestinal metaplasia.

Three main forms of chronic gastritis are identified

1. *Helicobacter*-**associated gastritis** is the most common form, arising at any age. It is associated with the presence of bacterial colonies of the organism *Helicobacter pylori*. The organisms colonize the surface of the epithelium beneath the thin layer of mucus. The presence of the organisms is associated with epithelial damage and a mixed acute and chronic inflammatory cell reaction in the lamina propria and superficial epithelium. The pyloric antrum is the most severely affected area, but damage is also seen in the fundus. Intestinal metaplasia is frequently seen, in which the normal gastric epithelium is replaced by a type similar to that seen in the small intestine.
   Helicobacter is also very important in the development of duodenal inflammation and ulceration.

2. **Autoimmune chronic gastritis** is associated with an autoimmune disease (**pernicious anemia**) and is generally seen in elderly patients, in whom severe atrophy of the mucosa develops. Those affected have antibodies against gastric parietal cells (90%) and intrinsic factor (60%). The autoimmune damage to the gastric cells is associated with reduced gastric production of hydrochloric acid (hypochlorhydria) and failure of absorption of dietary vitamin B_{12}. The vitamin B_{12} deficiency leads to interference with normal erythropoiesis in the bone marrow, and the patients develop a megaloblastic macrocytic anemia (**pernicious anemia**) (see Chapter 15). This pattern of gastritis particularly affects the body of the stomach.

3. **Reactive gastritis**, also known as chemical or reflux gastritis, occurs when alkaline duodenal fluid (containing bile) refluxes into the lower part of the stomach. It is common in people who have had previous gastric surgery to the pyloric area, which presumably causes incompetence of the pyloric sphincter. However, in most cases, there is no previous history of surgery and the cause of the incompetence is not understood. This pattern of gastritis is also seen with prolonged administration of non-steroidal anti-inflammatory drugs, the common factor probably being direct toxic damage to the mucus layer.

Peptic ulceration and intestinal metaplasia are complications of chronic gastritis

Intestinal metaplasia frequently develops from chronic gastritis (particularly the autoimmune form). The normal gastric pattern of epithelium is replaced by two patterns of metaplastic epithelium: a goblet-cell pattern, similar to that

Fig. 13.3 Acute erosive gastritis. Acute erosive gastritis is shown in the opened stomach. The mucosa appears hyperemic, and the foci of superficial ulceration are manifest as scattered, small red areas termed **erosions**.

Diagnosis of *Helicobacter* infection

1. **Urea breath test.** *Helicobacter* produces the enzyme urease. If radiolabeled urea is administered and *Helicobacter* urease is present, radioactive CO_2 can be detected in the breath.
2. **Serology.** Antibodies to *H. pylori* can be detected in serum.
3. **Histology.** Organisms can be seen in biopsy material, particularly if specially stained.
4. **Culture.** *H. pylori*, a curved microaerophilic organism, can be cultured from biopsy material.

seen in the small intestine, and a mucous cell pattern, similar to that seen in the pyloric antrum.

The importance of small intestinal metaplasia is its predisposition to undergo dysplastic change, with eventual transformation into carcinoma. An important part of the management of chronic gastritis is repeated endoscopic biopsy to detect dysplastic change before the development of malignancy.

Chronic gastritis may also be associated with the development of peptic ulceration, particularly in the presence of *H. pylori* infection.

Peptic ulcers may be acute or chronic

Peptic ulcers are caused by damage to the gastric or duodenal lining by gastric secretions, particularly acid. The vast majority (98%) occur in the first part of the duodenum.

Acute peptic ulcers usually develop from areas of erosive gastritis and are predisposed to by the same conditions as erosive gastritis. There is a strong association with *H. pylori* infection, and these organisms are found in up to 90% of patients with duodenal ulcers and in 70% of cases with gastric ulceration. Indeed, eradication of *H. pylori* infection promotes healing of the ulcers and leads to a reduced incidence of recurrence. Non-steroidal anti-inflammatory drugs (NSAIDs) are a major cause of peptic ulcer disease in patients without *H. pylori* infection, particularly those on long-term medication for chronic rheumatic conditions. Peptic ulcers may cause severe bleeding, heal without scarring, or progress to form a chronic peptic ulcer. Important

causes of acute peptic ulcers are severe stress or shock (e.g. after major trauma or burns), with hypotension; acute hypoxia of the surface epithelium may be an important pathogenic mechanism.

The histology and some of the complications of chronic peptic ulcers are discussed in Chapter 4.

The main sites of chronic peptic ulceration are the lower esophagus (due to gastric reflux), the stomach (*Fig. 13.4*), the duodenum, and gastroenterostomy sites.

The important complications of chronic peptic ulcer are:

- **Hemorrhage**.
- **Penetration**. The ulcer penetrates the full thickness of the stomach or duodenal wall, progressing into adherent underlying tissue, particularly the pancreas or liver. Penetration of the pancreas often manifests clinically as severe back pain.
- **Perforation**. This leads to peritonitis.
- **Fibrous stricture**. This is seen in peptic ulcer of the esophagus; fibrous thickening caused by healing leads to scarring of the esophagus and obstruction. In the stomach, ulcers may cause pyloric stenosis.
- **Malignant change**. This is extremely uncommon.

The most important tumor of the stomach is adenocarcinoma

Gastric adenocarcinoma is more common in men than in women, and is seen in patients over the age of 30, the incidence rising greatly after the age of 50 years.

Peptic ulceration is due to a breakdown of normal mucosal protective mechanisms

The gastric mucosa is normally protected by a mucous barrier containing acid-resisting neutral glycoproteins and buffering bicarbonate ions. Peptic ulceration occurs when protective mechanisms are deficient, and persists because of gastric acid.

In the **esophagus** the most important cause of ulceration is reflux of acid gastric secretions onto the unprotected esophageal mucosa, hypersecretion of acid by the stomach being the most important factor in ulceration of the **duodenum**. In the **stomach** the factors that predispose to peptic ulcers include regurgitated bile in pyloric incompetence, surface epithelial damage by *H. pylori* infection, and surface epithelial damage by non-steroidal anti-inflammatory agents (NSAIDs).

Other factors, such as chronic gastritis, smoking and genetic predisposition, are believed to play a role in the pathogenesis, although the mechanisms are poorly understood.

Fig. 13.4 Chronic peptic ulcer of the stomach. A large chronic peptic ulcer (**U**) is seen in the pylorus of the stomach. Chronic ulcers may be 1–7 cm in diameter, or even larger. They have sharply defined borders without any heaping up of the epithelium surrounding the ulcer crater. The floor of the ulcer is composed of fibrous scar tissue, overlaid by granulation tissue, inflammatory exudate and necrotic slough. The ulcer crater usually penetrates into the muscularis propria of the stomach, and complete healing of the ulcer leads to fibrous replacement of muscle, with regrowth of epithelium over the scar.

There is marked geographic variation in the incidence of gastric cancer; compared to western Europe and North America, it is seen more frequently in the Far East and certain parts of South America and Scandinavia. Because of the great variation in geographical distribution, dietary etiological factors have been sought, but none is firmly proven. Frequent ingestion of smoked and salted preserved foods has been implicated, particularly in the generation of nitrosamines. There is an association with blood group A. Recent studies have suggested a link between the development of gastric carcinoma and infection with *H. pylori*.

Conditions predisposing to the development of gastric carcinoma are chronic atrophic gastritis and gastric adenomatous polyps (see above). At-risk groups include patients with chronic gastritis and intestinal metaplasia, post-gastrectomy patients with persisting gastric inflammation, and patients in families with gastric cancer (rare).

The pathogenesis of gastric carcinoma in the fundus and antrum is believed to follow a sequence from normal mucosa, through chronic gastritis, intestinal metaplasia, dysplasia and intramucosal carcinoma, to invasive carcinoma.

Carcinomas in the cardia are infrequently associated with chronic gastritis and may have another pathogenesis.

Polyps of the stomach must be biopsied

There are several benign polyps of the stomach, all of which are uncommon compared to the incidence of carcinomas of this region. Polyps of the gastric mucosa must always be examined by biopsy to exclude the presence of a carcinoma. The main types are:

- **Hyperplastic polyps** (80–85%) formed by regeneration of mucosa, often at the edge of an ulcer.
- **Fundal polyps** (10%), which are cystic glandular lesions seen mainly in women.
- **Adenomatous polyps** (5%), which are true benign tumors of surface epithelium, ranging up to 5 cm in size. They carry a 25–70% risk of malignant change, but are very rare.
- **Hamartomatous polyps**, which occur in Peutz–Jeghers syndrome.

Other benign tumors of the stomach are derived from mesenchymal tissues, the most common being a leiomyoma. These appear as mucosal or intramural nodules and are usually asymptomatic.

Gastric adenocarcinoma has three main growth patterns

Gastric adenocarcinoma has three recognizable growth patterns: **exophytic**, **flat or depressed**, and **excavated** (*Fig. 13.5*). A further type involves diffuse infiltration of the stomach wall to produce widespread wall thickening. This pattern of spread is known as **linitis plastica** or, in the older literature, 'leather-bottle stomach.'

The **exophytic type** tends to present early because, as well as giving a feeling of gastric discomfort, the polypoid protrusion is traumatized and bleeds. Of the three types, it is the most amenable to surgical excision, and has the best prognosis.

Flat or depressed lesions appear only as an area of effacement of the underlying mucosal pattern, although some advanced lesions can ulcerate.

Excavated tumors mimic peptic ulcers but the margins are typically 'heaped-up' rather than 'punched-out;'

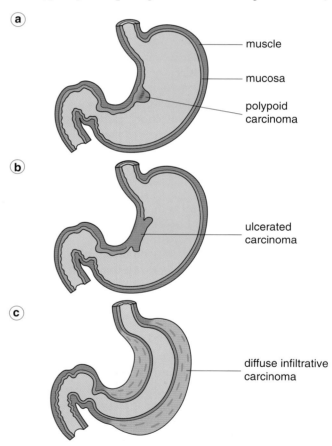

Fig. 13.5 Patterns of carcinoma of the stomach. (a) **Exophytic**. Tumor protrudes into the stomach lumen. (b) **Flat/depressed**. A thickened localized plaque of carcinoma undergoes central ulceration to mimic benign peptic ulcer. (c) **Excavated**. An erosive crater-like lesion is present in the stomach wall. (d) **Diffuse infiltrative**. There is extensive spread of tumor within the mucosa and submucosa, without extensive ulceration. This diffuse infiltration produces a shrunken inexpansible rigid stomach ('linitis plastica' or 'leather-bottle stomach').

however, histological examination is required to differentiate reliably between benign and malignant ulcers.

The **diffuse infiltrative pattern** tends to present very late. The symptoms are usually those of non-specific loss of appetite, and food intolerance due to both the small capacity of the stomach and its inability to distend under a food load. Because surface ulceration is not a prominent feature, hematemesis is not common until the late stage. Metastatic spread to lymph nodes and the liver is usually present at the time of clinical presentation and, of the three types, this pattern has the worst prognosis.

The term **early gastric cancer** has been used to describe tumors that are confined to the mucosa and submucosa. As these lesions may have metastases, the term 'early' can be misleading. Such tumors are generally of the polypoid type and have a better prognosis than other forms.

Histologically, adenocarcinoma of the stomach is divided into two main types. The **intestinal pattern** is composed of gland-like spaces, and the **diffuse infiltrative carcinoma** of the stomach is composed of sheets of anaplastic cells, many of which have a single vacuole of mucin, displacing

Molecular pathology of gastric cancer

Gastric cancer is associated with a number of molecular genetic abnormalities related to oncogenes. It has been proposed that accumulated molecular abnormalities have a role in the evolution of adenocarcinoma of the stomach.

In well-differentiated gastric carcinomas, several abnormalities are commonly documented:

- Inactivation of p53 tumor suppressor gene.
- Activation of *c-met*, a receptor for hepatocyte growth factor.

In poorly differentiated carcinomas there is:

- Amplification of *c-erb-B2*, a receptor-type tyrosine kinase.
- Amplification of *K-sam*, a receptor-type tyrosine kinase.

The significance of these events in relation to prognosis or treatment is still under evaluation.

the nucleus to one side (signet-ring cell). The histological features are shown in *Fig. 13.6*.

Spread of gastric carcinoma is by four main routes

Adenocarcinoma of the stomach spreads by local, lymphatic, hematogenous and transcelomic routes.

- **Direct invasion** through the wall of the stomach leads to involvement of adjacent viscera.
- **Lymphatic spread** (the main route) is to nodes on the greater and lesser curves of the stomach, then to other nodal groups. Involvement of the left supraclavicular nodal group is well recognized (**Virchow's node, Troisier's sign**).
- **Hematogenous spread** to liver, lung and brain is common. Spread to the ovaries leads to development of **Krukenberg tumors** (see page 433).
- **Transcelomic spread** through the peritoneum results in malignant ascites.

The prognosis of gastric adenocarcinoma in most cases is poor. The 5-year survival rate in gastric carcinoma is low and depends on the stage of the tumor. Many tumors are locally advanced at diagnosis and have spread to nodes or metastasized. Prognosis after surgery is 20% 10-year survival for advanced gastric cancer, but 90% 10-year survival for lesions confined to the mucosa and submucosa, as with small polypoid tumors.

Fig. 13.6 Histology of carcinoma of the stomach. (a) Intestinal type. (b) Diffuse type.

Lymphomas, neuroendocrine tumors and sarcomas are uncommon malignant tumors of the stomach

Lymphoma of the stomach accounts for about 3% of gastric tumors. This is an example of a tumor of mucosa-associated lymphoid tissue (MALT), discussed with others in Chapter 15.

Sarcomas of the stomach, which are mainly leiomyosarcomas, account for fewer than 2% of all gastric malignancies. Benign leiomyomas are more common. Derived from the smooth muscle of the stomach wall, these are smooth spherical tumors covered by stretched but intact mucosa.

Neuroendocrine tumors (carcinoid tumors) of the stomach are similar to those seen in the small bowel (see pages 262 and 266).

Gastrointestinal stromal tumors

Gastrointestinal stromal tumors (GIST) are tumors of the gastric submucosa that behave mostly in a benign manner but can show unpredictable malignant potential. The majority of GIST express the *c-kit* gene and some exhibit *PDGFα* mutations. Both of these protein receptors are linked to cytoplasmic tyrosine kinase signaling pathways. The tumors are thus responsive to tyrosine kinase inhibitors, e.g. imatinib (see Blue Box, Chapter 6).

DISEASE OF THE SMALL AND LARGE INTESTINE

Infective disorders of the intestine are common (see also Chapter 8)

Infective disorders of the bowel are common and are due to many classes of organism.

- **Viruses**: rotaviruses cause 50% of infantile diarrhea and account for some adult cases. Caliciviruses (Norwalk viruses) account for 30% of adult and some juvenile cases of gastroenteritis.
- **Bacteria**: some bacteria cause direct damage to the bowel (e.g. *Salmonella typhi* and *Campylobacter jejuni*), whereas others produce enterotoxins (e.g. in salmonellosis and enteropathogenic *Escherichia coli*). Tuberculosis may affect the gut, particularly the terminal ileum. *Yersinia* infection may cause ulceration and ileitis. *Campylobacter* infection is the commonest cause of bacterial diarrhea, mainly affecting the colon.
- **Protozoa**: *Entamoeba histolytica* causes dysentery-like symptoms and is spread by the feco-oral route. *Giardia* causes infection of the small bowel and gives rise to a malabsorption syndrome. *Cryptosporidia* may cause disease, particularly in immunosuppressed patients.
- **Fungi**: infection is virtually restricted to immunosuppressed patients.

- **Helminths**: parasitization of the bowel by helminths is widespread, especially in the tropics. Many of the clinical problems are causes by immune-mediated hypersensitivity causing hypereosinophilia syndromes.

Gastrointestinal infections are common in immunosuppressed patients, particularly those with AIDS. Most patients with AIDS have chronic diarrhea, which can be caused by a wide range of pathogens.

Some bacterial infections cause damage by invasion

Several bacterial infections of the gut cause infection by invasion of the mucosa. Many cause diarrhea with blood and pus in the stool, termed **bacterial dysentery**. The main organisms causing this type of infection are as follows:

- *Campylobacter* invades mucosa in the jejunum, ileum and colon, causing ulceration and acute inflammation.
- *Salmonella typhi*, *S. paratyphi A*, *B*, and *C* are transmitted in food and water contaminated by the feces or urine of a carrier. In *S. typhi* infection organisms initially proliferate in the reticuloendothelial system. A secondary bacteremia develops and Peyer's patches become ulcerated (see *Fig. 8.12*). Patients develop fever, diarrhea, splenomegaly (75%), and a skin rash consisting of rose spots (50%).
- *Shigella* infections are mainly seen in young children. The organism invades mucosa of the colon and distal ileum causing mucosal ulceration, most marked in the sigmoid colon and rectum.
- **Enteroinvasive and enterohemorrhagic** *E. coli* cause a hemorrhagic colitis similar to *Shigella*.

Most cases of **intestinal tuberculosis** are caused by ingestion of bacteria in food (commonly milk from infected cows) or by swallowing infected sputum. The disease particularly affects the terminal ileum and cecum, causing ulceration of the bowel mucosa, fibrous wall thickening and enlargement of regional lymph nodes which develop caseous graulomatous inflammation.

Whipple's disease is a rare condition caused by infection by an actinomycete called *Tropheryma whippelii*, the route of infection being unknown. It is a multisystem disorder affecting Caucasian men in the third and fourth decades with malabsorption due to small bowel involvement, lymphadenopathy, arthritis and CNS symptoms.

Some bacteria produce enterotoxins and cause disease without invasion

Bacterial enterotoxins cause disease in two circumstances. In the first, the toxin is formed in the food before it is eaten, resulting in vomiting and diarrhea about 12 hours after ingestion (e.g. staphylococcal food poisoning). In the second, the bacteria proliferate in the gut after ingestion and produce toxins which then cause intestinal disturbance;

this extra growth stage means that the disease takes about 24 hours to develop after contaminated food is eaten.

Salmonella enteritidis, *S. typhimurium*, *S. hadar* and *S. virchow* produce enterotoxin-induced fluid and electrolyte disturbance. Incubation is 24–48 hours, resulting in an enterocolitis with profuse diarrhea and vomiting lasting about 48 hours.

Vibrio cholerae is acquired through water contaminated with feces. Organisms grow in the small bowel and secrete a toxin which causes uncontrolled cAMP-stimulated secretion of fluid into the gut, producing severe watery diarrhea.

Pseudomembranous enterocolitis is caused by a clostridial toxin causing mucosal necrosis

In pseudomembranous colitis, *Clostridium difficile* overgrowth produces an enterotoxin that results in necrosis of the colonic mucosa. The condition is almost invariably associated with antibiotic therapy, but other diseases of the colon that allow clostridial overgrowth also predispose to its development (gastrointestinal surgery, ischemia, shock, burns). Patients develop fever, abdominal pain and diarrhea.

Important protozoans causing bowel infection are *Giardia*, *Cryptosporidia* and *Entamoeba*

The most important protozoa causing gut infection are:

- *Giardia lamblia*, which is a flagellate protozoan acquired from contaminated water. It infects the duodenum and upper jejunum and may cause diarrhea, abdominal pain, weight loss, or malabsorption.
- *Cryptosporidium parvum*, which is acquired from contaminated water, causing a self-limiting diarrheal illness which may be severe in patients with AIDS.
- *Entamoeba histolytica*, which is acquired through water or food contaminated by cysts and causes amebic colitis.

MALABSORPTION SYNDROMES

The small intestine provides an environment for absorption of nutrients from food. There are four main elements to absorption:

- The pancreas secretes digestive enzymes into the gut lumen, which are necessary for breakdown of macromolecules.
- The liver secretes bile acids needed for solubilization and absorption of fats.
- The mucosa is specialized for absorption: transverse mucosal folds and finger-like villi provide a vast surface area.

- The mucosa is the site of a set of enzymes, located on the brush border, which hydrolyze large molecules for absorption, especially complex sugars (e.g. sucrase and lactase).

Absence of any of these elements leads to impaired digestion of food and malabsorption. This manifests as weight loss, abdominal distension, and loose, bulky stools. If fat is not being absorbed, stools are pale, foul-smelling and characteristically float in water. Anemia is common. The main causes of malabsorption are shown in *Fig. 13.7*.

If the pancreas fails to produce or secrete the hydrolytic enzymes responsible for food breakdown, nutrients are not absorbed. The most common causes are cystic fibrosis, chronic pancreatitis, carcinoma of the pancreas, and pancreatic surgery.

The most important small intestinal cause of malabsorption in the western world is **celiac disease**; in the developing world it is probably severe **parasitic and worm infestation**.

Loss of absorptive surface of the bowel is common and is due to a number of diseases. Extensive resection of the small bowel (e.g. for infarction or Crohn's disease) reduces the absorptive area markedly. Crohn's disease, if very severe, leads to extensive submucosal edema and mucosal flattening, which reduces the surface area for absorption. Disease of the terminal ileum prevents absorption of vitamin B_{12}.

If secretion of bile into the gut is impaired, solubilization of fats cannot take place, resulting in impaired fat absorption. This is also manifest in malabsorption of fat-soluble vitamins A, D, E, and K.

Fig. 13.7 Causes of malabsorption

Common causes

Pancreatic insufficiency (e.g. chronic pancreatitis)
Celiac disease
Resection of ileum
Parasitic infestation of the gut

Less common causes

Resection of stomach
Crohn's disease
Liver disease causing failure of bile secretion into the gut

Uncommon causes

Bacterial overgrowth in blind loops or diverticula
Post-infective malabsorption (tropical sprue)
α-Chain disease
Giardiasis
Disaccharidase deficiency (e.g. lactase)
Abetalipoproteinemia
Intestinal lymphangiectasis
Whipple's disease

Damage to enterocytes in the bowel leads to replacement by cells that lack differentiation and fail to express brush-border enzymes such as lactase or sucrase (**disaccharidase deficiency**). Disaccharides in the diet cannot be broken down, and their presence in the gut causes diarrhea, as well as bacterial overgrowth. This may become manifest after an episode of infective diarrhea.

Congenital lack of disaccharidases is also seen in infants, in the absence of mucosal damage, and is a cause of failure to thrive.

Whipple's disease is a rare but important cause of malabsorption, in which the mucosa is infiltrated by macrophages full of infective actinomycete organisms.

Celiac disease is caused by hypersensitivity to a component of gluten

Celiac disease causes atrophy of small intestinal villi due to an abnormal sensitivity to gluten, a protein in wheat flour (**gluten enteropathy**). The disease can present at any age, and in infants and children it is an important cause of failure to thrive.

Celiac disease is caused by an immune response to the protein gliadin, a component of gluten. There is an increased incidence of disease in first-degree relatives of those affected, and linkage with certain HLA groups has been shown. There is a strong association with possession of the HLA-B8 antigen, a factor also linked with the itchy, blistering skin disease, dermatitis herpetiformis (see page 516), which may occur concurrently with celiac disease. The presence of serum antigliadin antibodies is seen in the majority of cases.

Diagnosis is by biopsy of small bowel mucosa. Histologically the immune-mediated damage causes heavy lympho-cytic infiltrate of lamina propria, and an increase in intraepithelial lymphocytes. There is also loss of villous architecture, ranging from blunting (partial villous atrophy) to complete flattening (total villous atrophy) (*Fig. 13.8*), and an increase in depth of crypts, which produce more epithelial cells to compensate for those lost through damage.

Complete withdrawal of gliadin from the diet (gluten-free diet) leads to gradual recovery of villous structure, which may be partial or complete.

Long-term complications of celiac disease include the development of primary T-cell lymphoma of the small intestine and, rarely, the development of adenocarcinoma.

Post-infective malabsorption histologically resembles celiac disease

Malabsorption may develop in travelers who return from tropical areas, lasting for at least 2 months after an episode of infective diarrhea. There is severe folate and vitamin B_{12} deficiency, as well as weight loss. Investigation reveals crypt

Fig. 13.8 Celiac disease. The normal surface pattern of the jejunal mucosa viewed through the dissecting microscope is shown in (a) as a series of ridges and finger-like projections. In celiac disease the surface becomes flattened, developing a mosaic-like pattern (b).

hyperplastic villous atrophy similar to that seen in celiac disease.

Microbiology shows colonization of the gut lumen by enterobacteria. Other causes of malabsorption in the tropics must be excluded, e.g. intestinal parasites, HIV enteropathy, and tuberculosis.

CHRONIC INFLAMMATORY BOWEL DISEASE

Idiopathic chronic inflammatory bowel diseases show primary inflammation of the intestinal wall

The idiopathic inflammatory bowel diseases, of which there are two main members, have no known cause. In **Crohn's disease** there is a granulomatous inflammatory pattern of disease that affects the full thickness of the bowel wall. It is most common in the terminal ileum, but may affect any part of the gastrointestinal tract in a discontinuous pattern from mouth to anus. With **ulcerative colitis**, a chronic

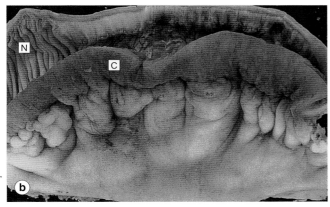

Fig. 13.9 Crohn's disease. The mucosa in Crohn's disease demonstrates a cobblestone pattern (a) as a result of fissured ulcers (**U**) with intervening areas of edematous mucosa (**M**). In (b), compared to normal small bowel wall (**N**) the Crohn's segment (**C**) shows wall thickening that has caused a stenosis.

inflammatory disease of the rectal and colonic mucosa, inflammation may extend proximally from the anus to involve the whole of the colon in continuity. The terminal ileum may also be involved in ulcerative colitis, but this is thought to be due to reflux of cecal inflammation and is known as 'backwash ileitis.' Importantly, both types of inflammatory bowel disease are associated with systemic manifestations outside the intestine.

In diagnosing idiopathic inflammatory bowel disease, infective causes of inflammation have first to be excluded. Investigation is by imaging and biopsy.

Established Crohn's disease has a cobblestone-pattern mucosa

Crohn's disease is more common in women than in men, patients usually being 20–60 years old. It particularly affects the terminal ileum (synonym: **regional ileitis**), but can occur anywhere in the gut, especially in the mouth, colon, and anus. For this reason, Crohn's disease can present as an acute appendicitis and can be confused with tuberculosis

of the cecum in regions where intestinal tuberculosis is endemic.

The macroscopic appearance of the bowel in Crohn's disease varies according to the stage of the disease.

In early disease the affected bowel shows marked swelling of submucosa and mucosa, mainly due to severe submucosal edema. This leads to loss of the pattern of normal transverse folds, and small superficial areas of hemorrhagic ulceration arise which, over time, develop into fissures.

In established chronic disease the bowel mucosa shows a **cobblestone pattern** due to a combination of submucosal edema and interconnecting **deep fissured ulcers** (*Fig. 13.9*). The bowel wall is thickened by edema and fibrosis and, commonly, there is **stricture formation**. Regional lymph nodes usually become enlarged. Disease is not continuous and areas of normal bowel may be present between the diseased segments (**skip lesions**). The normal bowel proximal to a segment of Crohn's disease is often dilated due to partial obstruction. The serosal surface of the bowel is often enveloped by mesenteric adipose tissue, a feature known as '**creeping fat**.'

Crohn's disease shows transmural inflammation with deep fissured ulcers

Crohn's disease is histologically characterized by inflammation of all layers, submucosal edema, ulcers that extend deep into the bowel wall and form fissures, and fibrous scarring. Non-caseating granulomas may be present (*Fig. 13.10*).

Inflammation in Crohn's disease is transmural, and serosal involvement leads to inflammatory adhesion to other loops of bowel, to the parietal peritoneum of the anterior abdominal wall, or to the bladder. Deep penetration of fissured ulcers, which may extend through the full thickness of the bowel wall into the adherent viscus, causes **fistulas** (an

Fig. 13.10 Crohn's disease histology. The inflammation in the wall is composed of lymphoid cells, macrophages and plasma cells. Small non-caseating granulomas (**G**), which occur in about 70% of cases, may be seen in any layer of the bowel, e.g. mucosa.

abnormal connection between two epithelial surfaces lined by granulation tissue) and **sinuses** (an abnormal, blind-ending track arising from an epithelial surface lined by granulation tissue). These are particularly seen in the perianal region.

The direct complications of Crohn's disease are:

- Stricture formation leading to intestinal obstruction.
- Fibrous adhesions leading to intestinal obstruction.
- Perforation of the bowel by the deep fissured ulcers causing intra-abdominal abscesses.
- Perianal fistulas, fissures and abscesses.
- Increased incidence of carcinoma of the bowel after many years.
- Rarely there can be significant bleeding from areas of ulceration.
- Short gut syndrome may develop as a result of multiple bowel resections for strictures etc.

Fig. 13.11 Active ulcerative colitis. In active disease (a) the ulcerated areas (**U**) are hemorrhagic, leading to bloody diarrhea. Intact mucosa remains as islands sitting above areas of ulceration (pseudopolyps). Histology of the intact mucosa (b) shows edema and an increase in numbers of lymphoid cells and plasma cells in lamina propria (**L**). Neutrophils are seen in lamina propria as well as in gland epithelium. Neutrophils migrate through the walls of glands to form collections, termed **crypt abscesses** (**A**), in the gland lumen. There is depletion of goblet cells and mucin from gland epithelium.

The natural history of Crohn's disease is one of remissions and relapses of inflammation, punctuated by complications caused by bowel disease. Surgery is often required to relieve intestinal obstruction and to close fistulas. Crohn's disease is also characterized by systemic complications similar to those seen in ulcerative colitis (see below).

Ulcerative colitis affects the rectum and variable amounts of colon

Ulcerative colitis starts at the rectum (proctitis) and may extend for a variable distance around the colon. In the most

Etiology of ulcerative colitis

The etiology of ulcerative colitis is unknown, but several hypotheses have been advanced, none of which is fully substantiated.

- **Psychosomatic cause**. Stress is believed to exacerbate disease in some individuals.
- **Infective cause**. Some evidence suggests that adhesive forms of enteropathogenic *E. coli* may trigger episodes of inflammation.
- **Immunological cause**. Lymphoid cells participate in inflammation.

Autoantibodies and immune complexes have been reported in some cases, but their role is uncertain. Steroids are effective in treatment of disease, suggesting that immune activation is important.

A unifying explanation is that some sort of infection triggers an inappropriate autoimmune response, which leads to destruction of colonic mucosa.

Involvement of the appendix as a 'skip lesion' in ulcerative colitis suggests that the appendix may represent an antigen-presenting site for distal luminal antigens.

Systemic complications of ulcerative colitis

- Erythema nodosum.
- Pyoderma gangrenosum.
- Iritis, uveitis, episcleritis
- Arthropathy of large joints, ankylosing spondylitis.
- Sacroiliitis.
- Ankylosing spondylitis.
- Chronic liver disease (4%).

extensive disease the whole colonic mucosa is affected. Patients typically develop diarrhea, the feces being mixed with blood, mucus and pus.

There are three clinical patterns of disease:

1. In **active acute disease** the mucosa in the rectum and affected colon shows areas of shallow ulceration, which become confluent (*Fig. 13.11*). In contrast with Crohn's disease, ulceration does not extend through the muscularis mucosae, and inflammation is limited to the mucosa and lamina propria.
2. In **chronic quiescent or treated disease** ulceration is not prominent and the mucosa appears red, granular, and thinned. Biopsy reveals chronic inflammation.
3. In **fulminant active disease** the colon shows extensive confluent mucosal ulceration. Edema and inflammation extend into the muscle layer of the colon, which progressively dilates (toxic dilatation – 'acute toxic megacolon').

Ulcerative colitis is complicated by bleeding and the risk of development of fulminant disease

Ulcerative colitis has local as well as systemic effects. The direct local complications of ulcerative colitis include blood and fluid loss from extensive ulceration, both of which may be severe. Acute disease may progress rapidly to toxic dilatation and perforation and, in long-standing disease, dysplasia and neoplastic change may occur.

The systemic complications of ulcerative colitis are listed in the blue box on page 260.

In some patients, ulcerative colitis is associated with migratory polyarthritis, sacroiliitis, ankylosing spondylitis, uveitis, erythema nodosum, and primary sclerosing cholangitis.

The natural history of ulcerative colitis can be divided into three main patterns:

- 10% of patients develop severe disease requiring early surgery.
- 10% of patients have persistent active disease despite treatment.
- 80% of patients have chronic quiescent colitis with infrequent episodes of relapse.

In establishing a diagnosis, ulcerative colitis must be distinguished from infective colitis, Crohn's disease, ischemic colitis, and proctitis caused by sexually transmitted diseases.

Long-standing extensive ulcerative colitis predisposes to colon cancer

In chronic ulcerative colitis, regenerative changes in the rectal mucosa lead to the development of dysplasia and to a risk of development of carcinoma of the colon (see pages 262–5), which is related to extent of disease (high risk for total colitis) and duration of illness (high risk for disease of over 10 years' duration). Patients in whom disease is limited

Comparison of clinical and histopathological features in ulcerative colitis and Crohn's disease

Feature	Crohn's disease	Ulcerative colitis
Involvement	Entire GI tract	Colon/rectum
Inflammation	Transmural	Mucosal
Disease pattern	Skip lesions	Continuous
Mucosal appearances	Cobblestone	Pseudopolyps
Strictures	Common due to scarring	Rare
Fissures	Common	None
Mucosal ulceration	Deep, fissured	Mucosal only
Granulomas	Yes	No
Bowel wall	Thickened wall Narrow lumen	Thin wall Dilated lumen
Serosal appearances	Creeping fat	Normal
Adhesions	Multiple due to fissuring inflammation and repeated surgery	None
MHC Class II	HLA-DR1/DQw5	HLA-DR2
Cancer risk	Raised	High
Complications	Short gut syndrome Fistula formation Bowel perforation Stricture formation	Haemorrhage Electrolyte loss Toxic megacolon Systemic effects See Blue Box (page 260)

to the left side of the colon are at small risk of developing cancer.

It has been recommended that all patients over the age of 50 with total colitis should have regular screening colonoscopy every 2 years, and rectal biopsy every 6 months, to detect dysplastic changes.

Symptomatic relief and reduction in cancer risk can be obtained by total colectomy with or without ileal (Parke's) pouch formation. Rectal surveillance, however, remains essential because cancer can still arise in the rectal stump.

TUMORS OF THE SMALL AND LARGE INTESTINE

Primary tumors of the small intestine are rare

The small intestine rarely develops primary tumors, but among those that do arise are **stromal tumors**; in particular, leiomyoma or lipoma may develop in the small bowel wall. Malignant smooth-muscle tumors (leiomyosarcomas) may also occur. An important complication of smooth-muscle or lipomatous tumors of the small intestinal wall is intussusception (see pages 272–3).

Carcinoid (neuroendocrine) tumors, derived from the neuroendocrine cells in the small intestinal crypts, are most common in the jejunum and ileum (see page 266).

Malignant lymphomas, derived from mucosa-associated lymphoid tissue of the small bowel, are usually B-cell lymphomas. Celiac disease is a major predisposing factor in T-cell lymphomas in the small bowel. Tumors may be multifocal, and spread is to local lymph nodes.

Primary adenocarcinoma of the small bowel is very rare. It usually presents as an ulcerating strictured lesion, producing small bowel obstruction. An occasional site for adenocarcinomas in the small intestine is the ampulla of Vater, the point at which the biliary and pancreatic drainage enters the duodenum.

Tumors of the large bowel are extremely common

The colon and rectum are frequently affected by both benign and malignant tumors.

Fig. 13.12 Patterns of colonic adenoma. (a) and (b) Tubular adenomata (**A**) are rounded lesions, 0.5–2 cm in size. They are generally red and sit on a stalk (**S**) of normal mucosa, which has been dragged up by traction of the polyp in the bowel lumen. Histologically they are composed of tubular-shaped glands. (c) Villous adenomata are frond-like lesions, about 0.6 cm thick, which occupy a broad area of mucosa, generally 1–5 cm in diameter. Rare lesions occupy very large areas of the whole circumference of the bowel. They have a velvety red appearance and, histologically, are composed of finger-like epithelial projections. (d) Tubulovillous adenomata are raised lesions, generally 1–4 cm in size. They are red and sit on a stalk of normal mucosa. Histologically they show a component identical to that of the tubular adenoma but also have a surface villous pattern that occupies between 25% and 50% of the lesion. This distinction is arbitrary as many tubular adenomata have a minor villous pattern but, by convention, are excluded from this category. Likewise, villous lesions may have a significant tubular pattern, but are excluded from a tubulovillous category if more than 50% of the lesion is villous.

- The most important and common tumors are derived from the surface epithelium of the bowel, forming **adenomata** and **carcinomas** of the colon.
- **Hyperplastic polyps** are small, flat, pale lesions, typically 5 mm in size, which occur most commonly in the rectum and sigmoid colon. They are considered to be a regenerative phenomenon and are non-neoplastic.
- **Hamartomatous polyps** occur in childhood and adolescence.
- **Neuroendocrine tumors** (carcinoid tumors) of the large bowel occur, similar to those seen in the small bowel (see page 266).
- **Lymphomas** of the large bowel may arise, particularly in the ileocecal region, but are uncommon.
- **Stromal tumors** derived from smooth muscle, adipose tissue or Schwann cells occur, but are uncommon.

Adenomata of the large bowel appear as polyps

Adenomata derived from the glandular epithelium of the large bowel manifest as one of three different patterns of polyp (*Fig. 13.12*), categorized as **tubular**, **villous** or **tubulovillous**. Such polyps are important because they frequently develop into a carcinoma. There is much evidence to suggest that most carcinomas of the colon develop from previous adenomata, and the well-established progression from adenoma to carcinoma is the basis of the **polyp–cancer sequence** for development of carcinoma of the colon. The risk of malignant change is greatest where large lesions are present.

Adenocarcinoma of the colon is common and may be sporadic or hereditary

Carcinoma of the colon is a most common cause of death from neoplasia. These tumors are adenocarcinomas derived from the glandular epithelium of the large bowel mucosa.

The epidemiology of carcinoma of the colon shows great geographic variation, which has been related to environ-

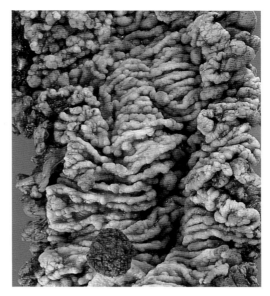

Fig. 13.13 Polyposis coli. In polyposis coli huge numbers of adenomatous polyps develop in the large bowel. They range from a few millimeters to several centimeters in size.

mental factors rather than genetic factors in local populations. Although there has been great interest in the role of dietary fats, fibre, processed sugar, and bile acids, none has been conclusively shown to be important in pathogenesis.

At the current level of knowledge there appear to be three types:

- Adenocarcinoma associated with familial adenomatous polyposis (FAP).
- Hereditary non-polyposis colorectal carcinoma (HNPCC).
- Sporadic colon cancer.

Carcinoma of the colon has a peak incidence in those aged between 60 and 70 years, and is rare under the age of 40. When young individuals develop the disease, inflammatory bowel disease or a genetic predisposition should be suspected.

Fig. 13.14 Inherited polyposis syndromes

Name	Clinical features	Carcinoma risk
Familial adenomatous polyposis	Adenomata in colon and rectum	High risk of carcinoma
Gardner's syndrome	Adenomata in colon, rectum, as well as small bowel Osteomas of bones Soft tissue tumors	High risk of carcinoma
Peutz–Jeghers syndrome	Hamartomas in small bowel, colon, and stomach Pigmented lesions around the mouth	Small risk of carcinoma

Familial adenomatous polyposis (FAP) is an important predisposing factor to colon cancer development

Familial adenomatous polyposis is a rare autosomal dominant condition in which large numbers of adenomatous polyps develop in the colon and rectum (*Fig. 13.13*). They may begin to develop in childhood, and by the age of 30–40 years there are hundreds, of varying sizes, throughout the entire length of colon and rectum. Inevitably, by the time the patient is aged 45 one or more of these many polyps will have converted into an invasive adenocarcinoma. Hence patients with this condition develop adenocarcinomas (often multiple) on average 20–30 years before the sporadic cases. Development of adenocarcinoma can only be prevented by a policy of frequent surveillance, with removal of the entire colon at an appropriate time.

FAP and other forms of inherited polyposis syndromes are listed in *Fig. 13.14*.

FAP has been found to be associated with a mutation in a tumor suppressor gene located on the long arm of chromosome 5 (5q21); this is known as the APC gene (adenomatous polyposis coli gene) and mutations can be detected in screening programs to provide early diagnosis before the polyps form.

Hereditary non-polyposis colorectal cancer (HNPCC) is much more common than FAP-associated cancer

This condition is also inherited in an autosomal dominant fashion, and is associated with an increased incidence of adenocarcinomas in the ovary, endometrium, and stomach. Around 90% of carriers will develop colon cancer in their lifetime and, as with FAP-associated colon cancer, the tumors develop on average 20–30 years before the sporadic cases. It is much more common than FAP, and estimates of the frequency in the USA range from 1% to 5%. The colon cancers that develop in patients with this inherited tendency are often poorly differentiated and highly aggressive, with a tendency to produce large quantities of extracellular mucin ('mucoid adenocarcinoma').

Currently, five gene mutations have been identified in this condition, all involving DNA mismatch repair genes. The two most important are mutations in *hMSH2* on chromosome 2p (6%) and *hMLH1* on chromosome 3p (30%). Screening for these and the three other, rarer, gene mutations in people with a strong family history of colorectal cancer enables carriers to be identified and placed under regular surveillance to detect colorectal abnormalities at an early stage.

Even 'sporadic' colon cancer may have a genetic basis

Studies on sporadic colon cancers show a mixture of gene abnormalities. For example, 35–65% of non-hereditary colon cancers show allelic loss of 5q21 (APC gene), and another gene, MCC (mutated in colorectal carcinoma), which is a tumor suppressor, is inactivated in 15% of tumors. These gene abnormalities are noted at the 'early adenoma' stage in the adenoma–carcinoma sequence, and it is believed that a further series of gene abnormalities, e.g. activation of *K-ras* oncogene, deletion of p53 tumor suppressor, etc, eventually lead to the development of invasive carcinoma. Mutations in mismatch repair genes (MMR) are also often detected in sporadic colon cancer cases.

Colorectal carcinoma has several morphological patterns

There are several well-recognized morphological types of carcinoma of the colon and rectum, each associated with different clinical patterns of presentation. The main presenting features are attributable to obstruction (colicky abdominal pain and distension with later vomiting) or blood loss (acute or chronic bleeding leading to the development of anemia).

Fig. 13.15 Morphology of adenocarcinoma of the colon.
Macroscopically carcinomas are raised red lesions (L) with a rolled edge (a) and frequent central ulceration. Lesions are composed of solid, white tissue, and invasion into the wall of the bowel may be seen. Histologically (b), the majority of lesions have a glandular pattern composed of pleomorphic neoplastic epithelial cells.

- 50% of tumors occur in the rectum and sigmoid.
- 30% of tumors occur in the cecum and right colon.
- 20% of tumors occur in the descending and transverse colon.

Because the feces are fluid in the right side of the colon, a lesion may grow to a large size before causing obstruction. **Carcinomas of the right side** are mainly large, polypoid exophytic lesions, which grow into the lumen of the bowel. **Carcinomas of the left side** cause obstruction early because the feces are more solid. Left-sided lesions are of two main types: annular carcinomas, which are small but cause stenosis; and ulcerating tumors, which present mainly with bleeding.

The macroscopic and histological appearances of colorectal carcinoma are shown in *Fig. 13.15*. On the basis of cytological and architectural features, lesions can be graded from well differentiated through to poorly differentiated. As poorly differentiated lesions frequently present at an advanced stage they are associated with a poorer prognosis. Lesions that display a vigorous lymphocytic inflammatory response at the invasive edge of the tumor are thought to have a better prognosis than lesions with no host response.

Spread of carcinoma of the colon is by three main routes. There is **local spread** through the bowel wall, when invasion of the serosa of adjacent bowel or bladder may occur; **lymphatic spread** to draining nodes; and **blood spread** to the liver and other sites such as lung.

Infiltrative carcinoma of the colon is a rare pattern caused by signet-ring cell carcinoma that is virtually identical to that seen in the stomach. It is often associated with carcinoma that develops in association with inflammatory bowel disease.

The prognosis of carcinoma of the colon is related to stage

The most significant prognostic indicator is the extent of spread (stage) of the tumor at the time of histological examination. The TNM classification is now the most commonly applied method of staging in colorectal cancer, but Dukes' staging is still used by some surgeons. Both are given for comparison in *Fig. 13.16*.

The spread of cancer is described in relation to depth of invasion through the various histological subdivisions of the bowel wall, adjacent organs, and organs distant to the site of tumor (T). Tis refers to carcinoma in situ, where only the mucosa is involved and the tumor has not spread beyond the muscularis mucosa.

The resection specimen is then carefully searched to find as many lymph nodes as possible in the pericolic fat and the mesentery. The number of nodes containing tumor deposits on histological examination are then documented (N).

Finally the surgeon's observations at the time of surgery and staging radiology are examined to detect any distant metastasis (M). The TNM scores are then combined to give a pathological stage, as shown in *Fig. 13.16*.

Following surgical resection, it is particularly important to determine the adequacy of resection margins, particularly lateral extension to pelvic side wall or adjacent structures, which is associated with a poor outcome.

Modern surgical techniques and advances in chemoradiotherapy are improving these survival times, but the most important factor is to detect the cancer early, thereby allowing complete surgical resection to be achieved.

TNM staging of colorectal cancers

Tumor (T)

0 =	None evident
is =	in situ carcinoma
1 =	invasion of the submucosa
2 =	invasion of the muscularis propria
3 =	invasion of the subserosa
4 =	invasion of adjacent structures

Lymph nodes (N)

0 =	None evident
1 =	1–3 positive pericolic nodes
2 =	4 or more positive pericolic nodes
3 =	any positive node with named blood vessel

Distant metastasis (M)

0 =	None evident
1 =	Any distant metastasis

STAGE	TNM	5-year survival	Duke's
0	Tis, N0, M0		
I	T1–2, N0, M0	93%	A
IIA	T3, N0, M0	85%	B
IIB	T4, N0, M0	72%	B
IIIA	T1–2, N1, M0	83%	C
IIIB	T3–4, N1, M0	64%	C
IIIC	Any T, N2, M0	44%	C
IV	Any T, Any N, M1	8%	(D)

Fig. 13.16 TNM staging of colorectal carcinoma. The first step in staging a colorectal cancer is to provide a TNM score by examining the surgical resection specimen. The TNM scores are then combined to give a pathological stage. Dukes' stages are given for comparison.

Molecular pathology of colonic epithelial neoplasms

As with many tumors, a sequence of molecular events in oncogenes has been identified in colonic epithelial malignancies that seems to relate to progression of lesions from adenomata through to invasive carcinomas. Adenomata show few molecular changes, whereas advanced carcinomas have many oncogene abnormalities.

This is referred to as the adenoma–carcinoma sequence, in which the progressive genetic defects are detailed below:

- Loss of the APC gene on chromosome 5q21 leading to upregulation of β-catenin.
- K-RAS on chromosome 12p12 is activated.
- Loss of p53 from chromosome 17p.
- Loss of DCC gene (deleted in colon cancer), a tumor suppressor gene, from chromosome 18q21.

In the above adenoma–carcinoma sequence, the APC/β-catenin pathway accounts for up to 80% of sporadic carcinomas. APC loss leads to upregulation of the activity of β-catenin, which in turn leads to increased cell cycle entry.

A second pathway involves dysfunction of DNA mismatch repair genes and accounts for approximately 15% of sporadic carcinomas. Currently, five gene mutations have been identified in this condition, all involving DNA mismatch repair genes. The two most important are mutations in *hMSH2* on chromosome 2p and *hMLH1* on chromosome 3p.

Loss of mismatch repair genes leads to microsatellite instability (MSI), which in turn leads to inappropriate cell cycle entry and defects in the apoptotic pathway.

Mutations in DCC give rise to familial adenomatous polyposis (FAP) and the Gardner syndrome.

Mutations in mismatch repair genes give rise to hereditary non-polyposis colon carcinoma (HNPCC).

Neuroendocrine tumors occur throughout the gut

Tumors derived from the neuroendocrine cells of the gut (carcinoid tumors) occur most commonly in the appendix and small bowel, but also arise in the stomach, colon, rectum, and esophagus. The biological behavior of the tumor appears to differ according to the site.

Lesions in the small bowel, colon and stomach are slow-growing, low grade, and malignant (*Fig. 13.17*). Some are multicentric. Tumors appear as yellow mucosal or mural masses, and metastasis is most commonly via the portal vein to the liver.

Lesions in the rectum and appendix almost never metastasize, appearing as tumor nodules composed of firm, yellow tissue.

A small proportion of lesions in the esophagus appear as small-cell anaplastic carcinomas that are histologically identical to oat-cell carcinoma of the lung.

Depending on the nature of the neuroendocrine cells in the tumor, patients may develop a syndrome caused by hormone secretion. Some of these tumors secrete 5-hydroxytryptamine (5-HT), and its breakdown product, 5-hydroxyindolacetic acid (5-HIAA), can be detected in excess in the urine. A primary carcinoid in the gut will secrete those substances into the hepatic portal vein to the liver, where they are broken down and rendered inactive. However, when there is metastatic spread to the liver, this detoxification is by-passed, and symptoms occur when the secretions enter the systemic circulation. Hepatic metastasis

Fig. 13.17 Neuroendocrine tumor of the gut. This is a carcinoid tumor of the ileum. It appears as a yellowish-white mural nodule, and in this instance caused intestinal obstruction. Histologically tumors are composed of cords and nests of cells that contain neurosecretory granules best detected by immunochemical and ultrastructural techniques.

can therefore produce the carcinoid syndrome, with symptoms due to excessive secretion of 5-HT (particularly facial flushing, bronchospasm and diarrhea). Tumors secreting gastrin may stimulate excess gastric acid secretion, causing peptic ulceration (Zollinger–Ellison syndrome).

VASCULAR DISEASE OF THE BOWEL

Vascular diseases of the intestine may affect small or large bowel

Interruption of the blood supply to the small bowel is most commonly seen in elderly patients with severe atherosclerosis. The arterial occlusion can be due to:

- **Emboli from intracardiac thrombosis**. E.g., mural thrombus following a myocardial infarct, thrombotic vegetations on mitral or aortic valves, or left atrial thrombosis. The emboli lodge in branches of the superior mesenteric artery, which supplies the entire small intestine apart from the first part of the duodenum. The extent of the bowel infarction depends upon whether the occlusion is in a proximal or distal branch (*Fig. 13.18*).

Fig. 13.18 Small bowel infarction. This segment of small bowel was surgically resected after infarction caused by an embolus from mural thrombus in the heart. The infarcted bowel is dilated and almost black in color.

- **Thrombosis in severely atherosclerotic mesenteric artery**. This is less common than embolic occlusion, but when it occurs it is usually located in the proximal part of the superior mesenteric artery, shortly after its origin from the aorta; the small bowel infarction is extensive and usually fatal.
- **Venous infarction due to strangulation**. Venous infarction results from occlusion of the thin-walled veins draining blood from the small bowel, and is usually due to extrinsic pressure. The bowel becomes deeply congested with venous blood, which is unable to drain out. This, in turn, prevents entry of oxygenated arterial blood, so that ischemic necrosis of the bowel wall ensues. In the small intestine this pattern of venous infarction due to strangulation results from strangulation of a loop of bowel in a narrow **hernial sac** (*Fig. 13.19*), **intussusception** (*Fig. 13.25*) or, occasionally, **volvulus**. In volvulus a loop of bowel twists on itself, usually in association with fibrous peritoneal adhesions which, in turn, are usually the result of previous abdominal surgery.

Fig. 13.19 Necrosis of bowel wall in hernia. A segment of small bowel has been entrapped in a hernial sac. It has been strangulated, undergoing ischemic discoloration and incipient necrosis.

Fig. 13.20 Sigmoid volvulus. This patient died as a result of twisting of the sigmoid colon causing venous congestion and necrosis. The affected sigmoid is greatly dilated and a dark plum color as a result of venous infarction.

- **Neonatal necrotizing enterocolitis** is discussed on page 272.

In the colon, acute ischemia is usually the result of volvulus, particularly in the sigmoid colon, where there is a large redundant sigmoid loop which twists upon itself to produce torsion of the mesentery (*Fig. 13.20*); volvulus of the cecum is usually secondary to a highly mobile cecum.

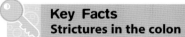

Key Facts
Strictures in the colon

The main causes of narrowing of the colon, resulting in a stricture are:

- Carcinoma of the colon.
- Diverticular disease.
- Ischemic fibrosis caused by ischemic colitis.

Chronic ischemic large bowel disease is most common in the elderly, but can occasionally occur in young people. Ischemic loss of the mucosa produces ulceration in the acute phase, and healing is followed by submucosal fibrosis and disruption of the fibers of the muscularis mucosae. There is frequently a chronic inflammatory infiltrate in the submucosa, in which macrophages filled with hemosiderin are a common feature. These features form the entity known as **ischemic colitis**. Fibrosis at the site of ischemia may result in stricture formation. The most common site is around the splenic flexure, at the overlap between vascular territories.

Localized ischemia in the rectal mucosa may be produced in the **mucosal prolapse syndrome** or **solitary ulcer syndrome**. Mucosal prolapse into the anal sphincter causes ischemic damage to the mucosa.

Angiodysplasia is a cause of large intestinal bleeding

Angiodysplasia is a condition in which abnormal vascular channels develop in the submucosa of the large bowel. The condition occurs in the elderly and is a cause of either occult or massive intestinal bleeding.

Clinical diagnosis is based on suspicion and is confirmed by angiography. Surgical resection of the affected bowel segment is required for treatment, and pathological diagnosis is assisted by radiographic examination of specimens after perfusion of vessels with contrast medium.

DISEASES CAUSED BY ABNORMAL GUT MOTILITY

Diverticular disease results in mucosal outpouching in the distal colon

Diverticular disease causes herniation of the mucosa of the colon through the muscularis propria, producing outpouching of the bowel lumen. There is thickening of the muscularis propria (*Fig. 13.21*).

Complications are related to stagnation of contents of the diverticula, with secondary inflammation. Acute diverticulitis is the result of acute inflammation of a diverticulum. Hemorrhage may result or the diverticulum may rupture, leading to peritonitis or the development of a paracolic abscess.

Chronic inflammation may occur, with walling-off of an area of inflammation by fibrous tissue. The resulting scarring and inflammatory changes form a **diverticular mass**, which may cause large bowel obstruction and may mimic the appearances of a carcinoma of the colon on imaging.

The pathogenesis of diverticular disease has been related to abnormally high intraluminal pressure in the colon, caused by abnormal contractility of the muscularis propria. The abnormal contractility is responsible for the muscle hypertrophy. Mucosal herniation occurs at sites of penetration of the muscularis propria by blood vessels supplying the colon, along lines between the tenia coli (longitudinal muscle layers).

Intestinal pseudo-obstruction is caused by defective bowel motility

Intestinal pseudo-obstruction is manifest by abdominal pain and distension, and is caused by abnormal gut motility rather than an organic obstructive lesion.

- Primary causes, which are rare, are due to abnormalities of smooth muscle or nerve plexuses in the gut.
- Secondary causes are common and include connective tissue diseases, particularly scleroderma, diabetic neuropathy, and amyloidosis of the gut.

Melanosis coli is associated with chronic laxative use

Patients who take laxatives for constipation sometimes develop black coloration of the mucosa of the large bowel, termed 'melanosis coli.' Histologically this is seen as accumulation of pigment-laden macrophages in the lamina propria of the colon (*Fig. 13.22*).

Fig. 13.21 Diverticular disease. In diverticular disease, the outpouchings of mucosa seen in the sigmoid colon appear as slit-like openings (arrows) from the mucosal surface of the opened bowel (a). On sectioning the bowel (b), the diverticula (**D**) extend through the thickened muscularis propria (**M**).

Fig. 13.22 Melanosis coli. In melanosis coli the bowel mucosa is macroscopically black. Histologically there is accumulation of brown pigment in macrophages in the lamina propria. The pigment is *not* melanin but rather a form of lipofuscin.

PATHOLOGY OF THE APPENDIX

Acute appendicitis results in severe acute inflammation of the appendix

Acute appendicitis is a common cause of abdominal pain. A predisposing factor is obstruction of the lumen of the appendix, sometimes by a fecolith, but such obstruction is not seen in all cases. The stages in the development of acute appendicitis are shown in *Fig. 13.23.*

The complications of acute appendicitis are:

- Necrosis of appendix wall (**gangrenous appendicitis**), leading to perforation, with subsequent generalized peritonitis.
- Involvement of adjacent bowel loops, causing perforation of small bowel.
- The omentum may become adherent, localizing the peritonitis to the right iliac fossa. Fibrosis and continued inflammation cause the development of a mass in the right iliac fossa (**appendix mass**). This may resolve with scarring, may form an abscess that drains to the surface, or may rupture, with the development of generalized peritonitis.
- Spread of infection by portal vein branches may propagate to the liver; this was formerly an important cause of portal pyemic abscesses in the liver.

Mucocele of the appendix is caused by obstruction of the lumen

A mucocele of the appendix is cystic dilatation of the appendix lumen, which contains clear mucus. There is fibrosis in the wall, and the lining is replaced by a layer of mucin-secreting goblet cells. This is caused by blockage of the proximal end of the appendix, most commonly the result of a previous episode of acute appendicitis.

Fig. 13.23 Acute appendicitis. In early acute appendicitis (a) there is acute inflammation of the mucosa of the appendix which undergoes ulceration (**U**). Pus (**P**) may be present in the lumen. At this stage the patient experiences an ill-defined central abdominal pain.

Macroscopically (b) the appendix, (this specimen taken from one of the authors), is usually swollen and serosal vessels are dilated. As the acute inflammation develops (c), it spreads through the full thickness of the appendix wall (**W**) to reach the serosal surface (**S**). This causes a localized acute peritonitis, which is perceived as a sharp pain, localized to the right iliac fossa. Macroscopically the appendix shows dilated serosal vessels and a rough, yellow, fibrinous exudate in the surface.

If the appendicitis progresses (d), there is necrosis of the wall (**W**) of the appendix (**gangrenous appendicitis**). The muscle layer is replaced by an acute inflammatory infiltrate and necrotic muscle. The resulting weakness leads to appendix perforation, liberating bowel contents into the peritoneal cavity. This causes a generalized peritonitis and leads to a severe deterioration in clinical condition. Macroscopically the appendix is typically plum-colored or black, and a site of perforation may be seen.

Tumors of the appendix are uncommon

Adenocarcinoma of the appendix is rare. However, adenocarcinoma of the cecum that extends into the proximal part of the appendix is not infrequent, and may be a cause of acute appendicitis in the elderly.

Carcinoid tumors may occur at the tip of the appendix and have an excellent prognosis, almost never metastasizing, mainly because of early detection.

An appendix mass may be caused by several disease processes

A mass localized to the region of the right iliac fossa and involving the ileum, cecum and appendix may be caused by several disease processes.

- **Inflammatory mass**
- Acute appendicitis
- *Yersinia* infection
- Ileocecal *Actinomyces* infection
- Ileocecal tuberculosis
- **Tumor mass**
- Cecal carcinoma
- Lymphoma
- Carcinoid tumor

DISEASES OF THE ANAL CANAL

The anal canal is lined by non-keratinizing squamous mucosa and opens to the exterior at the anal orifice, where the squamous epithelium becomes skin with keratinizing epidermis and skin appendages such as hair follicles and sweat glands.

Itching ('pruritus ani') and soreness are common anal symptoms in family practice

There are many causes of an itching anus, many of which are the result of skin diseases such as eczema and contact dermatitis affecting the anal region. An allergic reaction to topical applications such as anesthetic creams, deodorants, etc. is a common cause in adults, and these may also cause soreness and weeping of the skin. In children, itching and soreness around the anus should always raise suspicion of pinworm infestation (see page 138); the tiny worms may be visible on the perianal skin, particularly at night. Perianal soreness is a common transient symptom following acute diarrhea, but only persistent soreness requires medical investigation. Rare skin diseases such as Hailey–Hailey disease etc. may also occur in perianal skin, and often present as sore, swollen, red and weeping skin. These may be the presenting symptoms of anal fissures and fistulas. Soreness and pain are the symptoms of the most common

anal problem, **hemorrhoids**, which are due to varicose dilatation of the submucosal venous plexuses in the anal canal with prolapse, often producing tender palpable masses that protrude through the anus. Thrombosis in these is often associated with acute pain.

Infections may involve either perianal skin or the anal canal

In the perianal skin, the most common infections are fungal, mainly *Candida*, usually by local extension of candidal infection of the vulva and perineum, particularly in diabetic women. Infection with human papilloma virus may produce perianal fleshy warts (condyloma acuminata); the highly infectious fleshy perianal warts due to *Treponema pallidum* infection in secondary syphilis are now rarely seen.

The commonest cause of infection inside the anal canal is as the result of sexually transmitted diseases, mainly in homosexual men. Gonorrhea and amebic infections are important in this group, and primary syphilitic chancres still occasionally occur.

Infection occurring in a perianal gland, the drainage neck of which is blocked, may eventually lead to a large pus-filled **ischiorectal abscess** that requires drainage.

Anal fissure and anal fistula are common and important causes of persistent anal pain and discharge

An anal fissure is a triangular area of ulceration and inflammation at the lower end of the anal canal, mainly involving the anal mucosa, although associated inflammation may spread to the perianal skin. They are mostly located in the posterior half of the anus. Pain is particularly severe on defecation. In most cases the cause is not known, and the histological features are those of chronic ulceration with inflammation.

An anal fistula is an abnormal tract running between the anal canal at the pectinate line, passing through the perianal tissues and either ending as a blind tract in the perianal connective tissue or opening to the exterior at the perianal skin. The tract is surrounded by severe chronic inflammation, and parts of the fistula tract may contain remnants of inflamed epithelium. Again, pain is most severe on defecation.

Crohn's disease involving the colon is an important cause of both persistent anal fissure and anal fistula; anal involvement also occurs where the disease is limited to the small bowel, but it is far less common. In cases where fissure and fistula are due to Crohn's disease, the diagnosis can sometimes be made histologically by the presence of giant cell histiocytic granulomas in the chronic inflammatory tissue nearby, but foreign body giant cells are also often found when the lesions are not associated with Crohn's disease; the presence of distinct well-formed granulomas is the characteristic feature of Crohn's, not just the presence of giant cells.

The commonest tumor of the anus is squamous cell carcinoma

Squamous carcinomas at the anus may originate either in the perianal skin (in which case they are usually well differentiated and keratinizing) or from the lining of the anal canal (when they may be non-keratinizing and less well differentiated). Perianal skin carcinomas are more common in men, and tend to metastasize to inguinal lymph nodes, whereas squamous carcinomas of the anal canal are most common in women and spread to superior hemorrhoidal and lateral pelvic wall lymph nodes, as well as spreading locally into the soft tissues around the anal canal.

Carcinoma in situ of the perianal skin (**anal intraepithelial neoplasia – AIN**) presents as a red, scaly or weeping patch in perianal skin: it often represents local extension from similar intraepithelial neoplasia affecting the perineum and vulva (VIN – see page 415). Extramammary Paget's disease (adenocarcinoma cells invading the epidermis – see page 446) may also affect perianal skin, and clinically resembles AIN.

PATHOLOGY OF THE PERITONEUM

Peritonitis may be acute or chronic

Inflammation of the peritoneal cavity (peritonitis) may be acute or chronic. Acute peritonitis is most commonly caused by extension of inflammatory processes in the abdominal cavity, particularly after perforation of the gut. Less commonly, peritonitis may be a primary infection, seen in patients with nephrotic syndrome and cirrhosis.

Histologically there is acute inflammation of the peritoneum, with fibrinous and purulent exudation. Inflammation of the serosa of the small bowel causes paralysis of gut motility, leading to dilatation, termed **ileus**. Peritonitis may be localized by adherent loops of bowel and adherence of the omentum. Organization of fibrinous adhesion by granulation tissue leads to **adhesions** by fibrous tissue. Localization of infection in the peritoneal cavity may form local abscesses, particularly in the paracolic gutters and beneath the diaphragm (subphrenic abscesses).

Chronic peritonitis may be caused by infection with tuberculosis. Granulomatous inflammation leads to organization and fibrosis, with adhesions between bowel loops (plastic peritonitis). In patients treated by ambulatory peritoneal dialysis, there may be a chronic, low-grade peritonitis caused by a mixed flora of organisms.

Peritoneal tumors are most commonly the result of metastatic spread

The peritoneal cavity is most commonly affected by metastatic tumors that have spread from one of the abdominal organs, the main primary sites being stomach, ovary, uterus and colon. Deposits of metastatic tumor are seen as small nodules seeding the peritoneum, which often cause thickening of the omentum. In disseminated mucin-secreting carcinomas the peritoneal cavity may be filled with mucinous material (pseudomyxoma peritonei). Tumors may grow as larger nodules and cause adhesions between bowel loops, resulting in bowel obstruction. Infiltration of tumor in the peritoneum may also cause accumulation of fluid in the peritoneal cavity in the form of **ascites**.

Malignant mesotheliomas may develop as primary malignant tumors of the peritoneum. As with the pleural tumors (see page 220), these are also predisposed by exposure to asbestos. Tumor causes massive thickening of the peritoneum, leading to bowel obstruction and ascites.

Accumulation of fluid in the peritoneal cavity is termed 'ascites'

The principal causes of ascites are inflammation causing peritonitis, neoplasia in the peritoneal cavity, and increased transudation of fluid from vessels due to increased pressure in the portal venous system. The main cause of this increased pressure is cirrhosis of the liver (see page 294), portal vein thrombosis, or hepatic vein thrombosis (Budd–Chiari syndrome).

GASTROINTESTINAL DISEASE IN CHILDREN

Developmental abnormalities of the bowel

The most common congenital malformations affecting the alimentary tract are:

- **Esophageal atresia with tracheoesophageal fistula**. The most common pattern is that in which the upper end of the esophagus is intact but ends in a blind pouch (see *Fig. 5.7*). There is a central area of complete atresia and the lower esophagus is normal at the gastroesophageal junction, but tapers proximally and communicates with the trachea.
- **Omphalocele** is the result of failure of the intestine to return to the abdominal cavity during normal rotation of the midgut. Development of the whole gut outside the abdominal cavity is termed 'eventration.'
- **Gastroschisis** is due to a defect in the anterior abdominal wall, resulting in protrusion of the viscera into the amniotic cavity.
- **Failure of rotation of the gut** as it returns to the abdomen causes several patterns of malformation. In non-rotation, the small bowel lies on the right of the abdomen and the colon on the left. Other forms of malrotation lead to obstruction of bowel by twisting of the gut on itself (**volvulus**).
- **Intestinal atresia** is most common in the ileum, but also occurs higher in the bowel in the duodenum. It causes intestinal obstruction.

- **Meckel's diverticulum** is caused by an abnormality of the yolk stalk (*Fig. 13.24*). Other degrees of abnormality result in tethering of the ileum to the umbilicus by a fibrous band, development of a cyst in the fibrous band, or persistence of a sinus track between the ileum and the umbilicus.

Fig. 13.24 Meckel's diverticulum. This diverticulum (**D**) of the ileum (**I**), which occurs in 2–4% of the population, is caused by persistence of part of the yolk stalk. The diverticulum is 2–4 cm long, on the antimesenteric border of the bowel, 45 cm from the ileocecal valve. It has a muscular wall and is normally lined by small bowel epithelium, but may have gastric acid-secreting epithelium or heterotopic pancreatic tissue. If tethered to the umbilicus by a fibrous cord, the diverticulum may cause problems by acting as the apex of a volvulus. It may also be the site of inflammation similar to that seen in acute appendicitis. Alternatively, peptic ulceration may develop if acid-secreting epithelium is present.

- **Intestinal duplications** are caused by developmental abnormalities of canalization of the gut. There are two patterns: **closed cystic duplications** (most common) and **communicating tubular duplications** (unusual).
- **Imperforate anus** is more common in males than in females, and is often associated with other abnormalities. The anal canal may end blindly or, more often, opens into the urethra or vagina. A more common form is **anorectal agenesis**, in which the rectum ends blindly above the anal canal, with a fistula into the vagina or urethra. These defects are caused by defective separation of the cloaca by the urorectal septum.

Congenital pyloric stenosis is an important and common stomach disorder in infants

In pyloric stenosis, newborn infants, usually male, present with projectile vomiting, which is the result of narrowing at the pylorus due to an unusually hypertrophied pyloric sphincter muscle. It occurs in about 1 in 300 live births, and is relieved by surgical transection of part of the hypertrophied pyloric sphincter muscle.

Neonatal necrotizing enterocolitis is an important type of ischemic bowel disease

Necrotizing enterocolitis affects neonates and is rapidly fatal unless treated. Affected infants have bloody diarrhea and abdominal distension, often with vomiting. The bowel wall is thickened due to intense congestion, and there is extensive superficial mucosal ulceration. The pathogenesis is believed to be the result of poor perfusion of the mucosa of the bowel, followed by infection.

Predisposing factors are prematurity, ARDS (see page 220), Hirschsprung's disease (see below), and cystic fibrosis with meconium ileus (*Fig. 13.26*).

Intussusception occurs when one segment of bowel invaginates into another

Intussusception occurs when one portion of bowel invaginates into the adjoining segment. The most common site is at the ileocecal valve, with the ileum invaginating into the cecum. This pattern is most common in children. In the rare adult cases a structural abnormality of the small intestinal wall is almost invariably responsible for precipitating the invagination, and benign tumors such as leiomyoma or lipoma are important predisposing factors.

The structural lesion is carried by peristalsis into the adjoining bowel, and the bowel segment is invaginated. This leads to venous congestion of the invaginated portion, causing bleeding from the mucosa as well as intestinal obstruction. If the bowel remains invaginated infarction of the area takes place (*Fig. 13.25*).

Meconium ileus and rectal prolapse are manifestations of cystic fibrosis

One of the common manifestations of cystic fibrosis (see page 221) is meconium ileus, which occurs in 10–20% of cases. It is caused by abnormally viscid mucin forming a mass in the bowel lumen, which cannot be expelled (*Fig. 13.26*).

Intestinal obstruction may also occur after the neonatal period, mainly due to obstruction by thick mucus at the ileocecal valve.

Another common manifestation of cystic fibrosis is rectal prolapse, believed to be the result of bulky stools caused by malabsorption. Other gastrointestinal manifestations of cystic fibrosis are the result of pancreatic disease, which leads to failure of the production of digestive enzymes, causing malabsorption.

Hirschsprung's disease is caused by absence of normal myenteric plexus in the bowel wall

In Hirschsprung's disease there is failure of the normal motility of the bowel due to absence of the normal myenteric plexus.

The defect always involves the rectum and may be present in continuity for a variable distance along the bowel. Some cases involve just a short segment of rectum, others the

Fig. 13.25 Intussception. This segment of bowel has invaginated in on itself. Externally the affected segment is swollen and deeply congested. On cut surface the invagination (**I**) of the bowel from the proximal end (**P**) is seen. The invaginated portion of bowel has undergone venous infarction and is deeply congested.

Fig. 13.26 Meconium ileus. Microscopically the affected bowel is dilated and, on cut surface, is filled with dense gelatinous green mucoid material. Other associated complications are microcolon and intestinal atresia.

rectosigmoid segment and, in rare cases, there may be total colonic or total intestinal aganglionosis. Macroscopically the abnormally innervated bowel segment is narrowed, whereas the proximal bowel is dilated and shows hypertrophy of the muscle layers.

The disease usually presents in early childhood with failure to pass meconium, or later with persistent constipation. Diagnosis is made by biopsy of the rectal mucosa (*Fig. 13.27*).

One form of disease is caused by mutations in the *RET* oncogene on chromosome 10. Another is linked to mutations in the endothelin-B receptor gene on chromosome 13.

Rare cases of abnormal bowel motility in childhood are caused by primary abnormalities of visceral smooth muscle (visceral myopathies) or visceral axons (visceral neuropathies).

Fig. 13.27 Hirschsprung's disease (acetylcholinesterase histochemistry). In Hirschsprung's disease there is absence of normal myenteric and submucosal plexus ganglion cells. Nerve fibers in the submucosa and within the muscularis mucosa (M) are hypertrophied, and abnormal axons extend up into the lamina propria (L), visible as brown staining with histochemical stains for acetylcholinesterase.

Case-based questions

Case 1 – A young dancer with episodic bloody diarrhea and pain

A 25-year old talented ballet dancer presents with an intermittent, dull abdominal pain. She tells you that during the previous 6 months she has had several episodes of diarrhea, sometimes associated with the passage of fresh blood and mucus. This has, understandably, interfered with her work. She has also lost some weight and has recently developed joint pains.

On abdominal examination there is much voluntary guarding, with a suggestion of tenderness in the left iliac fossa. No lesions are palpated on rectal examination, but an anal fissure and skin tags are noticed.

A barium enema is performed which shows deep ulcers in the region of the sigmoid colon with tracking along the submucosa. A barium meal and follow-through demonstrate a long, irregular stricture in the terminal ileum.

On colonoscopy the rectum appears normal, but there are intermittent foci of congestion and irregularity of the mucosa, with a cobblestone appearance. The examination is extended round to the terminal ileum and multiple biopsies are taken.

1. What differential diagnoses should be considered with this presentation?

2. In view of the radiological and colonoscopic findings, what is the most likely final diagnosis?
3. What other disease processes of the small and large intestine show granulomatous histology?
4. What are the main non-gastrointestinal manifestations of chronic inflammatory bowel disease?
5. What are the long-term complications?

Case 2 – A woman with intermittent severe epigastric pain

A 49-year-old secretary presents to medical outpatients with a 7-month history of epigastric pain. She had been widowed in the last year, her husband having died of cancer. Her marriage had been unhappy and divorce proceedings were under way at the time of his death. The patient had been left to support two children and had recently moved to London from North Wales. She had recently become a vegetarian to cut down on meat costs. She smokes five cigarettes per day but does not drink alcohol. She has been treated with Gaviscon and antacids by her GP, but this has not controlled the symptoms. In the clinic, she complains of epigastric pains which are sharp and burning and radiate her subcostal margin to the right. The pain is worse at night and is relieved by food. She also describes several attacks of proctalgia fugax during the night over a period of 2 months which have convinced her she is dying of cancer. On examination, there is epigastric tenderness and clinical signs of anaemia.

1. What are the possible causes of this clinical presentation?
2. What are the predisposing causes?
3. What are the major complications?
4. What investigations should be performed?
5. What changes might an endoscopic biopsy show if there was ulceration of the gastric or duodenal mucosa?
6. What are the treatment options?

Case 3 – A man with retrosternal pain

A 57-year-old restauranteur presents with a history of a retrosternal burning sensation, particularly after large meals, and often on retiring to bed at night. Treatment with antacids has had little effect and he has been referred by his GP for endoscopy. Upper gastrointestinal tract endoscopy reveals reddening of the of the lower esophageal mucosa from the level of the gastroesophageal junction to a point 32 cm from the incisors. There is no evidence of a hiatus hernia. The proximal border of the reddened area is irregular, and this area is biopsied. The biopsy shows gastric and intestinal-type glandular mucosa.

1. What is the likely cause of the symptoms?
2. What is the final diagnosis?
3. What further information do you require from the biopsy report?

Case 4 – An underweight child with abdominal colic and distension

A 6-year-old boy has been brought to outpatients by his mother because he has abdominal pain after some meals. This has been getting increasingly frequent and it sounds, from his description, somewhat colicky in nature. You discover that he has always had very smelly, loose, pale bulky stools, which his parents have put down to the fact that he likes milk. On examination, he is pale, underweight, and of short stature. His abdomen is mildly distended.

1. What are the important differential diagnoses on presentation?
2. Blood tests reveal a mild macrocytic anemia with Howell–Jolly bodies. There is a low level of vitamin B_{12}, and folate is at the lower end of normal. Autoantibody screens reveal a positive reaction to antigliadin antibodies. Do these tests help to narrow down the diagnosis?
3. A duodenal biopsy shows villous atrophy with increased intraepithelial and lamina proprial lymphocytes. What is the final diagnosis?
4. What treatment options are available?

Case 5 – An old woman with a swollen abdomen and previous colonic polyps

A 68-year-old woman presents with intermittent constipation, weight loss, and a swollen abdomen. She has had two previous polypectomies: one showed a tubular adenoma and the other was a tubulovillous adenoma. Colonoscopy is performed and this gives good visualization of the colon round to the transverse colon only; no lesions are seen. Double-contrast barium enema shows an irregular stricture with shouldered edges approximately 4 cm long in the ascending colon. A tumor is diagnosed and surgery is advised. The tumor is resected and is found to have invaded through the thickness of the bowel wall, but is completely excised. Three of 15 lymph nodes identified contained metastatic tumor, but the 'high tie' node is free of disease.

1. What is the most likely diagnosis with this presentation?
2. What stage is this tumor and what is the prognosis?
3. What is the association between adenoma and carcinoma?
4. Where is the metastatic spread most likely?

Brief answers to these case-based questions are given on page 587. More detailed answers and other study resources are available online at www.studentconsult.com.

Liver, biliary tract, and pancreas

14

DISEASES OF THE LIVER

Functional differences in hepatocytes exist within the hepatic lobule

The liver is composed of hepatocytes, a form of epithelial cell, arranged in flat plates. Blood is supplied by branches of the hepatic artery as well as from the portal vein. After blood has passed between plates of hepatocytes in the sinusoidal spaces, it drains through branches of the hepatic vein. Bile produced by hepatocytes drains from the liver in branching bile ducts. The main connective tissue in the liver is a delicate framework of reticulin which supports hepatocytes. The portal tracts carry branches of the portal vein, hepatic artery and bile ducts, surrounded by collagen (*Fig. 14.1*).

All hepatocytes are not equal. Hepatocytes in different parts of the hepatic lobule have different metabolic properties, rendering each type vulnerable to different sorts of disease process.

Hepatocytes at the centre of the lobule near the veins (zone 3 of the acinus) are supplied by blood that is relatively depleted in oxygen, and these cells are most vulnera-

ble to damage by hypoxia or poor perfusion. Hepatocytes in this central zone also have a low level of oxidative enzymes, but a high level of esterases generating metabolic intermediate substances. These are vulnerable to certain toxins, e.g. paracetamol (acetaminophen).

In contrast, hepatocytes at the periphery of the lobule near portal tracts (zone 1 of the acinus) are well supplied with blood, and these cells resist damage by poor perfusion. Furthermore, they are not damaged by certain agents as they lack the enzymes for conversion to toxic intermediaries.

Fig. 14.1 Liver histology. In this preparation stained to show reticulin, hepatocytes (purple) are arranged in plates supported by reticulin (fine black). A portal tract (P) contains collagen (coarse black). A central vein (V) is also surrounded by some collagen.

> ### Key Facts
> #### Main functions of the liver
>
> - **Carbohydrate metabolism.** The liver is a storage site for glycogen and a main source of plasma glucose.
> - **Fat metabolism.** The liver is central in the processing of dietary fats to lipoproteins, which enter the blood for peripheral metabolism.
> - **Protein metabolism.** The liver is a major site of protein synthesis, particularly for plasma proteins. Important groups are albumin, coagulation factors, transport proteins for iron and copper, and most acute-phase proteins. Several of the signs and symptoms of chronic liver disease are a reflection of failure of synthesis of these vital plasma proteins. The liver is also a major site of protein catabolism resulting in the formation of urea.
> - **Bile synthesis.** The liver secretes bile containing bilirubin, cholesterol, electrolytes, and bile salts. In disease, abnormal bilirubin metabolism is the basis of jaundice.
> - **Storage.** The liver stores glycogen, iron, copper, and fat-soluble vitamins that may become pathologically excessive in disease.
> - **Detoxification.** The liver detoxifies certain drugs and many metabolites, particularly nitrogenous compounds and steroid hormones.

Liver disease – laboratory medicine and investigation

Biochemistry: liver function tests frequently give a good idea of the likely cause of liver disease. Certain patterns of abnormality suggest a particular type of liver disease, but none is specific.

Alkaline phosphatase: enzyme located on the cell membrane of biliary canaliculi. Very high levels indicate disease of the biliary system (intrahepatic cholestasis, extrahepatic biliary obstruction, or primary biliary cirrhosis). Moderate levels are less useful in predicting cause of liver disease.

Transaminases: enzymes located in the hepatocyte cytoplasm. High levels in blood reflect active necrosis of liver cells from any cause. ALT is more specific for the liver than AST. Low levels of increase in transaminases may be seen in cholestasis, as well as following induction of enzymes by drugs such as anticonvulsants. Elevated γ-glutamyl transpeptidase levels are a sensitive index of liver cell damage but are non-specific as to cause.

Conjugated bilirubin: secreted by liver cells. Obstruction of biliary canaliculi causes highest levels, but conjugated bilirubin also seen in association with liver cell destruction. Non-conjugated bilirubin levels increase in disorders causing excessive destruction of red cells.

Albumin: blood level reflects synthetic properties of the liver. Because of its half-life, low levels reflect long-standing liver disease, particularly cirrhosis. α-1-antitrypsin is reduced in disease caused by enzyme deficiency.

Ceruloplasmin: levels are reduced in Wilson's disease.

Transferrin: high saturation seen in hemochromatosis.

Immunology: several diseases are associated with abnormal immunological parameters. Primary biliary cirrhosis is associated with anti-mitochondrial autoantibodies and raised serum IgM levels. Autoimmune chronic hepatitis is associated with anti-smooth-muscle antibodies.

Clotting: abnormalities of clotting are commonly seen in liver disease with failure of hepatic synthesis of serum proteins. This is a feature of hepatic failure, as well as being the end-stage of chronic liver disease such as cirrhosis. The one-step prothrombin time is a sensitive index of vitamin-K-dependent clotting factors, particularly factor VII.

Imaging: imaging studies are valuable as primary investigations of patients with jaundice. Ultrasound examination may reveal dilatation of extrahepatic and intrahepatic bile ducts, or tumors as part of pre-operative assessment.

Biopsy: for the liver, percutaneous needle biopsy is usually performed. Blind biopsy of the right side of the liver is used to assess probable diffuse disease processes. CT- or ultrasound-guided needle biopsy may be used to sample discrete lesions.

Fig. 14.2 Investigation of liver disease. Liver disease may be investigated by imaging, blood tests and liver biopsy.

There are only a few main clinical patterns of liver disease

The liver has a relatively restricted set of pathological responses to disease and so there are relatively few main patterns of liver disease.

- **Cholestasis and obstructive jaundice** follow damage or blockage to either intrahepatic or extrahepatic bile ducts.
- **Acute hepatitis** occurs in diseases causing necrosis of liver cells with associated inflammation, and has several causes, the commonest being viral infection or toxic damage.
- **Chronic hepatitis** occurs when there is continued hepatic inflammation for over 6 months. This may also be due to many causes, including viral and immune-mediated diseases. This often progresses with the development of **hepatic fibrosis**.
- **Cirrhosis** is a common end-point of long-standing liver cell destruction and resulting fibrosis from any cause. The liver develops extensive scarring associated with nodules of regenerated liver cells. The development of this pattern of response causes distortion of liver architecture and leads to increased back-pressure in the portal blood vessels (**portal hypertension**)

Damage to the liver can be assessed by biochemical blood tests. The investigation of a patient with suspected liver disease is outlined in *Fig. 14.2*.

JAUNDICE

Jaundice is caused by abnormalities in bilirubin metabolism and excretion

The normal metabolism of bilirubin is shown in the Key Facts box below. Abnormalities in the metabolism or excretion of bile result in development of jaundice. Biochemical jaundice can be defined as an increase in the plasma bilirubin level above the normal level of about 18–24 μmol/L (1.2 mg/dL). Clinical jaundice is evident when levels are above 50 μmol/L (2.5 mg/dL), manifesting as a yellow discoloration of the sclera and skin. Different laboratories may have different reference ranges.

Jaundice is biochemically divided into conjugated and unconjugated types

Jaundice can be caused by impaired bilirubin metabolism at several levels. It can be divided into three main biochemical types.

In **unconjugated hyperbilirubinemia** there is excessive unconjugated bilirubin in the blood. Disorders causing this pattern of disease are mainly excessive generation of bilirubin, for example by red cell destruction, or abnormal hepatocyte metabolism.

In **conjugated hyperbilirubinemia** there is excessive conjugated bilirubin in the blood. The most common cause is obstruction of bile secretion.

Key Facts
Bilirubin metabolism

- Bilirubin is derived from breakdown of hemoglobin, entering the liver via the splenic vein and portal vein when derived from normal red cell destruction.
- Unconjugated bilirubin is bound to albumin (cannot be excreted in urine) and circulates to the liver, where it is normally internalized and conjugated to glucuronic acid.
- Conjugated bilirubin (water-soluble) is excreted in the bile to reach the gut. In the distal gut, bacteria split the conjugate into urobilinogen, most of which exits in the feces. However, 20% is resorbed into the blood and re-excreted by the liver (enterohepatic recirculation).
- A very small amount of resorbed urobilinogen is excreted in the urine.
- Unconjugated bilirubin is lipid soluble. In neonates high levels in the blood can enter the brain and cause damage (kernicterus).

Disease which causes generalized damage to hepatocytes results in a **mixed pattern** of conjugated and unconjugated hyperbilirubinemia. As the main rate-limiting step in bilirubin metabolism is excretion by the canaliculi, there is generally a predominance of unconjugated bilirubin in this type of jaundice.

Excessive generation of bilirubin is the most important cause of unconjugated hyperbilirubinemia

Increased bilirubin generation results from excessive destruction of red cells, the main causes of which are: hemolytic anemia (see page 321); breakdown of large hematomas; and abnormal formation of red cells (dyserythropoiesis) which is seen in megaloblastic anemia (see pages 319–20).

The amount of bilirubin generated exceeds the capacity of the liver to conjugate and excrete it. Bilirubin circulating in the blood is unconjugated, circulates complexed to albumin, and **does not appear in the urine**. The amount of conjugated bilirubin excreted into the intestine is increased because of the increased load; some is resorbed as urobilinogen, and this is excreted in increased amounts in the urine.

Reduced uptake of bilirubin by hepatocytes can also cause unconjugated hyperbilirubinemia. Drugs such as rifampin interfere with bilirubin uptake.

Many of the population have impaired conjugation of bilirubin

Between 5% and 10% of the population have an inherited mild unconjugated hyperbilirubinemia as a result of defective hepatic conjugation of bilirubin. **Gilbert's syndrome** is autosomal dominant and linked to mutations in the TATA box upstream of the uridine diphosphoglucose glucuronyltransferase gene resulting in impaired bilirubin glucuronidation. Bilirubin levels may increase in the presence of intercurrent disease, but the liver is structurally normal.

Impaired conjugation of bilirubin is also commonly seen in neonates, as activity of glucuronyl transferase is low in the first 2 weeks of life (neonatal jaundice) (see page 298). Hereditary lack of glucuronyl transferase activity is seen in the congenital **Crigler–Najjar syndrome**.

Conjugated hyperbilirubinemia is mainly caused by biliary obstruction

Abnormalities in the secretion or excretion of conjugated bilirubin results in the accumulation of conjugated bilirubin in the blood. The key clinical features, the combination of which is also known as **cholestatic or obstructive jaundice**, are as follows:

- Jaundice – usually pronounced (see Data Set).
- Bile is not able to enter the gut via the biliary system and is absent from the stools, which are pale as a result.
- Fat absorption is disturbed (development of steatorrhea) and, as a consequence, there is impaired absorption of vitamin K.

- Itching (pruritus) develops from accumulated bile salts.
- The urine contains bilirubin (dark urine), because conjugated bilirubin is soluble in water and can be excreted.

There are two main groups of causes of conjugated hyperbilirubinemia, as listed in *Fig. 14.3*.

Fig. 14.3 Causes of conjugated hyperbilirubinemia

Intrahepatic causes

Hereditary enzyme defects (Rare)
Intrahepatic cholestasis (*Fig. 14.7*)
Hepatocellular damage

Extrahepatic obstruction of bile ducts

Gallstones (see page 299)
Strictures of common bile duct
Carcinoma of the pancreas (see page 304)
Compression of bile ducts by extrinsic masses such as enlarged lymph nodes

---

Data Set
Obstructive jaundice

A 45-year-old woman with jaundice and right upper abdominal pain.

Plasma

Total bilirubin	163 µmol/L	(up to 70)
	9.5 mg/dL	(up to 1)
Albumin	42 g/L	(30–48)
Alanine transaminase (ALT)	38 U/L	(up to 50)
Alkaline phosphatase	354 U/L	(40–120)
γ-Glutamyl transferase (GGT)	356 U/L	(up to 70)

Urine

Bilirubin positive

This pattern of elevated plasma bilirubin, alkaline phosphatase and GGT is characteristic of obstructive jaundice. Bilirubin enters the liver cells and is conjugated with glucuronic acid. Because of the obstruction it cannot be excreted and is regurgitated into plasma. Conjugated bilirubin is water soluble and can therefore be excreted in urine.

In this patient, ultrasonography demonstrated a gallstone in the common bile duct.

LIVER DISEASE

Acute liver failure results in jaundice, coma, and bleeding tendency

Acute liver failure develops when there has been damage to the majority of hepatocytes and is seen in three main clinical situations (*Fig. 14.4*): following severe hepatocyte damage, e.g. extensive liver cell necrosis caused by viral infection or toxic damage; following systemic shock as part of multiorgan failure; as acute decline in slowly progressing but relatively stable chronic liver disease, usually caused by chronic hepatitis or cirrhosis.

Acute hepatic failure (*Fig. 14.5*) is a severe life-threatening condition, from which 80% of patients die.

Fatty change is most commonly caused by metabolic disease and alcohol

Fatty change (see pages 24–5) is a common hepatic response to several adverse stimuli (*Fig. 14.6*). The main causes are:

- **Metabolic** obesity, diabetes mellitus (see page 569) hypoxia, and kwashiorkor (see page 148).
- **Toxins** the most common being alcohol (see page 144).

Non-alcoholic fatty liver disease (NAFLD) is a complication of the metabolic syndrome, and is an increasingly recognized cause of chronic liver disease.

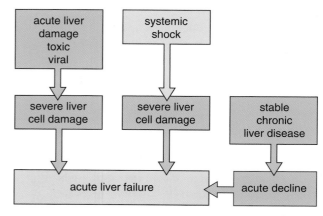

Fig. 14.4 The three main situations leading to acute liver failure.

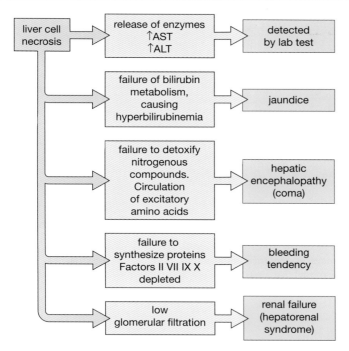

Fig. 14.5 **Features of acute liver failure.**

Fig. 14.6 Fatty liver. Macroscopically the fatty liver is enlarged and, instead of appearing deep red, is pale. Histologically, fat can be seen in hepatocytes.

Cholestasis may be intrahepatic or extrahepatic in origin

Many of the conditions that cause conjugated hyperbilirubinemia lead to the development of cholestasis. Clinically this is characterized by conjugated hyperbilirubinemia and a great increase in the serum levels of alkaline phosphatase, an enzyme normally located on the cell membranes of the biliary canaliculi. (This biochemical profile is often referred to as 'obstructive liver function tests – see Data Set). Two groups of cholestasis are recognized, according to whether blockage is within the liver or outside the liver in the biliary tract.

Intrahepatic cholestasis is caused by diseases affecting bile secretion in the liver, due either to abnormalities of liver cells and biliary canaliculi, or to disease of intrahepatic bile ducts (*Fig. 14.7*). Because they are generally managed by physicians, these conditions are sometimes loosely grouped as 'medical jaundice.' In this type of jaundice changes are apparent on liver biopsy (*Fig. 14.8*).

Extrahepatic cholestasis is caused by blockage of the main bile ducts outside the liver, discussed later in diseases of the biliary tract (pages 299–301). As many of the conditions responsible are amenable to operative intervention, this type of problem is sometimes referred to as 'surgical jaundice.' Liver biopsy shows cholestasis with edema in the portal tracts, proliferation of bile ducts, and some inflammatory changes (*Fig. 14.9*).

Fig. 14.7 Intrahepatic cholestasis
Intra-acinar
Viral hepatitis
Drug (e.g. chlorpromazine and estrogens)
Alcoholic liver disease
Pregnancy-related cholestasis
Septicemia
Extra-acinar
Primary biliary cirrhosis
Sclerosing cholangitis
Tumors within the liver

Fig. 14.8 Intrahepatic cholestasis. Bile (**B**) can be seen dilating canaliculi, predominantly in the centrilobular zones.

Fig. 14.9 Extrahepatic cholestasis. In addition to plugging of biliary canaliculi by bile, a characteristic feature of this type of cholestasis is edema of the portal tracts (**P**), which are expanded. In long-standing cases there is proliferation of small bile ducts around the periphery of portal tracts. Bile may leak from canaliculi associated with hydropic degeneration of hepatocytes to cause small so-called bile infarcts or lakes (**L**).

Fig. 14.10 Centrilobular (zone 3) necrosis caused by paracetamol (acetaminophen). Confluent necrosis (**N**) of centrilobular areas (zone 3) is seen, with surviving hepatocytes around portal areas (**P**) (zone 1).

Death of liver cells can be seen in several patterns

Six main patterns of liver cell death are seen:

1. In several diseases, single liver cells die by the process of apoptosis. Dead hepatocytes form brightly eosinophilic shrunken structures known as **Councilman bodies** (see *Fig. 14.14*).
2. Death of liver cells scattered throughout the lobule, both singly and in small groups (**spotty necrosis**) of about 20 cells, is seen with toxic damage and viral infections.
3. Death of liver cells confined to certain zones (**zonal necrosis**) is seen with certain diseases. For example, the centrilobular area (zone 3) is affected in paracetamol (acetaminophen) toxicity (*Fig. 14.10*) (see Data Set), and the periportal area (zone 1) is involved in phosphorus toxicity.
4. **Piecemeal necrosis** describes death of liver cells in a scattered pattern immediately next to the portal tract connective tissue. This pattern is a characteristic of chronic active hepatitis.
5. Extensive regions of necrosis that connect between central veins, or between portal tracts and central veins, are termed **bridging necrosis**.
6. **Massive necrosis** describes necrosis of the majority of hepatocytes. This occurs with fulminant hepatic damage and is seen in some cases of viral- and toxin-induced damage.

Data Set
Acute hepatic necrosis

A depressed 24-year-old man took an unknown number of paracetamol (acetaminophen) tablets. The following day he was admitted to hospital in coma following a convulsion.

Plasma

Total bilirubin	173 µmol/L	(up to 17)
	10 mg/dL	*(up to 1)*
Albumin	40 g/L	(30–48)
Alanine transaminase (ALT)	6831 U/L	(up to 50)
Alkaline phosphatase	89 U/L	(40–120)
γ-Glutamyl transferase (GGT)	82 U/L	(up to 70)
Prothrombin time	67.6 s	(control 9.5)

Urine

Bilirubin positive

Acute hepatic necrosis is characterized by markedly raised levels of ALT and AST, released from damaged hepatocytes. The prolonged prothrombin time indicates that the synthetic function of the liver is impaired; owing to its long half-life (3 weeks) plasma albumin is an insensitive test of liver synthetic function in acute disease. Further investigations in this severely ill man should include plasma glucose and creatinine, and acid–base status. Hypoglycemia should be treated with intravenous glucose.

Liver cell regeneration occurs following hepatocyte necrosis

There is normally a very low level of liver cell proliferation. After liver damage, including partial hepatectomy, regeneration of liver cells takes place in an orderly manner to restore liver function. In conditions causing repeated chronic damage to the liver, regeneration may become distorted by fibrosis, resulting in cirrhosis (see pages 294–6). In other instances, nodular hyperplasia may occur.

Stellate cells are the source of collagen-secreting cells in liver fibrosis

The development of fibrosis is an important complication of several liver diseases, and is one of the characteristic features of cirrhosis. It is thought that growth factors, produced as part of inflammatory responses, stimulate mesenchymal cells in the liver to proliferate and differentiate into collagen-secreting fibroblasts. The mesenchymal cells involved are the normally inconspicuous fat-storing stellate cells (cells of Ito), located in the space of Disse.

The liver may be involved in several storage diseases

The liver stores several substances that may become pathological in disease states. In hemochromatosis and hemosiderosis there is excessive iron storage, and excessive copper deposition is seen in Wilson's disease.

Abnormal storage of metabolic products in the liver may be seen in some of the inborn errors of metabolism. Glycogen deposition occurs in some of the glycogen storage diseases (*Fig. 14.11*), and lipids are stored in multisystem disorders of metabolism, e.g. Gaucher's disease and Niemann–Pick disease.

Fig. 14.11 Liver glycogenosis. In glycogenosis types IV, III, II and I, liver cells accumulate excess glycogen. Here, liver cells from a case of type II glycogenosis (debrancher deficiency) show striking vacuolation of hepatocytes and liver nuclei due to the accumulation of glycogen.

VASCULAR DISEASES OF THE LIVER

Blood is supplied to the liver via both arterial (hepatic artery) and portal venous circulations. It leaves the liver after passing through the sinusoids by the central and hepatic veins that enter the inferior vena cava. As each vascular component of the liver may be affected by disease, there are several distinct clinical and pathological syndromes.

True infarction of the liver is rare

True infarction of the liver is rare because of its dual blood supply and the rich anastomosis of blood flow through the sinusoids. True infarction may be seen in five conditions:

- Surgical trauma or accidental ligation of hepatic artery.
- Therapeutic arterial embolization of the liver or therapeutic hepatic arterial ligation (performed to treat isolated neoplastic masses).
- Bacterial endocarditis.
- Eclampsia.
- Polyarteritis nodosa.

Areas of infarction appear as geographic areas of yellow necrotic tissue.

Right-sided heart failure causes passive venous congestion of the liver

Right-sided cardiac failure causes back-pressure in the systemic venous system, which is transmitted back down the hepatic vein to the central veins, causing a mild increase in liver size. This is particularly seen in tricuspid valve incompetence, when the liver is pulsatile. The macroscopic appearance is described as nutmeg liver (see *Fig. 10.34*), properly called chronic passive venous congestion. The centrilobular sinusoids are dilated by blood, and the centrilobular hepatocytes are atrophic. If arterial hypotension complicates the right-sided cardiac failure, necrosis of the centrilobular hepatocytes may occur, with elevation of serum transaminase levels, termed ischemic hepatitis.

Portal hypertension is caused by obstruction of blood flow in the portal system

Portal hypertension is a continued elevation in portal venous pressure. This causes back-pressure in the portal vascular bed, leading to splenomegaly and ascites. New channels open up between the portal system and systemic venous system, taking the form of varicose venous channels. The main sites are the lower esophagus, where esophageal varices arise and may cause bleeding (see page 251); the umbilicus, where the channels are called 'caput medusae' and the anus, where they are known as hemorrhoids.

The causes of portal hypertension are best considered on an anatomical basis, according to the site of obstruction to flow (*Fig. 14.12*).

- Presinusoidal – blockage of vessels before the hepatic sinusoids.
- Sinusoidal – blockage in the sinusoids.
- Postsinusoidal – blockage in the central veins, hepatic veins or vena cava.

Sinusoidal obstruction in the liver is the most common cause of portal hypertension

Hepatic disease is the most common cause of portal hypertension.

- **Cirrhosis** causes distortion and destruction of the hepatic vascular architecture.
- **Portal tract fibrosis** caused by schistosomiasis is an important cause in endemic areas.

Presinusoidal portal hypertension is most often caused by portal vein thrombosis

Occlusion of the portal venous system at a point before the portal tracts is usually due to portal vein thrombosis. Predisposing factors are local sepsis, polycythemia (see page 323), and pre-existing sinusoidal portal hypertension due to cirrhosis. Occlusion of intrahepatic branches of the portal vein causes areas of venous infarction, which are seen as congested zones with a wedge-shaped pattern. Such areas are also termed **red infarcts** or **Zahn infarcts**.

Post-sinusoidal portal hypertension is caused by disease of hepatic veins and branches

Post-sinusoidal portal hypertension is caused by diseases that block central veins and hepatic venous branches.

Obliteration of central veins in the liver is seen in several diseases, and causes the gradual development of portal hypertension. For example, alcohol abuse may result in central venous obliteration with scarring, and some cytotoxic drugs may cause centrilobular scarring and obliteration of central veins.

Veno-occlusive disease of the liver is caused by ingestion of plants containing toxic alkaloids. These initially cause fibrosis around central veins, followed by obliteration of central veins by fibrosis. The problem is seen in Jamaica and certain areas of Africa, in those who drink herbal teas. Irradiation of the liver may also cause central venous fibrosis and development of portal hypertension.

Occlusion of the main hepatic vein produces the **Budd–Chiari syndrome**. Thrombosis is predisposed to by local compression of the hepatic vein, hepatocellular carcinoma,

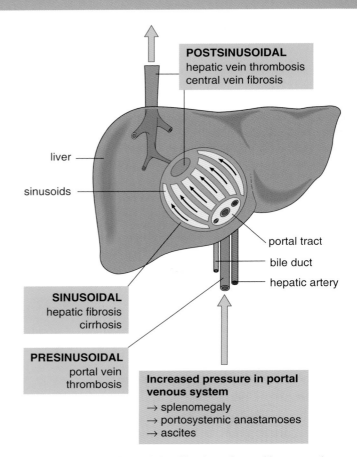

Fig. 14.12 Morphological classification of portal hypertension.
The three main groups of causes for portal hypertension are:

- Presinusoidal.
- Sinusoidal.
- Postsinusoidal.

The effects that are shown in the pink box are caused by increased portal venous pressure.

polycythemia, pregnancy, and estrogenic oral contraceptive therapy. In many cases, no predisposing factor is identified. Patients develop severe acute disease, with massive vascular congestion of the liver causing acute portal hypertension and jaundice. There is painful enlargement of the liver, with rapid development of ascites. Unless therapeutic portosystemic vascular anastomosis is performed, death results.

HEPATITIS

Inflammatory diseases of the liver are termed 'hepatitis'

Hepatitis, which may be acute or chronic, has several causes including viral infections, autoimmune disorders, drug reactions, and alcohol. In all types of hepatitis there are some common clinical features.

Viral infection is a common cause of hepatitis

The main hepatitis viruses are a group of **hepatotrophic viruses**. Although all cause a primary hepatitis, they are unrelated and belong to different viral types. The main viruses are hepatitis A and E (transmitted via the feco-oral route), and hepatitis B, C, D and G (transmitted via a parenteral route). Several non-hepatotrophic viruses may also cause hepatitis. Infection with a hepatitis virus is associated with a range of possible clinical manifestations, listed in *Fig. 14.13*.

The histology of acute viral hepatitis is similar for all types

Irrespective of the causative virus, the histological features of acute viral hepatitis are similar (*Fig. 14.14*):

- Hepatocytes are swollen and many undergo death by apoptosis, forming eosinophilic Councilman bodies.
- Focal infiltration of liver by lymphoid cells associated with liver cell necrosis.
- Increased number of lymphoid cells in portal tracts.
- Regeneration of liver cells produces lobular disarray.
- Mild cholestasis may be seen.

Hepatitis A is transmitted by the feco-oral route and does not lead to chronic liver disease

Hepatitis A is an RNA enterovirus of the picorna group. Clinically, disease is transmitted by the feco-oral route, and small epidemics may occur in institutions. Disease has also been contracted from recreational use of waters contaminated by sewage, and from eating sewage-contaminated shellfish. From the time of infection an incubation period

Clinical and biochemical features of acute viral hepatitis

Symptoms: nausea, anorexia, low-grade pyrexia, and general malaise.

Signs: liver may become palpably enlarged and tender. Jaundice 1 week after the onset of symptoms, peaking at around 10 days.
   Signs and symptoms generally recover over a period of 3–8 weeks.

Biochemical tests: bilirubin, which is mostly conjugated, is greatly elevated; levels of alanine transaminase (ALT) and aspartate transaminase (AST) are very high early in disease, reflecting liver cell necrosis, but fall with clinical recovery; serum albumin generally remains normal.
   The serum alkaline phosphatase level may become mildly elevated.

Coagulation tests: may become abnormal, the one-stage prothrombin time being a sensitive indicator of severity of liver disease.

Fig. 14.13 Clinical patterns following viral hepatitis

Pattern of disease	Viruses
Asymptomatic	A, B, C, D and E
Acute hepatitis without jaundice (anicteric hepatitis)	A, B, C, D and E
Acute hepatitis with jaundice (icteric hepatitis)	A, B, C, D and E
Massive necrosis of the liver with acute liver failure (rare)	A, B, C, D and E
One of the forms of chronic hepatitis (see page 285)	B, C and D
Chronic carrier state	B, C and D

Fig. 14.14 Histology in acute hepatitis. This is a liver biopsy from a patient with acute viral hepatitis. Many liver cells are swollen and vacuolated, termed 'ballooning degeneration' (**B**). Focal death of hepatocytes (**D**) occurs with associated inflammatory infiltration. Cells dying by apoptosis are seen as shrunken, eosinophilic Councilman bodies (**C**).

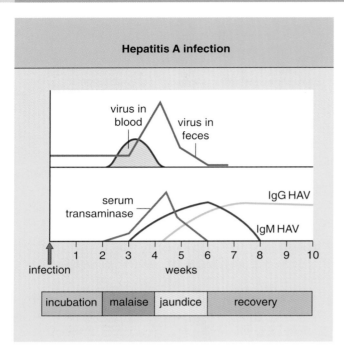

Fig. 14.15 Hepatitis A infection.

2. **Fulminant acute hepatitis** is very rare and causes massive necrosis of liver cells.
3. **Chronic hepatitis** affects 5–10% of cases. It may progress to cirrhosis or may recover (see *Fig. 14.16*).
4. **Asymptomatic chronic infection** (may later develop chronic hepatitis).

The importance of the chronic infective states is that patients are at risk of developing hepatocellular carcinoma. In adults, fewer than 10% of patients develop a chronic infection state, but virtually all neonates infected with HBV from the mother become chronically infected, possibly because of an immature immune response.

In diagnostic testing HBsAg is a surface protein component; HBeAg is a core component associated with viral replication. PCR detection of HBV-DNA is the standard for detection of viral replication on blood samples. Active infection has been defined as a minimum level of units detected on a standard PCR assay, below which infection is regarded as inactive.

of about 1–4 weeks is followed by fever, malaise, and anorexia (*Fig. 14.15*). Jaundice typically appears between weeks 5 and 6. Patients recover fully, with recovery of abnormal liver function tests. Virus is present in the stools of affected patients about 2 weeks before and 1 week after the onset of clinical jaundice. The disease does not cause chronic hepatitis, and infection confers subsequent immunity by development of serum anti-HAV antibodies, which are used in diagnosis. Histology of the liver shows features of acute hepatitis (see *Fig. 14.14*).

Hepatitis B infection is transmitted parenterally and may cause chronic liver disease

Hepatitis B virus (HBV) is a DNA virus of the hepadna group. Infective virus is transmitted in blood, semen and saliva through close physical contact, inoculation occurring through breaks in skin or mucous membranes. Hepatitis B can therefore be a sexually transmitted disease. Transmission by blood transfusion is now uncommon because of the screening of blood donations, but spread of infection among IV drug abusers via shared unsterile needles is an important mode of transmission. Vertical transmission from mother to child is also seen.

Infection causes four clinical patterns of infection (*Fig. 14.16*).

1. **Acute self-limited hepatitis** is a common outcome. Patients recover and have lifelong immunity.

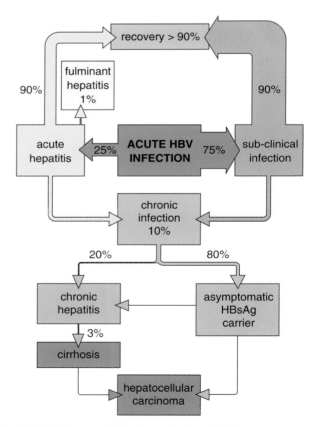

Fig. 14.16 Patterns of infection after hepatitis B infection. Flow diagram illustrating the probabilities of different clinical outcomes after hepatitis B infection. The width of the lines indicates the respective percentages. The timescales involved are not illustrated; some stages may last for many years, others a matter of weeks.

Acute hepatitis B infection is self-limiting in most patients

In symptomatic acute infection patients develop symptoms after an incubation period of 3–6 months. In the majority of patients, where the illness is self-limiting (*Fig. 14.18*), there is a rise in serum HBsAg that peaks just before the height of clinical disease, becoming undetectable after 6 months. Markers of active viral replication peak just before the height of clinical disease (HBcAg, HBeAg, HBV DNA). Serum transaminase levels begin to rise just before symptomatic disease and persist until resolution of the illness. With the fall in levels of HBeAg, anti-HBe appears in blood. Anti-HBs develops in blood after the acute phase of the illness is over and persists for life.

In chronic hepatitis B infection there is failure to eliminate virus from the liver

In some patients there is failure to eliminate HBV from the liver, with HBsAg persisting in the blood for 6 months after initial detection. There are two main possible consequences of this:

- Chronic carrier state associated with no active viral replication.
- Chronic liver disease associated with active viral replication.

The natural history of chronic HBV infection can be considered as four phases, the relationships shown in *Fig. 14.18*. Each phase may last many years, up to decades.

- **Immune tolerance phase** – the presence of HBsAg is associated with the presence of HBcAg, HBeAg and HBV DNA in the blood, indicative of active viral replication. Liver histology typically shows chronic hepatitis with a risk of developing cirrhosis
- **Immune clearance phase** – anti-HBe appears in blood (termed **HBeAg seroconversion**). HBeAg levels drop and there is an associated rise in serum transaminase levels, reflecting more active liver cell necrosis. Histology typically shows an active chronic hepatitis involving much of the hepatic lobule.
- **Immune control phase** – there is evidence that viral replication has been suppressed (HBcAg, HBeAg are not detected in the blood but low levels of HBV DNA can be found). The patient can be classed as a 'latent' state of infection in which the immune system is controlling HBV replication. Liver biopsy shown minimal evidence of inflammation, but hepatocytes can be seen packed with HBsAg (*Fig. 14.19*), as once viral DNA integration takes place surface antigen (HBsAg) can be produced without viral replication. HBsAg seroconversion is associated with the halting of disease progression.
- **HBe-negative phase** In some patients a further phase of disease can develop where viremia returns, but in the absence of HBe-antigen because of the emergence of a mutant (HBe-negative,) pre-core mutant strain of virus. The fact that there is viral replication is shown by levels of HBV DNA. HBeAg detection is therefore of less use than the detection of HBV DNA in predicting viral replication. There is development of renewed

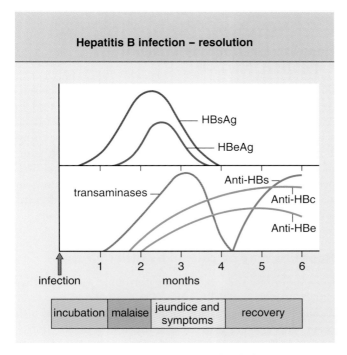

Fig. 14.17 Events in self-limiting hepatitis B infection.

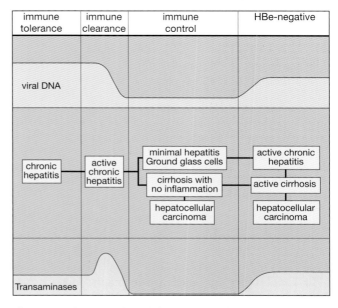

Fig. 14.18 Phases in chronic hepatitis B infection.

Fig. 14.19 Chronic hepatitis B infection. In chronic hepatitis due to hepatitis B infection, liver cells accumulate HBsAg in the cytoplasm, which appears homogeneous, pale and glassy (a). These so-called 'ground glass' hepatocytes may be immunostained by antibodies to HBsAg, as shown in (b), where they are stained brown.

inflammation and chronic hepatitis on liver histology, with the risk of developing cirrhosis.

Integration of HBV into the genome is oncogenic and chronic HBV infection is associated with an increased risk of development of hepatocellular carcinoma.

Hepatitis D virus can only cause infection in the presence of HBV

Hepatitis D virus (HDV) is a hepatotrophic RNA virus. It is a defective virus, requiring the presence of HBV infection for assembly. Consequently, it can cause disease only in the presence of hepatitis B infection. Its mode of transmission is the same as that for hepatitis B infection, and it is particularly prevalent in drug abusers and dialysis patients. Chronic HDV infection seldom resolves and over 60% of

affected patients will develop cirrhosis. In some patients there is rapid progression of disease over a few years.

Infection may be acquired simultaneously with HBV infection, or may occur later as a superinfection. Infection is confirmed by finding serum IgM anti-D in the presence of IgM anti-HBc. HDV RNA may also be detected in blood.

Hepatitis C is clinically similar to hepatitis B infection

Hepatitis C is an RNA flavivirus. There are six subtypes with different geographic incidences, and it is estimated that 3% of the world population harbors an infection. Its mode of transmission is the same as for hepatitis B, and it is an important cause of post-transfusion hepatitis. Although it accounts for many cases of sporadic acute hepatitis, often no recognized source of infection can be identified.

There is an incubation period of about 2 months, followed in some cases by acute hepatitis with fever, malaise, anorexia, and usually mild jaundice. The majority of patients have an asymptomatic acute infection. Some recover after a period of about 2 months with complete elimination of the virus; others have persistently abnormal liver function tests for over a year, developing a chronic hepatitis with periods of remission and relapse. Of the latter, most will develop chronic hepatitis, and many progress to cirrhosis, with a risk of hepatocellular carcinoma. The course of the disease is shown graphically in *Fig. 14.20*.

Extrahepatic manifestations of disease, such as arthritis and agranulocytosis, are common. Diagnosis can be confirmed by detection of antibodies to HCV and by detection of HCV RNA in blood by PCR tests.

Hepatitis E is clinically similar to hepatitis A infection

Hepatitis E infection is caused by an RNA calicivirus. Transmitted by the feco-oral route, it is often found in contaminated water supplies and causes epidemics of acute self-limited hepatitis. It has an incubation period of about 1 month, typically causing infection associated with jaundice which is generally more severe that that seen with hepatitis A. Infection in pregnant women may result in acute fulminant hepatitis in 20% of cases. There is no progression to chronic hepatitis. Immunity is not lifelong.

Hepatitis may be caused by other viruses

In addition to the specific hepatotrophic viruses, other viruses may also cause hepatitis. For example, yellow fever is caused by a group B arbovirus. Acute hepatitis may also occur with Epstein–Barr virus and cytomegalovirus infection. Rubella and herpes simplex infection may cause severe disease in childhood.

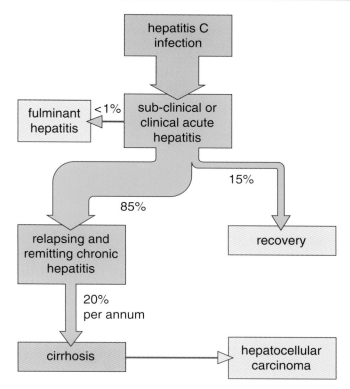

Fig. 14.20 Hepatitis C infection. Flow diagram illustrating the probabilities of different clinical outcomes after hepatitis C infection. The width of the lines indicates the respective percentages. The timescales involved are not illustrated.

NON-VIRAL INFECTIONS

The liver may be involved in several parasitic diseases

Parasitic infestation of the liver is an important problem worldwide. The main diseases involved are presented in *Fig. 14.21* and some are discussed in Chapter 8.

Bacterial infection of the liver is by three main routes

Bacterial infection of the liver occurs by three main routes:

- Ascending spread from colonization of the biliary tract by bacteria. This is almost always predisposed to by biliary obstruction.
- Infection ascending in the portal vessels (portal pyemia) into the liver from a focus of sepsis in the abdomen, e.g. abscess caused by complicated appendicitis (see page 269).
- Systemic blood spread in septicemia. This may cause severe acute liver failure.

An important complication of bacterial infection of the liver is the development of a **liver abscess**. This is a very serious condition with a high mortality if left untreated. Infection of the liver by *Leptospira* causes **Weil's disease**. There is fever, jaundice, a purpuric skin rash, and renal failure. The liver shows focal hepatocyte necrosis and cholestasis. Syphilis may affect the liver in congenital infection,

Fig. 14.21 Parasitic diseases affecting the liver	
Protozoa	
Amebiasis *Entamoeba histolytica*	Amebic abscess contains necrotic material resembling anchovy paste. May rupture into the abdomen or perforate the diaphragm to cause disease in the chest
Malaria	Causes enlarged liver. Kupffer cells are hyperplastic and contain malaria pigment
Visceral leishmaniasis	Liver is enlarged. Kupffer cells contain *Leishmania* which appear as Donovan bodies
Helminthic infection	
Ascariasis *Ascaris lumbricoides*	Eggs and worms in the biliary tract cause cholangitis. Hepatic abscesses are reported
Schistosoma	Eggs from worms cause fibrosis in portal tracts
Liver flukes *Clonorchis sinensis*	Flukes colonize the biliary tree and cause chronic inflammation, as well as biliary obstruction. Predispose to development of carcinoma of biliary tree
Hydatid disease *Echinococcus granulosus*	Liver cysts develop, containing the scolices of developing worms

causing diffuse fibrosis of the parenchyma. In tertiary syphilis gummatous necrosis may develop (see page 109), leading to deep scars (hepar lobatum). Tuberculous infection of the liver is seen in miliary tuberculosis (see page 197).

CHRONIC INFLAMMATORY LIVER DISEASE

Chronic inflammatory liver disease is caused by many different agents

Several diseases of the liver that are characterized by progressive hepatic damage over a period of many months or years can be grouped together as chronic inflammatory liver diseases. The most important long-term consequences of such diseases are progressive liver cell loss, fibrosis, and regeneration of hepatocytes. When this process is diffuse and progressive, it may develop into cirrhosis.

Chronic hepatitis is defined as inflammation of the liver persisting for more than 6 months

Chronic hepatitis it is not a single disease but a syndrome with several causes. It is clinically defined as persistent abnormal liver function tests of hepatitic type of 6 months' duration. The diagnosis of chronic hepatitis is usually made in three main situations:

- A patient is under medical follow-up (involving repeated liver function tests and serology) after an episode of acute viral hepatitis. Instead of recovering, liver function tests show continued elevation of serum transaminase levels for more than 6 months.
- A patient develops non-specific features of anorexia, malaise, and weight loss, and is discovered to have abnormal liver function tests suggestive of hepatitis, with raised transaminase levels. A cause of liver disease is found on investigation (viral, autoimmune or toxic/metabolic) and, as the disease persists for 6 months, a liver biopsy is performed to establish the pattern of chronic inflammation of the liver.
- Many patients are completely asymptomatic and come to medical attention only because they test HBV- or HCV-positive on routine screening, e.g. when donating blood. Investigations may then suggest a chronic hepatitis.

The classification of chronic hepatitis is based on etiology is shown in *Fig. 14.22*.

Chronic hepatitis can be staged and graded according to histology of the liver

Chronic hepatitis is characterized by variable degrees of liver cell necrosis with inflammation and associated fibrosis (*Figs 14.23* and *14.24*).

Fig. 14.22 Classification of chronic hepatitis

Caused by viral infections

Chronic hepatitis B
Chronic hepatitis C
Chronic hepatitis D

Caused by autoimmune disease

Autoimmune hepatitis
Primary biliary cirrhosis
Primary sclerosing cholangitis

Caused by toxic/metabolic damage

Chronic drug hepatitis
Wilson's disease
α_1-Antitrypsin deficiency

Fig. 14.23 Variation in severity of inflammation in chronic hepatitis. (a) Grade 2 inflammation in portal tract (**P**), which spills over into the adjacent parenchyma with liver necrosis (**N**) (b) Grade 1 lymphoid infiltration limited to the portal tract with no necrosis of liver cells.

- Inflammation may be in the portal tracts, around the edges of portal tracts, or within the hepatic lobule. Increasing severity of inflammation is associated with necrosis of liver cells. The assessment of the severity of inflammation and liver cell necrosis in a liver biopsy is used to assess the grade of disease, active inflammation being an adverse prognostic factor (*Figs 14.25* and *14.26*).
- Fibrosis initially develops around the portal tracts, then progresses to bridge between portal tracts and later may be associated with true cirrhosis (see below). The degree of fibrosis in a liver biopsy is used to assess the stage of disease.

Chronic viral hepatitis is mainly caused by hepatitis B and C

Chronic hepatitis B infection is due to failure of elimination of virus from the liver and leads to biochemical tests showing liver cell damage lasting longer than 6 months (see Data Set). Markers of active viral infection are present (see *Fig. 14.18*). Inflammatory activity varies, with predominantly lymphocytic inflammation in the lobules associated with liver cell necrosis. Liver cell necrosis can also be seen adjacent to portal tracts. In severe disease bridging fibrosis is seen. This may progress to cirrhosis.

Chronic hepatitis C infection causes continued liver cell necrosis lasting longer than 6 months. Serological markers of active viral infection are present. In contrast to HBV, inflammation is characterized by the presence of lymphoid follicles in the liver and fatty change in hepatocytes.

Data Set
Chronic viral hepatitis

A 35-year-old man with a history of intravenous drug abuse contracted hepatitis B infection. Eight months later he remained unwell.

Plasma

Total bilirubin	41 µmol/L	(up to 17)
	2.4 mg/dL	*(up to 1)*
Albumin	30 g/L	(30–48)
Alanine transaminase (ALT)	261 U/L	(up to 50)
Alkaline phosphatase	360 U/L	(40–120)
γ-Glutamyl transferase (GGT)	233 U/L	(up to 70)
Total protein	97 g/L	(63–78)

Chronic hepatitis produces a variable profile of liver function tests as a result of continuing inflammation. Raised alkaline phosphatase, GGT and bilirubin indicate cholestasis; the raised ALT level is due to liver cell necrosis. Impaired liver synthetic function contributes to the hypoalbuminemia. The total protein level is nevertheless raised, due to high immunoglobulin production. Additional tests should include tests for hepatitis B and C, and assessment of clotting function.

Fig. 14.24 Grading and staging of chronic hepatitis

Grade of necroinflammatory lesions

Grade score	Portal	Lobular
0	None or minimal	None
1	Portal inflammation	Inflammation but no necrosis
2	Mild necrosis of periportal hepatocytes	Focal necrotic cells with acidophil bodies
3	Moderate necrosis of periportal hepatocytes	Severe focal cell damage
4	Severe necrosis of periportal hepatocytes	Damage includes necrosis of liver cells that bridges between portal tracts

Stage of fibrosis

Stage score	Severity
0	None
1	Enlarged fibrotic portal tracts
2	Fibrosis extends to periportal areas
3	Fibrosis extends into septa but no distortion of liver architecture
4	Fibrosis associated with architectural distortion corresponding to cirrhosis

Autoimmune chronic hepatitis is associated with anti-Sm and antinuclear antibodies

Autoimmune chronic hepatitis typically occurs in women between the ages of 20 and 40 years. It is associated with hypergammaglobulinemia, autoantibodies in the serum, and other autoimmune disorders such as thyroiditis, arthritis and Sjögren's syndrome. There is an insidious onset of anorexia, malaise and fatigue, and investigation reveals raised bilirubin, moderately raised transaminase levels, and slight elevation of alkaline phosphatase. ESR is commonly elevated, and normochromic anemia occurs in some cases. The disease may run a relapsing and remitting course, or may progress inexorably to cirrhosis.

The etiology is unknown. Anti-smooth muscle antibodies SMA (80% of cases), antinuclear autoantibodies ANA (40–60% of cases), anti-liver/kidney microsomal LKM-1 antibodies (4% cases) and soluble liver antigen (anti SLA) antibodies (25% cases) are found in the serum but are not specific for this disease and are often seen in HCV infection. In 10% cases autoantibodies are not detected. None of the autoantibodies is thought to cause liver cell damage. T-cell mediated cytotoxicity directed against liver cells is thought to play a role in disease.

In establishing a diagnosis of autoimmune chronic hepatitis, other causes of chronic inflammatory liver disease (e.g. viral infection, alcoholic liver disease, sclerosing cholangitis, primary biliary cirrhosis, drug-related hepatitis and Wilson's disease) need to be excluded. Liver biopsy is part of the routine patient evaluation.

Drug-related chronic hepatitis must be excluded by clinical history

Certain drugs can cause chronic hepatitis, the most common being methyldopa, nitrofurantoin, minocycline, lisinoprol and diclofenac. Many other drugs have been implicated, albeit rarely, so it is important to consider any drug or herbal remedy as a potential cause of chronic hepatitis.

The mechanism is uncertain, but direct hepatotoxicity and induced autoimmune responses have been suggested.

Other forms of liver disease may result from drug ingestion, including acute liver cell necrosis (see page 280).

Primary biliary cirrhosis is associated with antimitochondrial antibodies

Primary biliary cirrhosis (PBC) is characterized by chronic destruction of intrahepatic bile ducts. The incidence is 10 times higher in women than in men, and it is an important cause of chronic liver disease and cirrhosis in women over the age of 50.

Although immune phenomena are involved, the etiology of primary biliary cirrhosis is uncertain. Autoantibodies are found in the blood but are not believed to be directly responsible for disease. Antimitochondrial antibodies AMA are directed against inner mitochondrial enzymes. ANA directed against nuclear pore protein gp120 is also seen.

An asymptomatic phase is recognized in which patients are found to have abnormal liver function and circulating autoantibodies. This group of patients typically develop symptomatic disease within 5 years.

In the early symptomatic stages of disease patients develop pruritus, tiredness and mild hyperbilirubinemia (see Data Set). Symptomatic patients typically develop advanced disease over a period of 6–10 years.

Some patients present with advanced decompensated disease with clinical evidence of complicated cirrhosis, having a poor prognosis without liver transplantation.

Liver biopsy is performed to evaluate the stage of the disease; early disease reveals obliteration of bile ducts from portal tracts, associated with small granulomas. Later, there is infiltration of portal tracts by lymphoid cells, with extension into the liver and destruction of adjacent hepatocytes in a manner similar to that seen in chronic hepatitis. As the disease progresses there is loss of large bile ducts and progressing fibrosis. In the final stages cirrhosis develops. There is gradual progression over about 10 years. Treatment using ursodeoxycholic acid may improve liver function, but liver transplantation is often necessary.

Data Set
Primary biliary cirrhosis

A 51-year-old woman complained of increasing generalised itching over a 12-month period.

Plasma

Total bilirubin	24 µmol/L	(up to 17)
	1 mg/dL	*(up to 1)*
Albumin	30 g/L	(30–48)
Alanine transaminase (ALT)	78 U/L	(up to 50)
Alkaline phosphatase	531 U/L	(40–120)
γ-Glutamyl transferase (GGT)	421 U/L	(up to 70)
Total protein	91 g/L	(63–78)

The high alkaline phosphatase and GGT indicate cholestasis. Jaundice is not a constant finding in primary biliary cirrhosis; this patient was not visibly jaundiced. IgM levels are usually elevated, as indicated by the high total protein concentration. Further laboratory tests should include antimitochondrial antibody titers, which are characteristically high in primary biliary cirrhosis.

Primary sclerosing cholangitis is the result of inflammation and fibrosis of bile ducts and leads to cirrhosis

Primary sclerosing cholangitis (PSC) causes progressive obstructive jaundice and is characterized by chronic inflammation and fibrosis of bile ducts. It is a condition with a male preponderance and a peak incidence between the ages of 25 and 40 years. It is associated with the presence of inflammatory bowel disease: 60% of patients with PSC have ulcerative colitis. However, only about 5% of patients with ulcerative colitis develop PSC. The autoantibodies seen in PBC are not found in cases of PSC.

PSC affects both intrahepatic and extrahepatic bile ducts. Large intrahepatic and extrahepatic ducts develop fibrous strictures with segmental dilatation. Radiological examination after the injection of contrast agent up the common bile duct back into the liver (endoscopic retrograde cholangiogram) reveals a 'beaded' appearance of affected ducts (*Fig. 14.25a*).

Medium-sized ducts, and ducts in portal tracts, show inflammation and a pattern of concentric fibrosis around the ducts (*Fig. 14.25b*), whereas small bile ducts in portal tracts are replaced by collagenous scar (vanishing bile ducts).

Patients develop cholestatic jaundice with progression to cirrhosis over a period of about 10 years. There is an increased risk of developing cholangiocarcinoma (see page 297).

TOXIC LIVER DISEASE

Drugs are an important and common cause of liver disease

Drugs are a very common cause of liver disease, and a careful drug history is a vital part of the assessment of any patient with abnormal liver function. Hepatotoxic drugs may be divided into two main groups: intrinsic hepatotoxins, which are dose dependent, predictable, and responsible for a high incidence of toxic damage to liver; and idiosyncratic hepatotoxins, which cause liver disease in a small percentage of exposed individuals, because of either hypersensitivity or abnormal drug metabolism.

All types of liver pathology may be caused by drugs, the main forms being given in *Fig. 14.26*. In view of the fact that almost any drug can cause liver disease, it is advisable to consult a specialist text when relating a drug history to potential hepatic damage.

Alcohol is the most common cause of chronic liver disease

Alcohol abuse is the most common cause of liver disease in western countries, and women are more prone to alcohol-induced liver damage than men.

Alcohol is a hepatotoxin and liver damage is related to daily intake. There is no safe lower limit for alcohol inges-

Fig. 14.26 Drug-induced liver damage	
Liver pathology	**Drugs causing damage**
Fatty change	Methotrexate, tetracyclines, sodium valproate
Hepatic granulomas	Sulphonamides, allopurinol
Acute hepatitis	Isoniazid, halothane
Chronic hepatitis	Isoniazid, methyldopa
Cholestasis	Steroids, chlorpromazine
Central vein occlusion	Cytotoxic drugs
Tumors	Oral contraceptives (adenomata) Anabolic steroids (carcinomas)
Acute necrosis	Paracetamol

Fig. 14.25 Sclerosing cholangitis. A beaded appearance of dilatation and stricture is seen on retrograde cholangiography (a). Histologically (b) ducts in the liver (**D**) are surrounded by a pattern of concentric fibrosis (**E**) and associated chronic inflammation, which leads to later duct obliteration.

tion, but maximum advised daily intakes have been defined when the risk of liver damage is thought to be small (50–60 g/day in males; 30–40 g/day in females).

The toxicity of ethanol is probably due to several factors: generation of its metabolic breakdown product acetaldehyde; generation of reactive oxygen species causing oxidative damage to hepatocytes; and activation of the endoplasmic reticulum stress response in hepatocytes.

Alcohol causes fatty liver, acute hepatitis and cirrhosis

Alcoholic liver damage may lead to fatty liver (*Fig. 14.6*), in which the accumulation of fat in hepatocytes is reversible with abstinence.

In **acute alcoholic hepatitis the** ingestion of large amounts of alcohol causes a true hepatitis, with focal necrosis of liver cells. The illness resembles acute viral hepatitis, and liver function tests show raised levels of transaminases and γ-glutamyl transpeptidase (*Fig. 14.27*).

If a patient with alcoholic hepatitis abstains, the inflammation resolves without harm. With continued ingestion of alcohol, fibrosis develops around central veins, and in response to continued hepatocyte necrosis. The result is hepatic fibrosis that may progress to cirrhosis.

Alcoholic cirrhosis affects fewer than 10% of patients suffering from chronic alcoholism. It may develop after episodes of acute alcoholic hepatitis, or may be insidious in its onset, presenting only as end-stage liver disease.

METABOLIC LIVER DISEASE

Hemochromatosis is caused by excessive deposition of iron in tissues

In hemochromatosis, excessive iron accumulation causes chronic damage to liver cells. Two types of disease are distinguished.

Primary hemochromatosis is inherited as an autosomal recessive trait and leads to excessive absorption of iron from the gut. The gene is located on chromosome 6, close to the HLA locus, called HLA-H. Iron accumulates as hemosiderin in many tissues, including the liver (*Fig. 14.28*), pancreas, pituitary, heart and skin. Accumulation of iron in the liver causes death of hepatocytes (possibly from the generation of free radicals) and leads to cirrhosis. Accumulation in the pancreatic islets causes diabetes mellitus, and in the cardiac muscle gives rise to a cardiomyopathy with heart failure.

Macroscopically, the liver and other affected tissues appear rusty brown due to hemosiderin in cells (hepatocytes, Kupffer cells, and biliary epithelium in the liver).

Fig. 14.28 Hemochromatosis. Perls' stain reveals iron deposition in tissues as a blue color. In (a) iron is seen in liver cells, as well as in biliary epithelium. Macroscopically, affected tissues look rusty brown, as illustrated by the pancreas in (b), taken from a patient with primary hemochromatosis.

Fig. 14.27 Alcoholic hepatitis. Liver biopsy shows fatty change (**F**) and focal necrosis of liver cells associated with neutrophil infiltration adjacent to dead cells (**N**). Mallory's hyaline (**H**) accumulates in a small proportion of hepatocytes. Composed of cytokeratin intermediate filaments, ubiquitin and P62, it appears as brightly eosinophilic globules in liver cell cytoplasm.

Diagnosis can be made on the finding of an extremely high saturation of transferrin in the blood, with high serum iron and ferritin levels, and is usually confirmed by liver biopsy.

Secondary hemochromatosis (also called **hemosiderosis**) is the result of excessive iron accumulation caused by other primary diseases (e.g. alcoholism) and by repeated blood transfusions for diseases with abnormalities of red cell formation, particularly thalassemia (see pages 321–2).

Wilson's disease is an inherited disease of copper metabolism

Wilson's disease is a rare but treatable cause of chronic destructive liver disease. An inherited autosomal recessive disorder of copper metabolism, it causes excess copper to accumulate in the liver and brain. This defect is a mutation in a copper-transport ATPase gene, ATP7B, located on chromosome 13. The carrier rate is about 1:90 in the population, with about 300 mutations now described. As most cases represent compound heterozygotes with so many potential mutations, genetic diagnosis is limited and reliance is placed on biochemical testing.

Excess copper in the liver initially causes a chronic hepatitis picture clinically, and pathologically progresses to cirrhosis. Some patients have significant fatty change as the dominant feature in Wilson's disease.

Accumulation in the brain leads to psychiatric disorders that account for about 20% of presenting cases, as well as a neuological presentation with abnormal eye movements, and a movement disorder resembling Parkinson's disease.

Diagnosis can be made by finding a low level of ceruloplasmin, the copper-binding protein, in the serum (as it is not released from the liver). Excess copper is demonstrable in liver biopsy material by special staining.

Copper accumulation in Wilson's disease

In normal circumstances dietary copper is taken to the liver, complexed to ceruloplasmin, and secreted into the plasma. Circulating ceruloplasmin is recycled by the liver in the endosome–lysosome system, free copper being re-excreted into the bile. In Wilson's disease the liver fails to secrete the copper–ceruloplasmin complex into the plasma, thereby accumulating copper in hepatocyte cytoplasm. Free copper overspills into the blood and is deposited in the brain and cornea (Kayser–Fleischer rings).

α₁-Antitrypsin deficiency causes chronic liver disease and cirrhosis

α_1-Antitrypsin deficiency (*Fig. 14.29*) is an important heritable cause of chronic liver disease, and also causes panacinar emphysema (see page 204). Affected individuals fail to produce the normal active extracellular protease inhibitor α_1-antitrypsin. Many alleles for this protease inhibitor (**Pi**) gene are known, each of which has been given a letter. The normal phenotype is known as **PiMM**. The most significant abnormal allele is termed Z. Heterozygotes (**PiZM**) carry an increased risk of lung damage if they smoke, developing emphysema. Homozygotes (**PiZZ**) develop emphysema and liver disease.

Disease may be manifest in neonates as a neonatal hepatitis (see page 298), although this is not an inevitable consequence of the PiZZ genotype. In adult life, disease may be discovered following investigation of abnormal liver function tests. Investigation may reveal either a chronic hepatitis or cirrhosis.

Fig. 14.29 α₁-Antitrypsin deficiency. Liver biopsy shows accumulation of α_1-antitrypsin in hepatocytes as globules (**G**) which stain with PAS (a) and can also be specifically stained by immunoperoxidase methods using antibodies to α_1-antitrypsin (b).

CIRRHOSIS OF THE LIVER

In cirrhosis the liver is diffusely replaced by nodules of hepatocytes separated by fibrosis

In cirrhosis the normal architecture of the liver is diffusely replaced by nodules of regenerated liver cells, separated by bands of collagenous fibrosis (*Fig. 14.30*). An irreversible form of chronic liver disease, cirrhosis is the end-stage of many processes. It has three key characteristics: long-standing destruction of liver cells, associated chronic inflammation that stimulates fibrosis, and regeneration of hepatocytes to cause nodules.

Fibrosis is caused by growth factors liberated from inflammatory cells, Kupffer cells, and hepatocytes. The inflammatory cells may be part of the disease process (e.g. in chronic hepatitis) or may be recruited in response to liver cell necrosis (for example in chronic alcoholism). Myofibroblast-like cells, termed stellate cells, are responsible for secreting collagen.

Nodules of hepatocytes form as part of the normal capacity of hepatocytes to divide and regenerate in response to damage, but lack normal vascular and bile drainage connections.

The best way to classify cirrhosis is by its etiology. The main causes of cirrhosis (*Fig. 14.31*) are conditions known to result in chronic liver cell necrosis with fibrosis and regeneration.

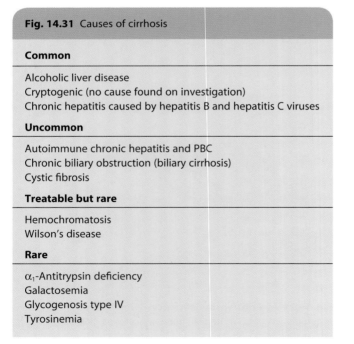

Fig. 14.30 Cirrhosis. Macroscopically (a, b) the external surface of the cirrhotic liver has a bosselated appearance. On cut surface (c) the parenchyma is replaced by nodules of regenerated hepatocytes, separated by fine fibrosis. Histologically (d), nodules of hepatocytes (stained yellow in this preparation) are separated by bands of collagenous tissue (stained red). Bile ducts and portal vessels run in the fibrous septa. Some of the nodules contain a central vein, others do not. This distortion of vascular architecture leads to portal hypertension. In some cases the cause of cirrhosis can be determined from liver biopsy, e.g. alcoholic cirrhosis is frequently characterized by fatty change in hepatocytes, as shown in (e).

Fig. 14.31 Causes of cirrhosis
Common
Alcoholic liver disease
Cryptogenic (no cause found on investigation)
Chronic hepatitis caused by hepatitis B and hepatitis C viruses
Uncommon
Autoimmune chronic hepatitis and PBC
Chronic biliary obstruction (biliary cirrhosis)
Cystic fibrosis
Treatable but rare
Hemochromatosis
Wilson's disease
Rare
α_1-Antitrypsin deficiency
Galactosemia
Glycogenosis type IV
Tyrosinemia

In early classifications two types of cirrhosis were described, based on the size of the regenerative nodules: **micronodular cirrhosis** nodules are small, ranging in size up to 3 mm; **macronodular cirrhosis** nodules are larger than 3 mm, ranging in size up to 2 cm. This classification has little clinical relevance.

Cirrhosis results in liver failure and portal hypertension

The main consequences of cirrhosis are:

- Reduced hepatocyte function (decreased synthesis of proteins, failure of detoxification).
- Disturbance of blood flow through the liver, causing portal hypertension with all its attendant complications (see pages 281–2). In particular sudden deterioration caused by bleeding from esophageal varices.
- Reduced immune competence and increased susceptibility to infection.
- Increased risk of development of hepatocellular carcinoma.
- Increased risk of development of portal vein thrombosis.

These consequences are manifest by a group of distinctive clinical features in a typical patient with cirrhosis (*Fig. 14.32*). In clinical practice, cirrhosis is encountered in one of two ways. It may develop in patients who are under follow-up for known chronic liver disease (e.g. chronic hepatitis or alcoholic liver disease), or it may first present as end-stage disease, having been entirely subclinical in its evolution.

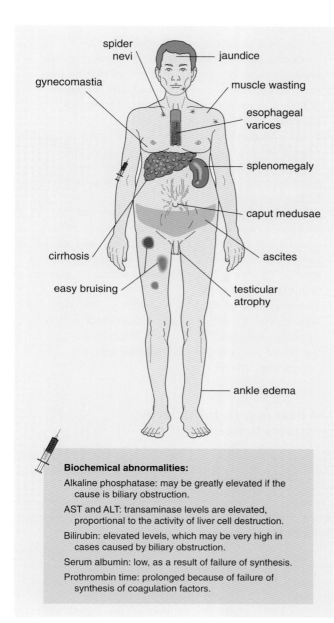

Biochemical abnormalities:

Alkaline phosphatase: may be greatly elevated if the cause is biliary obstruction.

AST and ALT: transaminase levels are elevated, proportional to the activity of liver cell destruction.

Bilirubin: elevated levels, which may be very high in cases caused by biliary obstruction.

Serum albumin: low, as a result of failure of synthesis.

Prothrombin time: prolonged because of failure of synthesis of coagulation factors.

Fig. 14.32 Clinical stigmata of cirrhosis. Cirrhosis gives rise to clinical stigmata caused by failure of liver metabolism as well as those caused by portal hypertension. Testicular atrophy, spider nevi and gynecomastia are the result of impaired metabolism of endogenous estrogens. Ascites and edema are caused by low serum albumin. Varices, splenomegaly and caput medusae are caused by portal hypertension. Bruising is caused by failure to synthesize clotting factors.

Data Set
Cirrhosis

A 54-year-old man with a history of alcohol abuse presented with jaundice.

Plasma

Total bilirubin	283 µmol/L	(up to 17)
	16.4 mg/dL	*(up to 1)*
Albumin	28 g/L	(30–48)
Alanine transaminase (ALT)	76 U/L	(up to 50)
Alkaline phosphatase	193 U/L	(40–120)
γ-Glutamyl transferase (GGT)	549 U/L	(up to 70)

The liver function tests in patients with cirrhosis can be very variable, and are never diagnostic. In the early stages of the disease liver function tests may be normal. As the disease progresses cholestasis may occur, as in this patient, and liver cell necrosis may result in raised transaminase levels. Albumin levels are often low, due to impaired synthesis. Further tests should include plasma urea, creatinine and electrolytes, as derangements of fluid balance are common in patients with cirrhosis.

Pathogenesis of ascites in cirrhosis

Ascites is the accumulation of fluid in the peritoneal cavity that exceeds the expected volume of about 25 mL. The most common reason for ascites in association with portal hypertension is cirrhosis. Three mechanisms are involved:

1. Portal hypertension leads to vasodilatation in the splanchnic vessels, reducing blood volume and activating the renin–angiotensin–aldosterone system. This causes sodium and water retention.
2. Increased transudation of fluid takes place because of increased hydrostatic pressure in the splanchnic vascular bed.
3. Increased transudation of fluid is predisposed to by low plasma oncotic pressure (associated with hypoalbuminemia due to reduced albumin synthesis by damaged liver cells).

Acute liver failure frequently develops in cirrhosis

Signs of chronic liver failure are seen in association with cirrhosis (see *Fig. 14.32*), and this is usually a fairly stable clinical state. Importantly, patients with chronic liver failure are at risk of an abrupt deterioration in condition that leads to acute liver failure. The main precipitating factors are alcohol binge, the development of intercurrent infection, gastrointestinal bleed (e.g. from esophageal varices), portal vein thrombosis, and the development of carcinoma of the liver (see page 297).

Cirrhosis may develop as a consequence of chronic biliary obstruction

Biliary cirrhosis is the result of long-standing obstruction of bile ducts, leading to the development of obstructive jaundice, liver cell necrosis, and fibrosis with regenerative nodules. The main causes are **primary biliary cirrhosis**, unrelieved obstruction of the main extrahepatic bile ducts (also termed **secondary biliary cirrhosis**), and **sclerosing cholangitis** (see pages 291 and 294).

Early in the course of biliary obstruction there is edema and expansion of intrahepatic portal tracts, with portal tract fibrosis. Bile plugs develop in biliary canaliculi, which may rupture and cause the death of adjacent hepatocytes (so-called bile infarcts, see *Fig. 14.9*). Over a long period, liver cell death, regeneration and fibrosis result in cirrhosis.

TUMORS OF THE LIVER

Benign tumors of the liver are derived from several cell types. Some are better considered as hamartomas rather than neoplasms.

- **Hepatic adenomata** are true neoplasms, arising as well-circumscribed nodules up to 20 cm in size. Seen in women in the reproductive period, they are predisposed to by estrogen-containing oral contraceptives. The histological appearances closely resemble those of normal liver, except that no portal structures are seen. These lesions cause problems as they may rupture and cause intra-abdominal bleeding.
- **Focal nodular hyperplasia** is seen in under 1% of the population, 90% being in women. It represents hyperplasia of hepatocytes, often around an area of zonal scarring. Lesions may be detected as incidental findings on imaging.
- **Bile duct adenomata** are very common and are probably hamartomas. They appear as small white nodules, often beneath the liver capsule, and are composed of abnormal bile ducts in a collagenous stroma. They may be mistaken for metastatic tumor deposits at laparotomy.
- **Hemangioma of the liver** is common. It is seen beneath the capsule as a dark, almost black, lesion (typically 2–3 cm in size) which, histologically, is composed of abnormal vascular channels in a collagenous stroma.

The liver may be involved by secondary tumors

The most common malignant tumor of the liver is **metastatic tumor**. Spread to the liver is via the bloodstream, either from the portal vein in the case of tumors in the gastrointestinal tract, or by the systemic circulation for other tumors (see page 77). Clinically the liver is enlarged, and feels hard and craggy on palpation.

The colon, rectum, stomach, pancreas, breast and lung are the most common primary sites of tumors that metastasize to the liver. Many other tumors also spread to the liver, but they are numerically less frequent. There is often involvement by tumors of the lymphoreticular system, **malignant lymphomas** (see page 309), and by malignant tumors of the bone marrow, **leukemias** (see pages 324–7).

Small deposits of tumor in the liver have little clinical effect but, when extensive, metastases cause compression of the intrahepatic bile ducts and lead to jaundice (see page 301). Partial hepatic resection, chemotherapy or percutaneous ablation are increasingly used for management.

Primary hepatocellular carcinoma is predisposed to by cirrhosis, hepatitis B infection and mycotoxins

Primary carcinomas derived from hepatocytes are termed **hepatocellular carcinomas**, often referred to as hepatomas (*Fig. 14.33*). Worldwide this is the fourth commonest malignant tumor because of its causation by hepatitis B and C infection. The marked geographic variation seen in the incidence of this condition (very high in Africa and the Far East) is due to the regional high hepatitis virus carrier rates. These are also associated with cirrhosis from other causes, especially due to hemochromatosis and alcohol.

Serum α-fetoprotein (AFP) levels may be raised in cases of hepatocellular carcinoma and it is demonstrable by immunochemistry in tumor cells. The prognosis is very poor, with a median survival of less than 6 months from diagnosis. Fibrolamellar carcinoma is a form that occurs in young adults, in normal liver, and with a better prognosis.

Cholangiocarcinoma is predisposed to by chronic inflammatory diseases of bile ducts

Adenocarcinomas arising from the intrahepatic bile duct epithelium are termed **cholangiocarcinomas**. They may be predisposed to by chronic inflammatory diseases of the intrahepatic biliary tree, particularly sclerosing cholangitis (see page 291) and disease caused by liver flukes (see page 287). Macroscopically, lesions may be single or multifocal and are associated with a very poor prognosis, most patients being dead within 6 months of diagnosis.

Angiosarcomas of the liver are caused by exposure to environmental agents

Derived from vascular endothelium, angiosarcomas are highly malignant tumors that appear as multifocal hemor-rhagic nodules within the liver. Such tumors are rare unless there has been exposure to thorotrast (a radiological contrast agent used until the 1950s), vinyl chloride monomer (used in the plastic industry to make PVC), arsenic (administered in the past in certain 'tonics'), or anabolic steroids.

MULTISYSTEM DISEASE AND TRANSPLANTATION

The liver is frequently involved in multisystem disease

Liver enlargement or deranged liver function tests are commonly caused by liver involvement in systemic disease processes.

- **Amyloidosis**: the liver may be involved in deposition of the abnormal protein, amyloid (see Chapter 25).
- **Sarcoidosis**: the liver is frequently involved by granulomatous inflammation as part of systemic sarcoidosis (see Chapter 25).
- **Extramedullary hemopoiesis** occurs in the liver when diseases efface the bone marrow. This is particularly seen in the myeloproliferative diseases (see page 327).
- **Cardiac failure** (see page 171–3).
- **Diabetes mellitus**: fatty liver and glycogen accumulation.

Liver transplants are prone to rejection as well as recurrence of original disease

Liver transplantation is being performed with increasing frequency to treat chronic liver disease, particularly that

Fig. 14.33 Hepatocellular carcinoma. Macroscopically hepatocellular carcinomas may be single or multifocal. As in (a), they usually develop in a liver already affected by cirrhosis. Tumor appears as an abnormal mass (**M**) within the liver. Histologically (b) tumor is composed of liver cells with atypical nuclear cytology and abnormal architectural arrangement. Bile secretion (**B**) by tumor cells may be seen.

which has progressed to cirrhosis. It is also used to treat cases of fulminant hepatic failure due to extensive liver cell necrosis.

The pathological complications of transplantation are acute rejection, affecting 60% of patients in the first few weeks (treatable with steroids), and chronic rejection, affecting 15% of patients within the first year. Immune-mediated destruction of intrahepatic bile ducts and obliteration of intrahepatic vessels leads to progressive cholestatic jaundice. This is unresponsive to immunosuppression. Bile duct strictures at anastomosis sites may also complicate transplantation, and recurrent disease is seen in hepatitis B and C, and in primary biliary cirrhosis.

LIVER DISEASE IN CHILDHOOD

Biliary atresia is a cause of neonatal jaundice

In biliary atresia there is destruction of bile ducts that leads to severe jaundice in neonates. Two patterns are seen:

- **Intrahepatic atresia**, in which ducts within the liver are absent.
- **Extrahepatic atresia**, in which the main extrahepatic ducts are not patent.

These syndromes are believed to be due to intrauterine inflammatory diseases, which can also cause neonatal hepatitis, discussed next.

Liver biopsy shows striking proliferation of small bile ducts at the margins of portal tracts. Affected children develop severe jaundice. Extrahepatic atresia may be treated by surgical bypass operations. Children with severe disease develop unremitting jaundice and secondary biliary cirrhosis.

Neonatal hepatitis is a syndrome with many causes

Neonatal hepatitis is a clinical condition with many causes, presenting as neonatal jaundice.

Histologically there is hepatocyte damage, parenchymal inflammation and, in many cases, **giant-cell transformation** of hepatocytes (so-called giant cell hepatitis). The main causes are:

- Idiopathic (no cause found), accounting for 50% of cases.
- α_1-Antitrypsin deficiency, responsible in about 30% of cases (see page 293).
- Viral hepatitis.

- Hepatitis due to **to**xoplasma, **r**ubella, **cy**tomegalovirus or **h**erpes simplex (TORCH group).
- Metabolic causes (galactosemia, hereditary fructose intolerance).
- Extrahepatic biliary atresia.
- Congenital hepatic fibrosis.

With the exception of cases associated with biliary atresia who require a surgical bile-drainage operation, children with neonatal hepatitis generally recover from the acute jaundice, although the underlying condition may persist.

Jaundice in neonates can cause brain damage termed 'kernicterus'

Unconjugated hyperbilirubinemia in neonates may lead to kernicterus. Unconjugated bilirubin, which is lipid soluble, enters the brain to cause damage to neurons, particularly in the basal ganglia. Affected children develop spasticity, choreoathetosis and mental deficiency. The most common causes are hemolysis due to rhesus incompatibility, or functional immaturity of hepatic conjugating enzyme systems.

Cystic fibrosis leads to cirrhosis in adult life in about 10% of cases

In cystic fibrosis (see page 221) affected neonates may develop obstructive jaundice due to blockage of bile ducts by abnormally viscous bile. Of those who survive to adult life, 10–15% develop chronic liver disease. This is a form of secondary biliary cirrhosis due to chronic obstruction to bile ducts by viscid bile.

Reye's syndrome is associated with microvesicular fat in liver cells

Reye's syndrome results in acute liver failure associated with cerebral edema and encephalopathy. It is seen in children and may be triggered by preceding viral infection or salicylate administration. Histologically the liver shows microvesicular fatty change. The condition is fatal in about 50% of cases.

Hepatoblastoma is a rare malignant childhood tumor

Rare malignant tumors of childhood, hepatoblastomas often replace large portions of the liver. They are composed of several cell types including fetal-pattern liver cells and mesenchymal elements. The serum α-fetoprotein is elevated.

DISEASES OF THE GALLBLADDER AND EXTRAHEPATIC BILE DUCTS

Gallstones

Stones in the gallbladder and bile duct system (**cholelithiasis**) are the most common cause of disease affecting the biliary tree. Stones form from the constituents of bile, the main components being variable proportions of cholesterol, calcium salts (phosphates, carbonates) and bilirubin (in the form of calcium bilirubinate).

Although it is recognized that most stones have several constituents, two main types of stone have been defined according to the major constituent of each: **cholesterol stones** (80% of all stones) and **pigment stones** (20% of all stones). Mixed stones also form, being composed of cholesterol, pigment and calcium salts.

Cholesterol stones are predisposed to by changes in cholesterol solubility in bile

Cholesterol stones (*Fig. 14.34*) occur in 20% of women and 8% of men, usually causing no problems. They form when bile becomes supersaturated with cholesterol, there being insufficient bile salts to keep the cholesterol in solution. In most cases the reasons for these changes are unclear.

The main risk factors associated with cholesterol stone formation are:

- Reduced bile acids in bile, caused by estrogen or excessive loss from gut (leading to reduced enterohepatic recirculation) due to malabsorption, in Crohn's disease or cystic fibrosis.
- Increased cholesterol in bile caused by obesity, female gender, increasing age.

Cholesterolosis of the gallbladder occurs when the submucosa of the gallbladder is focally infiltrated by macrophages laden with cholesterol. This condition is frequently associated with the development of cholesterol stones and is believed to be predisposed to by the same conditions that cause reduced solubility of cholesterol in bile. Understanding of the pathogenesis of cholesterol stone formation has led to medical treatment by oral therapy with bile salts to dissolve the stones.

Pigment stones are predisposed to by increased hepatic secretion of bilirubin

Several clinical situations are associated with the development of pigment stones (*Fig. 14.35*), which are largely composed of calcium bilirubinate, with lesser amounts of other calcium salts and mucoproteins. It is easy to understand why patients with abnormal red-cell breakdown, generating large amounts of conjugated bilirubin, develop pigment stones. The association of pigment stones with cirrhosis and ileal resection is believed to be related to disturbance of the enterohepatic recycling of factors that regulate the solubility of factors secreted in bile. Chronic biliary infections predispose to pigment gallstones by bacterial production of glucuronidases, which unconjugate secreted conjugated bilirubin.

Gallstones may obstruct the biliary tract and predispose to the development of carcinoma of the gallbladder

Over 70% of gallstones remain clinically silent. The main clinical complications of cholelithiasis arise from obstruction of the cystic duct or common bile duct by a stone.

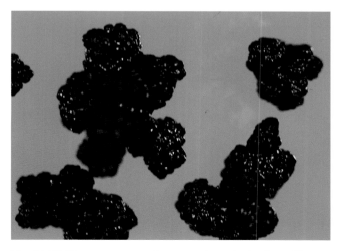

Fig. 14.34 Cholesterol stones. Stones are round, faceted and can be 0.5–3 cm in size, but are typically large. Biochemical analysis reveals over 50% cholesterol composition, with lesser amounts of calcium salts so, strictly, most such stones are of mixed composition.

Fig. 14.35 Pigment stones. Stones are irregular in shape. They measure up to 1 cm, being typically smaller than cholesterol stones.

The presence of stones in the biliary tract leads to muscle hypertrophy and thickening of the wall of the gallbladder (**obstructive cholecystopathy**). Stones impacted in the cystic duct predispose to inflammation of the gallbladder (**cholecystitis**), which may be acute or chronic (see below), and those forming in the bile ducts (**choledocholithiasis**) predispose to obstructive jaundice, cholangitis and acute pancreatitis. Stones in the gallbladder predispose to the development of carcinoma of the gallbladder (see below).

Fig. 14.36 Chronic cholecystitis. In chronic cholecystitis there is thickening of the gallbladder wall (**W**). Histologically this is due to muscular hypertrophy, submucosal fibrosis, and chronic inflammation. Outpouchings of mucosa into the wall form small cystic spaces termed 'Aschoff–Rokitansky sinuses.' In this example, stones (**GS**) are seen in the fundus, and the mucosa is inflamed.

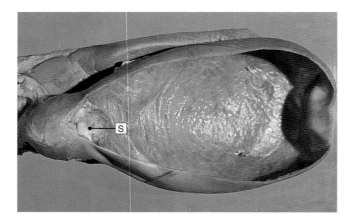

Fig. 14.37 Mucocele of the gallbladder. Mucocele of the gallbladder is caused by obstruction of the cystic duct by stones (**S**). The bile is resorbed and the epithelium changes type to a mucin-secreting pattern, filling the gallbladder with clear mucus (emptied from this specimen). The mucosal surface is smooth and the wall is thinned.

Gallstones may cause acute cholecystitis

Acute inflammation of the gallbladder causes pain in the right upper quadrant of the abdomen. The affected gallbladder is enlarged, red and edematous, and histologically there is acute inflammation of the wall, with focal epithelial ulceration.

Most cases are associated with gallstones, and there is often obstruction of the cystic bile duct by a stone. Inflammation is precipitated by the chemical effects of concentrated bile in the gallbladder, but secondary infection may develop with enteric organisms such as *Escherichia coli*. Primary bacterial infection of the gallbladder, e.g. with *Salmonella*, is rare.

Acute cholecystitis can occur in critically ill patients in the absence of gallstones, when septicemic spread of infection is postulated. Complications of acute cholecystitis include perforation into the abdomen (causing **biliary peritonitis**), and secondary infection which, in severe cases, may cause **empyema** of the gallbladder, filling the lumen with pus.

Chronic cholecystitis is associated with the presence of gallstones

Chronic cholecystitis is caused by the chronic effects of gallstones. There is thickening and fibrosis of the wall, with variable chronic inflammatory infiltration of mucosa and submucosa (*Fig. 14.36*).

The pathogenesis of chronic cholecystitis is probably multifactorial. As many gallbladders that have been removed show muscle thickening and fibrosis without inflammatory changes, it may be more appropriate to call such cases **obstructive cholecystopathy**. Other cases have associated chronic inflammation, and these may truly be called **chronic cholecystitis**. The development of disease has been related to contractile abnormalities of the gallbladder (stimulated by the presence of stones), to direct chemical injury to the mucosa by bile, or to the effects of repeated episodes of acute cholecystitis.

Secondary changes include extensive **calcification** of the wall of the gallbladder (porcelain gallbladder) and the development of a **mucocele** of the gallbladder (*Fig. 14.37*).

Carcinoma of the gallbladder is associated with gallstones

Carcinoma of the gallbladder is the most common tumor of the gallbladder and is usually associated with the presence of gallstones and chronic cholecystitis. Most cases are seen in women over the age of 70.

Most tumors arise in the fundus and, histologically, are moderately differentiated adenocarcinomas (*Fig. 14.38*). The prognosis is poor, with a 5-year survival rate of under 5%. Infiltration of local structures, mainly the liver, makes curative surgery difficult.

Fig. 14.38 Carcinoma of the gallbladder. Adenocarcinoma of the gallbladder is seen as a raised, ulcerated area (**T**) in the fundus. Most tumors have invaded through the wall at the time of diagnosis.

Blockage of the main bile ducts causes obstructive jaundice

Obstruction of the common bile duct is most commonly due to a gallstone. Other causes include pancreatic carcinoma (see page 304), carcinoma of the ampulla of Vater (see page 262), fibrous stricture (often postoperative), and bile duct carcinoma (predisposed by chronic inflammation and liver flukes).

Microscopically, the common and intrahepatic bile ducts become dilated, and are detected by ultrasound examination.

DISEASE OF THE EXOCRINE PANCREAS

The normal exocrine pancreas comprises over 80% of the gland. Digestive enzymes are secreted and travel by pancreatic ducts to the duodenum.

Developmental defects in the pancreas are uncommon. Heterotopic pancreatic tissue may be found in the wall of the duodenum, the stomach, and in Meckel's diverticulum (see page 272).

Chronic pancreatitis is mainly caused by chronic alcohol abuse

Chronic pancreatitis results from chronic inflammation and fibrosis in the gland. The main associations of chronic pancreatitis are shown in *Fig. 14.39*. The four pathological features of chronic pancreatitis are continued chronic inflammation, fibrous scarring, loss of pancreatic parenchymal elements, and duct strictures and ectasia with the formation of intrapancreatic calculi (*Fig. 14.40*).

Patients have recurrent bouts of severe abdominal pain, with the eventual development of malabsorption (see page

257) and diabetes mellitus as the pancreatic parenchyma is destroyed. Episodes of acute pancreatitis may complicate chronic pancreatitis.

Severe pancreatic atrophy occurs with cystic fibrosis

In cystic fibrosis (see pages 221–2) viscid mucin occludes pancreatic ducts. Blockage results, with duct dilatation and atrophy of pancreatic acini. With time, both exocrine and endocrine parts of the pancreas are destroyed. Patients develop pancreatic insufficiency, with malabsorption and diabetes mellitus.

Fig. 14.39 Main associations of chronic pancreatitis	
Common	
Chronic alcoholism	Accounts for the majority of cases. Protein plugs form in ducts and become calculi. Ducts become obstructed, inflamed and scarred
Idiopathic chronic pancreatitis	Onset in old age. Often associated with peripheral vascular disease. Pathogenesis uncertain
Rare	
Cystic fibrosis	Protein plugs in ducts
Idiopathic juvenile pancreatitis	Uncertain etiology
Tropical pancreatitis	Prevalent in India and Africa. Uncertain cause

Fig. 14.40 Chronic pancreatitis. In chronic pancreatitis the pancreas (**P**) is atrophic and replaced by rubbery, fibrous tissue, in which dilated ducts (**D**) are seen. In many cases calculi are present in the dilated ducts. In this example the duodenum is attached (**A**).

Acute pancreatitis results in enzymatic necrosis of tissues

Acute pancreatitis is an important cause of severe abdominal pain and enters the differential diagnosis of the acute abdomen (see Data Set). Severe acute inflammation and necrosis of the pancreas leads to liberation of the powerful digestive enzymes, resulting in extensive enzyme-mediated local tissue necrosis, particularly **fat necrosis** (*Fig. 14.41*). The main predisposing factors for pancreatitis are summarized in *Fig. 14.42*, and its pathogenesis is illustrated in *Fig. 14.43*. A complication of the development of acute pancreatitis is the conversion of the necrotic pancreas into a cyst filled with serosanguinous fluid (**pancreatic pseudocyst**).

Fig. 14.41 Acute pancreatitis. In acute pancreatitis (a) the pancreas appears edematous and is commonly hemorrhagic (**H**). Pancreatic tissue becomes necrotic and may become semi-liquid. Lipase released from the pancreatic acini causes the development of foci of fat necrosis. This is seen in (b) as white spots (**F**), typically 0.5 cm in diameter, in mesenteric and retroperitoneal fat. Histologically (c) these foci are composed of necrotic adipose tissue (**F**), with adjacent reactive inflammation (**I**).

Data Set
Acute pancreatitis

A 42-year-old man with a history of alcohol abuse presented with severe abdominal pain and abdominal rigidity.

Plasma

Amylase   6470 U/L   (30–110)

Elevated levels of amylase in plasma are seen in a range of intra-abdominal emergencies in addition to acute pancreatitis, including perforated peptic ulcers, intestinal obstruction, and biliary obstruction due to gallstones. Amylase is rapidly cleared from plasma, with a half-life of around 12 hours, and returns to normal within a few days of an attack of acute pancreatitis.

Serum amylase levels of this magnitude are only seen in acute pancreatitis.

Fig. 14.42 Predisposing factors in acute pancreatitis

Mechanical obstruction of pancreatic ducts
Gallstones
Trauma
Postoperative (e.g. ERCP)
Metabolic/toxic causes
Alcohol
Drugs (e.g. thiazide diuretics, azathioprine, steroids)
Hypercalcemia
Hyperlipidemia
Vascular/poor perfusion
Atherosclerosis, vasculitis
Hypothermia
Infections
Mumps and other viruses (EBV, CMV)

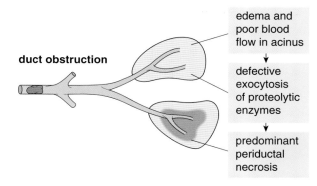

duct obstruction

edema and poor blood flow in acinus
↓
defective exocytosis of proteolytic enzymes
↓
predominant periductal necrosis

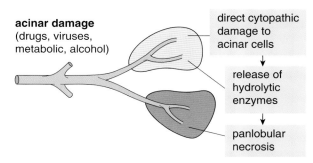

acinar damage
(drugs, viruses, metabolic, alcohol)

direct cytopathic damage to acinar cells
↓
release of hydrolytic enzymes
↓
panlobular necrosis

hypoperfusion
(shock, hypothermia, vascular disease)

reduced perfusion to acinar cells
↓
cell necrosis with release of hydrolases
↓
predominant perilobular necrosis

Fig. 14.43 Pathogenesis of pancreatitis. Three patterns of pancreatic necrosis have been defined, although in the advanced state it is hard to tell which pattern was present at the initiation as massive necrosis supervenes.

1 Periductal necrosis: necrosis takes place in acinal cells adjacent to ducts. This form is seen in conditions caused by duct obstruction, particularly associated with gallstones and alcohol.

2 Panlobular necrosis: necrosis is found affecting all portions of the pancreatic lobule. Conditions which cause direct acinar damage may initiate this pattern of damage, for example drugs, viruses, toxins and metabolic causes. Panlobular necrosis may be due to spread from initial periductal or perilobular necrosis.

3 Perilobular necrosis: necrosis takes place in the periphery of lobules. The pathogenesis is poor vascular perfusion of this zone, leading to acinar necrosis. This pattern is seen in shock and hypothermia.

The outcome of acute pancreatitis relates to severity

Episodes of mild acute pancreatitis may resolve. In severe acute pancreatitis systemic metabolic complications may develop, such as adult respiratory distress syndrome (ARDS) or disseminated intravascular coagulation. Shock associated with such severe complications may lead to multiorgan failure.

Laboratory medicine

Acute pancreatitis

Full blood count: neutrophil leukocytosis.

Serum amylase: greatly elevated.

Serum albumin: falls in severe disease, due to loss in acute inflammatory exudate.

Serum calcium: falls in severe disease, due to complexing with necrotic fat and loss in exudate.

Blood sugar: hyperglycemia in severe disease, due to loss of pancreatic endocrine cells.

Alkaline phosphatase: mild elevation from edema and obstruction of lower end of bile duct.

Bilirubin: mild elevation due to oedema and obstruction of lower end of bile duct.

Key Facts
Pancreatitis

- Caused by necrosis of pancreatic acinar cells which release hydrolytic enzymes.
- Macroscopic hemorrhagic necrosis of the pancreatic tissue associated with fat necrosis in adjacent tissues.
- Commonest predisposing factors are gallstones and alcohol-related disease.
- Three main pathogenic mechanisms are related to duct obstruction, direct acinar damage, and hypoperfusion.
- Serum amylase is elevated in acute disease and is a key feature in establishing a diagnosis.
- Local complications: pancreatic pseudocyst.
- Systemic complications: ARDS, DIC, glucose intolerance, hypocalcemia.

TUMORS OF THE PANCREAS

Benign tumors of the pancreas are uncommon

Benign tumors of the pancreas are rare. Cystadenomata are the most common benign tumors of the exocrine pancreas. These well-circumscribed masses are composed of multiple cystic cavities lined by serous or mucin-secreting epithelium.

Carcinoma of the pancreas is increasing in incidence

Carcinoma of the pancreas is one of the most common causes of death from cancer, with an increasing incidence in western countries. Although it is predominantly seen after the age of 60 years, there are occasional cases in younger patients.

The only environmental factor that is firmly associated with carcinoma of the pancreas is smoking. It has been speculated that dietary factors and exposure to chemical carcinogens may be contributory, but no definite risks have been determined. Diabetic women have an increased risk of developing pancreatic carcinoma.

Most carcinomas of the pancreas are adenocarcinomas. They arise with different frequencies in different parts of the pancreas (*Fig. 14.44*).

Carcinoma in the head of the pancreas tends to present early with obstructive jaundice. As a result, tumors are, on average, smaller at diagnosis than in other sites (*Fig. 14.45*).

Histologically most tumors are moderately differentiated adenocarcinomas with a prominent fibrous stroma. Less common histological variants are also described.

The main routes of spread are:

- **Local**, causing obstructive jaundice, or invasion of the duodenum.
- **Lymphatic**, spreading to adjacent lymph nodes.
- **Hematogenous**, spreading to the liver.

Pancreatic carcinoma is associated with several clinical syndromes:

- Weight loss, anorexia and chronic persistent pain in the epigastrium, radiating to the back.
- Obstructive jaundice with painless palpable dilatation of the gallbladder (Courvoisier's sign).
- Migratory thrombophlebitis, in which there is development of multiple thrombosis in superficial and deep leg veins (Trousseau's syndrome).

The prognosis for carcinoma of the pancreas is extremely poor, 90% of patients dying within 6 months of diagnosis. Palliative surgery is often performed to bypass obstruction of the bile duct (relieving jaundice) and obstruction of the duodenum. Islet-cell tumors, neoplasms derived from the pancreatic neuroendocrine cells, are discussed in the context of endocrine pathology in Chapter 16.

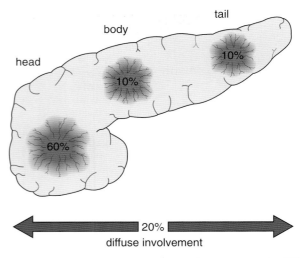

Fig. 14.44 Frequency of carcinoma of the pancreas in different parts of the gland.

Fig. 14.45 Carcinoma of the head of the pancreas. Tumors appear as gritty, gray, hard nodules (**T**), irregularly invading the adjacent gland and local structures (a). Histologically (b) they are usually moderately differentiated adenocarcinomas, which are composed of gland spaces in a fibrous stroma.

Case-based questions

Case 1 – Rough drinking

A 29-year-old former estate agent whose business has collapsed and who is now living rough presents because he has been feeling nauseous and generally unwell for 3 days. On examination he has a mild pyrexia and is tender in the right upper quadrant of his abdomen. He has been drinking one or two bottles of spirits a day. This started off as single malt whisky, but since the loss of his savings he now drinks a bottled blend of whisky, white wine and ginger as sold in his local supermarket.

A diagnosis of alcoholic hepatitis is made. After a period of time in hospital during which he is treated with vitamins, a needle biopsy of the liver is performed.

1. **What pathological changes may alcohol produce in the liver?**
2. **You will need to use your understanding of the pathology of liver disease to give him advice on his drinking. What proportion of patients with chronic alcoholism develop cirrhosis?**
3. **Given your understanding of the functions of the liver and how these can be compromised in disease, how do you prepare such a patient with liver disease for biopsy?**

Case 2 – A man with a swollen abdomen

A 60-year-old retired stockbroker is seen because he has bilateral parotid enlargement, a right Dupuytren's contracture, and has developed increasing abdominal swelling. On examination it is apparent that the cause of his abdominal swelling is ascites. He also has spider nevi, mild ankle edema, splenomegaly, and a firm, slightly enlarged liver. Further investigations are performed.

After ensuring that his blood clotting was nomal, a liver biopsy is performed which shows established cirrhosis with features consistent with an alcoholic causation.

1. **What are the histopathological features seen in cirrhosis?**
2. **What histological features would have been seen in the biopsy to suggest an alcoholic causation?**
3. **What are the complications of cirrhosis and how do these relate to the clinical features seen in the patient?**

Case 3 – A woman with itching

A 52-year-old bakery assistant presents to her family doctor because of increasingly troublesome generalized itching. On examination she is not jaundiced, and there are no stigmata of chronic liver disease. Investigations are performed.

Investigation

Full blood count and ESR	Normal
Blood sugar	Normal
Alkaline phosphatase	Very high
Bilirubin	Moderately elevated
AST and ALT	Mildly elevated
Albumin	Normal
Prothrombin time	Mildly prolonged
Immunology	Antimitochondrial autoantibodies (titre > I: 40) elevated levels of serum IgM

1. **What is the most likely diagnosis?**
2. **What are you going to tell the patient about her likely progress?**

Case 4 – A man with an acute abdomen

An unemployed 49-year-old security guard is admitted to hospital as an emergency, accompanied by a friend. He had recently been dismissed from his job after several prisoners escaped from his custody. His personal circumstances had not improved and he had recently separated from his wife because of several episodes of domestic violence. He and his friend had been having a drinking session which had been going on for about 5 days. His friend had called round to go out and had found the patient collapsed in the kitchen, hunched forward over a chair with severe abdominal pain. As part of the investigations he is found to have a greatly elevated serum amylase level and a diagnosis of acute pancreatitis is made.

1. **What are the main causes of acute pancreatitis, and which is most likely in this case?**
2. **What is the pathogenesis of acute pancreatitis?**
3. **What complications of acute pancreatitis may develop in this patient?**

Brief answers to these case-based questions are given on pages 587–8. More detailed answers and other study resources are available online at www.studentconsult.com.

Lymphoid and hemopoietic tissues

15

DISEASES OF THE LYMPH NODES

REACTIVE CHANGES

Reactive lymphadenopathy is the most common cause of enlarged lymph nodes

The main function of lymph nodes is to allow the interaction of antigen, antigen-presenting cells and lymphoid cells in the generation of an immune response. Different types of stimulus generate different patterns of response in lymph nodes, identification of which may be helpful in diagnosing the cause. The most common reason for patients to develop enlargement of lymph nodes is as a reaction to antigenic stimuli (reactive lymphadenopathy).

There are five main patterns of reactive response, but in most diseases a mixed pattern of responses is seen:

- **Follicular hyperplasia**: increase in B-cell germinal centres.
- **Paracortical hyperplasia**: increase in T-cell paracortical region.
- **Sinus hyperplasia**: increase in histiocytic cells in cortical and medullary sinuses.
- **Granulomatous inflammation**: formation of histiocytic granulomas in nodes.
- **Acute lymphadenitis**: acute inflammation and suppuration in lymph nodes.

Follicular hyperplasia shows increase in size and number of germinal centres

Follicular hyperplasia is a common response to most types of antigen exposure (*Fig. 15.1*). The main situations associated with this reaction are nodes draining sites of chronic inflammation (see pages 50–3), and nodes in rheumatoid disease (see page 549). The pattern is also seen in nodes enlarged in the early stages of persistent generalized lymphadenopathy in HIV infection (see page 308).

Paracortical hyperplasia shows increase in size of T-cell areas

Expansion of the T-cell paracortical zone is associated with follicular hyperplasia as part of a reaction to chronic inflam-

mation (*Fig. 15.2*). Relatively pure expansion of the paracortex is seen in drug hypersensitivity reactions (e.g. lymphadenopathy with phenytoin treatment) and viral infections, particularly infectious mononucleosis (caused by Epstein–Barr virus).

Fig. 15.1 Follicular hyperplasia. In follicular hyperplasia there is an increase in the size and number of B-cell germinal centers (**G**) in the node.

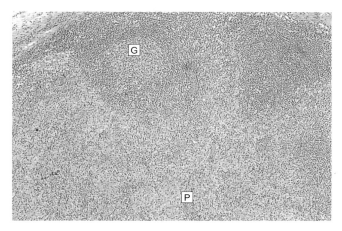

Fig. 15.2 Paracortical hyperplasia. This lymph node shows expansion of the T-cell paracortex (**P**). Germinal centers (**G**) are pushed to the margin of the node. This example was taken from a patient with infectious mononucleosis (glandular fever).

Histiocytic cells accumulate in medullary sinuses and may store phagocytosed material

An increase in the number of histiocytic cells in the medullary sinuses is seen in many non-specific reactions to chronic inflammation, and in nodes draining tumors. Histiocytes in sinuses may also store exogenous materials within nodes, e.g. carbon in peribronchial and hilar nodes draining the lungs.

A particular type of lymph node enlargement is seen in nodes draining inflamed skin. In these cases the medullary region is expanded by histiocytic cells that often contain melanin pigment and lipid (**dermatopathic lymphadenopathy**).

Acute lymphadenitis occurs with acute bacterial infections

Acute inflammation of lymph nodes (acute lymphadenitis) is almost exclusively seen with bacterial infections, in nodes draining the infected focus. Affected nodes enlarge rapidly and are tender. Histologically there is reactive hyperplasia of follicles, and focal infiltration of the node by neutrophils. With pyogenic organisms there may be necrosis and suppuration in the node, which may develop into an abscess.

Granulomatous inflammation in nodes may be seen in several diseases

Granulomatous inflammation in lymph nodes can present with generalized or localized lymphadenopathy; lymph node biopsy is performed to establish the cause. The main causes are:

- **Tuberculosis**: granulomas typically undergo caseous necrosis. TB must be confirmed by culture of biopsy tissue in all cases of undiagnosed lymphadenopathy.
- **Sarcoidosis** may affect regional nodes or be part of a generalized lymphadenopathy (see Chapter 25).
- **Cat scratch disease** is caused by a Gram-negative bacterium *Bartonella henselae*, transmitted by cat scratches. It leads to a self-limited febrile illness with localized lymphadenopathy (*Fig. 15.3*).
- **Crohn's disease**: granulomas are a frequent finding in the enlarged nodes draining the bowel in Crohn's disease.
- **Toxoplasmosis**. Numerous small aggregates of histiocytic cells forming 'mini granulomas' are seen within enlarged nodes (*Fig. 15.4*).
- **Reaction to tumor**: granulomas may be found in lymph nodes draining malignant tumors.

Less common causes are infections with fungi (histoplasmosis, coccidioidomycosis), *Chlamydia* (lymphogranuloma venereum) and other bacteria (*Yersinia* infection, *Brucella* infection).

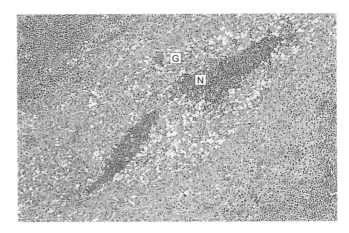

Fig. 15.3 Cat scratch disease. In this condition, nodes show large histiocytic granulomas (**G**), which contain central necrosis and neutrophilic infiltration (**N**) ('suppurating granulomas').

Fig. 15.4 Toxoplasmosis. In toxoplasmosis, small granulomas (**G**) form within the lymph node and may encroach on germinal centers.

Patients with HIV infection may develop lymphadenopathy at several stages of disease

At the time of seroconversion, many patients with HIV infection develop lymphadenopathy. Later in the disease, lymphadenopathy is common (**persistent generalized lymphadenopathy**), with hematological and serological evidence of impaired cell-mediated immunity and reduced T-cell numbers.

As clinical AIDS develops, generalized follicular hyperplasia gradually gives way to loss of follicles and depopulation of nodes of lymphoid cells.

Patients with HIV infection and AIDS are predisposed to the development of lymphomas and Kaposi's sarcoma, both of which may affect nodes and cause lymphadenopathy. Immune suppression also increases risk of development of opportunistic infections and mycobacterial infection that may cause lymphadenopathy.

NEOPLASTIC DISEASE IN LYMPH NODES

Metastatic tumor is a common cause of lymphadenopathy

The lymph nodes are a major site for metastasis of tumor by lymphatic spread. This is most commonly seen with carcinomas and melanomas, less frequently with sarcomas. Clinically, the development of enlarged lymph nodes may be the presenting sign of the tumor, the diagnosis being made only after histological examination of a lymph node biopsy.

Tumor cells are first seen in the subcapsular sinus; they later form solid areas, replacing the nodal structure (see page 77). With time, tumor extends outside the nodal capsule, tethering nodes to adjacent structures.

Typically, nodes involved by metastatic tumor are very hard and, in advanced cases, fixed to other structures.

Lymphomas are neoplasms derived from lymphoid cells

The malignant lymphomas are primary neoplastic diseases of lymphoid cells, which have been divided into two main groups on the basis of clinical and pathological features.

Hodgkin's disease is characterized by neoplastic proliferation of an atypical form of lymphoid cell eponymously termed the Reed–Sternberg cell.

Non-Hodgkin's lymphomas are characterized by neoplastic proliferation of B lymphocytes, T lymphocytes or, very rarely, histiocytic cells. Disease typically starts in the lymph nodes, spreading to involve the spleen, liver and bone marrow. Other organs are commonly involved in advanced disease.

Immunohistochemistry is essential in diagnostic assessment of lymphoid neoplasms

The diagnosis of lymphoid tumors and delineating them from reactive conditions requires that lymphocyte markers be used to discriminate between different types of lymphoid neoplasm. Markers used in diagnosis correspond to the CD system.

- The classic reagents used to show a B-cell lineage detect CD19, CD20, CD22 and CD79a.
- Identification of cells as being of T-cell lineage relies on detection of one or more pan-T-cell markers such as CD2, CD3, CD5, or CD7.
- CD30 (TNF receptor superfamily) and CD15 mark Reed–Sternberg cells seen in Hodgkin's disease.
- CD1a detects Langerhans' cells characteristic of histiocytoses.
- Antibodies that detect granzyme, perforin or TIA1 can be used to characterize cells as being of NK lineage. Such cells may also express CD56, CD57 and CD16.
- Antibodies that specifically detect the product of fusion oncogenes produced by translocations can also be used to characterize certain types of lymphoid tumor.

HODGKIN'S DISEASE

Hodgkin's disease is caused by proliferation of Reed–Sternberg cells

Hodgkin's disease involves proliferation of an atypical form of lymphoid cell that, until the routine use of immunohistochemistry, was difficult to categorize; it was therefore named the Reed–Sternberg cell, after the two workers who identified its significance. This neoplastic cell is derived from transformed B cells.

Clinically, disease presents as enlargement of a single lymph node or group of nodes, or enlarged nodes may be discovered following investigation for non-specific systemic symptoms such as weight loss, fever, or pruritus.

Macroscopically, affected nodes are enlarged (generally up to cm in diameter) and are replaced by firm, rubbery, pinkish-white tissue (*Fig. 15.5*). The natural history of untreated disease is of spread to adjacent lymph nodes, with involvement of spleen, liver, and bone marrow.

Fig. 15.5 Lymph nodes in Hodgkin's disease. These lymph nodes are enlarged and replaced by firm, creamy white tissue. Although this example was taken from a case of Hodgkin's disease, nodes in non-Hodgkin's lymphomas may appear identical.

Five histological subtypes of Hodgkin's disease are defined according to the histological pattern of disease

Histologically, five types of Hodgkin's disease have been defined (**WHO classification**) (*Fig. 15.6*).

Common to all types of Hodgkin's disease is the presence of Reed–Sternberg cells, the morphology of which varies in different subtypes of disease (*Fig. 15.8*). The difference between the types is in the extent and vigor of the host immune response associated with neoplastic transformation. The response is marked in lymphocyte-predominant disease, moderate in mixed cellularity, variable in nodular sclerosis, and in lymphocyte-depleted disease it is virtually non-existent.

Nodular lymphocyte-predominant disease is mainly seen in young men. Histologically the nodes are replaced by reactive lymphoid cells, among which are a small population of Reed–Sternberg cells of the lymphocytic/histiocytic type. Importantly, and in contrast with the other types of Hodgkin's disease, the neoplastic cells express immuno-chemical markers of B-cell origin. Most patients present with stage I or II disease.

Mixed cellularity disease mainly affects adults in later life, but any age can be affected. Lymph nodes are replaced by an infiltrate of Reed–Sternberg cells of the classic and mononuclear types, with a cellular response composed of lymphoid cells, eosinophils, plasma cells and histiocytes. Over 50% of patients present in stage III or IV.

Nodular sclerosis is the most common type of Hodgkin's disease, mainly affecting young adults. In most cases the mediastinal nodes are involved at presentation. The key feature is that the infiltrate is divided into nodules by broad bands of collagen. In nodular sclerosis grade I the infiltrate is cytologically the same as in mixed-cellularity disease. In nodular sclerosis grade II the infiltrate contains pleomorphic Reed–Sternberg cells in high density.

Lymphocyte-rich Hodgkin's disease is characterized by classic Reed–Sternberg cells set in a diffuse background of lymphoid cells. The Reed–Sternberg cells do not mark as B cells and hence are separated from nodular lymphocyte-predominant disease.

Lymphocyte-depleted disease is rare and seen mainly in elderly adults. The infiltrate is composed of many pleomor-phic Reed–Sternberg cells, and shows few reactive lymphoid cells. Most patients with this pattern present with stage III or IV disease, which is associated with the poorest prognosis. Re-examination of cases previously classified as this form of disease has reclassified most as large-cell ana-plastic non-Hodgkin's lymphomas, often expressing a specific ALK oncogene product (see later).

EBV integration has been associated with a significant proportion of cases of classic Hodgkin's disease, and this is regarded as a significant etiological factor.

Diagnosis and staging of Hodgkin's disease

Disease is initially diagnosed on lymph node biopsy. Next, the extent of disease is assessed by staging. CT scanning or MR imaging is used to detect enlarged lymph node groups and infiltration of spleen and liver. Liver biopsy enables assessment of hepatic involvement, and bone marrow aspiration is used to determine marrow infiltration.

The clinical stage of disease is described using the Ann Arbor system (*Fig. 15.7*).

Fig. 15.7 Ann Arbor clinical staging for Hodgkin's disease

Stage	Description
I	Disease confined to one lymph node group or Involvement of a single extranodal site (I$_E$)
II	Disease confined to several nodal groups on the same side of the diaphragm or With limited involvement of adjacent extranodal site (II$_E$)
III	Disease is present in lymph node groups on both sides of the diaphragm or With limited involvement of adjacent extranodal site (III$_E$) or With involvement of the spleen (III$_S$)
IV	Disseminated involvement of one or more extranodal tissues, such as the liver or bone marrow, with or without nodal involvement.

Notes: Disease is subclassified according to the presence or absence of systemic symptoms (e.g. fever, night sweats, weight loss)

Systemic symptoms absent – A
Systemic symptoms present – B

Fig. 15.6 WHO classification of Hodgkin's disease

Nodular lymphocyte-predominant Hodgkin's disease	3%
Classic Hodgkin's disease	
Nodular sclerosis	67%
Lymphocyte-rich	3%
Mixed cellularity	25%
Lymphocyte-depleted	<1%

Fig 15.8 Reed–Sternberg cell

- classical Reed–Sternberg cell
- nucleolus
- reactive cells

a

- mononuclear Reed–Sternberg cell

- nucleolus

c

b

Fig. 15.8 Reed–Sternberg cells. Several types of Reed–Sternberg (RS) cell have been described and these are found in different subtypes of Hodgkin's disease (HD). Immunohistochemistry shows that RS cells in classic Hodgkin's disease label with CD15 and CD30. Although derived from B cells they do not express B-cell markers.

- Classic RS cells are binucleate, resembling owl eyes, and are seen in mixed-cellularity (a, b) and in nodular sclerosis grade I Hodgkin's disease.
- Mononuclear RS cells may be seen in any type of Hodgkin's disease but are mainly encountered in mixed cellularity disease (c and b).

Prognosis in Hodgkin's disease is related to stage and subtype

The best outcome is seen in lymphocyte-predominant and nodular sclerosis grade I types, the worst prognosis being seen in lymphocyte-depleted disease and nodular sclerosis grade II. Mixed-cellularity disease has a varied prognosis, which is largely dependent on the stage at the time of diagnosis.

Overall, the 10-year survival rate for patients with Hodgkin's disease is >80% for the nodular lymphocyte-predominant type, 75% for nodular sclerosis type I, 60% for the mixed-cellularity type, 55% for nodular sclerosis grade II, and 5% for the lymphocyte-depleted type (40% have a 5-year survival).

Within each subgroup, factors associated with reduced survival and early death are advanced stage, advanced age of patient, and the presence of systemic symptoms (type B disease – see *Fig. 15.6*).

NON-HODGKIN'S LYMPHOMAS

The non-Hodgkin's lymphomas can be grouped according to the site of origin

Non-Hodgkin's lymphomas may be classified as **nodal** (tumors originating in lymph nodes, which account for the vast majority of cases) or **extranodal** (tumors originating in specialized groups of lymphoid cells). Most extranodal lymphomas arise in specialized epithelial-associated lymphoid cells (mucosa-associated lymphoid tissue – **MALT**), and cases are seen in the gut and lung. Other examples develop in tissues that have been the seat of chronic lymphocytic inflammation in organs not normally noted to have a lymphoid population (e.g. testis and thyroid). Lymphomas may also develop in the brain and skin as a primary disease.

Non-Hodgkin's lymphomas originate from either B or T lymphocytes

Non-Hodgkin's lymphomas can be derived from either B or T lymphocytes. They are composed of a predominant cell type, which can be related to one of the stages of differentiation of normal T or B cells.

In very general terms, the growth of these tumors is related to the cytology of the malignant cells: cells with small nuclei have a low rate of proliferation and are associated with a slow pace of growth; cells which have large nuclei and large nucleoli are associated with rapid proliferation and aggressive biological behavior.

Characterization of lymphomas gives an assessment of clinical behavior

As chemotherapy regimens differ for each pattern of lymphoma, pathological evaluation of tumor type is required for the purposes of treatment. The division of lymphomas

Fig. 15.9 WHO classification of lymphomas

B-cell neoplasms

Precursor B-cell lymphoblastic leukemia lymphoma
Mature B-cell neoplasms
  B-cell chronic lymphocytic leukemia small lymphocytic lymphoma
  B-cell prolymphocytic leukemia
  Lymphoplasmacytic lymphoma (lymphoplasmacytoid lymphoma)
  Mantle cell lymphoma
  Follicular lymphoma (follicle center lymphoma)
  Marginal zone B-cell lymphoma of mucosa-associated lymphoid tissue (MALT) type
  Nodal marginal zone lymphoma with or without monocytoid B cells
  Splenic marginal zone B-cell lymphoma
  Hairy cell leukemia (page 326)
  Diffuse large B-cell lymphoma
  Subtypes mediastinal (thymic), intravascular, primary effusion lymphoma
  Burkitt lymphoma
  Plasmacytoma
  Plasma cell myeloma

T-cell neoplasms

Precursor T-cell lymphoblastic leukemia lymphoma
Mature T-cell and NK-cell neoplasms
  T-cell prolymphocytic leukemia
  T-cell large granular lymphocytic leukemia
  NK-cell leukemia
  Extranodal NK/T-cell lymphoma, nasal-type (angiocentric lymphoma)
  Mycosis fungoides
  Sézary syndrome
  Angioimmunoblastic T-cell lymphoma
  Peripheral T-cell lymphoma (unspecified)
  Adult T-cell leukemia lymphoma (HTLV1+)
  Systemic anaplastic large cell lymphoma (T- and null-cell types)
  Primary cutaneous anaplastic large cell lymphoma
  Subcutaneous panniculitis-like T-cell lymphoma
  Enteropathy-type intestinal T-cell lymphoma
  Hepatosplenic γ/δ T-cell lymphoma

into prognostic-related entities for clinical purposes has resulted in the REAL and the latest WHO classifications (*Fig. 15.9*).

The main divisions in classification are into B- and T-cell types. Within each main type a division into precursor and mature lymphoid types has been made. In general, precursor lymphoid tumors are confined to childhood and adolescence. This classification scheme has developed over many years. Within it are some entities which are extremely rare, and would only be recognized by lymphoma specialists ('lymphomaniacs').

On the basis of their cytology, phenotype and clinical behavior, non-Hodgkin's lymphomas can be divided into four main groups:

1. Slow-growing, indolent B-cell lymphomas (50% of cases).
2. Rapid-growing, aggressive B-cell lymphomas (30% of cases).
3. Slow-growing T-cell lymphomas (10% of cases).
4. Rapid-growing aggressive T-cell lymphomas (10% of cases).

In older classifications, histiocytic lymphomas were included. However, modern investigative techniques have reclassified most such cases. True histiocytic lymphomas are remarkably rare.

B-CELL LYMPHOMAS

B-cell small lymphocytic lymphoma is seen in elderly patients

B-cell small lymphocytic lymphomas are low-grade tumors composed of cells that cytologically resemble small lymphocytes; there is an overlap with chronic lymphocytic leukemia, which is composed of virtually identical cells (see page 326).

The disease typically occurs in the elderly, and in most cases runs an indolent course over many years. It can present with enlarged nodes or anemia secondary to infiltration of bone marrow (seen in 80% cases). Immune deficiency secondary to hypogammaglobulinemia is seen in many patients, frequently leading to death by predisposing to infection. The 5-year survival is better than 60% with this type.

Histologically, lymph nodes are replaced by sheets of small lymphoid cells with little cytoplasm (*Fig. 15.10*). It is common for overspill of cells into the bloodstream to give a picture similar to chronic lymphocytic leukemia.

Lymphoplasmacytic lymphoma is seen in the elderly and runs an indolent course

Lymphoplasmacytoid lymphoma is a form of disease which, like B-cell lymphocytic lymphoma, is seen mainly in the elderly and generally runs an indolent course. Histologically it is characterized by cells with plasmacytic features which often secrete immunoglobulin and produce a monoclonal band on serum electrophoresis. If there is production of IgM, patients may develop a hyperviscosity syndrome with poor blood flow in small vessels and a bleeding tendency. This syndrome is termed **Waldenström's macroglobulinemia**.

Follicular lymphomas are B-cell lymphomas in which the lymphocytes resemble normal follicle-center cells

Lymphomas formed from B cells which recapitulate normal follicle-center cells arrange themselves into follicles to form a follicular pattern of lymphoma.

Follicular lymphoma (*Fig. 15.11*) occurs most commonly after the sixth decade and represents one of the commonest types of disease. It is usually extensive at presentation, with involvement of bone marrow and liver. Although it is an indolent disease with slow progression over many years, it is difficult to cure, even with aggressive chemotherapy. Median survival is about 7–10 years. As part of the natural history of this disease, many cases transform into a high-grade diffuse lymphoma. Follicular lymphomas frequently show a chromosomal translocation t(14;18) that activates the Bcl-2 oncogene.

B-cell lymphomas composed of large cells in a diffuse pattern are aggressive but respond well to therapy

Diffuse large B-cell lymphomas are common (*Fig. 15.12*). Histologically, nodes are replaced by sheets of large atypical lymphoid cells with prominent large nucleoli. Because this type of lymphoma grows so fast, enlargement of nodes is very obvious and patients notice the signs early. As a result, disease is often localized at the time of diagnosis. Presentation with extranodal disease is common, for example with gut involvement.

This type of lymphoma affects all ages, including children, but is most common in later adult life. Even when advanced, the disease is curable with aggressive chemotherapy. A distinct t(14;18) translocation is seen in about 30% of cases.

Marginal zone B-cell lymphomas occur as extranodal disease arising in mucosal associated lymphoid tissue

The marginal zone lymphomas are believed to be the neoplastic counterpart of the marginal zone lymphoid cells that are normally present in lymph nodes and the spleen. These tumors characteristically arise in association with glandular epithelial tissues often in the setting of a pre-existing lymphocytic inflammatory process, being classified as lymphomas of mucosa-associated lymphoid tissue (**MALT lymphomas**) (*Fig. 15.13*). Such lymphomas may arise in the tonsils, gut, bronchi, salivary glands, lacrimal glands or thyroid. The cells that become neoplastic continue to have the same specialized homing functions, recirculating only to the site of origin and the draining local nodes. Clinically such tumors run an indolent course. They tend not to become systematized, as it has been proposed that neoplastic cells lack adhesion molecules that would allow them to home in on other sites.

Fig. 15.10 B-cell small-cell lymphoma. Neoplastic cells are arranged in diffuse sheets which efface the normal nodal architecture. Nuclei are small and cells have little cytoplasm.

Fig. 15.11 B-cell follicular lymphoma. In follicular lymphoma, neoplastic cells form follicles (**F**) resembling normal germinal centers.

Fig. 15.12 Diffuse large B-cell lymphoma. Neoplastic cells are large and have open nuclei with very prominent nucleoli.

Fig. 15.13 B-cell marginal zone lymphoma. Neoplastic cells are small to medium-sized and have irregular nuclei and variable nucleoli. This pattern is seen in MALT lymphomas.

Fig. 15.14 B-cell mantle zone lymphoma. Neoplastic cells have irregularly shaped nuclei with clefts and grooves and prominent nucleoli.

Fig. 15.15 Burkitt's lymphoma. In Burkitt's lymphoma a characteristic feature is the presence of large macrophagic cells (**M**) scattered through the tumor, likened to a 'starry sky'.

Mantle cell B-cell lymphomas occur in adults and tend to run an aggressive course

The neoplastic cells in this form of lymphoma are believed to resemble the normal mantle zone lymphocytes found in relation to follicles in normal lymph nodes (*Fig. 15.14*). Disease typically presents as lymphadenopathy in adults and runs an aggressive course even with treatment.

Precursor B-cell lymphoblastic lymphomas are high-grade tumors mainly seen in childhood

Precursor B-cell lymphoblastic lymphomas are composed of cells resembling transformed lymphocytes. There is a great overlap with B-cell acute lymphoblastic leukemia, and extensive involvement of nodes and extranodal sites. This is an aggressive disease but is often curable. Cells express markers of early B-cell lineage.

Burkitt's lymphoma is an aggressive but curable disease seen mainly in childhood

Burkitt's lymphoma is a type of lymphoma that is endemic in Africa but arises sporadically elsewhere, particularly affecting the jaw, ovaries, and gut (*Fig. 15.15*). In endemic Burkitt's lymphoma, Epstein–Barr virus genome is found in over 90% of cases, contrasting with under 20% of cases in sporadic disease. t(2;8), t(8;14), t(8;22) or rearrangement of the cMYC oncogene is seen in 80% of tumors.

Plasma-cell neoplasms cause lytic lesions in bone and secrete immunoglobulin

Three tumors can be considered plasma cell neoplasms. These tumors retain the immunoglobulin-secreting property of mature plasma cells.

Multiple myeloma is most commonly seen after the age of 50 years. It is due to neoplastic proliferation of a single clone of bone-marrow-derived plasma cells. There are several main effects:

- Plasma cells grow within marrow, diffusely replacing normal hemopoietic tissue. Expansion may cause lytic lesions and bone pain (see *Fig. 24.11*, page 545). Bone destruction may cause hypercalcemia and pathological fractures. Lesions are most common in the vertebrae, ribs, skull and pelvis.
- Cells synthesize monoclonal immunoglobulin chains, which accumulate in the blood and may be detected by serum electrophoresis as a monoclonal band. In most cases the monoclonal immunoglobulin is IgG. When the immunoglobulin is IgM, patients may develop hyperviscosity of blood.
- Free light chains from excess monoclonal immunoglobulin may be filtered by the glomerulus to enter the urine, where they can be detected as Bence–Jones protein.

- Increased protein concentration in the blood is responsible for an elevated ESR as a result of rouleaux formation.
- Patients develop immune paresis and are susceptible to infection.
- In some cases the light chains form amyloid (see Chapter 25), which is deposited in tissues, particularly the renal glomeruli and heart.
- Renal dysfunction is common as a result of light-chain protein casts, with secondary damage to tubules and amyloid.

Diagnosis is based on examination of bone marrow aspirates, which show an excess of plasma cells (*Fig. 15.16*). It is supported by finding a monoclonal immunoglobulin band on serum protein electrophoresis, and Bence–Jones protein in urine.

Plasmacytomas are also composed of neoplastic plasma cells and may be associated with the secretion of monoclonal immunoglobulin. In contrast to multiple myeloma, they are solitary circumscribed lesions. In bone they may form osteolytic lesions. They may also develop in soft tissue. Many cases develop multiple myeloma after a period of years.

Benign monoclonal gammopathy is a term applied to patients who have a monoclonal immunoglobulin band on serum electrophoresis, but no demonstrable plasma-cell abnormality. The natural history is for many patients to develop myeloma after a period of years.

Fig. 15.16 Bone marrow in multiple myeloma. The bone marrow shows replacement by plasma cells, many of which show cytological abnormalities with nuclear irregularities.

T-CELL LYMPHOMAS

T-cell lymphomas commonly affect the skin or other extranodal tissues

Mycosis fungoides and **Sézary syndrome** are two types of indolent, slowly progressing T-cell lymphoma which affect the skin and draining lymph nodes. The T cells have been termed cerebriform because the nuclear membrane is very convoluted, resembling the gyri of the brain. In mycosis fungoides and Sézary syndrome neoplastic T cells migrate into the epidermis, causing an erythematous rash (see page 530). In Sézary syndrome these atypical cells also circulate in the blood. Lymph nodes can become affected. With disease progression the skin develops thick plaques of lymphoma and there is visceral involvement.

Angio-immunoblastic T-cell lymphoma presents in the elderly, with systemic features of malaise, fever and skin rashes. There is generalized lymphadenopathy. Investigations reveal polyclonal hypergammaglobulinemia and hemolytic anemia. Histologically, nodes show proliferation of small T cells, which attract a considerable population of reactive cells (plasma cells, eosinophils, histiocytes) through the secretion of lymphokines. The disease pursues an aggressive course and may transform into a high-grade T-cell lymphoma.

One form of T-cell lymphoma, termed **angiocentric lymphoma**, grows by invading the walls of blood vessels. This type of disease is common in Asia and often presents as disease affecting the nose or skin. Histologically atypical T cells can be seen invading and occluding vessels, leading to the common finding of necrosis of both normal and neoplastic tissues. Immunochemistry may show that these cells have a T-cell/NK-cell phenotype.

Enteropathy-type intestinal T-cell lymphomas are especially seen as a complication of celiac disease (page 258). The small bowel shows thickening of the mucosa by neoplastic T cells. There is frequent ulceration of the bowel, and this may be complicated by perforation. This type of disease runs an aggressive course.

Peripheral T-cell lymphomas have diverse clinical and pathological patterns

With the wider use of immunohistochemistry peripheral T-cell lymphomas have been increasingly recognized, but even so such tumors only account for a small proportion of lymphomas. For practical purposes the peripheral T-cell neoplasms are grouped together under the term **peripheral T-cell lymphoma, unspecified**. In addition to the presence of atypical neoplastic T cells (*Fig. 15.17*), such tumors often recruit a substantial population of reactive cells, presumably related to the ability of neoplastic T cells to secrete appropriate cytokines.

In addition to the group of 'unspecified' peripheral T-cell lymphomas there is a group of distinctive types:

- In children and adolescents, **precursor T-cell lymphoblastic lymphoma** is an aggressive but curable form of disease. Characteristically there is dominant involvement of the mediastinal nodes or thymus gland, and disease usually presents with leukemic features. Extensive colonization of nodal and extranodal sites dictates the use of aggressive therapy, including irradiation of the neuraxis.

- Although uncommon in the western world, in the Caribbean and Asia T-cell lymphoma is more common due to causation by human T-cell leukemia virus type 1 (HTLV-1). In resulting **adult T-cell lymphoma/ leukemia** (*Fig. 15.17*) there is frequent extensive disease, with skin involvement, hypercalcemia and leukemia.

- **Large-cell anaplastic lymphoma** is composed of large cells with a superficial resemblance to epithelial cells in that they have abundant, pale eosinophilic cytoplasm. Tumor cells express CD30 (formerly called Ki-1) as well as epithelial membrane antigen. The term 'Ki-1 **anaplastic lymphoma**' has been used for these tumors. Cells have either a T-cell or a null cell phenotype. A t(2;5) translocation has been seen in many cases, leading to expression of the ALK oncogene. Detection of this oncogene product is possible using immunohistochemistry, and this has led to increased recognition of such lymphoid tumors. The term '**ALKoma**' has been used to group such tumors. This group of lymphomas has been found to be the true diagnosis in many cases that in the past would have been called lymphocyte-depleted Hodgkin's disease.

Investigation of lymphomas

The management of lymphoma has developed into a specialized area of clinical practice. It is essential that the oncologist, surgeon, radiologist and pathologist discuss cases at all stages in the diagnostic process.

Histological evaluation of biopsy tissue is central to diagnosis and subsequent management. The mainstay of diagnosis is surgical removal of an entire lymph node for examination.

In cases of suspected lymphoma, tissue removed for biopsy should be sent fresh to the laboratory, where it is divided to allow a detailed morphological and molecular analysis.

In addition to conventional histological assessment it is essential to use immunohistochemical markers for different lymphoid cell types, especially for B and T cells, as previously described (page 309). In some circumstances, establishing that a lesion is malignant depends on showing that a cell proliferation is monoclonal by demonstrating clonal immunoglobulin gene rearrangement (B lymphocytes) and clonal T-cell receptor gene rearrangement (T lymphocytes). Cytogenetic investigation may demonstrate the presence of a specific chromosomal marker, e.g. the translocations seen in follicular lymphomas (see page 313) and Burkitt's lymphomas (see page 314).

Fig. 15.17 Peripheral T-cell lymphoma. In this peripheral T-cell lymphoma neoplastic cells are large, with moderate amounts of cytoplasm. Although cells superficially resemble histiocytes (which in the past caused such tumors to be incorrectly classed as histiocytic lymphomas), immunohistochemical techniques reveal them to be T-cells.

Etiological factors in lymphomas

Although several factors have been implicated in the development of lymphomas, e.g. they may be caused by Epstein–Barr (EBV) virus or HTLV-1, in most cases a cause is not known.

Lymphomas may develop in the setting of long-standing chronic immune-mediated disease. This may be autoimmune disease (thyroiditis, see page 335, Sjögren's disease, or a reaction to exogenous antigen, e.g. celiac disease). It is thought that continued immune activation predisposes to neoplastic change.

The incidence of lymphomas increases in patients with immune deficiency, be it congenital or acquired, when they are associated with EBV infection.

SURVIVAL AND PROGNOSIS IN LYMPHOMA

Survival in non-Hodgkin's lymphoma evens out after 10 years because low-grade disease is hard to cure

Survival for patients with non-Hodgkin's lymphoma varies according to grade and stage. Paradoxically, patients with rapidly growing aggressive tumors may be cured, whereas many with slow-growing lesions suffer late relapses.

Patients who have clinically aggressive disease may be cured by chemotherapy. Patients with slow-growing, indolent tumors often may be controlled by therapy, but cure is less often achieved.

Although there is around a 70% 5-year survival for the indolent types of non-Hodgkin's lymphoma, with a 40% 5-year survival for initially aggressive disease, survival at 10 years is still about 40% for both types, reflecting continued deaths in patients with indolent forms of disease.

Patients who tend to die early with non-Hodgkin's lymphoma include the elderly, those who have extensive dissemination with hematological abnormalities, and those with systemic symptoms or weight loss and fever.

> ### Key Facts
> #### Lymphoma
>
> - **Lymphomas** usually originate in the lymph nodes and spread to other areas, especially bone marrow, spleen and liver.
> - **Hodgkin's disease** is due to a neoplastic proliferation of modified B cells, termed Reed–Sternberg cells.
> - **Hodgkin's disease** is divided into five histological subtypes, the commonest of which is nodular sclerosing pattern.
> - **Hodgkin's disease** is staged using the Ann Arbor system. Low stage equates with better prognosis.
> - **Non-Hodgkin's lymphomas** are caused by neoplastic proliferation of B or T cells. B-cell types are commonest.
> - **B-cell lymphomas** vary from small cell types with indolent behavior to large cell types with aggressive behavior.
> - **T-cell lymphomas** commonly affect the skin (peripheral) as well as nodal forms.
> - **MALT lymphomas** arise in mucosal sites and are B-cell in type.

DISEASES OF THE THYMUS

The normal thymus

The thymus is composed of lymphoid cells and specialized epithelial cells. It is the site of development and maturation of T lymphocytes, as well as clonal deletion of self-reactive T lymphocytes. Normally the thymus regresses after puberty. Failure of development of the thymus results in deficient T-cell mediated immunity (see page 98).

The thymus is a site of development of several different types of tumor

Several different types of tumor occur in the thymus, usually presenting as an anterior mediastinal mass. These may be detected on chest radiographs as an incidental finding, or may produce disease by compression of adjacent structures. Occasionally attention is drawn to the thymus because of an autoimmune disease such a myasthenia gravis (see Chapter 21). The main tumors of the thymus are as follows:

- **Lymphomas**, particularly T-lymphoblastic lymphoma, nodular sclerosing Hodgkin's disease, and some B-cell lymphomas.
- **Germ-cell tumors** (teratoma and seminoma) account for about 20% of mediastinal tumors. They display a similar histological spectrum to that seen in the testis (see page 402).
- **Neuroendocrine tumors** are composed of neuroendocrine cells and resemble those seen elsewhere. Clinically they may be associated with Cushing's syndrome.
- **Thymomas** are derived from thymic epithelial cells (spindle-cell or round-cell types) with an infiltrate of reactive lymphoid cells. They may be associated with myasthenia gravis, red cell aplasia, and non-organ specific autoimmune diseases (see pages 104–5). Although 80% of thymomas are benign, 20% behave as low-grade malignant tumors, infiltrating local structures with metastatic spread in about 10% of cases.

Thymic hyperplasia can be associated with autoimmune disease

Thymic hyperplasia is uncommon. Histologically, lymphoid follicles composed of B cells develop in the thymic medulla, and there may be associated increase in the size of the thymus. This may also be associated with the development of autoimmune disease, particularly myasthenia gravis (see page 492).

DISEASES OF THE SPLEEN

The normal spleen weighs 100–200 g. Its two main functions are trapping and presenting antigens circulating in the blood, and culling effete red cells from the circulation.

Hypersplenism is associated with enlargement of the spleen

A common physical sign, enlargement of the spleen may have many causes, summarized in *Fig. 15.18*. Irrespective of its cause, enlargement may result in the development of hypersplenism. This syndrome is associated with two main problems: sequestration of red cells, white cells and platelets; and premature destruction of red cells. Hypersplenism therefore leads to a reduction in the numbers of cells in the blood (pancytopenia) and, as a compensatory response, hyperplasia of the bone marrow. Splenectomy leads to hematological improvement.

Hyposplenism increases the risk of serious bacterial infection by capsulated organisms

Lack of splenic function is encountered clinically in three main circumstances: surgical removal (for disease or trauma), sickle-cell disease (microvascular occlusion causes multiple microinfarcts, known as 'autosplenectomy'), and celiac disease (splenic atrophy).

As a consequence, patients become susceptible to recurrent bacterial infections, particularly by capsulated bacteria (*Streptococcus pneumoniae*, *Haemophilus influenzae*, *Neisseria meningitidis*, *Escherichia coli*), and may develop severe septicemia, intravascular coagulation, and multiorgan failure.

There are also abnormalities of red cells, which develop inclusion bodies (Howell–Jolly bodies) and abnormal shape (schistocytes and target cells). Usually, abnormal red cells are removed from the spleen as they squeeze through the splenic sinusoids.

Fig. 15.18 Causes of splenomegaly

Infective causes	
Bacterial	For example, typhoid, tuberculosis, brucellosis, infective endocarditis
Viral	Infectious mononucleosis
Protozoal	Malaria, leishmaniasis, trypanosomiasis, toxoplasmosis
Vascular causes	
Portal hypertension	Main cause is cirrhosis (see page 281)
Neoplastic causes	
Lymphomas	Hodgkin's disease and non-Hodgkin's lymphoma
Leukemias	Particularly chronic leukemias, less common in acute types
Extramedullary hemopoiesis	Seen in myeloproliferative diseases and diseases with diffuse marrow replacement by tumor
Metastases	Splenic metastases from solid tumors are rare
Hematological causes	
Hemolytic anemias	Hereditary spherocytosis, β-thalassemia, autoimmune hemolysis
Autoimmune thrombocytopenia	Destruction of platelets in spleen results in accumulation of foamy histiocytes in sinuses
Immunological causes	
Felty's syndrome	Follicular hyperplasia in the spleen associated with hypersplenism with rheumatoid disease
Sarcoidosis	Spleen infiltrated by granulomas (see Chapter 25)
Amyloidosis	Spleen infiltrated with amyloid (see Chapter 25)
Metabolic causes	
Storage disorders	Due to heritable enzyme deficiencies, e.g. Gaucher's disease and Niemann–Pick disease, which result in storage of material in splenic macrophagic cells

DISEASES OF THE BLOOD

RED CELL DISORDERS

Reduction in the mass of circulating red cells is termed anemia

Anemia can be defined as a reduced hemoglobin level; it is detected by analysis of peripheral blood (low hemoglobin, low red cell count, low hematocrit). This is the commonest blood disorder worldwide and affects about 30% of the global population. There is a high prevalence in developing countries because of social factors and poor medical care. Dietary deficiency and parasitic infection of the gut are important contributions.

To compensate for the lack of oxygen-carrying capacity, several changes take place in anemia. Biochemical changes in red cells reduce the affinity of hemoglobin for oxygen, and there is increased cardiac output, together with attempted increased red cell production.

The causes of anemia can be classified according to etiology (*Fig. 15.19*). In clinical practice the most common cause is iron deficiency, followed by the anemia of chronic disorders and deficiency of vitamins B_{12} and folate. All of the other causes are much less common.

Fig. 15.19 Pathological classification of anemia

Reduced production of red cells

Deficiency of hematinics
Iron deficiency
B_{12} and folate deficiency

Dyserythropoiesis (production of defective cells)
Anemia of chronic disorders
Myelodysplasia
Sideroblastic anemia

Marrow infiltration

Aplasia (failure of production of cells)
Aplastic anemia
Red-cell aplasia

Increased destruction or loss of red cells

Bleeding

Hemolytic anemia
Red-cell abnormalities (membrane, enzymes, hemoglobinopathies)
Abnormalities outside red cells (immune, microangiopathic, parasitic)

Hypersplenism

ANEMIA DUE TO DEFICIENCY OF HEMATINICS

Iron deficiency is the most common cause of anemia

The main causes of iron-deficiency anemia are impaired intake, excessive blood loss (most common cause in adults), or increased demand (e.g. pregnancy and lactation).

The peripheral blood shows a hypochromic microcytic pattern (*Fig. 15.20*). There is a low total serum iron and increased total iron-binding capacity; a reduced serum ferritin level reflects reduced total body iron stores.

In addition to signs and symptoms of anemia, some patients with iron-deficiency anemia may develop angular cheilitis, atrophic glossitis, esophageal webs, koilonychia and brittle nails.

Chronic blood loss is the most common cause of iron-deficiency anemia

If blood loss has been slow, anemia can be severe. The most important causes are diseases of the gastrointestinal tract, particularly peptic ulceration, carcinoma of the stomach and carcinoma of the colon (especially cecum), menorrhagia, and loss of blood from lesions in the urinary tract.

Patients with unexplained iron-deficiency anemia require careful screening for an occult cause of blood loss.

Deficiency of vitamin B_{12} and folate causes macrocytic megaloblastic anemia

Megaloblastic anemia is the result of impaired DNA synthesis in marrow precursor cells. This type of anemia is due to deficiency of vitamin B_{12} and folic acid. Vitamin B_{12} is normally absorbed from the diet by binding to intrinsic factor (IF), a glycoprotein secreted by gastric parietal cells. The B_{12}–IF complex binds to cells in the terminal ileum, where B_{12} is absorbed. The most common cause of B_{12} deficiency is lack of production of IF, resulting in

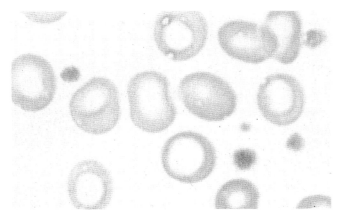

Fig. 15.20 Hypochromic, microcytic red cells.

pernicious anemia. In the stomach this is associated with autoimmune atrophic gastritis, or can occur after surgical gastrectomy. Disease or surgical removal of the absorption site in the terminal ileum may also cause B₁₂ deficiency.

Folic acid deficiency is most commonly due to inadequate dietary intake (folic acid is normally found in vegetables, meat and eggs). Deficiency is commonly encountered in alcoholics and in patients with malabsorption.

In the marrow, lack of B₁₂ or folate causes development of abnormally large red-cell precursors (megaloblasts), which develop into abnormally large red cells (macrocytes). Because much erythropoiesis results in the formation of defective cells that are prematurely destroyed, the marrow compartment is expanded and normally fatty marrow in the long bones becomes active. Patients have anemia, neutropenia and thrombocytopenia. In vitamin B₁₂ deficiency, but not in folate deficiency, neurological disease may occur, with the development of subacute combined degeneration of the spinal cord. Patients may also develop impaired cardiac function.

ANEMIA DUE TO FAILURE OF PRODUCTION

Aplastic anemia is due to failure of hemopoietic stem cells

In aplastic anemia there has been 'bone marrow failure.' Patients develop a pancytopenia and have a severe life-threatening disease. The marrow is depopulated of cells, which are replaced by fat. Many cases are idiopathic, but others follow a known insult to the marrow (*Fig. 15.21*).

ANEMIA DUE TO DYSERYTHROPOIESIS

Anemia of chronic disorders is the second most common cause of anemia

Patients with underlying diseases such as non-organ specific autoimmune diseases (e.g. rheumatoid disease and SLE), chronic infective diseases (e.g. tuberculosis, malaria, schis-

Fig. 15.21 Factors associated with development of aplastic anemia

Radiation

Antineoplastic chemotherapeutic agents

Drugs: chloramphenicol, gold, NSAIDs

Toxins: benzene

Viruses: papovavirus, HIV-1

Antibodies: autoimmune pancytopenia

Fanconi's anemia: autosomal recessive

tosomiasis), or neoplasia (lymphoma and some carcinomas) may develop a normochromic or hypochromic anemia.

There are three main abnormalities found in such anemias: iron stored in macrophages is not released for use in bone marrow, circulating red cells have a reduced lifespan, and the marrow shows a lack of response to erythropoietin.

Serum iron and total iron-binding capacity (TIBC) are low, but serum ferritin is normal or raised (compare with iron-deficiency anemia, see page 319).

Myelodysplastic syndromes cause refractory anemia and predispose to leukemia

Myelodysplastic syndromes are diseases of late adult life, in which there is production of abnormal clones of marrow stem cells. The products of abnormal clones are defective and prematurely destroyed; thus, depending on severity, anemia and pancytopenia may develop. The presence of genetically abnormal clones in the marrow predisposes to the development of leukemia in about 40% of cases. The main problem is an indolent anemia that requires treatment with transfusions over several years but does not respond to administering hematinics (refractory anemia).

Histologically the marrow shows normal or increased cellularity with megaloblastic cells. Abnormal red-cell precursors containing iron (ringed sideroblasts) may be seen, and abnormal myeloblasts may be found. Based on the numbers of myeloblasts and abnormal red-cell precursors, five subtypes of myelodysplasia have been defined in a French–American–British (FAB) classification (*Fig. 15.22*). Once 30% of marrow cells are composed of blasts, patients are regarded as having transformed to leukemia.

Marrow infiltration may result in leukoerythroblastic anemia

Extensive infiltration of the bone marrow may cause obliteration of normal hemopoietic elements. Extramedullary hemopoiesis then commonly develops. Patients develop leukoerythroblastic anemia, which is characterized by circulating erythroblasts and primitive white cells. The main conditions causing extensive infiltration of bone marrow are disseminated carcinoma, disseminated lymphoma and myelofibrosis (see page 327). A leukoerythroblastic picture

Fig. 15.22 FAB classification of myelodysplastic syndromes

Refractory anemia

Refractory anemia with ring sideroblasts

Refractory anemia with excessive blasts

Refractory anemia with excessive blasts in transformation

Chronic myelomonocytic leukemia

may also develop after massive hemorrhage, severe hemolysis and severe infections.

ANEMIA DUE TO DESTRUCTION OF RED CELLS

Hemolytic anemia is characterized by reduced red-cell survival in the blood

In hemolytic anemia, chronic increased red-cell destruction causes the development of anemia, with increased reticulocytes in blood, splenomegaly, erythroid hyperplasia resulting in expansion of bone marrow, and unconjugated hyperbilirubinemia. There are two main groups of factors causing hemolysis. Intrinsic defects in red cells result in abnormal erythrocyte fragility.

- **Membrane defects**, e.g. hereditary spherocytosis.
- **Enzyme defects**, e.g. glucose-6-phosphate dehydrogenase.
- **Defects outside red cells** causing red cell lysis, autoimmune and mechanical trauma to cells.

Red-cell destruction takes place in the spleen and by reticuloendothelial cells in the liver.

HEMOLYSIS DUE TO DEFECTS IN RED CELLS

The most common red-cell membrane defect causing hemolysis is hereditary spherocytosis

Hemolytic anemia may be caused by membrane defects in red cells. The most common disease is hereditary spherocytosis. Red cells have an abnormal cell membrane-associated cytoskeleton, which is caused by abnormalities

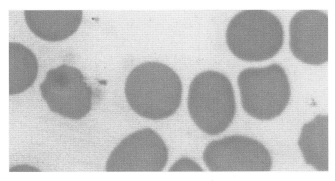

Fig. 15.23 Hereditary spherocytosis. Spherocytes are abnormal red cells which have a convex instead of a biconcave shape. In a normal blood film, the center of red cells is slightly paler than the periphery. In spherocytes, the center of the cell is darker than the periphery. Such cells are abnormally fragile and prone to hemolysis.

of the red-cell membrane-bracing proteins ankyrin, spectrin or band 4.2 protein. In some cases a defect in one of the spectrin genes has been documented.

Patients with this disease have jaundice, splenomegaly and hemolytic anemia. Red cells are spherical on blood film (*Fig. 15.23*) and are abnormally fragile, undergoing lysis in the spleen. There is expansion of the hemopoietic marrow and splenomegaly. Splenectomy is performed to prevent hemolysis.

Enzyme defects in red cells may predispose to hemolysis

Hemolytic anemia may also be caused by enzyme defects that render red cells susceptible to damage by oxidant stress. Glucose-6-phosphate dehydrogenase deficiency is an X-linked condition in which hemolytic crises are precipitated by infections or administration of certain drugs (quinine, phenacetin, aspirin). Pyruvate kinase deficiency causes a chronic hemolytic anemia.

Thalassemia is the result of quantitative abnormalities of globin production

Thalassemia syndromes are caused by defective synthesis of the α- or β-globin chains of hemoglobin. Disease is inherited and is common in the Mediterranean, Middle and Far East, and Southeast Asia, where carrier rates of 10–15% are found. The main pathological features are the consequence of increased requirements for red-cell production (caused by red-cell destruction):

- Increased intramedullary hemopoiesis causes deformed bones (increased size and bossing of the skull).
- Increased extramedullary hemopoiesis causes hepatosplenomegaly.
- Consequences of excess iron deposition in tissues, derived from transfusions with hemolysis (affects heart, liver and pancreas).

In severe forms of disease there is a hypochromic microcytic anemia associated with hemolysis of red cells. The most severe form of disease is that which results from abnormality of the β-globin chain.

Normal adult hemoglobin (HbA) is composed of two α-globin chains and two β-globin chains ($\alpha_2\beta_2$). In thalassemia, one or more of the genes responsible for synthesis of α- or β-globin chains is abnormal. Depending on which chain is affected, an α thalassemia or a β thalassemia results.

In β thalassemia over 90 different mutations have been described, leading to either reduced or absent synthesis of β-globin chain, one of which is present on each copy of chromosome 11. Heterozygotes develop a mild disease termed '**thalassemia minor**' (thalassemia trait), whereas homozygotes develop '**thalassemia major**', which is associated with a severe hemolytic anemia. In some instances no β-globin is produced ($β^0$) whereas in others β-globin chains are markedly reduced ($β^+$).

In α thalassemia, disease is mainly caused by deletion (rather than mutation) of parts of the globin genes. Each individual has four α-globin genes (a pair of α-globin genes is present on each of the copies of chromosome 16), thus there are four possible degrees of α-thalassemia, depending how many genes are abnormal. Hemolysis is less severe in α-thalassemia than in β-thalassemia. Features of thalassemia syndromes are summarized in *Fig. 15.24*.

Sickle-cell disease causes increased destruction of red cells associated with an abnormal hemoglobin

In sickle-cell disease a point mutation in the gene coding for the β-globin chain results in an abnormal form of hemoglobin, termed HbS ($α_2βS_2$). This form of hemoglobin polymerizes at low oxygen saturations, causing abnormal rigidity and deformity of red cells, which assume a sickle shape. As a result, red cells are abnormally fragile (undergoing hemolysis), and sludge in small vessels (causing vascular occlusion).

In sickle-cell trait individuals are heterozygous for the β-globin gene abnormality and 30% of the hemoglobin is HbS, resulting in no significant clinical abnormality.

In patients with sickle-cell disease (homozygous for the abnormal β-globin gene) over 80% of hemoglobin is HbS, the rest being HbF and HbA_2. There are three patterns of acute deterioration, termed sickle-cell crises:

1. **Sequestration crises**. In the early years of sickle-cell anemia sudden pooling of red cells in the spleen may develop, causing a rapid fall in hemoglobin concentration, which can lead to death.
2. **Infarctive crises**. Obstruction of small blood vessels occurs, leading to infarcts. Commonly affected tissues are bone (especially the femoral head), spleen (leading to splenic atrophy, *Fig. 15.25*), and skin (leading to ankle ulcers).
3. **Aplastic crises**. Splenic atrophy caused by infarction predisposes to infection, leading to depression of red-cell production. This precipitates a rapid fall in hemoglobin concentration in the face of continued hemolysis.

In addition to development of crises, abnormalities occur in many organs (*Fig. 15.26*). Other mutations of the β-globin gene form hemoglobins C, D and E, which also result in hemolysis.

HEMOLYSIS CAUSED BY DEFECTS OUTSIDE RED CELLS

Hemolysis may be caused by immune or mechanical destruction

Antibodies binding to antigens on red cells may cause premature destruction of red cells. The three main types of disease in which this happens are warm-antibody hemolytic anemia (80% of cases), cold-antibody hemolytic anemia

Fig. 15.24 Summary of thalassemia

Clinical disease	Globin chains present	Features
β-Thalassemia		
Thalassemia major	Homozygous $β^0/β^0$ Homozygous $β^+/β^+$	Hypochromic microcytic anemia. Severe hemolysis, hepatosplenomegaly, marrow hyperplasia causing skeletal deformities. Iron overload develops with repeated transfusions
Thalassemia minor	Heterozygous $β^+/β$ Heterozygous $β^0/β$	Moderate reduction in HbA, increase in HbA2 ($α_2δ_2$). Mild anemia with hypochromic cells
α-Thalassemia		
Silent carrier	$-α/αα$	Asymptomatic with no structural blood abnormality
α-Thalassemia trait	$--/αα$ $α-/α-$	Asymptomatic but mild hemolytic anemia with some microcytic cells
Hemoglobin H disease	$--/α-$	Moderate hemolytic anemia with hypochromia and microcytosis, HbH forms from tetramers of β chain
Lethal (hydrops fetalis)	$--/--$	Lethal in utero

(20% of cases) and isoantibody hemolytic anemia (rare) (*Fig. 15.27*).

Mechanical damage to red cells may lead to reduced lifespan and hemolysis. There are three main groups of mechanical hemolysis:

- **Macroangiopathic.** Prosthetic cardiac valves.
- **Microangiopathic.** Fragmentation by fibrin strands in small vessels, as seen in disseminated intravascular coagulation. In this condition there is activation of the

Fig. 15.25 Sickle cell disease – spleen. The spleen is shrunken as a result of scarring due to multiple episodes of microinfarction in the past. Recent microinfarcts are arrowed.

coagulation system in small vessels, causing microthrombi. This results in depletion of coagulation factors and platelets (increased risk of bleeding) and in mechanical fragmentation of red cells (hemolysis).

- **Splenic.** Hypersplenism caused by enlargement of the spleen is associated with hemolysis. Red cells are sequestered in the spleen and are prematurely destroyed.

Increase in the red cell mass is termed polycythemia

Polycythemia, also termed erythrocytosis, is characterized by an absolute increase in the mass of circulating red cells, detectable by a rise in the hematocrit.

Secondary polycythemia occurs in conditions that give rise to arterial hypoxia, the two main causes being chronic lung disease and cyanotic congenital heart disease. In these circumstances, hypoxia stimulates expansion of red cell mass. A similar phenomenon is seen in people who live at high altitudes, such as in the Andes. Uncommonly, abnormal secretion of erythropoietin causes polycythemia, e.g. in renal disease or cerebral hemangioblastoma.

Primary polycythemia occurs in a condition termed **polycythemia rubra vera**, which is one of the myeloproliferative disorders (see page 327).

At a hematocrit above 50%, hyperviscosity of blood predisposes to vascular thrombosis, for example causing cerebral infarction.

Fig. 15.26 Systemic complications of sickle-cell disease	
Lungs	Pulmonary infarction, development of acute chest syndrome (characterized by decreased pulmonary function, which may be fatal).
Brain	Cerebral infarction.
Kidneys	Papillary necrosis caused by vascular occlusion in vasae rectae.
Bone	Salmonella osteomyelitis is predisposed by small infarcts in bone caused by vascular occlusion.
Immune	Hyposplenism increases susceptibility to bacterial infection.
Hepatobiliary	Pigment gallstones due to hemolysis. Secondary hemosiderosis due to iron overload in transfused patients.
Eye	Blindness caused by small vessel occlusion and ischemic retinopathy.

Fig. 15.27 Causes of immune hemolytic anemias
Warm-acting antibodies   IgG class, destruction of red cells in spleen
Idiopathic (50%)   CLL   Lymphocytic lymphoma   SLE   Viral infections   Drug-induced hemolysis (α-methyl-dopa, quinidine)
Cold-reacting antibodies   IgM class, destruction of red cells by Kupffer's cells in liver
Idiopathic   Lymphoma-related   *Mycoplasma* pneumonia   Infectious mononucleosis
Isoimmune
Hemolytic disease of the newborn (Rhesus incompatibility)   Transfusion reactions

DISORDERS OF CIRCULATING WHITE BLOOD CELLS AND MARROW

The two main reasons for an increase in numbers of white blood cells (leukocytosis) are **reactive changes** in the number of circulating white cells (associated with different types of disease, see Key Facts), and **neoplastic diseases** of white cells.

White cell function may be impaired because of too few cells or because of abnormal function

White cell function may be qualitatively impaired or there may be reduced numbers of circulating cells. Reduced neutrophil function predisposes to bacterial infections, particularly those causing ulceration in the mouth and oropharynx. The main causes of reduced numbers of neutrophils (**neutropenia**) are:

- Generalized abnormalities of marrow function (associated with disorders of red cells and platelets).
- Marrow hypoplasia, which is commonly acquired due to therapeutic irradiation or chemotherapy, B_{12} or folate deficiency, and some overwhelming infections. Reduced marrow cellularity is seen on bone marrow biopsy.
- Abnormal destruction of neutrophils (drug-induced, autoimmune, hypersplenism). This is associated with increase in neutrophil precursors on bone marrow biopsy.

Among the main causes of defective neutrophil function are systemic disturbances, particularly diabetes mellitus, corticosteroid therapy, renal failure and alcoholism. Rare congenital causes may lead to defects in phagocytosis and bacterial killing.

Numbers of lymphoid cells are reduced (**lymphopenia**) with age, but this is also seen in association with SLE (see Chapter 25), steroid therapy, and immunodeficiency states (see Chapter 7).

NEOPLASTIC DISEASES OF WHITE CELLS

Neoplastic diseases of white blood cells are divided into four main groups:

- **Malignant lymphomas** are diseases of tissue-based and nodal lymphocytes (see page 309).
- **Leukemias** and myeloproliferative disorders are malignant neoplasms derived from cells of the bone marrow. Neoplastic cells may circulate in the blood, secondarily colonizing other tissues.
- **Plasma cell tumors** are neoplasms derived from terminally differentiated B cells derived from bone marrow (see page 314).
- **Histiocytoses** are neoplasms derived from histiocytic (macrophagic) cells, particularly Langerhans' cells.

Certain of these diseases overlap with each other: for example, some lymphomas also have a leukemic pattern.

Leukemias are the most common neoplastic diseases of white cells

The most common neoplastic disease of white cells is leukemia, the incidence of which is 9 per 100 000. The disease may be acute or chronic. The general characteristics of leukemias include: neoplastic proliferation of marrow cells, forming one or more cell lines; circulation of neoplastic cells in peripheral blood in most (but not all) cases; and suppression of other marrow elements, leading to symptoms caused by lack of normal red cells, white cells and platelets. Common to all leukemias is expansion of the bone marrow and infiltration by neoplastic white cells (*Fig. 15.28*).

Acute leukemias are characterized by proliferation of immature cells known as blast cells, which form a high proportion of the bone marrow cells. Typically there is rapid progression of disease which, without treatment, is fatal in a short period of time.

Chronic leukemias are characterized by proliferation of blasts, but they form a smaller proportion of the total marrow than in acute leukemia. Typically there is slow progression of disease, but this type may also transform into a more aggressive pattern.

> ### Key Facts
> ### Changes in circulating white cells in blood
>
> - **Neutrophil leukocytosis** most commonly occurs as a response to bacterial infection or to tissue necrosis (infarction).
> - **Eosinophilia** is seen as a response to parasitic infections, in hypersensitivity responses, associated with neoplasia (chronic granulocytic leukemia and Hodgkin's disease) and in hypereosinophilia syndromes, with vasculitis and pulmonary infiltration.
> - **Lymphocytosis** is seen in viral infections, particularly glandular fever (infectious mononucleosis), and less commonly in infections such as typhoid and brucellosis.
> - **Monocytosis** is uncommon, but may be seen in infective endocarditis and with some protozoal infections (malaria, trypanosomiasis).

Acute leukemias are divided into lymphoblastic or myeloid groups

Acute leukemias are divided into those derived from lymphoid cells, **acute lymphoblastic leukemia** (ALL), and those derived from myeloid, monocytic, erythroid, and megakaryocytic cells, which are grouped as **acute myeloblastic leukemia** (AML).

In acute leukemia, replacement of the bone marrow by blast cells causes anemia due to loss of red cells, susceptibility to infection due to loss of normal white cells, and susceptibility to bleeding due to loss of platelets.

Patients develop fever, malaise, bleeding (petechial hemorrhages), and mouth ulcers due to infections. The peripheral blood shows an increased white cell count (including blast cells) in about 50% of cases; importantly, in many cases the white cell count may be normal or reduced.

The diagnosis of acute leukemia is based on examination of bone marrow aspirate and histology (*Fig. 15.29*). Acute leukemias frequently show infiltration of many organs, especially the brain and gonads. Splenomegaly and lymphadenopathy are not usually prominent, except in some cases of acute lymphoblastic leukemia.

Acute lymphoblastic leukemia (ALL) most commonly affects children, only rarely occurring in young adults. The prognosis is related to the type of leukemia as defined by the FAB classification (*Fig. 15.30*).

Fig. 15.28 Leukemic infiltration of marrow. In leukemia, neoplastic cells replace normal red (hemopoietic) and yellow (inactive) bone marrow. Vertebrae, ribs and long bones show diffuse replacement of marrow space by pale, cellular, neoplastic cells (a). Histologically (b), the normal marrow is replaced by abnormal, monotonous, leukemic cells.

Fig. 15.29 Acute leukemia histology. Marrow in acute leukemia is extensively replaced by neoplastic cells, which efface normal marrow. There is hypercellularity, large numbers of blast cells characterized by large nuclei and mitoses, and reduced amounts of normal hemopoietic elements. This example is from a case of acute lymphoblastic leukemia.

Fig. 15.30 ALL classification. ALL is classified by morphology into groups L1–L3. Using immunochemistry, the nature of the cells can be further defined, and this is related to prognosis. Patients with L3 morphology, a high white count, and mature B-cell type have worst prognosis.

FAB type	Cytology	Phenotype	Incidence (%)	Prognosis
L1	Small lymphoid cells	Null cell ALL (early B-cell)	12	intermediate
L2	Large lymphoid cells	Common ALL (pre-B-cell)	75	good
		T-cell ALL	12	intermediate
L3	Large lymphoid cells with vacuolated cytoplasm	Mature B-cell ALL	1	poor

Acute myeloblastic leukemia (AML) is most commonly seen in adults and encompasses several different types of disease, as categorized by the FAB classification (*Fig. 15.31*). M1–M3 are myeloblastic in type. They are separated according to the degree of differentiation, which is assessed by cytochemical detection of myelocyte markers. M5 is composed of monoblasts, and M4 is an overlap between myeloblastic and monoblastic types. Although M6 is termed 'erythroblastic leukemia' both myeloblastic and erythroblastic cells are seen.

Chronic leukemias are divided into lymphocytic, myeloid and hairy-cell types

Chronic leukemias are mainly seen in adults over the age of 40 years, but can develop in childhood.

Accounting for about 25% of all cases of leukemia, **chronic lymphocytic leukemia** (CLL) is mainly seen in patients over the age of 50 years. It is characterized by neoplastic proliferation of small mature lymphocytes (*Fig. 15.32*). The vast majority of cases of CLL are of the B-cell type, with only about 5% of cases of T-cell type. The bone marrow is infiltrated by abnormal clusters of lymphocytes, initially sparing normal hemopoietic elements but later effacing the marrow. The peripheral blood contains large numbers of circulating abnormal lymphoid cells. Lymphadenopathy is common and is often a presenting feature of disease; affected nodes show the same histological picture as small-cell diffuse lymphocytic lymphoma (see page 312). Splenomegaly is also commonly seen. Autoimmune hemolytic anemia and thrombocytopenia are present in about 10% of cases, and a paraproteinemia is found in about 5% of cases. Prognosis is related to clinical staging (*Fig. 15.33*).

Hairy-cell leukemia is a form of B-cell leukemia in which cells have many fine surface projections. Typically, there is diffuse marrow involvement and the spleen is very large, with hypersplenism and pancytopenia, but lymphadenopathy is uncommon. Increase in circulating white cells is not marked. As several of the clinical problems are derived from hypersplenism, splenectomy may alleviate many of the symptoms. Many cases also respond to interferon treatment.

Chronic myeloid (granulocytic) leukemia (CML) is also considered one of the myeloproliferative disorders (see page 327). It is most common in adults between 30 and

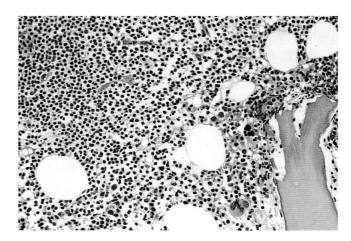

Fig. 15.32 Bone marrow in CLL. The bone marrow is replaced by small mature lymphoid cells. In early stages of disease this replacement is focal, allowing normal platelet and red-cell production.

Fig. 15.31 FAB Myeloblastic leukemia classification		
FAB type	**Cytology**	**Incidence**
M0	Undifferentiated myeloblastic	Uncommon
M1	Acute myeloblastic leukemia (>90% blasts)	50% of all cases
M2	Acute myeloblastic leukemia (granulocytic differentiation)	
M3	Acute promyelocytic leukemia	Uncommon
M4	Acute myelomonoblastic leukemia	30% of all cases
M5	Acute monocytic leukemia	Uncommon
M6	Acute erythroblastic leukemia	Uncommon
M7	Acute megakaryocytic leukemia	Uncommon

Fig. 15.33 Clinical staging of CLL. Poor prognosis, with survival of about 2 years, is associated with low hemoglobin <11 g/dL or platelet count <100 ∞ 10⁹/L at presentation	
Stage 0	Lymphocytosis of blood and marrow.
Stage 1	Lymphocytosis and enlarged nodes.
Stage II	Lymphocytosis and enlarged liver or spleen.
Stage III	Hemoglobin <11 g/dL, with features of stage 0, I or II.
Stage IV	Platelet count <100 × 10⁹/L, with features of stage 0, I, II or III.

Fig. 15.34 Bone marrow in CML. The bone marrow is replaced by myeloid cells in varying stages of differentiation.

Cytogenetic changes in chronic myeloid leukemia

Patients with chronic myeloid leukemia commonly have an abnormal chromosome in leukemic cells, termed the **Philadelphia chromosome** (Ph1). This is a reciprocal translocation between the long arms of chromosome 9 and 22 t(9;22)(q34;q11). It results in the formation of the *bcr-abl* fusion gene, which produces a protein with tyrosine kinase activity, involved in cell transformation as part of the neoplastic phenotype. Around 90% of cases of CML are Ph-positive-associated, with a better median survival than the remaining 10% of cases, which are Ph negative. A drug, imatinib, acts as an abl-specific tyrosine kinase inhibitor and can be effective in this disease.

40 years of age, accounting for about 20% of all cases of leukemia. Affected patients develop hepatosplenomegaly, with massive enlargement of the spleen due to infiltration by leukemic cells. The peripheral blood shows a leukocytosis with an excess of neutrophils, myelocytes and metamyelocytes. There is usually a moderate anemia, but thrombocytopenia is not marked. Basophils may be increased in number. The bone marrow shows increased cellularity, with marrow replaced by neutrophil precursors (*Fig. 15.34*). The natural history of the disease is for treated disease to remain stable for around 5 years (chronic phase), followed by transformation to an acute leukemia with large numbers of blasts (advanced phase). Treatment with stem cell bone marrow transplantation is generally advised, with some patients having benefit from imatinib (see pink box).

MYELOPROLIFERATIVE DISEASES

Myeloproliferative diseases are caused by abnormal marrow stem-cell proliferation

Myeloproliferative disorders are characterized by proliferation of marrow stem cells, which differentiate into erthyroid, granulocytic, megakaryocytic or fibroblastic. There is frequent overlap between diseases, with transformation of one into another, and termination of disease as AML.

Included in this group of diseases is **polycythemia rubra vera**, which occurs mainly after the age of 40 years, causing polycythemia with all its complications, particularly vascular thrombosis. The marrow contains increased numbers of erythroid precursors, as well as increased numbers of megakaryocytes and fibroblasts. Splenomegaly is common, and 15% of patients develop myelofibrosis, 10% developing AML. With treatment, overall survival is about 10 years.

In **primary thrombocythemia** there is thrombocytosis associated with a bleeding tendency or thrombosis. Splenic infarction and secondary hyposplenism are common.

Myelofibrosis is characterized by proliferation of fibroblasts in the marrow, which is a response to growth factors secreted by abnormally proliferating myeloid cells. As the marrow is replaced by fibroblasts and collagen, extramedullary hemopoiesis develops in the spleen and liver, causing hepatosplenomegaly. Clinically, patients develop anemia and the signs and symptoms of a massively enlarged spleen. The peripheral blood shows anemia with abnormally shaped red cells and a leukoerythroblastic picture. Patients typically survive for about 3 years, and approximately 10% develop AML.

Chronic myeloid leukemia is also a form of myeloproliferative disease with splenomegaly, anemia, and neutrophilia.

HISTIOCYTOSES

The Langerhans'-cell histiocytoses are proliferations of histiocytic cells

The Langerhans'-cell histiocytoses are a group of diseases characterized by proliferation of histiocytic cells with markers and structural features of Langerhans' cells. These disorders were formerly called histiocytosis-X. Normal Langerhans' cells are found in the skin and lymph nodes, where they act as dendritic antigen-presenting cells. The spectrum of severity in this condition has three main clinical patterns (overlaps are also seen).

Eosinophilic granuloma (unifocal Langerhans' histiocytosis) is a localized collection of Langerhans' cells associated with many reactive eosinophils (*Fig. 15.35*). Lesions may develop in bone (pathological fractures, bone pain, radiographic finding) or soft tissues (swelling). Local removal of lesions is curative.

Hand–Schuller–Christian disease (multifocal Langerhans' histiocytosis) is characterized by multiple deposits of Langerhans' cells associated with reactive cells (principally eosinophils) in bone, lung, skin and pituitary gland. Deposits cause local tissue destruction and, in the lung, restrictive lung disease.

The classic clinical triad is diabetes insipidus, exophthalmos, and bone defects on skull radiograph.

Letterer–Siwe disease (acute disseminated Langerhans' cell histiocytosis) is seen mainly in young children. It is manifest by skin rash, lymphadenopathy and hepatosplenomegaly. Infiltration of bone marrow causes thrombocytopenia, anemia and predisposition to infections. It is rapidly fatal unless treated.

Fig. 15.35 Langerhans' cell histiocytosis. (a) Langerhans' cells are large, with pale-stained bean-shaped nuclei. Typical lesions show infiltration by numerous eosinophils, as here. (b) Immunochemistry shows expression of CD1a by the Langerhans' cells, stained brown

DISEASES OF COAGULATION AND PLATELETS

Reduced platelets in blood lead to increased susceptibility to bleeding

Reduced platelet numbers or defects in function result in a bleeding tendency. Patients develop petechial hemorrhages and bruising in skin, bleeding into mucosal surfaces and, sometimes, severe bleeding into tissues after trauma. The main causes are reduced platelet production due to marrow disease, or increased destruction of platelets.

Defective production is seen in megaloblastic anemias, marrow infiltration, and after marrow suppression by chemotherapy.

Idiopathic thrombocytopenia (ITP) is due to autoimmune destruction of platelets, which are coated with antiplatelet antibodies. Disease may be acute or chronic, the acute form being seen mainly in children after viral infection that generally recovers spontaneously. The chronic form is seen mainly in women and is associated with autoimmune disease or drugs. Platelet destruction occurs in the spleen, and splenectomy prolongs platelet survival.

Consumption of platelets and coagulation factors is seen in **disseminated intravascular coagulation, thrombotic thrombocytopenic purpura**, and **hemolytic uremic syndrome**. The common mechanism is the formation of microvascular thrombi that consume platelets.

Platelet dysfunction is seen in several systemic disturbances, e.g. uremia, chronic liver disease, myeloma, and with the administration of antiplatelet drugs. Congenital disorders of platelet function are uncommon.

Increase in platelet numbers may be due to neoplasia (thrombocythemia) or a reactive process (thrombocytosis). **Primary thrombocythemia** is one of the myeloproliferative diseases, patients developing both a thrombotic as well as a bleeding tendency. **Reactive thrombocytosis** is seen after splenectomy, in association with systemic neoplasia, and with systemic inflammatory responses.

Coagulation disorders lead to increased risk of serious bleeding

Abnormalities of coagulation lead to increased risk of serious bleeding. The main causes are iatrogenic administration of anticoagulants, hereditary defects in coagulation factors (e.g. hemophilia, von Willebrand's disease), and liver disease causing impaired production of clotting factors.

The main pathological consequences of poor blood coagulation are bleeding after surgical procedures such as biopsy, bleeding into joints after minor trauma, and intracranial hemorrhage; the predisposition to subdural hemorrhages is particularly increased.

Disseminated intravascular coagulation results in tissue ischemia, hemorrhage, and red-cell hemolysis

Disseminated intravascular coagulation results from activation of the coagulation system in small vessels throughout the body. This has several main effects:

- Platelets are consumed, resulting in a low platelet count.
- Fibrin/platelet thrombi are deposited in small vessels in brain, kidney, lungs and other organs, causing ischemic changes.
- Coagulation factors are consumed and there is activation of the fibrinolytic system; fibrin-degradation products acting as inhibitors of coagulation are generated.
- Red cells are fragmented by passage through vessels occluded by thrombi, and there is destruction of red cells (microangiopathic hemolysis).

Patients develop ischemia and dysfunction of major organs, bleeding into tissues, and hemolytic anemia. The main precipitating causes of this syndrome are:

- septicemia (see page 108)
- systemic shock (e.g. major surgery and transfusion)
- obstetric catastrophes (eclampsia, placental abruption, amniotic fluid embolism).

BONE MARROW TRANSPLANTATION

The graft-versus-host reaction is a problem in bone marrow transplantation

In bone marrow transplantation, commonly used to treat hematological malignancies, the patient's own immune system is destroyed following cytotoxic or radiotherapeutic destruction of bone marrow cells. When healthy bone marrow cells are transplanted into the recipient, there is a danger of a **graft-versus-host reaction** (**GVH**), which may be acute or chronic.

In the GVH reaction, transplanted immunologically competent bone marrow cells (including T lymphocytes) may mount an immune response against various components of the recipient's tissues, which bear antigens that the transplanted immune cells recognize as foreign.

Acute GVH occurs within 3 months of grafting in up to 70% of recipients. It produces features of diarrhea, dermatitis, malabsorption, and jaundice. The proliferating transplanted immunocompetent cells destroy epithelial cells in the gut, liver and skin. This is a potentially life-threatening condition, the risk of which is minimized by careful HLA matching. Although recent efforts to remove T cells from donor marrow have reduced the risk of GVH reactions, they have increased the risk of graft failure.

Chronic GVH occurs 3–15 months after transplantation in about 40% of recipients. It produces a syndrome similar to progressive systemic sclerosis (see Chapter 25).

Problem-based learning

Case 1 – A man with enlarged neck nodes

A 72-year-old retired steel erector has recently undergone biopsy of one of a group of enlarged cervical lymph nodes which have been present for about 6 weeks. You phone the laboratory for a report and the pathologist dictates a preliminary report as follows:

- Macroscopic findings: lymph node, 2 cm in maximum extent with a focally yellow cut surface.
- Microscopic findings: the lymph node contains multiple well-formed granulomata.

1. **From the preliminary report, what is the differential diagnosis?**
2. **What other investigations would be appropriate?**
3. **Describe a typical granuloma and the mechanisms important in its formation.**

Case 2 – Lymphadenopathy detected on a chest X-ray

A 26-year-old hospital kitchen worker has a chest X-ray as part of her occupational health surveillance. This is reported as showing mediastinal lymphadenopathy. When she is questioned further she says that she has had occasional bouts of fever and night sweats, and has lost one stone in weight over the preceding 6 months. A routine physical examination reveals cervical lymphadenopathy and a node is removed for histological assessment. The report confirms the presence of Hodgkin's disease (HD).

1. **What is necessary for the histological diagnosis of Hodgkin's disease, and how are the different forms of the disease classified?**

▶ **2. What is the Ann Arbor Staging System?**
3. What factors are important in the prognosis of HD?

Case 3 – An old man with back pain

A 72-year-old retired man is admitted to hospital as an emergency. He lives alone and is confused and complaining of severe back pain. His daughter tells you that when she saw her father a week ago he was complaining that he was drinking a lot and could not stop going to the toilet to pass urine. Physical examination reveals pallor, but otherwise nothing. The results of the initial investigations are as follows:

Investigation	Result
Hb	9 g/dL
WBC	6.8×10^9/L
ESR	60 mm/h
Creatinine	120 mmol/L
Platelets	150×10^9/L
Corrected Ca^{2+}	3.8 mmol/L
Lumbar-spine X-ray	Multiple punched-out lytic lesions seen in ribs and vertebral bodies

A diagnosis of myeloma is confirmed by further investigations. In the subsequent months the patient's renal function gradually declines.

1. How is the diagnosis of myeloma confirmed?
2. What are the possible causes of a decline in renal function?
3. This patient's symptoms were caused by destruction of bone and hypercalcemia. What is the other major cause of symptoms in myeloma?

Case 4 – A sick child with a rash

A 2-year-old boy has been brought to see you because his mother is worried about his health. Over the previous 4 days the child, who had been previously well, has had a temperature, been off his food, and today has come out in red spots with bleeding gums. Examination reveals a petechial skin rash and mild splenomegaly. A diagnosis of acute leukemia is made.

1. How might one disease process explain this complex of symptoms?
2. How is a specific diagnosis achieved?
3. How are acute leukemias classified?

Brief answers to these case-based questions are given on pages 588–9. More detailed answers and other study resources are available online at www.studentconsult.com.

Endocrine system 16

The endocrine system produces hormones, which act as chemical messengers, passing in the bloodstream to their target tissues

In clinical practice, endocrine dysfunction normally presents either as a consequence of over- or underproduction of hormones, commonly due to genetic, metabolic or neoplastic disease, or from mass effects due to compression of surrounding structures. In addition, the endocrine system also has a significant burden of autoimmune disease. To complicate matters further, endocrine disease can also result from disturbances in the frequency and amplitude of hormone release, rather than simple extremes of over- or underproduction, for example failure to coordinate ovulation in the female menstrual cycle. This can make diagnosis difficult, as 'one off' measurements of hormone levels may well be within the normal range. Disease in one endocrine gland often has secondary effects on other endocrine target organs; thus, it is essential to consider downstream effects when interpreting endocrine abnormalities, particularly in organs subject to control by the hypothalamopituitary axis, e.g. the androgen insensitivity syndrome.

Hormones fall into three major groups: peptide hormones, steroid derivatives, and metabolites of tyrosine (adrenaline, noradrenaline, dopamine and the thyroid hormones). Hormone receptors are found either on the epithelial surface (peptide hormones), where they are linked to a variety of second messenger cascades, or in the nucleus (steroids/thyroid hormones), where hormone-bound receptor molecules bind to, and regulate, promoter regions of target genes. Thus, disturbances in endocrine function can originate at multiple levels in the endocrine pathway, from synthesis, packaging and storage of the hormone, through mechanisms of release and secretion, and finally to deficiencies in the target organ.

The most important diseases of the endocrine glands are associated with over- or underproduction of hormones

The control of hormone secretion by the various components of the endocrine system is normally finely tuned by a combination of neural and chemical feedback mechanisms. Loss of this control, due to either primary or secondary disease affecting the endocrine organ, produces metabolic and structural abnormalities. Tumors occurring within endocrine glands may be hormonally active (functioning) or inactive (non-functioning).

PITUITARY

The pituitary gland has two components, the adenohypophysis and the neurohypophysis

The **adenohypophysis** (**anterior pituitary**) synthesizes and secretes six principal hormones, most of which act on other endocrine glands. The main anterior pituitary hor-

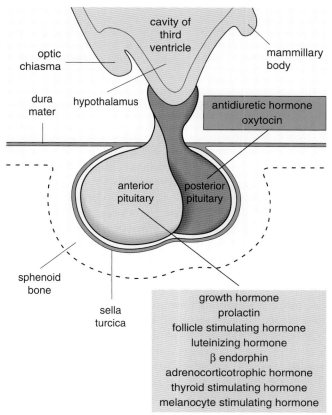

Fig. 16.1 Pituitary and hypothalamus and their hormones. The hormones secreted by the anterior pituitary (adenohypophysis), hypothalamus and posterior pituitary (neurohypophysis) are shown.

331

mones are: growth hormone, prolactin, adrenocorticotrophic hormone (ACTH), thyroid-stimulating hormone (TSH) and the gonadotropins luteinizing hormone (LH) and follicle-stimulating hormone (FSH). The pathological consequences of anterior pituitary disease are related either to **over- or underproduction** of the above hormones, or related to compression of surrounding structures (**mass effects**) by tumors. The intimate relationship of the pituitary fossa (sella turcica) to the optic chiasm, cranial nerves III–VI as they traverse the cavernous sinus, and the pituitary stalk and hypophyseal portal blood supply explains many of the clinical presentations of pituitary disease due to expansion of the lesion.

The **neurohypophysis** (posterior pituitary) is in direct continuity with the hypothalamus, storing and secreting antidiuretic hormone (ADH) and oxytocin synthesized in the neurons of the hypothalamus (*Fig. 16.1*).

Many of the functions of the pituitary gland are controlled by neural and chemical stimuli from the hypothalamus, diseases of which cause secondary abnormalities in pituitary function.

The most common and important diseases of the pituitary gland are tumors of the adenohypophysis (pituitary adenomas)

Pituitary adenomas, albeit benign in that they do not metastasize, can be life-threatening by virtue of their position and ability to secrete excess hormone. As a group, they represent about 10% of intracranial neoplasms, of which 3% are associated with **multiple endocrine neoplasia (MEN) type 1** (see below). Many pituitary adenomas are associated with mutations in components of the G-protein signaling mechanism, resulting in dysregulation of hormone synthesis and secretion.

Non-functioning (or silent) adenomas progressively enlarge until they break out of the sella turcica in an upwards direction, often compressing the optic chiasm. This produces a characteristic visual disturbance known as **bitemporal hemianopia** (*Fig. 16.2*). The tumor may destroy the normal functioning adenohypophysis, producing symptoms and signs of hypopituitarism. As these adenomas are clinically 'silent' they tend to present late, with symptoms of raised intracranial pressure or local mass effects.

Functioning adenomas (*Fig. 16.3*) may, in theory, produce any of the adenohypophyseal hormones, but the majority produce either prolactin or growth hormone (*Fig. 16.4*); a few produce ACTH.

In general, functioning pituitary tumors present earlier than the non-functioning variety, their presence being revealed by the effects of excess hormone production. Sometimes these functioning adenomas may be very small, despite producing significant metabolic abnormality. Pituitary adenomas less than 1 cm in diameter are arbitrarily designated **microadenomas**.

Other rare causes of hyperpituitarism include pituitary hyperplasia, pituitary carcinoma and some hypothalamic disorders.

Reduced output of all anterior pituitary hormones is termed 'panhypopituitarism'

Defective production of anterior pituitary hormones (panhypopituitarism), which may result from either pituitary or hypothalamic disease, is rare. The most important **pituitary causes** are:

- Surgical removal of a pituitary tumor or radiation therapy.
- Obliteration of normal pituitary by a primary pituitary tumor or metastatic tumor, e.g. metastatic breast carcinoma.
- Ischemic necrosis of adenohypophysis, due to hypotensive shock. This may occur as a result of intrapartum or postpartum hemorrhage (**Sheehan's syndrome**).
- Hemorrhage into a pituitary adenoma (**pituitary apoplexy**). This causes an acute expansion in the volume of the pituitary gland and may lead to sudden death. This represents a neurosurgical emergency.

Fig. 16.2 CT scan (a) of a large pituitary adenoma (A) expanding upwards to compress optic chiasma (arrows). This large tumor presented with visual disturbance and was not hormone-producing. Macroscopically (b), adenomas are soft fleshy tumors (**A**). This is in a postmortem specimen of pituitary fossa.

Fig. 16.3 Functioning pituitary adenomata

	Clinical features
Prolactin-producing (30%)	Menstrual disturbances and infertility in women
	Impotence, loss of libido and depression in men
Growth-hormone-producing	Before puberty: gigantism
	After puberty: acromegaly
ACTH-producing	Adrenal cortical hyperplasia (Cushing's disease) (see page 344)

Fig. 16.4 Pituitary adenoma. (a) H & E. (b) Immunochemistry. Pituitary adenomas have solid and trabecular patterns (a). Immunochemistry can be used to ascertain hormone production; here, growth hormone is stained brown (b).

Very rare causes of hypopituitarism include inflammation (autoimmune adenohypophysitis, sarcoidosis) and traumatic disruption following skull fracture.

Hypothalamic causes of panhypopituitarism include destruction of the hypothalamus by:

- Primary brain tumor, e.g. glioma or craniopharyngioma.
- Infarction.
- Inflammation, e.g. sarcoid (see Chapter 25).
- Infection, e.g. encephalitis or meningitis.

Diseases of the neurohypophysis are very rare

Most failures of ADH and oxytocin production are the result of damage to the hypothalamus, usually due to tumor invasion or infarction.

Failure of ADH production leads to **diabetes insipidus**, in which lack of ADH prevents resorption of water from the glomerular filtrate in the renal collecting ducts. Large quantities of very dilute urine are excreted (polyuria), and the risk of body water depletion must be counteracted by greatly increasing water intake (polydipsia). The main causes of diabetes insipidus are: surgical extirpation of pituitary or its stalk – usually in the course of tumor removal – and inflammatory or neoplastic lesions in the hypothalamus, the most common inflammatory cause being sarcoidosis. In about 30% of cases of diabetes insipidus, no structural cause is found.

Inappropriate ADH secretion, independent of disease in the pituitary or hypothalamus, may occur in association with some tumors, particularly oat-cell carcinoma of the lung, and some neuroendocrine tumors. It is also a frequent transient phenomenon after head injury, neurosurgery for tumor, and some lung diseases, producing a low serum sodium and water imbalance, with the risk of water intoxication.

Key Facts
Acromegaly

- Due to excessive growth hormone production from a pituitary somatotroph cell adenoma **after** epiphyseal fusion.
- Conspicuous growth of soft tissues, skin and viscera.
- Growth of bones and soft tissues in hands and feet gives a 'spade-like' appearance, with 'sausage' fingers.
- Enlargement of the jaw results in prognathism (protrusion of the lower mandible), enlargement of the face, and separation of the teeth.
- Metabolic disturbances include: abnormal glucose tolerance, diabetes mellitus, hypertension, osteoporosis and congestive cardiac failure.

THYROID GLAND

The thyroid gland secretes two different types of hormone from two cell types

The thyroid gland is a pure endocrine gland composed of two cell types, which secrete two types of hormone. The **thyroid follicle cells**, which make up the bulk of the gland, are arranged in a follicular pattern. They produce the hormone **thyroxine** (T_4) and its more potent deiodinated product **tri-iodothyronine** (T_3). Most T_3 is produced by removal of an iodine atom from T_4 in the peripheral tissues. Both hormones affect many metabolic processes, almost always by increasing their activity, thereby increasing the basal metabolic rate. There is a rich lymphatic drainage and adrenergic and cholinergic innervation.

The **parafollicular or 'C' cells** are a minority population of cells that occur mainly in small clusters in the interstices between follicles. They produce the hormone **calcitonin**, which is involved in **calcium homeostasis**, possibly inhibiting osteoclastic bone resorption (compare with parathormone, page 538).

The thyroid follicle cells synthesize and secrete T_4 and T_3 under the control of thyroid-stimulating hormone (TSH) from the pituitary

T_4 is synthesized by the thyroid follicle cells, which preferentially take up iodine and link it to tyrosine. The iodotyrosines are then stored in the follicle acini and linked with protein to form **thyroglobulin** (**thyroid colloid**). This is removed as required from the colloid store, as a result of pinocytosis by the same follicle cells, which then split off the linked protein by lysosomal breakdown and convert the hormone into active components T_3 and T_4. These are then secreted into the adjacent thyroid capillaries to pass into the circulation.

The term 'goiter' is used to describe any swelling of the thyroid gland

Traditionally the word 'goiter' has been used to describe any enlargement of the thyroid. Thyroid enlargement can have many causes, and may sometimes be associated with metabolic disorder due to decreased or increased thyroid hormone output. The term 'toxic goiter' is sometimes used to describe enlarged thyroids associated with increased thyroid hormone output (thyrotoxicosis), and the term 'non-toxic goiter' is applied to an enlarged thyroid when thyroid hormone levels are normal. As both terms are imprecise and imply no specific pathology, they are best avoided.

Increase in size of the thyroid may be diffuse or nodular

Enlargement of the thyroid gland produces a palpable and often visible swelling in the front of the neck. The increase in size may be diffuse or nodular, and nodular enlargement may involve all or part of the gland. The distribution and palpation characteristics of the swelling often give valuable clues to the underlying pathology:

- **Irregular multinodular enlargement of the entire thyroid** is the most common cause of thyroid enlargement, and is particularly seen in the elderly. This pattern is also called **multinodular goiter**.
- **Focal nodular enlargement within the thyroid** may be due to a thyroid tumor. This pattern of enlargement must be investigated (usually by excision and histological examination), as the tumor may be either benign or malignant.
- **Symmetrical slightly nodular (bosselated) firm enlargement of the whole thyroid** is characteristic of Hashimoto's disease (see page 338).
- **Symmetrical diffuse enlargement of the thyroid** is usually associated with evidence of hyperthyroidism, e.g. in Graves' disease (see below), and is sometimes called **parenchymatous goiter**. This pattern of enlargement is also seen as a physiological response in women at puberty and in pregnancy.

With the exception of tumors and Hashimoto's disease, most forms of thyroid enlargement are due to **hyperplasia** of the thyroid follicles and their cells. The increase in cell numbers may also be associated with an increase in cell function, with excessive production and secretion of T_4 and T_3, leading to the clinical features of **hyperthyroidism**.

Multinodular goiter is the most common cause of thyroid enlargement in the elderly

At postmortem examination many elderly people are found to have nodular distortion of thyroid architecture. However, only in cases in which the enlargement is great do patients seek treatment, usually for **cosmetic reasons** (the thyroid enlargement producing an unsightly swelling in the neck) and because **compression symptoms** may develop due to pressure on the trachea. Compression symptoms are particularly likely when the main enlargement is in the thyroid isthmus, with the large nodule passing behind the manubrium (**retrosternal goiter**).

Multinodular goiter produces irregular hyperplastic enlargement of the thyroid owing to the development of well-circumscribed nodules of varying size. As many of the larger nodules are filled with brown gelatinous colloid, the larger goiters are often called **multinodular colloid goiters** (*Fig. 16.5*). A few nodules may show evidence of hemorrhage and fibrous scarring. Sometimes, there are smaller, creamy coloured, fleshy nodules, which contain little colloid and are composed mainly of thyroid follicle cells.

Most patients with multinodular goiter have normal thyroid function, but occasionally one of the nodules becomes functionally as well as structurally hyperplastic and

Fig. 16.5 Multinodular colloid goiter. (a) Gross. (b) Low-power histology. The nodules in multinodular goiter are composed of hyperplastic thyroid acini. Many contain gelatinous colloid, others are solid and cream coloured. Cystic degeneration and fibrosis are common.

secretes excess T_3 and T_4. The cause of multinodular colloid goiter is uncertain, but it may represent the uneven responsiveness of various parts of the thyroid to fluctuating TSH levels over a period of many years.

An extremely rare cause of thyroid enlargement is **Riedel's thyroiditis.** In this condition there is dense fibrosis that often extends into adjacent muscles. On clinical examination the condition can mimic thyroid carcinoma.

Diffuse smooth enlargement of the thyroid is usually due to follicle-cell hyperplasia

The structural hyperplasia responsible for enlargement of the organ as a whole may be associated with normal (**euthyroid**), increased (**hyperthyroid**) or reduced (**hypothyroid**) secretion of thyroid hormones, according to the stimulus producing the hyperplasia.

The symmetrical diffuse pattern of enlargement may be caused by **dietary thyroid deficiency** (**endemic goiter**), which is the result of low iodine levels in the local water and soil. Iodine deficiency leads to low levels of T_3 and T_4 in the blood, initiating increased TSH secretion from the pituitary gland. This stimulates compensatory hyperplasia of the thyroid follicular cells throughout the organ, produc-

ing the characteristic pattern of enlargement. Formerly seen in small communities in the inland mountainous areas of parts of Europe (giving rise to names such as 'Derbyshire neck'), this is now rare in the western world but can still be seen in the mountain populations of the Himalayas and Andes. Despite the attempted compensatory hyperplasia, patients are hypothyroid.

Congenital enzyme deficiency may also be responsible for parenchymatous goiter. It arises in certain very rare disorders in which there is failure of normal T_3 and T_4 synthesis. Patients are thus hypothyroid despite the attempted compensatory hyperplasia.

The most common cause, however, is **autoimmune thyroiditis**. There are two patterns, one of which (**Graves' disease**) is particularly associated with hyperthyroidism. The other pattern (**Hashimoto's disease**) is associated with eventual reduced secretion of hormone, often after passing through transient hyperthyroid and euthyroid states. These two important diseases are discussed in more detail later.

Thyroiditis is usually due to either viral or autoimmune inflammation

Inflammation of the thyroid gland, which is termed **thyroiditis**, may be viral or autoimmune.

Viral thyroiditis is rare, the most common clinical pattern being **de Quervain's thyroiditis**. Seen in young and middle-aged women as a slight diffuse tender swelling of the thyroid, it usually occurs in association with a transient febrile illness, often during various viral epidemics. Many of the patients are young mothers whose children are concurrently suffering with or recovering from mumps, measles or other viral illnesses. Inflammatory destruction of follicles is often associated with a giant-cell granulomatous reaction to leaked colloid, hence the synonym 'giant cell thyroiditis' or 'granulomatous thyroiditis.'

Autoimmune thyroiditis encompasses Graves' disease and Hashimoto's disease, both of which are discussed in more detail below. Progressive lymphocytic infiltration of the thyroid is noted in patients as they age, and may be a normal change of aging. However, some patients have focal lymphocytic infiltration in excess of what would be expected for their years, and this condition has sometimes been called **focal lymphocytic thyroiditis**.

Excessive secretion of thyroid hormones produces hyperthyroidism

Hyperthyroidism is caused by excessive secretion of thyroid hormones. The disease is common, with a prevalence of 1–2% in women in non-iodine deficient countries, most having autoimmune thyroid disease (**Graves' disease**). Most of the clinical features (collectively known as **thyrotoxicosis**) (*Fig. 16.6*) are manifestations of a permanently raised metabolic rate, and the pathological changes that occur include loss of subcutaneous fat, reduction of skeletal muscle bulk and, sometimes, cardiomyopathy. In addition,

Fig. 16.6 Clinical features of hyperthyroidism

Feeling hot
Increased sweating
Weight loss, despite increased appetite
Proximal muscle weakness ± tremor
Rapid heart rate, palpitations
Atrial fibrillation (occasionally)
Bowel hypermotility, malabsorption, diarrhoea
Anxiety and restless hyperactivity
Wide, staring gaze and lid-lag

there may be a visible or palpable enlargement of the thyroid gland (goiter).

Thyrotoxicosis may result from an autonomous nodule of hyperactive thyroid tissue that is out of TSH control. This autonomous 'hot' nodule may be a solitary thyroid adenoma, or may be a component of a multinodular enlargement of the thyroid (multinodular goiter; *Fig. 16.5*).

Graves' disease is the most important cause of hyperthyroidism

Graves' disease is a form of autoimmune thyroiditis (*Fig. 16.8a*), presenting with diffuse enlargement of the thyroid gland, exophthalmos (protuberant eyes due to expansion of retro-orbital structures by adipose tissue and fibroblasts aberrantly expressing surface TSH receptors), pretibial myxoedema and finger clubbing. The disease is more common in young adults, particularly women.

In patients with **Graves' disease** a variety of autoantibodies can be detected in the serum, including antibodies against the thyroid receptor, thyroid peroxisomes or thyroglobulin. Of these, antibodies against various epitopes of the TSH receptor are probably the most important. The most frequently detected antibody, **thyroid-stimulating immunoglobulin (TSI)**, binds the TSH receptor to acti-

Fig. 16.7 Thyrotoxic hyperplasia. The epithelial cells are increased in number and size, and the edges of the colloid (**C**) are scalloped, indicating active removal of stored colloid for processing into thyroxine.

Fig. 16.8 Graves' disease. (a) Clinical photo showing exophthalmos. **(b) Histology.** In this disease the thyroid is focally infiltrated by lymphoid cells (**L**). Antibody-stimulated hyperplastic thyroid acini are enlarged, with large nuclei and a scalloped appearance to the colloid (**C**).

vate adenylate cyclase, thereby constitutively activating thyroid hormone production. The disease appears to be the result of B-cell expansion driven by aberrant T-helper cells that have escaped normal regulatory processes. There is a high incidence of the HLA antigen HLA-DR3 in patients with Graves' disease and polymorphisms of the cytotoxic T-lymphocyte antigen 4 (CTLA4) occur, the latter being postulated to have a suppressor function on T cells. A second group of antibodies, also directed against the thyroid receptor, result in proliferation of the thyroid follicular epithelium, this group being known as the thyroid growth-stimulating immunoglobulins (TGI). The third group of anti-thyroid receptor antibodies are known as TSH-binding inhibitor immunoglobulins (TBIIs). These inhibit the binding of TSH to its receptor and, depending on the site of binding, can either mimic the action of TSH or inhibit hormone secretion; thus they can produce either hyper- or hypothyroidism, depending on the binding site.

Data Set
Hyperthyroidism

A 34-year-old shop assistant complained of night sweats and palpitations. She had lost 10 kg in weight over the previous 6 months.

Free thyroxine	42 pmol/L	(12–26)
Free tri-iodothyronine	12 pmol/L	(3.3–7.5)
Thyroid-stimulating hormone	<0.1 mU/L	(0.4–6.3)

This patient has Graves' disease, characterized by high free thyroxine levels which suppress pituitary secretion of thyroid-stimulating hormone. The condition is caused by autoantibodies that bind to TSH receptors in the thyroid gland. It is seldom necessary to measure the titer of these antibodies in order to make the diagnosis. Autoantibodies to thyroid microsomes and thyroglobulin are simpler to measure, and are frequently present at high titers in Graves' disease, although they are not specific for this condition.

Data Set
Hypothyroidism

A 44-year-old woman was seen by her GP complaining of lack of energy.

Free thyroxine	4 pmol/L	(12–26)
Thyroid-stimulating hormone	56 mU/L	(0.4–6.3)

This patient has primary hypothyroidism, with low levels of thyroid hormone secretion in spite of the massively raised output of TSH from the pituitary gland. A raised plasma TSH is a sensitive early marker of thyroid insufficiency, and measurement of TSH is valuable in monitoring the adequacy of thyroid hormone replacement therapy.

Autoimmune stimulation in Graves' disease results in division of thyroid follicle cells, stimulating them to divide (hyperplasia) and to synthesize and secrete thyroid hormone continuously, out of the control of TSH from the pituitary. Thyroid hormone is therefore synthesized and secreted and the normal feedback mechanism is bypassed. The thyroid shows diffuse, fleshy enlargement, and the follicles are lined by large, active follicle cells, the follicle lumina containing virtually no stored colloid (*Figs 16.7 and 16.8b*). Another histological feature of the disease is the presence of increased numbers of lymphoid aggregates, including some lymphoid follicles. This infiltrate, in keeping with the mechanism proposed above, is composed predominantly of T cells admixed with B cells and mature, antibody-secreting plasma cells.

Reduced output of thyroid hormone produces the symptoms and physical signs of hypothyroidism (myxoedema)

In infants, hypothyroidism produces the clinical syndrome called **cretinism**, which produces a puffy face and enlarged tongue, coarse features, a protuberant abdomen, and delayed physical and mental development. The main causes of cretinism are:

- **Untreated maternal hypothyroidism.** This is now rare, thanks to better prevention, recognition and treatment of maternal hypothyroidism. It is still a problem in some areas of the world where endemic goiter due to dietary iodine deficiency is seen.
- **Inherited enzyme defect.** This produces sporadic cretinism due to failure of normal T_3 and T_4 synthesis.

In adults, hypothyroidism is almost always due to autoimmunity or previous treatment of thyrotoxicosis. It occurs in 1–2% of women, with a 5–10 times lower prevalence in men. Hypothyroidism in adults manifests as the syndrome called **myxedema**, which is due to reduced metabolic rate and the accumulation of mucopolysaccharides in the dermal connective tissues. There is progressive slowing of physical and mental activity, increasing lethargy and sensitivity to cold, puffy face, coarse dry skin, thinning of hair (particularly of the eyebrows), hoarseness and deepening of the voice, and various internal abnormalities, particularly heart failure and a predisposition to hyperlipidemia and hypothermic coma. The main causes of myxedema are:

- **Surgical ablation of the thyroid gland**, normally the result of total thyroidectomy for malignant disease, or aggressive subtotal thyroidectomy for hyperthyroid Graves' disease.
- **Hashimoto's disease** (see below).
- **Some drug therapies**, e.g. lithium, sulfonylureas, and amiodarone.

However, many patients with myxedema present for the first time in old age, and only a few have a history of previous thyroid surgery or disease. At postmortem examination these patients have a uniformly shrunken fibrous gland with very little residual follicular tissue and often only a scanty lymphocytic infiltrate, representing an end-stage thyroid.

There are no clues in either the history or the histology as to the etiology of the thyroid shrinkage, but some patients have demonstrable anti-thyroid antibodies. These cases are sometimes called **primary atrophic thyroiditis**. It is speculated that some patients with so-called focal lymphocytic thyroiditis may progress to this state, as may patients with subclinical Hashimoto's disease or previous de Quervain's thyroiditis.

Hashimoto's disease is a destructive autoimmune thyroiditis that leads to hypothyroidism

Hashimoto's disease is most common in middle age and is up to 20 times more common in women. It is the most common cause of hypothyroidism in Europe and the US, and is an example of an organ-specific autoimmune disease that has both cellular and humoral components. The cellular component, largely responsible for destruction of the gland parenchyma, is composed of cytotoxic T cells. The humoral component is derived from a population of B cells secreting inhibitory TSH receptor-binding immunoglobulins. These antibodies inhibit activation of the thyroid epithelium, resulting in hypothyroidism. Antibodies against thyroglobulin and thyroid peroxidase are also produced, probably as a consequence of exposure of antigens previously subjected to immune sequestration. Hashimoto's disease is particularly seen in association with HLA-DR5 and HLA-B8.

The initial clinical manifestations include diffuse enlargement of the thyroid, occasionally with a preliminary phase of hyperthyroidism, but by the time most patients seek medical attention they have passed through hyperthyroid and euthyroid phases and are becoming progressively hypothyroid.

On clinical examination, the thyroid is usually symmetrically enlarged and firm, with a bosselated surface. As a result of the disappearance of brown (iodine-rich) colloid, and its replacement by lymphocytes, the cut surface (*Fig. 16.9*) is white rather than the normal brown.

It may be that some Hashimoto thyroids proceed to primary atrophic thyroiditis. Laboratory demonstration of the anti-thyroid antibodies forms the basis of the diagnosis of Hashimoto's disease, rendering biopsy unnecessary.

Patients with Hashimoto's disease (and Graves' disease) show a high incidence of other autoimmune diseases (e.g. vitiligo, SLE, etc.).

Solitary nodules in the thyroid usually require excision to confirm their nature

Because most malignant epithelial tumors of the thyroid initially present as a solitary thyroid nodule, complete surgical excision with a safe margin of normal thyroid tissue is usually necessary. However, an accurate preoperative

Fig. 16.9 Hashimoto's disease. The thyroid is diffusely enlarged and slightly bosselated (a), with a fleshy, white cut surface due to the lymphocytic infiltrate and the replacement of brown colloid. Histology (b) shows follicular and diffuse lymphocytic infiltration, with destruction of thyroid follicles.

Fig. 16.10 Solitary thyroid adenoma. A single, well-circumscribed, ovoid nodule, partly brown but with flecks of white calcification, occupies one pole of the thyroid (a). Histology from the edge of the nodule (b) shows at least part of the adenoma to be composed of large colloid-filled acini (colloid adenoma). Other variants may be more cellular.

diagnosis can often be made after cytological examination of cells obtained by **fine-needle aspiration** of the nodule.

Solitary palpable thyroid nodules may be due to a:

- Disproportionately prominent nodule in a multinodular goiter.
- Solitary thyroid adenoma (*Fig. 16.10*), which may either be full of colloid or have a more cellular follicular pattern. The latter may appear fleshy on cut surface.
- Malignant thyroid tumor (mainly carcinomas derived from the follicle epithelium). Only histological examination can distinguish these tumors from solitary thyroid adenomata with the more cellular follicular pattern.

There are three main types of malignant tumor derived from thyroid follicle cells

The three main types of malignant tumor derived from thyroid follicle cells (*Fig. 16.11*) have very different natural histories, behaviors and prognoses. The most common type is **papillary carcinoma (70–80% of all cases)**, a well-differentiated tumor that arises most frequently in young adults. Histologically, the cells are arranged in papillary configurations and individual epithelial cells are large, with a clear central nuclei. The tumor is often multifocal within the thyroid, and tends to metastasize via lymphatics to nodes in the neck. It is slow growing and has an excellent prognosis; even metastatic tumors grow slowly and can be cured by surgical resection.

Fig. 16.11 Thyroid carcinoma. (a) This gross specimen shows a thyroid carcinoma which is showing extensive local spread. The upper arrow shows its upwards extension to involve the larynx, and the lower arrow shows its backward growth to infiltrate, compress and distort the trachea. This pattern of growth is characteristic of anaplastic carcinoma in the elderly. This patient had symptoms for only 8 weeks before death. (b) This photomicrograph shows typical papillary carcinoma of the thyroid with the tumor cells on a vascular core producing the characteristic papillary pattern. Sometimes the stromal core contains small calcific spherules ('psammoma bodies'). (c) This photomicrograph shows typical follicular thyroid carcinoma in the upper half. Although the tumor attempts to reproduce the follicular pattern of the normal thyroid, it is much more cellular with less colloid (pink) being formed. The arrow shows where the tumor has invaded into a nearby blood vessel, an important indication that the tumor is malignant rather than a benign adenoma. (d) Histology anaplastic carcinoma. The tumor is composed of undifferentiated small round cells arranged in sheets, with no evidence of follicular or papillary differentiation. Histologically it may be difficult to distinguish this type of tumor from a lymphoma without the aid of immunocytochemistry.

Follicular carcinoma (10–25% of all cases) most commonly affects middle-aged people. Metastasizing via the bloodstream, it is one of the tumors that characteristically spreads to bone. Patients may occasionally present with a spontaneous fracture due to metastatic disease, before the primary tumor is detected. It has a good prognosis.

Entirely confined to the elderly, **anaplastic carcinoma** (<5% of all cases) grows very rapidly, extensively invading tissues near the thyroid, such as the trachea and soft tissues of the neck. It may present with a rapidly enlarging thyroid mass causing tracheal compression or jugular vein invasion. The prognosis is very poor. The cells of the tumor, which are usually small, undifferentiated and round, must be distinguished histologically from **malignant lymphoma**; the latter can also affect the thyroid in the elderly, but is more responsive to treatment.

The only significant abnormality of the parafollicular or 'C' cells of the thyroid is the tumor known as 'medullary carcinoma'

Medullary carcinoma (5% of all cases) has the features of a neuroendocrine tumor, being composed of small cells containing neuroendocrine granules. An unusual feature is

Fig. 16.12 Medullary carcinoma of the thyroid. The tumor in (a) presented as a solitary nodule in the thyroid, but there was metastatic tumor in a neck lymph gland at the time of presentation. Histology (b) shows a neuroendocrine pattern of growth, with tumor cells and large masses of amyloid in the stroma (**A**).

the occasional presence of amyloid in the supporting stroma. Occurring in the middle-aged and elderly, these tumors are occasionally seen in children and young adults as a component of the multiple endocrine neoplasia (MEN) types IIa and IIb syndrome (see below).

The tumors are slow-growing, metastasize to local lymph nodes (*Fig. 16.12*), and generally have a good prognosis. Those arising in patients with the MEN syndrome are sometimes more aggressive and are associated with a poorer prognosis. However, the poor prognosis is usually due to the adverse affects of the other endocrine tumors rather than that in the thyroid. The tumors secrete calcitonin, and the diagnosis can be supported by the demonstration of raised plasma calcitonin levels. The increased calcitonin produces no systemic manifestations.

PARATHYROIDS

The parathyroid glands are small endocrine glands whose sole function is the secretion of parathormone

There are usually four, and sometimes up to eight, parathyroid glands, which are usually located close to the thyroid gland. Two glands are close to the upper poles of the right and left lateral thyroid lobes, and the others are situated near to the lower poles, but their position is variable; there may be parathyroid glands within the thyroid gland tissue and in the thymic fat remnant below the thyroid and in the mediastinum. This variable location is clinically important because the most important parathyroid diseases are treated surgically, and the glands may be difficult to find, particularly as normal parathyroids are so small (approximately $5 \times 3 \times 2$ mm).

Parathormone (PTH), the parathyroid hormone secreted by chief cells, is important in calcium balance, acting at two main sites:

- **The bone surface**, where it mainly stimulates the resorption of mineralized bone, initially by stimulating osteoblasts to produce osteoclast activating factor, thereby indirectly liberating calcium into the bloodstream by inducing osteoclast activation.
- **The renal tubules**, where it stimulates the preferential resorption of calcium ions from the urine, minimizing phosphate ion resorption. It also catalyses the production of 1,25-dihydroxyvitamin D from a less active precursor (see page 538). In addition, PTH inhibits the resorption of sodium and bicarbonate; thus, it has diuretic effects and may provoke hyperchloremic acidosis. It also reduces renal clearance of uric acid, and therefore hyperparathyroidism is associated also with hyperuricemia and gout.

The production of 1,25-dihydroxyvitamin D by the kidney is vitally important in controlling **intestinal** absorption of calcium and phosphorus.

Overall, increased PTH secretion increases serum calcium levels, and reduced secretion lowers serum calcium levels. Variations in serum calcium level are usually kept within the normal physiological range by limited variation in PTH secretion; an inappropriate increase or reduction in PTH secretion leads to a pathological increase (**hypercalcemia**) or reduction (**hypocalcemia**) in serum calcium levels. The bone changes produced by excess PTH activity are discussed in Chapter 24.

Hypercalcemia

Fig. 16.13a Causes of hypercalcemia

Widespread metastatic tumor in bone	Destruction of cancellous bone by tumor releases calcium
Parathyroid adenoma	Increased PTH secretion releases calcium from bone by osteoclastic resorption
Multiple myeloma	Plasma-cell tumors in medullary bone release calcium by eroding bone
Ectopic PTH secretion	Some tumors, e.g. oat-cell carcinoma of bronchus, secrete PTH
Vitamin D intoxication Sarcoidosis Milk–alkali syndrome	Rare

Fig. 16.13b Pathological effects of hypercalcemia

Deposition of calcium in kidney tubules (nephrocalcinosis)
Renal calculi
Excessive calcification of blood vessels
Corneal calcification

Data Set
Primary hyperparathyroidism

A 42-year-old man with recurrent renal calculi.

Plasma

Calcium	2.92 mmol/L	(2.2–2.6)
	11.6 mg/dl	(8.5–10.3)
Phosphate	0.51 mmol/L	(0.7–1.4)
Albumin	43 g/L	(35–50)
	4.3 g/dl	(3.5–5.0)
Alkaline phosphatase	270 U/L	(80–280)
Parathyroid hormone	75 ng/L	(10–55)

Hyperparathyroidism and malignant disease are the two most common causes of hypercalcemia, and can be distinguished by measurement of parathyroid hormone (PTH) in plasma. Levels are suppressed in hypercalcemia due to malignant disease, and high or high-normal in patients such as this man with hyperparathyroidism. Plasma phosphate may be low in either condition, but phosphate levels are raised in patients with renal impairment of any cause. Alkaline phosphatase levels are raised in a minority of patients with primary hyperparathyroidism.

Increased PTH secretion is usually due to the presence of a benign parathyroid adenoma

Parathyroid adenoma is usually a solitary tumor that affects only one of the parathyroids, the other parathyroids often showing atrophy. The tumors are usually small and are very rarely palpable in the neck, the main presenting symptoms being due to excessive secretion of parathyroid hormone (**primary hyperparathyroidism**), which produces the symptoms and signs of **hypercalcemia**. The histological features of parathyroid adenoma are shown in *Fig. 16.13b*.

Malignant parathyroid tumors, with invasion and metastatic spread, are very rare, although some parathyroid adenomas may show considerable pleomorphism and nuclear and cytoplasmic atypia.

Primary parathyroid adenoma is only one of the possible causes of hypercalcemia (see *Fig. 16.14a*). Rarely, primary hyperparathyroidism is the result of diffuse hyperplasia of the parathyroids rather than a solitary tumor.

Diffuse hyperplasia of all parathyroid glands is usually a compensatory response to persistently low serum calcium levels

The most common cause of compensatory parathyroid hyperplasia is renal failure, in which excessive urinary loss of calcium leads to a persistent serum hypocalcemia (*Fig. 16.15*).

The parathyroid hyperplasia produces increased PTH secretion, which mobilizes calcium from bone by stimulat-

Fig. 16.14 Parathyroid adenoma. (a) A 1 cm parathyroid adenoma removed at operation from a patient with hypercalcemia. (b) The edge of a parathyroid adenoma showing a solid mass of parathyroid cells. (c) The normal parathyroid shows that the hormone-producing cells normally comprise only a small part of the gland, the rest being adipose tissue.

Fig. 16.15 Parathyroid hyperplasia. (a) A photograph of the posterior aspect of the thyroid gland taken at postmortem examination of a man who died of untreated chronic renal failure, showing enlargement of all parathyroids (arrows). (b) The hyperplastic parathyroid is histologically almost identical to the parathyroid adenoma in *Fig. 16.13(b)*; compare the cellularity with that of the normal parathyroid shown in *Fig. 16.13(c)*.

Data Set
Secondary hyperparathyroidism

An 83-year-old man who lived alone seldom cooked for himself, eating mainly bread and biscuits.

Plasma

Calcium	1.97 mmol/L	(2.2–2.6)
Phosphate	0.50 mmol/L	(0.7–1.4)
Albumin	36 g/L	(35–50)
Alkaline phosphatase	410 U/L	(80–280)
PTH	85 ng/L	(10–55)

Hypocalcemia, due in this patient to dietary vitamin D deficiency, causes secondary hyperparathyroidism. The resulting increase in osteoblastic activity is reflected in the raised alkaline phosphatase levels. Suppression of renal phosphate resorption causes hypophosphatemia.

Hypocalcemia

Fig. 16.16 Causes of hypocalcemia

Chronic renal failure	Due to excessive calcium loss and phosphate retention by the failed kidney. This is often compensated by secondary hyperparathyroidism and bone disease (see page 538)
Hypoparathyroidism	Surgical removal, autoimmune disease
Vitamin D deficiency	Leads to osteomalacia and rickets (see Chapter 24)

ing increased osteoclastic activity. However, the calcium so released only brings the serum calcium level closer to normal, never producing hypercalcemia. This compensatory device is called **secondary hyperparathyroidism** and is associated with normal or low serum calcium levels. Very rarely, an autonomous parathyroid adenoma may arise in one of the hyperplastic parathyroids (**tertiary hyperparathyroidism**).

Primary hyperparathyroidism is normally clinically silent

Hyperparathyroidism commonly produces a clinically silent increase in serum ionized calcium levels that can mimic the hypercalcemia commonly seen in association with bone infiltration by tumor metastasis. The conditions can be distinguished biochemically, because the hypercalcemia produced by hyperparathyroidism is accompanied by a corresponding elevation of PTH, whereas in malignancy PTH levels are barely detectable.

As a consequence of early detection of hypercalcemia, the traditional symptoms of bone pain due to trabecular bone erosion and fracture, and 'brown tumors' (see page 540), are now rarely encountered. However, there may be several symptoms and signs that are not unique to hyperparathyroidism, including constipation and nausea, peptic ulcer disease, pancreatitis, gallstones, and muscle weakness and hypotonia. There may also be psychiatric presentations, including depression. It is therefore essential that thyroid/parathyroid function tests and serum calcium are measured in all patients presenting with depression and other psychiatric disorders.

Hypoparathyroidism is most commonly the result of surgical removal of the parathyroid glands

The parathyroid glands may be removed inadvertently or deliberately during surgery on the thyroid gland. If not surgically excised, they may be severely damaged by operative trauma or by interference with their blood supply.

Much less commonly, the parathyroid glands may be damaged by an autoimmune disease process (autoimmune parathyroid disease) associated with the presence of an autoantibody; this usually occurs in patients who have another autoimmune endocrine disease, e.g. Hashimoto's disease (see page 338) or Addison's disease (see page 345).

Reduced PTH secretion leads to a reduction in the serum calcium, with a corresponding increase in serum phosphate levels. Hypoparathyroidism is only one of the causes of hypocalcemia (see *Fig. 16.16*).

Hypoparathyroidism commonly presents with signs of neuromuscular irritability, including tingling, muscle spasms, facial twitching, and sustained carpopedal spasm. Patients can also present with cardiac arrhythmias and/or seizures. Dystrophic calcification in tissues can also be detected.

ADRENAL

The adrenal gland has two distinct endocrine components: the cortex and the medulla

The adrenal cortex (*Fig. 16.17*) synthesizes, stores and secretes three main groups of hormone, all of which are steroid hormones synthesized from cholesterol:

- **Glucocorticoid hormones**, e.g. hydrocortisone from zona fasciculata and zona reticularis.
- **Mineralocorticoid hormone** (aldosterone), from the zona glomerulosa.
- **Sex steroids**, from zona reticularis.

The adrenal medulla is derived embryologically from neural crest ectoderm and is part of the sympathetic nervous system. It synthesizes and secretes the vasoactive amines, **adrenaline** and **noradrenaline** (**epinephrine** and **norepinephrine**).

Excessive production of adrenal cortical hormones usually results from hyperplasia or tumor

The production of adrenal cortical hydrocortisone and sex steroids is controlled by ACTH secreted by the pituitary gland; aldosterone secretion is controlled by renin production by the juxtaglomerular apparatus in the kidney (see

Fig. 16.17 Normal adrenal cortex. Micrograph showing the three distinct zones of the adrenal cortex: the zona glomerulosa (**ZG**), the zona fasciculata (**ZF**) and the zona reticularis (**ZR**). They are enclosed by a capsule (**C**).

Fig. 16.18 Adrenal cortical hyperplasia. The adrenal on the right is normal, that on the left shows hyperplasia.

> ### Key Facts
> #### Cushing's syndrome
>
> - Due to excess glucocorticoids, with the most common cause being therapeutic administration of corticosteroids. May also result from pituitary adenoma (causes excess ACTH secretion), adrenal adenoma, ectopic ACTH secretion (e.g. from bronchial carcinoma), and adrenal cortical carcinoma.
> - Affects most systems, including: typical facies (moon face), with acne and hirsutism; severe osteoporosis, with vertebral collapse common, myopathy (muscle weakness and wasting); skin fragility and poor wound healing; trunk obesity with striae; peptic ulceration, hypertension and diabetes; hypokalemia; and psychiatric disturbances.
> - Diagnosis is based on clinical features and demonstration of raised plasma cortisol level.
> - Elucidation of cause is through dexamethasone suppression test, MRI and CT scan visualization of pituitary and adrenal glands, and through analysis of blood ACTH level (high – pituitary adenoma or ectopic ACTH source; low – primary adrenal tumor).

page 356). Excessive ACTH production, for example by an ACTH-secreting adenoma of the pituitary, stimulates an increase in the number, size and secretory activity of the adrenal cortical cells, leading to adrenal cortical hyperplasia (*Fig. 16.18*), which may be diffuse or nodular.

The uncontrolled excessive production of adrenal cortical hormones may produce Cushing's or Conn's syndromes (see Key Facts).

Adrenal cortical adenoma is a well-circumscribed, yellow tumor (*Fig. 16.19*) in the adrenal cortex which is usually 2–5 cm in diameter. The color of the tumor, as with the adrenal cortex as a whole, is due to the stored lipid (mainly cholesterol), from which the cortical hormones are synthesized. These tumors are frequent incidental findings at postmortem examination, and appear to have produced no significant metabolic disorder; only a very small percentage produce Cushing's syndrome. Nevertheless, these apparently 'non-functioning' adenomata are most often encountered in elderly obese people, who are often hypertensive. There is some debate that they may really represent nodules in diffuse nodular cortical hyperplasia.

Very occasionally, a true adrenal cortical adenoma is associated with the clinical manifestations of Conn's syndrome, and can be shown to be excreting mineralocorticoids.

Adrenal cortical carcinoma is rare, and virtually every case is associated with excessive production of hormones,

> ### Key Facts
> #### Conn's syndrome
>
> - Due to excessive secretion of the mineralocorticoid aldosterone, which is autonomous (primary aldosteronism). Excessive secretion of aldosterone due to excess plasma renin levels (secondary aldosteronism) is more common, e.g. in hepatic cirrhosis, nephrotic syndrome.
> - Primary aldosteronism almost invariably caused by adrenal cortical adenoma.
> - Effects include retention of sodium and water (in combination this leads to systemic hypertension), and excessive urinary potassium loss (leads to risk of cardiac arrhythmias).
> - Diagnosis is based on establishing the presence of hyperaldosteronism by blood electrolyte estimations (high Na$^+$, low K$^+$, metabolic alkalosis), and is confirmed by detection of raised plasma aldosterone levels and by visualization of adrenal cortical adenoma by CT scan or MRI. Plasma renin level is low in Conn's syndrome and high in secondary aldosteronism.

Fig. 16.19 Adrenal cortical adenoma. The adrenal contains a solitary, well-circumscribed, yellow adenoma derived from the cortex.

usually glucocorticoids and sex steroids. As a result, patients usually have features of Cushing's syndrome mixed with androgenic effects, which are particularly noticeable in women. The tumors are usually large and yellowish white, and local invasion and metastatic spread are common.

Ectopic ACTH secretion may be associated with non-adrenal tumors, particularly oat-cell carcinoma of the bronchus and some carcinoid tumors. In cases of the highly malignant bronchial tumor the symptoms are mainly metabolic, with hypokalemia, alkalosis, and impaired glucose tolerance. The patient rarely survives long enough to develop the physical features of Cushing's syndrome, although these and hypertension may develop if the inappropriate secretion is due to a less rapidly fatal tumor.

Chronic adrenal cortical insufficiency produces Addison's disease

Addison's disease is caused by chronic adrenal cortical insufficiency leading to lack of glucocorticoids and mineralocorticoids. The main features of the disease are low serum sodium and high serum potassium with chronic dehydration; hypotension, often markedly postural; lethargy and weakness; vomiting and loss of appetite; and brownish pigmentation of skin and buccal mucosa.

The most common cause is destruction of the cortex of both adrenals by autoimmune adrenalitis, often associated with autoimmune thyroid disease (see pages 337–8 and 343), autoimmune gastritis and other endocrine organ autoimmune disease. Other causes are bilateral adrenal

tuberculosis, fungal infections, and adrenal destruction by tumor, but all are rare.

Acute adrenal cortical failure is usually due to hemorrhagic infarction, but may be iatrogenic

Bilateral hemorrhagic necrosis of the adrenals is usually associated with disseminated intravascular coagulation. It is a feature of severe septicemia, particularly meningococcal septicemia, in which it is known as the 'Waterhouse–Friderichsen syndrome' (*Fig. 16.20*). There is hypovolemic

Fig. 16.20 Waterhouse–Friderichsen syndrome. Taken from a child with meningococcal septicemia, both adrenals show acute hemorrhagic necrosis leading to acute adrenal failure.

Data Set
Chronic adrenal cortical failure

A 45-year-old woman with a history of progressive lassitude and weight loss over a period of months was seen by her general practitioner.

Plasma

Sodium	129 mmol/L	(135–145)
Potassium	6.2 mmol/L	(3.5–5.3)
Urea	9 mmol/L	(1.0–6.5)
Creatinine	125 µmol/L	(60–120)
Plasma cortisol	4–22 µg/dL	(110–607 nmol/L) am
	3–17 µg/dL	(83–469 nmol/L) pm

Mineralocorticoid deficiency due to adrenal cortical failure causes loss of sodium from the distal renal tubules, resulting in hyponatremia. Associated loss of

water leads to dehydration and reduced renal blood flow, reflected in the mild uremia. Potassium and hydrogen ions are retained in the distal tubules, and hyperkalemia and metabolic acidosis are common findings. Glucocorticoid deficiency may result in hypoglycemia.

A short Synacthen test was performed:

Basal	Plasma cortisol	54 nmol/L

Synacthen 250 µg given intramuscularly

30 minutes post-Synacthen	Plasma cortisol	71 nmol/L

Synacthen is a synthetic analog of ACTH. A normal response to Synacthen shows a rise in plasma cortisol of at least 200 nmol/L above baseline. The absence of an adequate response in this patient confirms the diagnosis of adrenal insufficiency.

and hypotensive shock, with hypoglycemia, and a high risk of sudden death.

Iatrogenic acute adrenal cortical failure may occur when prolonged high-dose therapeutic corticosteroid therapy is stopped abruptly. Prolonged corticosteroid therapy leads to suppression of normal endogenous steroid production by the adrenal cortex, which becomes markedly atrophied. Sudden cessation of exogenous steroid therapy produces acute adrenal cortical failure (**adrenal crisis**), with hypovolemic and hypotensive shock, hypoglycemia, and risk of sudden death.

Tumors of the adrenal medulla may produce excess adrenaline/noradrenaline or their breakdown products

The two principal types of tumor of the adrenal medulla are **pheochromocytomas** (occurring in adults) and **neuroblastomas** (occurring in children). Neuroblastomas are dealt with in a later section on pages 350–1.

Data Set
Pheochromocytoma

A 38-year-old woman complained of panic attacks. Her blood pressure was high (170/105), and was not controlled by conventional doses of β-blocking antihypertensive medication.

24-hour urinary catecholamine excretion

Adrenaline (epinephrine)	170 nmol/day	(up to 200)
Noradrenaline (norepinephrine)	2967 nmol/day	(up to 530)
VMA	47 μmol/day	(up to 35)

Excessive catecholamine secretion from a pheochromocytoma results in increased urinary excretion of noradrenaline and/or adrenaline, and the catecholamine metabolite VMA (vanillylmandelic acid, or 3-methoxy-4-hydroxymandelic acid). Measurement of catecholamines in plasma is useful if the sample can be obtained during an attack.

Fig. 16.21 Pheochromocytoma. (a) The adrenal contains a well-circumscribed, spherical, brown tumor with small foci of hemorrhage. (b) Histology shows a typical neuroendocrine tumor with cells resembling those of the normal adrenal medulla.

Pheochromocytoma is a tumor of the adrenaline- and noradrenaline- (epinephrine- and norepinephrine-) secreting cells of the adrenal medulla. It produces high levels of one or both hormones and their breakdown products vanillylmandelic acid (VMA) and homovanillic acid (HVA), both of which are excreted in the urine and can be estimated as a diagnostic test.

The tumor is usually spherical (*Fig. 16.21*) and less than 5 cm in diameter. It has a pale, creamy cut surface that changes to dark brown almost instantly when exposed to air, owing to oxygenation of tumor pigments. Despite the fact that the tumor is usually small and non-metastatic, it is a hazardous condition with high perioperative mortality.

The excessive amine production produces hypertension that is often initially paroxysmal and associated with severe headaches, but the hypertension eventually becomes constant. There may be intractable, often unexplained, cardiac failure. Pheochromocytoma is one of the causes of surgically treatable systemic hypertension.

Bilateral tumors are more commonly seen in patients with MEN syndromes types IIA and IIB (see page 349).

Pheochromocytoma may rarely occur in extra-adrenal sympathetic tissue, mainly in the retroperitoneal area alongside the abdominal aorta (organ of Zuckerkandl).

PANCREATIC ENDOCRINE TISSUE

Most of the endocrine tissue in the pancreas is located in discrete islands

Islands of endocrine cells, the **islets of Langerhans**, are scattered throughout the head, body and tail of the pancreas, embedded in the enzyme-secreting exocrine component. The islets are nests of endocrine cells with pink granular cytoplasm containing neuroendocrine granules; each nest has an intimate capillary network, into which the secretions of the islets are discharged. There is a minor non-islet endocrine component, with scattered endocrine cells in the ducts leading from the exocrine acini, particularly the smaller ducts.

The endocrine cells secrete the following hormones:

- **Insulin**, which permits transfer of blood glucose into cells and stimulates the synthesis of glycogen in liver and skeletal muscle. Insulin lowers the blood sugar level, and in the absence of insulin the blood glucose level rises and cells become depleted of glucose.
- **Glucagon**, which opposes the functions of insulin.
- **Somatostatin**, which has many functions and is found widely throughout the body. In the pancreas it inhibits the release of insulin and glucagon from the islets; in other organs, e.g. the stomach and hypothalamus, it has other functions.
- **Pancreatic polypeptide**, which is a minor secretion, the function of which is not known.

Well over 60% of the cells in the islets are associated with insulin production; about 20% are associated with glucagon secretion. The nomenclature of the islet cells has been complex. However, as the use of immunocytochemical techniques allows the identification of the product of an individual cell, it is now best to label the cell types by their secreted product, e.g. 'insulin-secreting.'

The most common and important disease associated with the endocrine pancreas is a form of diabetes mellitus

Diabetes mellitus due to autoimmune damage to the insulin-secreting cells of the islets is a common and significant disease associated with the endocrine pancreas.

Diabetes mellitus is a clinical syndrome resulting from disorders in carbohydrate, lipid and protein metabolism due to an intracellular lack of glucose. This lack can be due to either severe primary insulin deficiency in the blood, leading to failure of transport of glucose into the cells, or to failure of glucose to enter the cells as a result of resistance of the cell membranes to the effects of what may be normal levels of circulating insulin.

The former pattern is termed **type I (insulin-dependent) diabetes mellitus (IDDM)**, and the latter is called **type II (non-insulin-dependent) diabetes mellitus**

Fig. 16.22 Islet-cell tumor of the pancreas. This surgically resected specimen of the pancreas (a) was taken from a patient with MEN I syndrome, and shows a number of separate islet-cell tumors (T). Histologically (b), tumors are composed of cords and nests of neuroendocrine cells in contact with adjacent pancreatic tissue. Immunohistochemistry (c) showed that the neuroendocrine cells were producing insulin (brown color). In this case, the patient presented with recurrent hypoglycemic attacks (**see text on page 348**).

(NIDDM). Type I is the pattern associated with autoimmune damage to the insulin-secreting cells of the islets of Langerhans, which leads to a deficiency of insulin secretion, producing high blood glucose levels.

Although some of the features of both types of diabetes mellitus are the result of gross biochemical disturbance, many of the clinical features producing severe morbidity and mortality are structural complications that affect many tissues and organs throughout the body. A detailed description of diabetes mellitus is therefore given in the chapter concerned with systemic disease processes (Chapter 25).

The only other important condition resulting from abnormality in the endocrine component of the pancreas is islet-cell tumor

Tumors of the islet cells of the pancreas are examples of neuroendocrine tumors. Most are benign, producing their symptoms through excess secretion of a specific hormone, usually insulin. The tumors are usually solitary, but in the MEN syndromes most are multiple (*Fig. 16.22a*).

Insulinoma produces hypersecretion of insulin, leading to hypoglycemic attacks that are often severe enough to produce coma; pre-coma symptoms include confusion and behavioral disturbance (sometimes aggressiveness).

Glucagonoma is very rare. The excess secretion of glucagon is often asymptomatic, although patients may be anemic and develop an unexplained secondary diabetes. A bizarre characteristic skin rash called necrolytic migratory erythema sometimes occurs.

Very rarely, islet-cell tumors may secrete unusual hormones such as vasoactive intestinal peptide (VIP) and gastrin (producing the Zollinger–Ellison syndrome of recurrent and multiple peptic ulcers in stomach and proximal small intestine), or may even produce ACTH.

OVARY AND TESTIS

The ovary is an important endocrine organ, producing oestrogens and progesterones

The ovary cyclically produces oestrogen and progesterone under the influence of cyclical production of follicle-stimulating hormone (FSH) and luteinizing hormone (LH) by the pituitary gland, which in turn is stimulated by hypothalamic gonadotropin-releasing hormones. Complex feedback loops involving estrogen, progesterone and the polypeptide inhibin act at both hypothalamic and pituitary levels to regulate gonadotropin synthesis and release.

- **Estrogens**, produced by the ripening **ovarian follicle**, stimulate the proliferation of the endometrium and are responsible for the development and maintenance of secondary sexual characteristics. Estrogens are also produced in small amounts by other components of the ovary, e.g. the stroma and the hilar cells.

- **Progesterones**, produced by the **luteinized follicle (corpus luteum)**, stimulate secretory changes in the endometrium. Persistence of the corpus luteum after conception leads to persistence of progesterone secretion, which is essential for the development of the decidua and for the maintenance of pregnancy. It also has an influence on breast structure and function.

An imbalance of estrogens and progesterones can have significant pathological effects on the uterus and breasts, leading to menstrual abnormalities, infertility, spontaneous abortion, irregular breast enlargement, and breast lumps. Imbalance has been implicated in the development of breast cancer and endometrial cancer. Many of these conditions are discussed in Chapters 19 and 20.

The ovary can sometimes produce abnormal amounts of androgens, leading to masculinization

Although the ripening follicles mainly produce estrogens, they (and the hilus cells) can also produce androgens. These are normally produced in such minute amounts that there is no significant clinical impact, but some rare diseases of follicles or hilus cells (Stein–Leventhal syndrome and Sertoli–Leydig cell tumors; see Chapter 19) can be associated with excessive androgen secretion. This leads to masculinization, with cessation of menstruation, infertility, loss of female secondary sexual characteristics, and the acquisition of male characteristics such as hirsutism. Excess estrogens are also secreted, but they are usually overwhelmed by the androgen effects.

The endocrine component of the testis secretes testosterone

The interstitial or **Leydig cells** form the endocrine component of the testis. These cells secrete testosterone, the hormone responsible for the initiation of spermatogenesis in childhood and for its maintenance in adult life. It is also responsible for the maintenance of structure and function of the male genital ducts (e.g. vas deferens) and the accessory secretory glands (e.g. the prostate), and for the development and maintenance of the male secondary sexual characteristics.

Testosterone depletion is rare, although the amount secreted decreases in old age

Pathological testosterone depletion produces loss of masculine characteristics and reduction of spermatogenesis. It is rare as a spontaneous disease, but will inevitably follow bilateral orchidectomy, which is sometimes undertaken medically to control advanced cancer of the prostate (see Chapter 18). The undescended testis continues to produce testosterone, even though it may be incapable of spermatogenesis (see page 398). The Leydig cells are also capable of secreting estrogens, but normally do so in such small amounts that they are overwhelmed by the testosterone effect. However, rare tumors of the Leydig cells (interstitial cell tumor, see page 407) frequently secrete abnormal quantities of estrogens, and may present with features of feminization, such as loss of libido, loss of body hair, and gynecomastia.

The pineal gland and thymus both secrete hormones

Although the pineal gland and thymus both secrete hormones, diseases of these organs that produce hormone effects are very rare. The thymus gland is discussed in Chapter 15.

The most common disease of the diffuse neuroendocrine system is tumor formation

Through advances in immunocytochemical methods, many scattered cells in epithelial surfaces and solid organs have been identified as being neuroendocrine in nature. In addition, many of their peptide and protein hormones have been identified. Under normal circumstances these cells are **paracrine**, i.e. produce hormones that act locally and do not enter the blood circulation. However, some tumors pass excessive amounts of the hormone into the circulation and can produce systemic effects, e.g. carcinoid tumor of the small intestine and the **carcinoid syndrome** (see page 266, Chapter 13).

MULTIPLE ENDOCRINE NEOPLASIA SYNDROMES

In the multiple endocrine neoplasia (MEN) syndromes patients develop tumors in a number of endocrine organs

In those affected by the MEN syndromes there is usually a strong family history of multiple endocrine tumors with autosomal dominant inheritance. Patients are younger than those who develop single sporadic tumors. The tumors arise in multiple organs, either synchronously or metachronously, and are often multifocal.

MEN type I is inherited in an autosomal dominant pattern and the *MEN1* gene is a tumor suppressor gene located on chromosome 11q13. In **MEN I syndrome** patients usually show a combination of parathyroid hyperplasia (95%), pancreatic islet-cell tumors (>40%) (often multiple), and pituitary adenomas (>30%). These are the most common features, but there may also be parathyroid adenomas, hyperplasia of the parafollicular calcitonin-secreting cells in the thyroid, and adrenal cortical hyperplasia.

Patients with the **MEN II syndromes** have activating mutations of the *RET* proto-oncogene. MEN II syndromes are inherited in an autosomal dominant pattern and the *RET* proto-oncogene is located on chromosome 10q,11.2. **MEN IIA (Sipple syndrome)** patients have a combination of pheochromocytoma (50%) (sometimes bilateral) and medullary carcinoma of the thyroid (almost 100%) which may be multifocal. Occasionally there is hyperparathyroidism due to parathyroid hyperplasia (30%). A small subgroup of the MEN syndromes, **MEN IIB (William syndrome)** (sometimes called **MEN III**), also shows large numbers of neuromas and ganglioneuromas in the dermis and submucosal regions throughout the body. Unlike with MEN IIA, these patients do not develop primary hyperparathyroidism.

The medullary carcinoma of the thyroid in *Fig. 16.12* and the islet-cell tumor in *Fig. 16.22* were from patients with MEN II and MEN I syndromes, respectively.

ENDOCRINE DISEASE IN CHILDREN

Deficiency of growth hormone in children leads to pituitary dwarfism

Children with pituitary dwarfism are perfectly formed but very small, and fail to grow at the usual rate. Bone age is delayed, the voice is high-pitched, and the genitalia are small (most noticeable in boys). Those affected are prone to recurrent attacks of hypoglycemia. The pituitary abnormality may be a familial deficiency of growth hormone, or there may be a tumor replacing the pituitary (e.g. a large pituitary adenoma or a craniopharyngioma); in the case of tumors, there is a deficiency of other anterior pituitary hormones.

Hypothyroidism in children leads to cretinism

Cretinism is discussed earlier in this chapter (see page 337). It may be endemic, and is due either to maternal hypothyroidism associated with lack of iodine, or to a congenital enzyme deficiency.

Transient hyperthyroidism is common in girls at the time of puberty

Transient hyperthyroidism is usually associated with a mild, diffuse enlargement of the thyroid gland. It occurs so frequently that it may almost be regarded as a transient physiological response. Symptoms of hyperthyroidism are usually minimal and disappear within a short time, but the thyroid enlargement occasionally persists, and the hyperthyroid state may become permanent.

Adrenal cortical disorders in children are rare

Adrenal cortical tumors are very uncommon in children, most children with Cushing's syndrome having a pituitary tumor, or resulting from exogenous steroid therapy. An important condition that occurs in children is **congenital adrenal hyperplasia**, an autosomal recessive disorder associated with lack of 21-hydroxylase in the adrenal cortex. 21-hydroxylase is involved in the production of both aldosterone and cortisone from precursors; in its absence the precursors are instead converted into testosterone. The patients thus have cortisone and aldosterone deficiency but testosterone excess; this manifests as precocious sexual development in boys, and as virilization in girls (with masculinization of the female external genitalia, e.g. clitoral hyperplasia). Because the plasma cortisone levels are low, the anterior pituitary is stimulated by the feedback mechanism to secrete excess ACTH, which leads to marked adrenal cortical hyperplasia. The clinical features are called the **adrenogenital syndrome**. Patients may also develop electrolyte abnormalities, including excessive salt loss, due to aldosterone deficiency.

Neuroblastoma of the adrenal medulla is an important malignant tumor in children

Neuroblastoma is an example of an 'embryonal tumor' and is derived from primitive neuroblasts. Tumors arise from the adrenal medulla and from the sympathetic ganglia of the autonomic nervous system (75% arise in the abdomen). It is one of the group of peripheral primitive neuroectodermal tumors (PNETs). Most tumors occur in children under the age of 3 years, the majority occurring in children under the age of 1 year. Neuroblastoma accounts for approximately 15% of childhood cancer deaths.

Macroscopically, neuroblastomas range from small nodules to enormous masses (*Fig. 16.23a*), although in most cases the tumor is already large at first diagnosis, the most common presenting symptom being a palpable abdominal mass. Metastatic spread is via the bloodstream, and the tumor has a predilection for spread to bone. Some cases present with symptoms due to bone metastasis. In some cases the tumor spreads along the renal vein to extend into the inferior vena cava.

Histologically the tumors are composed of mitotically active small primitive neuroblastic cells which exhibit variable degrees of neuronal maturation (*Fig. 16.23b*); occasionally, characteristic 'rosettes' can be seen comprising a

Fig. 16.23 Neuroblastoma. (a) An advanced neuroblastoma which has arisen from the adrenal at the upper pole of the kidney and has spread to produce a large mass on one side of the aorta, with para-aortic lymph nodes. The brown, hemorrhagic cut surface appearance is characteristic. (b) Histology showing predominantly small, undifferentiated cells (neuroblasts), with a small amount of intervening stroma in the form of nerve fibers.

Neuroblastoma – laboratory medicine

- Neuroblastomas secrete catecholamines and so elevated levels of metabolites may be found in the urine. Markers measured are vanillylmandelic acid (VMA), homovanillic acid (HVA) and dopamine (see Data Set below).
- Diagnosis of neuroblastoma must always be based on tissue diagnosis: either biopsy of primary tumor, or based on cells seen in bone marrow aspiration or trephine biopsy.

ring of neuroblasts with fine neurofilaments in the lumen. These characteristic histological arrangements are known as '**Homer Wright**' rosettes. Some tumors even contain mature ganglion cells in addition to the primitive neuroblastic areas, in which case they are called **ganglioneuroblastomas**. Still better differentiated tumors contain mature ganglion cells in the absence of primitive neuroblasts. These tumors are known as **ganglioneuromas**. These tumors exhibiting advanced maturation usually also show spindle-cell areas mimicking **Schwann cells**. Ganglioneuromas have a more favorable prognosis.

Data Set
Neuroblastoma

A 3-year-old boy had been unwell for several weeks. On examination, a large mass was palpable on the right side of the abdomen and flank.

Urinary catecholamines

Adrenaline (epinephrine)	18 nmol/mmol of creatinine (up to 30)
Noradrenaline (norepinephrine)	360 nmol/mmol of creatinine (up to 120)
Dopamine	96 165 nmol/mmol of creatinine (up to 900)

Neuroblastomas commonly secrete dopamine, which is excreted in urine. Alternatively, the dopamine metabolite HVA (homovanillic acid) can be measured in urine.

Genetic analysis of neuroblastoma has shown frequent presence of deletion of the short arm of chromosome 1, or amplification of the N-*myc* oncogene on chromosome 2p, or loss of alleles from chromosome 14, or a combination. Tumors with N-*myc* amplification have a worse prognosis

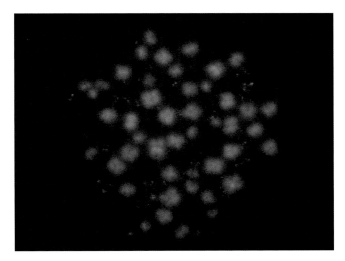

Fig. 16.24 Neuroblastoma – Double minutes. Chromosome spread showing amplified DNA as extrachromosomal, dumbell-shaped or 'double minute' segments.

Neuroblastoma – Prognostic factors

- **Prognosis in neuroblastoma** is highly dependent on the age of onset of disease, with survival rates 2 years after diagnosis as follows: neonates (70%), aged under 1 year (30%), aged between 1 and 2 years (20%), and aged over 2 years (5%).
- **Tumor stage** also has an important bearing on prognosis. Staging is based on whether tumor is confined to the adrenal, on whether it crosses the midline, on evidence of lymph node involvement, and on evidence of bloodstream spread. An important stage of neuroblastoma is defined as **stage IV-S**, in which there is a localized primary tumor with metastasis to skin and liver, and minimal marrow involvement; this is confined to children under the age of 1 year. Paradoxically, **stage IV-S** is associated with a very good prognosis and **spontaneous regression of tumor** with little or no treatment. Staging criteria are as follows:

Stage	Spread
I	Confined to organ of origin
II	Direct spread from organ of origin but does not cross midline
III	Tumour extends in continuity beyond midline
IV	Metastatic disease to solid organs, distant lymph nodes, soft tissues or bone.
IV-S	Patients aged less than one year who would otherwise be stage I or II but have distant spread to liver, skin or bone marrow but WITHOUT lytic bone involvement on imaging.

(10% 3-year survival) than those with one copy of this gene (50–90% 3-year survival). N-*myc* gene amplication can be detected by fluorescence *in situ* hybridisation on chromosome metaphase spreads cultured from tumour cells (*Fig. 16.24*). These amplifications can occur as homogeneously staining regions on single chromosomes or as double minutes, the latter representing small dumbell-shaped fragments of chromatin (*Fig. 16.24*).

Case-based questions

Case 1 A man with headaches and impaired vision

A 42-year old salesman who works for a company selling microscopes and optical equipment comes to see you, his GP, because he has been getting increasingly severe headaches for about a month. He also complains of feeling very tired. He confesses that the day before he had backed his car into a wall which he hadn't noticed, and he thinks there is something wrong with his vision. He has never suffered from migraine.

On examination, you find the presence of a visual field defect which you discover to be bitemporal hemianopia. No papilledema is present. You refer him to the neurosurgery department at the local hospital where a MRI scan reveals the presence of a large mass in the pituitary fossa. The mass is treated by trans-sphenoidal hypophysectomy, and histology reveals a non-functioning pituitary adenoma.

1. What clinical signs, biochemical tests and radiological investigations are useful in the preoperative assessment of a patient presenting with bitemporal hemianopia?
2. What is the cause of the visual defect?
3. What are the main histological subtypes of pituitary adenoma and what are the clinical symptoms of patients presenting with each of these adenomas?

Case 2 An irritable housewife with weight loss

A 30-year-old housewife presents to her GP because her sister has told her she was looking a bit thin and has become unusually irritable and hyperactive. She tells you that she has indeed lost weight despite a good appetite. When you question her, you notice she has exoph-thalmos. On examination, her thyroid gland is diffusely enlarged and her pulse is 100/min with atrial fibrillation.

1. What is the likely diagnosis?
2. What single investigation would be most useful?
3. What is the most likely pathogenesis of her condition?

Case 3 A young woman with a hard lump in the neck

A 25-year-old woman, who recently set up in a small business refurbishing old rocking horses and other large pieces of nursery equipment, presents to outpatients because her family doctor is worried about a lump in her neck. The lump had become obvious as a vague discomfort when she was applying skin cream, and had been increasing in size over the previous 2 months. She appears well otherwise.

On examination, a hard 3 cm nodule is felt in the left lobe of her thyroid gland, together with adjacent cervical lymphadenopathy.

Investigations are performed and a papillary carcinoma of the thyroid gland is diagnosed and treated.

1. What is the differential diagnosis of a nodule in the thyroid gland?
2. What investigations would you have performed to assess the thyroid nodule?
3. What features in the history are suggestive of carcinoma?
4. What is her prognosis?

Case 4 A man with an odd mixture of symptoms

A 40-year-old assembly worker in a car plant presents to outpatients complaining of several 'odd episodes' over the previous 3 weeks. He describes attacks, each lasting approximately 20 minutes, where he develops severe headaches, thumping of the heart, sweating, nausea, tremor, and feeling faint. His past medical history includes a parathyroid gland adenoma which was removed 10 years previously.

On examination, the only positive finding is hypertension (BP = 180/100).

1. What is the likely diagnosis?
2. How would you confirm the diagnosis?
3. What is the significance of the patient's previous parathyroid adenoma?

Case 5 An old woman with diabetes

An 83-year-old woman presented to casualty after falling in the street. She had pain in her wrist, particularly when pressure was applied over the radial fossa. X-ray investigations showed a fracture of the wrist and there was a suspicion of a scaphoid fracture, even though this was not visible on the film. It was decided that she was not a good candidate for anesthesia because she was overweight and suffered from angina. The wrist was therefore splinted to effect a natural repair.

Analysis of her blood and urine showed an elevation in blood glucose and glycosuria. A subsequent glucose tolerance test showed that she was suffering from

▶ diabetes mellitus. She also complained that her vision was becoming worse, particularly at night, and she had fallen because she had not seen the kerb stone. Ophthalmoscopy revealed the presence of cataracts and some evidence of retinopathy. There were no other physical signs.

1. **Document the multiple pathologies present in the above patient.**
2. **Do you suspect any others?**
3. **What are the complications of non-insulin dependent diabetes mellitus (NIDDM)?**
4. **What symptoms may raise a suspicion of NIDDM in elderly patients?**

Case 6 An old woman with a swollen hairy face

A 64-year-old woman, a lifelong smoker, presents to clinic complaining of increasing weight and hair loss. She also complains of facial swelling and hirsutism.

On examination, you find central obesity with striae, and she is hypertensive. Blood tests reveal elevated blood glucose.

1. **What is the differential diagnosis?**
2. **What further tests would you perform?**
3. **What are the systemic effects of excess glucocorticoids?**
4. **What is the negative dexamethasone suppression test?**

Brief answers to these case-based questions are given on pages 590–1. More detailed answers and other study resources are available online at www.studentconsult.com.

Diseases of the urinary system

INTRODUCTION

The urinary system can be divided into the upper and lower urinary tracts.

The **upper urinary tract** comprises the kidney, which is responsible for the ultrafiltration of blood (to remove the waste products of the body's metabolic processes in the form of urine), and for the maintenance of water and electrolyte homeostasis. Impaired kidney function is evident as a variety of metabolic disturbances and, according to the severity, is termed either **partial renal failure** or **total renal failure**.

The **lower urinary tract** comprises the pelvicalyceal systems, ureters, bladder and urethra, which are responsible for the collection, transportation, storage and ultimate voiding of urine.

The kidney develops from part of the mesodermal mass, the metanephric blastema, high on the posterior abdominal wall on either side of the midline. The pelvicalyceal system and ureters are derived from the ureteric bud, which is an outgrowth of the primitive mesonephric duct. The bladder and urethra develop from the urogenital sinus.

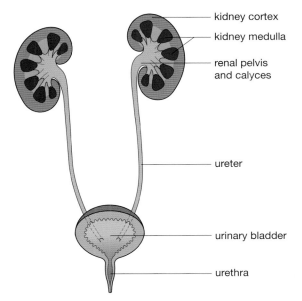

Fig. 17.1 Diagram of the urinary system. This diagram shows the upper (red) and lower (green) urinary tracts.

KIDNEY

Brief revision of kidney structure

The kidneys are paired organs situated retroperitoneally high on the posterior abdominal wall on either side of the vertebral column, embedded in a mass of adipose tissue (perinephric fat). They are ovoid, but somewhat flattened anteroposteriorly, and have a concavity at their medial border (the renal hilum) which is the site of entry of the main renal artery and emergence of the renal vein and pelvicalyceal system. The surface is covered by a thin fibrous capsule and is smooth, except in babies, where some lobulation can be seen. The cut surface shows an outer cortex and an inner medulla, the latter in the form of cones, the pointed tips of which (renal papillae) open into the calyces, which are the first part of the lower urinary tract (*Figs 17.1, 17.2*). The **cortex** contains all the glomeruli, the pre- and post-glomerular vasculature, the proximal and distal tubules,

Fig. 17.2 Kidney: cut surface. This photograph of part of the kidney shows the outer cortex (C) and the medulla (M), which comes to a point at the papilla (P) where it drains into one of the calyces (Ca) of the pelvicalyceal system.

and part of the loop of Henle component. The **medulla** contains the rest of the loop of Henle, and collecting tubules and ducts (*Fig. 17.3*).

The main functioning unit of the kidney is the nephron

The structure of the nephron is given in simplified diagrammatic form in *Fig. 17.3*. The main components are:

- **The pre-glomerular blood vessels**, which are responsible for supplying blood to the glomerulus.
- **The glomerulus**, which is a highly specialized capillary system. The basement membrane of the lining endothelium is fused to that of surrounding epithelium to create a highly selective filtration barrier. The glomerular capillary tuft is situated within **Bowman's capsule**, which collects the ultrafiltrate and passes it into the next component of the nephron:
- **The tubular system**, which is divided into several parts. The **proximal tubules** are mainly involved in the selective resorption of various components of the glomerular filtrate, the **loop of Henle** is involved in creating an ionic concentration gradient in the renal medulla, and the **distal tubule** is mainly involved in acid–base balance and resorption of sodium and potassium ions.
- **The collecting tubules and ducts**, which are responsible for the resorption of water from the dilute urine under the control of antidiuretic hormone (ADH).
- **The post-glomerular vasculature** has two main functions: it provides oxygenated blood for the tubular epithelium, and also participates in homeostasis; ions, water, and other small molecules pass between the tubular and ductular parts of the nephron and the post-glomerular vasculature. The post-glomerular (peritubular) capillaries are therefore in very close association with the tubular and ductular system.

The kidney has numerous metabolic functions

The **glomerulus** is responsible for filtration of urine, retaining proteins and other large molecules in the blood. The property of selective filtration lies in the structure and ionic charge of the glomerular basement membrane (GBM). Structural abnormalities in the membrane and neutralization of anionic sites cause it to lose this property.

The **tubular and ductular systems** have several main functions, each of which is dependent on normal cellular function of tubular epithelial cells. These systems are responsible for the resorption of glucose and amino acids filtered by the glomerulus, selective resorption of water under the control of ADH, and selective resorption or secretion of sodium, potassium, calcium, phosphate and hydrogen ions to maintain homeostasis.

Erythropoietin is secreted by the kidney and is essential for the normal production of red blood cells by the marrow.

Renin is secreted by the juxtaglomerular apparatus and is responsible for activating angiotensin, which stimulates

VASCULAR COMPONENT

intralobular artery

afferent arteriole

glomerular capillary system

efferent arteriole

mesangium

peri-tubular capillary system

tubule and collecting duct system

TUBULAR/DUCTAL COMPONENT

Bowman's capsule
Collection of glomerular filtrate

Proximal convoluted and straight tubule
Re-absorption of water, proteins and aminoacids, glucose and carbohydrates

Loop of Henle
Creation of hypertonicity gradient between collecting ducts and interstitium

Distal straight and convoluted tubule
Acid–base and water balance Absorption of water, Na^+ and HCO_3^- Excretion of K^+ and H^+

Collecting tubule and collecting ducts
Controlled reabsorption of water under influence of ADH

Fig. 17.3 The nephron. The main functional unit of the kidney is the nephron. Arterial blood enters the glomerular capillary system by an afferent arteriole and leaves it by an efferent arteriole, which then provides an intimate capillary system for the tubules. Ultrafiltration of the blood occurs in the glomerular capillary system, with water, salts, nitrogenous waste products, and some small protein molecules passing through the glomerular filtration barrier into Bowman's (urinary) space. The filtrate then passes down the tubular system where there is reabsorption of some components to maintain water and electrolyte homeostasis, and then into the collecting tubule and duct system where further reabsorption of water occurs to produce a concentrated urine rich in nitrogenous waste products.

the secretion of aldosterone by the adrenal cortex. Aldosterone then acts on tubules to reabsorb sodium ions and water from the glomerular filtrate, thereby maintaining plasma volume and blood pressure.

AA   JGA   EA   MC   MM

Fig. 17.4 a&b Glomerular structure. The detailed structure of the glomerulus is beyond the scope of this book, and normal histology books should be studied if the reader is confused. It can best be regarded as an anastomosing knot of capillaries invaginating a bulbous end of a proximal convoluted tubule **PCT** so that the outer surface of the glomerular capillaries is invested in a layer of epithelium continuous with that of the tubule. Thus, the afferent arteriole **AA** enters the structure at its vascular hilum and divides into branches which further divide to form a complex network of specialized small vessels lined internally by a fenestrated endothelium **E** and covered externally by epithelial cells (podocytes) **P**, which do not lie directly on the vessel basement membrane **BM** but contact with it by foot processes **FP**. The glomerular vessels have a thick basement membrane, and have a specialized support structure, acting as a sort of mesentery, called the mesangium **M**, which is composed of acellular matrix **MM** and mesangial cells **MC**. The anastomotic vessels eventually join to form the efferent arteriole **EA** which leaves the glomerulus at the vascular hilum. The entire vascular structure is contained within the bulbous distension of the proximal convoluted tubule, called Bowman's capsule, and the space between the glomerular tuft and Bowman's capsule is called the urinary space **US**. The juxtaglomerular apparatus **JGA** is situated at the vascular hilum of the glomerulus.

Fig. 17.5 Cortical tubules (H&E). The renal cortex contains glomeruli and proximal **P** and distal **D** convoluted tubules, together with the vessels supplying the glomeruli, and the intimate tubular capillary network **CN**. The luminal surface of both types of tubule shows microvilli which are prominent in proximal tubules but scanty in distal tubules. Both types show extensive basolateral interdigitations (see a histology text).

Fig. 17.6 Medullary tubules (H&E). The medulla contains vertically arranged collecting tubules and ducts **CD**, together with some parts of the loops of Henle **HL**. They are embedded in a loose interstitium **I** within which also run vertically arranged capillaries, the vasa recta **VR**.

DISEASES OF THE KIDNEY

Damage to one component of the nephron usually leads to damage in the other components

Glomerular function tends to be disrupted by diseases that alter glomerular structural arrangements (seen with structural damage to basement membrane, endothelium, epithelium or mesangium), and tubular function tends to be disrupted by metabolic insult to the tubular cells (e.g. hypoxia or toxins).

As both glomerular and tubular functions are highly dependent on adequate perfusion by blood, if this is disrupted both functions are impaired. Once function is disturbed in one part of the nephron, secondary abnormalities often develop in other parts because of the close structural and functional relationships in the nephron.

The kidneys have a considerable degree of functional reserve, but when disease processes damage sufficient numbers of nephrons to exceed the compensatory ability of those remaining, renal failure ensues.

Partial renal failure syndromes affect only some elements of renal function

There are four main types of partial renal failure:

- **Asymptomatic hematuria** is usually discovered during routine urine examination for health checks, insurance or occupational medical examinations. If it is persistent, it suggests minor glomerular damage as an early stage of a progressive glomerular disease such as IgA nephropathy (see page 375).
- **Persistent proteinuria** is also usually asymptomatic, and discovered on urinalysis. It is usually indicative of the early stages of glomerular abnormality involving the basement membrane or mesangium, or both. In the early stages, only small molecular weight proteins leak through the glomerulus into the urine, but as the glomerular abnormality worsens, larger quantities of higher molecular weight proteins are lost; this minor abnormality may progress to the nephrotic syndrome.
- **Nephrotic syndrome** is the result of abnormality in the glomerular basement membrane or mesangium, such that the glomerulus loses the capacity for selective retention of proteins in the blood. This leads to loss of very large amounts of protein, mostly albumin, in the urine (**proteinuria**), with consequent loss of protein from the blood (**hypoalbuminemia**) leading to **edema**. There is **susceptibility to infections** because of low levels of immunoglobulins and complement, **susceptibility to thrombosis** because of increased levels of fibrinogen in the blood, and **hyperlipidemia.**
- **Nephritic syndrome** is the result of disturbance of glomerular structure that involves reactive cellular proliferation. This causes reduced glomerular blood flow (leading to reduced urine output – **oliguria**), leakage of red cells from damaged glomeruli (**hematuria**), and consequent retention of waste products (**uremia**). The low renal blood flow activates the renin–angiotensin system, with fluid retention and mild hypertension. Small amounts of proteins are also lost in the urine, but this is usually trivial. The hematuria is not gross and is usually manifest as a smoky brown discoloration of urine.

In total renal failure syndromes, all functions of the nephron are impaired

In partial renal failure only some of the functions of the glomeruli and tubules are impaired, but in total renal failure all functions of the nephron are impaired although some are not manifest clinically or biochemically for a time. There are two total renal failure syndromes:

- **Acute renal failure,** in which there is sudden cessation of nephron function, affecting all nephrons at the same time.
- **Chronic renal failure,** in which the nephrons are destroyed one by one over a long period. Because the deterioration in nephron function is slowly progressive, for many years the patient may be asymptomatic as residual undamaged nephrons work harder to compensate for the lost nephrons, although the deterioration may be detected by laboratory testing of glomerular filtration rate (*Fig. 17.7*).

Acute renal failure is characterized by widespread abrupt cessation of nephron function

Acute renal failure is a form of total renal failure in which the majority of nephrons suddenly and simultaneously stop working. Clinically this causes a dramatic fall in urine production (**oliguria**), which is often total (**anuria**). With little opportunity for metabolic compensation, problems of disturbed fluid and electrolyte balance and failure of elimination develop rapidly. There is an increase in serum potassium level and metabolic acidosis, and nitrogen retention with uremia (see Data Set).

Several diseases can produce acute renal failure, all operating by causing sudden generalized cessation of all functions of all nephrons. There are many causes, which can be divided into:

- **Central perfusion failure** – conditions such as hypovolemic shock, sudden and profound hypotension (due, for example, to massive hemorrhage or central pump failure in myocardial infarction) lead to inadequate perfusion of the kidneys. The most sensitive component of the nephron to poor perfusion and consequent anoxia are the epithelial cells of the proximal and distal convoluted tubules, which may undergo extensive necrosis (**acute tubular necrosis**). Combined with insufficient glomerular perfusion for ultrafiltration to take place, this leads to failure of the entire nephron. This is the most common cause of reversible acute renal failure.

- **Tubular and interstitial disease** – due to hypoxic, toxic or infective damage, for example acute pyelonephritis (see page 382).
- **Glomerular diseases** – immune-mediated damage to glomeruli sometimes causes acute renal failure when all glomeruli are damaged severely at the same time. Occlusion of glomerular capillaries prevents ultrafiltration, and also prevents blood flowing through the efferent arterioles to the peritubular capillary system to provide vital oxygen for the highly oxygen-dependent tubular epithelial cells.

In many cases, acute renal failure is reversible

Depending on the cause, patients with acute renal failure may make a complete recovery, with re-establishment of full renal function, provided the initiating damaging stimulus is removed. Fortunately, this is the case in the commonest cause of acute renal failure, **acute tubular necrosis** (see page 384). The destroyed tubular lining is replaced by regenerated tubular epithelial cells, and normal function is generally regained, provided glomerular perfusion of blood is adequate to perfuse the tubular capillary network. Clinically, recovery is heralded by the establishment of urinary flow which, for a while, may be excessive (polyuria) as re-established glomerular perfusion occurs before the regenerating tubular epithelial cells have fully regained their ability to concentrate urine.

When the acute renal failure is due to sudden severe glomerular damage, complete recovery may not be possible and the patient develops chronic renal failure (see below). This may also occur with severe tubulointerstitial damage, for example in severe acute bilateral pyelonephritis (see page 384).

Chronic kidney disease can be detected at an early stage by measuring the glomerular filtration rate (GFR)

In chronic kidney disease there is progressive destruction of individual nephrons over a long period, often many years. As more and more nephrons are irrevocably destroyed, renal function becomes progressively more impaired. However, in contrast to acute renal failure, there is the opportunity for some metabolic compensation.

Because the kidneys contain so many nephrons there is an immense reserve of renal excretory function, and urea and creatinine continue to be excreted at normal levels for a long time during the natural history of any slowly progressive kidney disease in which only a few nephrons are destroyed at a time. However, a true picture of the status

Data Set
Acute renal failure

A 24-year-old man sustained severe intra-abdominal injuries in a motor cycle accident. At laparotomy he was found to have a ruptured spleen and liver and extensive intraperitoneal hemorrhage. Over the next 24 hours he passed only 200 mL of urine.

Plasma

Sodium	135 mmol/L	(135–145)
Potassium	6.1 mmol/L	(3.5–5.3)
Bicarbonate	15 mmol/L	(23–33)
Urea	32 mmol/L	(1.0–6.5)
Creatinine	427 mmol/L	(60–120)
Osmolality	309 mmol/kg	(285–295)

Urine

Na	58 mmol/L
Osmolality	310 mmol/kg

Acute renal failure is associated with raised levels of urea and creatinine in plasma, owing to decreased filtration at the glomeruli. Retention of potassium and hydrogen ions results in hyperkalemia and metabolic acidosis, reflected in the low plasma bicarbonate. Tubular damage impairs sodium resorption, resulting in urinary sodium loss, usually at concentrations in excess of 20 mmol/L. The plasma osmolality is high, due mainly to the high urea concentration. The ability of the damaged renal tubules to dilute or concentrate urine is impaired, and consequently the urinary osmolality approximates that of plasma.

of renal function can be obtained by measuring the GFR which, in clinical practice, is achieved by measuring the **creatinine clearance**, using a calculation based on the creatinine content of a 24-hour collection of urine and a single blood creatinine estimation. The normal ranges are 90–140 mL/min for men, and 80–125 mL/min for women. The blood levels of urea and creatinine do not usually rise above normal until the GFR (creatinine clearance) has fallen below 50%, and for many years of a chronic progressive kidney disease the patient may be asymptomatic or show only minor symptoms or signs. It is important to detect these early stages and to investigate the cause and monitor rate of progression. The stages, and their implications, are tabulated in *Fig. 17.7*. Stages 4 and 5 are considered to equate to **irreversible chronic renal failure**, and are marked by increasing severity and number of symptoms as the kidneys' capacity for nitrogenous waste excretion and metabolic compensation fail.

Fig. 17.7 Staging of chronic kidney disease

Stage	GFR (mL/min)	Descriptive term	Comment
1	90–140	Normal kidney excretion	Despite normal excretory function, there is other evidence of renal abnormality, e.g. proteinuria, or imaging evidence of abnormal kidney structure e.g. polycystic kidney disease
2	60–89	Reduced renal reserve	May be other evidence of renal disease as above but with early impairment of glomerular filtration. Indication for further investigation, perhaps renal biopsy
3	30–59	Renal insufficiency	If cause is not established by other means, biopsy strongly indicated. Raised blood urea and creatinine appear during this stage
4	15–29	Chronic renal failure	Increasing uremia and homeostatic control failure
5	14 or less	End stage renal failure	Terminal stage of uremia

Chronic renal failure produces many symptoms

The clinical features of chronic renal failure are due to a combination of the effects of:

- Progressive retention of toxic nitrogenous metabolites (azotemia), particularly urea (uremia). These features include cerebral intoxication with clouding of consciousness and eventual coma, polyneuropathy, and autonomic disturbance, gastrointestinal symptoms including gastro-esophagitis and colitis, uremic pericarditis, and a muddy brownish discoloration of the skin with severe itching.
- Progressive failure of tubular function producing abnormalities in biochemical homeostasis, including salt and water retention, metabolic acidosis and other electrolyte imbalances, particularly hyperkalemia and hyponatremia in the end stages. Sodium and fluid retention may cause hypertension in earlier stages.

Failure of renal activation of vitamin D, combined with excessive calcium loss in urine, causes secondary hyperparathyroidism and bone disease (renal osteodystrophy; see page 540). Destruction of renal parenchyma leads to reduced erythropoietin levels which, together with the direct suppressive effect of uremia on bone marrow, results in anemia. Uremia also causes defective platelet function and a bleeding tendency.

Chronic renal failure has many causes

Several diseases can lead to chronic renal failure, all of which cause slow, progressive, irreversible generalized destruction of nephrons. The main groups of causes are:

- Chronic vascular disease (e.g. long-standing hypertension (see page 164).

- Disease of glomeruli, e.g. glomerulonephritis (see page 368) and diabetic glomerular disease (see page 380).
- Disease of tubules and interstitium – infective (see page 383), toxic and obstructive damage to tubules and renal papillae.
- Some congenital kidney diseases, e.g. autosomal dominant polycystic kidney disease (ADPKD, see page 389).

A kidney in which virtually all nephrons have been destroyed is called an end-stage kidney (*Fig. 17.8*).

An end-stage kidney is small and shrunken

After many years of nephron destruction, virtually all glomeruli are converted into acellular spheres of hyaline material (formed from mesangial matrix) devoid of patent capillaries, and their associated tubules are severely atrophied and functionless. The medullary interstitium is shrunken and often fibrotic These changes lead to a considerable reduction in the bulk of the kidney, and an end-stage kidney is usually small and shrunken, with fine granularity of the subcapsular surface.

At this stage the cause of the disease is not usually apparent on histological examination of the kidney, but the presence of irregular cortical scars suggests that the cause may be vascular, or due to repeated episodes of kidney destruction by infection (pyelonephritis – see page 383). However, in most cases the cause has usually been established before the kidney reaches this state, either on clinical grounds or by renal biopsy at a much earlier stage in the long natural history of the progressive kidney disease.

Fig. 17.8 shows the naked-eye appearances of a selection of end-stage kidneys of various causes.

On the following page is a Data Set of a typical case of end-stage chronic renal failure.

Data Set
Chronic renal failure

A 46-year-old man with insulin-dependent diabetes mellitus since the age of 16.

Plasma				24-hour urine		
Sodium	133 mmol/L	(135–145)		Protein	1.1 g/day	(up to 0.1)
Potassium	5.5 mmol/L	(3.5–5.3)				
Bicarbonate	16 mmol/L	(23–to 33)				
Urea	44 mmol/L	(1.0–6.5)				
Creatinine	637 mmol/L	(60–120)				

Proteinuria is an early indicator of renal damage in patients with diabetes. Chronic renal failure develops over months to years, with progressive rises in plasma urea and creatinine as glomerular filtration falls. Regular monitoring of the rising plasma creatinine level enables the physician to anticipate the need for dialysis or renal transplantation. Electrolyte imbalance causing hyperkalemia and hyponatremia is a relatively late development. Metabolic acidosis due to impaired renal hydrogen ion excretion causes hypobicarbonatemia.

Fig. 17.8 End-stage kidneys. The normal kidney is 10–12 cm long, so these kidneys are less than half-size and the distinction between cortex and medulla is lost. The center and bottom right kidneys are irregularly shrunken, suggesting a vascular or infective cause.

Key Facts
Patterns of renal failure

Six patterns, four partial and two total.

Partial renal failure patterns are:

- **Asymptomatic hematuria** implies minor or early damage to the glomerulus, usually endothelial and/or mesangial cells.
- **Persistent proteinuria** implies minor or early damage to the glomerulus, usually basement membrane and mesangium. As the proteinuria becomes more severe, the patient may develop:
- **Nephrotic syndrome** (heavy proteinuria, hypoalbuminemia and edema) – implies severe damage to glomerular basement membrane and mesangial matrix.
- **Acute nephritic syndrome** (oliguria, hematuria, uremia and facial edema) implies occlusion of glomerular capillary lumina by endothelial and mesangial proliferation.

Total renal failure patterns are:

- **Acute renal failure** implies acute global nephron failure; sometimes recoverable.
- **Chronic renal failure** implies permanent, slowly progressive destruction of almost all nephrons, and is irreversible. With progression of glomerular damage, all types of partial failure can progress to chronic renal failure.

VASCULAR DISEASE AND THE KIDNEY

As has been emphasized, renal function is dependent on a normal vascular supply. Vascular disease therefore has a great impact on renal function. The main problems stem from ischemic changes induced by **hypertension**, and from occlusion of renal vessels by emboli, causing **infarction**.

Several vascular diseases have a major impact on the capillaries of the glomerular tuft, particularly vasculitis and conditions associated with intravascular thrombosis.

Reduction in blood flow to the kidneys, for example in prolonged hypotension, commonly results in necrosis of renal tubular epithelium, termed **acute tubular necrosis**. This is discussed in the later section on tubulointerstitial diseases (see page 382).

Diseases affecting pre-glomerular vessels may produce either chronic or acute renal failure

Normal renal function is dependent on adequacy of renal blood supply, with sufficient flow to maintain glomerular filtration, as well as oxygenation of the tubular and ductal parts of the nephron. Diseases of pre-glomerular vessels, or central pump failure, have a major impact on the function of the kidney.

In general, **slowly progressive disease of the vessels** leads to slowly progressive destruction of nephrons, ischemic glomerular filtration failure and ischemic tubular atrophy, culminating in chronic renal failure and a small, shrunken end-stage kidney.

The initial effect of **rapidly progressive disease of vessels** or **severe central pump failure** is sudden reduction of glomerular filtration, and the development of hypoxic necrosis of tubular epithelium. This leads to acute renal failure with oliguria or anuria, and the affected kidney is usually swollen.

Renal artery stenosis causes renal ischemia and may result in secondary hypertension

Generalized atherosclerosis particularly affects the aorta and the origin of the renal artery, but in severe cases may extend into the main renal arteries and the major branches. In most cases the atherosclerotic occlusion of the renal artery is most severe at its origin from the aorta. This **renal artery stenosis** can lead to chronic ischemia of the affected kidney, with reduction in function of all nephrons on that side, producing an end-stage shrunken kidney. The unaffected kidney undergoes compensatory hypertrophy, so renal function is largely unaffected in most cases (*Fig. 17.9*). Renal artery stenosis is also caused by **arterial fibromuscular dysplasia**.

Renal artery stenosis may lead to **renovascular hypertension**, thought to result from abnormal activity in the renin–angiotensin system in the chronically ischemic kidney. It is important in that it is one of the recognized causes of hypertension that is amenable to surgical correction.

Fig. 17.9 Renal artery stenosis. Severe atheroma of the aorta (**A**) has occluded the origin of the left main renal artery, causing ischemic atrophy of the kidney (**S**). Loss of function of this irreversibly damaged kidney is compensated by the right kidney undergoing hypertrophy and taking on double the workload. Over-secretion of renin by the damaged kidney can cause systemic hypertension.

Large renal infarcts are usually due to thromboemboli in the systemic circulation

The most common cause of renal infarction is the passage of emboli down branches of the renal arteries. Typical embolic infarcts in the kidney are usually wedge-shaped subcapsular areas of necrosis, with the broad base at the capsular surface. Infarcts initially appear red and slightly raised above the capsular surface, but after 4–5 days they develop a yellowish-white centre with a rim of hyperemia. Old infarcts appear as narrow, wedge-shaped, depressed scars. The most common causes are emboli from a mural thrombus formed over a recent myocardial infarct, thrombotic vegetations on mitral and aortic valves, thrombus on a mitral or aortic valve prosthesis, or thrombus from the left atrium of patients with atrial fibrillation.

Complete occlusion of a renal artery due to thrombosis leads to infarction of the whole kidney. However, except as a complication of arterial surgery during renal transplantation, this is a rare occurrence.

Fig. 17.10 Renal infarct. This photograph shows recent renal infarcts (**I**): the necrotic tissue is yellow, surrounded by a zone of hyperemia (arrows).

Benign hypertension produces thickening of the wall of renal vessels, with persistently reduced flow

In long-standing benign hypertension, changes in muscular renal arteries and renal arterioles lead to reduced flow of blood to glomeruli (*Fig. 17.11*).

- Renal artery branches within the kidney show thickening of the wall due to a combination of fibroelastic intimal proliferation, elastic lamina reduplication, and muscular hypertrophy of the media (see page 164).
- Afferent arterioles undergo hyalinization, their muscular walls being replaced by an amorphous material, which is rigid and inelastic (see page 164).

These thickenings of the vessel wall lead to reduction in the size of the lumen and reduced blood flow.

Chronic and progressive reduction in blood flow to the nephron leads to chronic ischemia, with slow conversion of individual glomeruli into a mass of hyaline tissue devoid of capillary lumina. As the blood supply to the tubule is derived from flow through the glomerulus into the efferent arteriole and peritubular capillaries, ischemic destruction of the associated tubule occurs. This process picks off individual nephrons over a period of many years, with no initial clinical symptoms but with reducing GFR (creatinine clearance rate, see page 360) until gradually the blood levels of creatinine and urea begin to rise.

Eventually, sufficient numbers of nephrons become non-functioning for the patient to develop manifestations of chronic renal failure. This sequence of changes, called **benign hypertensive nephrosclerosis**, is an important complication of long-standing benign hypertension, chronic renal failure being one of the important sequelae of benign hypertension.

In accelerated 'malignant' hypertension the renal vessel walls are acutely damaged

In accelerated hypertension the rise in blood pressure is very rapid, causing a pattern of renal damage different from that seen in benign hypertension. Larger muscular vessels respond with a loose fibroelastic proliferation of the intima, but the afferent arterioles exposed to the sudden high pressures frequently undergo necrosis, often with fibrin in their damaged walls (**fibrinoid necrosis**, see pages 27 and 165). Similarly, the glomerular capillary network may also undergo **segmental tuft necrosis**. When sufficient nephrons are rendered non-functional because of damage to glomerular tufts and afferent arterioles, the patient may develop acute renal failure.

The renal changes seen in benign and accelerated hypertensive nephrosclerosis are summarized in *Fig. 17.11*.

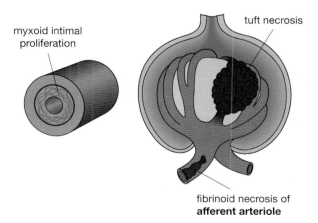

Fig. 17.11 Hypertensive renal disease. In hypertensive damage to the kidneys, the main initial effects are on the small muscular renal arteries, the afferent arterioles, and the glomerular capillaries. These changes lead to structural damage to the glomerular capillary walls, with reduction of blood flow through them, and eventual destruction of the glomerulus as a functioning unit. The associated tubular system undergoes ischemic and disuse atrophy.

The glomerulus is particularly vulnerable to diseases affecting small vessels

Diseases in which there is destruction of the walls of small vessels and occlusion of the vessel lumen, such as accelerated hypertension (see page 165), microscopic polyarteritis and other patterns of small vessel vasculitis (see page 521), produce multiple **micro-infarcts** in the kidney ('flea-bitten kidney'). When the disease is limited to very small vessels, the necrosis is confined to segments of the glomerular capillary tuft (**tuft necrosis**). Destructive small vessel disease is often associated with occlusion of the vessels by microthrombosis ('**thrombotic microangiopathy**').

Thrombotic microangiopathy and disseminated intravascular coagulation often lead to renal failure

When disseminated intravascular coagulation occurs (see pages 328–9), platelet and fibrin microthrombi form in small vessels throughout the body ('thrombotic microangiopathy'). When this occurs in the kidney, many glomerular capillaries are occluded by microthrombi (*Fig. 17.12*).

Degranulation of the platelet component of the microthrombi releases factors that stimulate mesangial cell proliferation and may produce necrosis of capillary walls, leading to tuft necrosis (see pages 367 and 377). Widespread microthrombosis produces intravascular hemolysis of red cells. The combination of intravascular hemolysis, and acute renal failure due to microthrombotic occlusion of the capillary networks of all glomeruli is termed the **hemolytic–uremic syndrome**.

Hemolytic–uremic syndrome has many causes

In children, most cases of hemolytic–uremic syndrome follow gastroenteritis due to certain forms of *Escherichia coli* (e.g. type 0157) which produce a toxin that damages capillary endothelial cells (see page 114).

In adults, hemolytic–uremic syndrome may also be caused by septicemias, including *E. coli*, and in patients with antiphospholipid antibody syndrome (see page 154), as well as being a rare side effect of some cytotoxic and immunosuppressive drugs. An important related cause is profound shock associated with obstetric catastrophes such as severe intrapartum and postpartum hemorrhage, and in some cases of eclampsia.

In this, and in other causes of hemolytic–uremic syndrome, the kidneys may show the changes of **renal cortical necrosis**, in which there is necrosis of the outer cortex of both kidneys. To the naked eye the affected cortex is pale with focal small hemorrhages; if extensive, acute renal failure develops, progressing rapidly to chronic renal failure. If patchy, some renal function can be preserved.

Fig. 17.12 Hemolytic–uremic syndrome (H&E). This glomerulus from a child shows many glomerular capillaries to be occluded by homogenous red-stained microthrombi **M** composed of platelets and fibrin. The child developed acute renal failure (with uremia) and hemolytic anemia.

GLOMERULAR DISEASES

The glomerulus is the target of many disease processes, leading to temporary or permanent impairment of function

As a highly specialized component of the blood circulatory system, responsible for ultrafiltration, the glomerulus can be damaged by: **generalized vascular disease**, particularly hypertension (see page 164), vasculitis, and diabetes mellitus (see page 569); **immunological disorders**, particularly where immune complexes are deposited in glomerular capillary walls; and **depositions of foreign material**, e.g. amyloid (see Chapter 25).

The term **glomerulonephritis** is traditionally used to describe the group of diseases in which the primary pathology is some sort of structural abnormality in the glomerulus. In most cases of primary glomerulonephritis, and in many of those in which glomerulonephritis occurs as a component of another disease (e.g. systemic lupus erythematosus, see pages 561–4), the initial insult to the glomerulus is immunological, with antigen–antibody complexes forming, or being deposited within, various components of the glomerulus (see pink box, page 365).

Despite the suffix-*itis*, most are not characterized by inflammatory changes. Damage to the glomerulus may be severe, leading to permanent scarring, in which case the associated tubule atrophies. Alternatively, some conditions produce temporary abnormality and, following resolution, there is restoration of nephron function.

Glomerular disease is classified according to the histological pattern of damage seen on renal biopsy, hence a knowledge of this aspect of histopathology is needed to understand disease. This arrangement is supplemented by further classification according to etiology of disease. In many cases the cause of glomerular disease is uncertain and some types of glomerular disease are considered idiopathic.

Immune mechanisms in glomerular disease

Many glomerular diseases are caused by immune-mediated damage, with three main mechanisms involved.

1. **Circulating immune complexes.** In the most common pattern of immunological disease, immune complexes circulating in the blood are trapped or deposited at the basement membrane or the mesangium, or both. The pattern of glomerular disease depends on the nature, quantity and distribution of the immune complexes, and the pattern of the reaction to their presence (cell proliferation, necrosis and membrane thickening). In some cases the reason for the circulating immune complexes is known (e.g. response to a recent infection or tumor); in others it is undetermined.

2. **Trapped circulating antigen.** It is speculated that in some diseases a circulating antigen becomes trapped in the glomerulus, subsequent circulating antibodies then binding to the trapped antigen. This is believed to occur in certain cases of the autoimmune disease systemic lupus erythematosus (SLE) (see page 561), when free DNA in the blood is trapped in the glomerular basement membrane (GBM), subsequently binding to anti-DNA antibodies. It is also thought to occur in cases of hepatitis B viral infection, in which viral DNA is deposited in the glomerular basement membrane, predisposing to immune complex formation.

3. **Anti-GBM antibodies.** In an uncommon form of immune-mediated damage there are autoantibodies directed to a component of the GBM (anti-GBM disease). This is the basis of Goodpasture's syndrome, in which antibodies cause direct damage to the basement membrane (see page 375). The nature of the antigen involved has been determined. Type IV collagen, a major constituent of basement membrane, is composed not of a single protein but of a family of at least five chains (termed $\alpha 1-\alpha 5$), each of which contains a non-collagenous domain. The Goodpasture antigen is the non-collagenous domain of the $\alpha 3$ type IV collagen chain, which is the target for anti-GBM autoantibodies in patients with Goodpasture's syndrome.

In some of these immune-mediated glomerular diseases there is secondary activation of complement, leading to attraction of neutrophils and activation of the coagulation system.

In other types the reason for the cellular reaction to immune complex is uncertain. In assessing renal disease it is important to identify the site, type, and pattern of immune complexes and complement within the glomerulus by immunohistochemistry and electron microscopy. The different patterns point to different diagnoses, discussed in descriptions of the main types of glomerulonephritis.

Renal biopsy is important in the assessment and diagnosis of renal disease

The diagnosis and management of renal disease has been greatly enhanced by the routine use of percutaneous needle biopsy of the kidney, carried out under local anesthetic and under radiological control. A core of renal tissue, 2 cm long and 0.2 cm wide, is removed. Using a combination of light microscopy, immunofluorescence or immunocytochemistry, and electron microscopy, the distribution of immune complexes within the glomerulus, and their composition (which immunoglobulins and complement factors are present) can be determined, as can the pattern of glomerular reaction to the presence of immune complexes. The pattern present usually allows an accurate diagnosis to be made. Almost all the other causes of renal failure (e.g. hypertensive disease, diabetes, amyloid, tubulointerstitial disease etc.) can be diagnosed on renal biopsy.

The renal biopsy

The biopsy core is divided into three main portions; one is snap-frozen to provide frozen sections for immunohistochemistry, one is specially fixed in glutaraldehyde for electron microscopy, and the rest is routinely fixed for paraffin sectioning.

Histological examination of glomeruli and tubules is performed to identify structural abnormalities and to characterize patterns of glomerular, tubular and interstitial damage.

Immunohistochemical examination is required to identify immunoglobulins and complement components in immune glomerular disease, and electron microscopic examination is required for fine detail of glomerular structure, including the site of immune complexes within the glomerulus.

Most glomerular diseases are due to abnormalities at the glomerular filtration barrier

Ultrafiltration of the blood occurs in the glomerulus, producing an ultrafiltrate which passes into Bowman's capsule and thence into the tubular system, where selective absorption and secretion of various components take place, followed by concentration to produce urine. Ultrafiltration occurs across the **glomerular filtration barrier,** which is composed of:

- The fenestrated thin **endothelial cell layer,** which forms the internal lining to the glomerular capillary (red in *Fig. 17.13*).
- An unusually thick **glomerular capillary basement membrane** (blue in *Fig. 17.13*).
- The **epithelial cells** or 'podocytes,' which form an outer coating to the glomerular capillary. These cells (green in *Fig. 17.13*) are in contact with the outer surface of the basement membrane via a series of foot processes. At the vascular hilum of the glomerulus these epithelial cells are continuous with the flattened epithelial cells lining Bowman's capsule.
- A high **polyanionic charge** on the epithelial surface of the basement membrane and on the inner surfaces of the podocytes (indicated by minus signs in *Fig. 17.13*).

Another important component of glomerulus structure is the **mesangium**, which is the supporting 'mesentery' to the capillary (*Fig. 17.14*). It comprises mesangial cells (phagocytic support and secretory cells) and their amorphous secretory product, the mesangial matrix. The role of the mesangium in ultrafiltration is not known, but abnormalities of the mesangium are an important component of acute and chronic glomerular disease.

The glomerulus has a limited set of histological responses to damage

Five main patterns of response to damage are seen in the glomerulus, combinations of which describe all types of glomerular disease.

Proliferation of endothelial cells leads to occlusion of capillary lumina, often with neutrophils present. This proliferation reduces the flow through glomeruli and correlates with oliguria and uremia.

Proliferation of mesangial cells, which is usually associated with increased production of matrix, is a common feature of many glomerular diseases. In some cases this may regress once the acute episode is over; in others the production of excess mesangial matrix over many years eventually leads to sclerosis (hyalinization) of all or part of the glomerular tuft, with loss of capillary lumina.

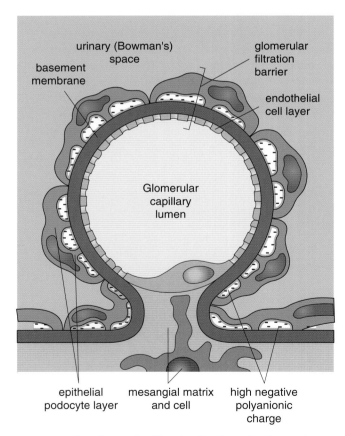

Fig. 17.13 The glomerular filtration barrier. The glomerular filtration barrier comprises the fenestrated endothelial cell layer (red), the glomerular capillary basement membrane (blue), the endothelial podocyte layer (green) and the high polyanionic charge on the outer surface of the basement membrane and the inner layers of the podocytes (indicated by minus signs).

Fig. 17.14 The normal glomerulus. 1 μm resin section, Toluidine blue. The glomerulus has four main components: the basement membrane **BM** lined internally by endothelial cells **En** and coated externally by epithelial popocytes **Ep**. The capillary network is supported on the mesangium **M**. Red blood cells **RBC** can be seen in capillary lumina.

Basement membrane thickening may be due to the deposition of an abnormal substance (immune complexes or amyloid), synthesis of excess basement membrane material, insinuation of mesangial cytoplasm and matrix, or a combination of these.

Alteration in epithelial podocytes is a commonly observed abnormality in a wide range of glomerular diseases, usually in the form of loss or fusion of the foot processes. In one pattern of disease (minimal change nephropathy, see page 376), fusion and loss of foot processes is the only structural abnormality. In more severe glomerular disease podocytes may be lost, the remaining cells being stretched to cover the capillaries.

Capillary wall necrosis, usually fibrinoid necrosis (see *Fig. 17.27*), occurs in diseases in which there is severe acute capillary wall damage, e.g. necrotizing vasculitis and accelerated (malignant) hypertension. Capillary wall necrosis often permits blood components to pass from the capillary lumen into Bowman's (urinary) space, stimulating the formation of epithelial crescents partly derived from the epithelial cells lining Bowman's capsule (see below and page 373).

Crescent formation occurs when breaks in the capillary wall permit leakage of fibrin and blood, including macrophages, into the urinary space. This stimulates the proliferation of epithelial cells lining Bowman's capsule. The macrophages and epithelial cells crush the glomerulus and lead to loss of the entire nephron (see *Fig. 17.22*). The presence of widespread crescents is a poor prognostic sign.

Glomerular disease may not affect all glomeruli in a uniform manner

Most glomerular diseases affect different glomeruli to varying degrees, with only a small number of diseases affecting all glomeruli in a uniform manner. This explains how some glomerular diseases cause sudden acute renal failure (disease affects all glomeruli in a uniform manner), whereas others cause a selective partial renal failure syndrome (disease affects small areas in a small proportion of glomeruli). A nomenclature has been agreed for the various patterns of disease (*Fig. 17.15*).

- Diffuse – all glomeruli in both kidneys are involved.
- Focal – only some glomeruli are involved.
- Global – all parts of each individual glomerulus are involved.
- Segmental – only some segments of each glomerulus are involved, the other segments being normal.

Thus a glomerular disease may be described as:

- Diffuse global.
- Diffuse segmental.
- Focal global.
- Focal segmental.

The vast majority are either 'diffuse global' or 'focal segmental.'

Fig. 17.15 Patterns of glomerular disease. (a) Global: affecting the whole of the glomerulus uniformly. (b) Segmental: affecting one glomerular segment, leaving other segments unaffected. (c) Diffuse: affecting all glomeruli in both kidneys. (d) Focal: affecting a proportion of glomeruli, with others unaffected.

Clinical features of glomerulonephritis relate broadly to histological findings

Although learning the clinical patterns of disease that relate to each of the several types of glomerulonephritis seems daunting, there are four general rules of thumb which, albeit not absolute, explain the vast majority of cases.

1. Structural change in the glomerular basement membrane (usually thickening) or deposition of excessive mesangial matrix leads to increased loss of protein in urine, which if severe leads to the **nephrotic syndrome**.
2. Glomerular damage associated with proliferation of endothelial or mesangial cells is associated with the development of microscopic hematuria or **nephritic syndrome**.
3. If there is both damage to basement membrane and cell proliferation, a **mixed nephritic/nephrotic syndrome** is likely.
4. If damage to glomeruli is rapid and widespread, features of acute renal failure develop.

Another common conceptual hurdle is understanding how someone with a partial renal failure syndrome, such as a nephrotic syndrome, eventually develops total chronic renal failure. In most glomerular diseases the damage causing the nephritic or nephrotic syndrome also eventually causes glomeruli to become completely scarred (hyalinized), leading to loss of individual nephrons.

Glomerular hyalinization is the result of excessive production of mesangial matrix by the mesangial cells over a long period of time. The expanding mesangial matrix mass slowly but progressively crushes the sophisticated glomerular architecture out of existence, until no blood flows through the glomerular capillaries, and no oxygenated blood passes into the efferent arterioles and peritubular capillary systems. The tubules are deprived of oxygenated blood, and tubular epithelial cells die irrevocably and become atrophic. Thus the destruction of the glomerulus leads to destruction of the entire nephron unit.

As more and more nephrons are destroyed, the partial renal failure syndrome (nephritic or nephrotic) develops into the total renal failure syndrome of chronic renal failure. This is associated with progressive shrinkage of the kidney to form a small, scarred organ termed 'end-stage kidney.'

IMPORTANT TYPES OF GLOMERULONEPHRITIS

Acute diffuse proliferative glomerulonephritis usually presents as the nephritic syndrome

Acute proliferative glomerulonephritis is a diffuse global disease of glomeruli. It is caused by deposition of immune complexes in glomeruli, which is stimulated by a preceding infection. Although infection is most commonly strepto-coccal, a range of bacterial, viral and protozoal infections can also stimulate this pattern of disease.

Histologically, there is increased cellularity of the glomerulus, with four main features (see *Fig. 17.17*):

- **Proliferation of endothelial cells** produces occlusion of capillary lumina, leading to reduced glomerular filtration, with rising blood pressure and blood levels of nitrogenous components (urea and creatinine).
- **Presence of immune complexes** in lumps on the epithelial side of the GBM.
- **Presence of neutrophil polymorphs** in capillaries.
- **Mild mesangial cell proliferation.**

In children the illness is usually clinically mild and transient. As there has been cell proliferation, patients develop features of the nephritic syndrome, with oliguria, hematuria, hypertension and periorbital edema. Supportive treatment is required until the nephritic syndrome resolves, usually over 3–6 weeks, as the immune complexes are cleared from the GBM. With resolution of disease, the proliferating endothelial cells are shed, mesangial cell increase regresses, capillary lumina become patent again, and renal function returns to normal.

A small percentage of cases do not resolve completely but persist, with evidence of **rapid progression to renal failure**. These cases develop epithelial crescents, which compress the glomeruli, and rapidly progressive renal failure ensues (**rapidly progressive glomerulonephritis**). This is more common in adults than in children. The pathology is presented on page 373.

Alternatively, in rare cases there is **slow inexorable deterioration in renal function** over a period of many years.

Fig. 17.16 Acute diffuse glomerulonephritis (H&E). The glomerulus is hypercellular due to proliferation of endothelial and mesangial cells. Glomerular capillary lumina cannot be identified because they are obliterated by the proliferating cells. The immune complexes can only be seen by electron microscopy (see *Fig. 17.17b*).

Although the patient appears to recover from the acute nephritic syndrome, urine testing reveals persistent proteinuria. This is associated with persistent enlargement of the mesangium, which fails to regress when the endothelial proliferation regresses. Over the years the mesangial cells produce excess matrix, eventually producing large hyaline masses that compress the glomerular capillaries and ultimately replace the entire tuft. Throughout this period the patient is asymptomatic until the increasing urinary protein loss leads to the nephrotic syndrome. When all glomeruli have become hyalinized by this diffuse global process, chronic renal failure develops.

Fig. 17.17 Acute diffuse glomerulonephritis. (a) In diffuse acute proliferative glomerulonephritis there is endothelial proliferation with neutrophils (1), subepithelial lumpy immune complex deposits (2), and mesangial cell increase (3). (b) Electron micrograph showing typical large immune complex deposits **D** on the epithelial side of the basement membrane **BM. L** is the capillary lumen, not yet obliterated by proliferation of endothelial (E) cells.

Pathogenesis of acute diffuse proliferative glomerulonephritis

The most common cause of acute diffuse glomerulonephritis is pharyngeal infection with β-hemolytic streptococci of Lancefield group A. Not all strains cause this disease, and there are certain so-called 'nephritogenic' strains (Griffith's types 12, 4, 1, 25 and 49). Children are most commonly affected, with onset 1–2 weeks after the primary infection. Immune complexes develop and circulate in the blood, to be filtered out in the glomerulus. Immunofluorescence shows granular deposition of IgG and C3 in the GBM and mesangium. Ultrastructurally these deposits are sited beneath the epithelium. The activation of complement is the reason for attraction of neutrophils into the glomerulus. These degranulate and damage endothelial cells, stimulating their proliferation. Mesangial cell proliferation is mediated by factors derived from complement and platelets, and is accompanied by increased expression of PDGF and PDGF-receptor proteins, resulting in an autocrine mechanism of cell proliferation.

If damage to the glomerular capillaries is severe, fibrin and blood leak into Bowman's space and stimulate epithelial cell proliferation, resulting in a crescent which permanently effaces the glomerulus. If 80% of glomeruli have crescents, this is associated with rapid progression to renal failure with a poor prognosis (see page 373).

Membranous nephropathy presents with proteinuria and the nephrotic syndrome

Characterized by the presence of immune complex deposits in the basement membrane of all segments of all glomeruli, membranous nephropathy is diffuse and global. The etiology of immune complexes in membranous disease is uncertain (see pink box on page 365). Unlike diffuse proliferative glomerulonephritis, there is no inflammation or associated endothelial or epithelial proliferation, although the mesangium may be increased. The disease passes through three pathological stages (see *Fig. 17.9*):

1. Immune complex deposited on epithelial side of basement membrane.

2. New basement membrane deposited around immune complex deposits.

3. Immune complex deposits disappear, leaving thickened 'lacy' basement membrane.

The abnormality of the basement membrane renders it unusually permeable; it no longer selectively retains proteins, leading to heavy proteinuria and the **nephrotic syndrome**. With time, the abnormal glomeruli develop increase in mesangial matrix produced by the mesangial cells. This, together with membrane thickening, causes gradual hyalinization of the glomeruli and death of individual nephrons. This process takes place over many years and, from a nephrotic syndrome the patient may develop chronic renal failure with uremia. The natural history of the disease is

membranous nephropathy | late-stage membranous nephropathy

Fig. 17.18 Membranous nephropathy.
(a) In membranous nephropathy there are electron-dense deposits on the epithelial side of the basement membrane (1), and slight mesangial increase (2). In late-stage disease there is removal of deposits, leaving a thick 'lacy' membrane (3), and increasing mesangial matrix deposition (4). (b) Electron micrograph of a basement membrane thickened by deposition of antigen–antibody complexes **C** on the epithelial side of the basement membrane, from a patient with membranous nephropathy who presented with the nephrotic syndrome. (c) Methenamine silver staining shows mesangial matrix and basement membrane material. In membranous nephropathy, new basement membrane material is deposited around immune complexes, and can be seen as spaced black spikes and dots on the outer surface of the membrane (arrows).

variable. In crude figures, about 25% of patients develop remission, 25% develop stable, persisting proteinuria, and 50% develop chronic renal failure over a period of about 10 years.

Membranous nephropathy is one of the most important causes of the nephrotic syndrome in adults, and patients can be divided into two groups:

- 80–90% of cases have no apparent reason for development of immune complexes, and are classed as primary or idiopathic membranous nephropathy.
- 10–20% of cases have a reason for development of immune complex disease, as they have abnormal circulating antigens:
  - **Infective**: hepatitis B, malaria, syphilis.
  - **Drug-related**: gold therapy, penicillamine, captopril, heroin.
  - **Tumor-associated**: lung cancer and lymphomas.
  - **SLE**: 10% of renal involvement in lupus is of the membranous pattern.

In some cases, where there is a recognizable cause, successful treatment of the cause (e.g. withdrawal of drug or the complete excision of the lung tumor) leads to spontaneous remission of the membranous nephropathy.

Pathogenesis of membranous nephropathy

In membranous nephropathy, subepithelial immune complexes develop in the glomeruli (mainly IgG with a small amount of complement). In most cases circulating immune complexes cannot be demonstrated in the blood, and the concept that preformed circulating complexes are filtered out in the glomerulus seems doubtful in this pattern of disease. It is more likely that the immune complexes form in situ, with a circulating antigen becoming trapped in the glomerulus, followed by deposition of antibody. This in situ formation may explain why, in contrast to diffuse proliferative glomerulonephritis, there is little complement and no inflammatory or proliferative responses. The precise reason why the presence of immune complexes causes basement membrane thickening is, at present, unknown. The basement membrane becomes abnormally leaky as its composition changes, and there is reduction in the normal polyanionic sites, which normally 'repel' proteins and keep them from filtering into urine.

In cases with a drug-related, neoplastic or infective cause, treatment of the underlying condition removes the source of circulating antigen and may cause remission of renal disease.

Diffuse membranoproliferative ('mesangiocapillary') glomerulonephritis often presents as a nephrotic or a mixed nephritic/nephrotic syndrome

Membranoproliferative glomerulonephritis (MPGN), also called **mesangiocapillary glomerulonephritis**, is a pattern of glomerular reaction to complement abnormalities. Some are secondary to systemic disorders, such as SLE, infective endocarditis, malaria and infected ventricular CSF shunts, but the major group is idiopathic, divided by clinical and pathological features into two types (type I and type II), each with a particular pathogenesis.

As the name implies, the common factors in this process are **mesangial proliferation** and **basement membrane thickening** as the main structural abnormalities.

The basement membrane abnormality is responsible for the clinical symptoms of proteinuria or a full nephrotic syndrome. Because there is cellular proliferation, patients may also develop hematuria or a nephritic syndrome. A mixed nephrotic/nephritic syndrome is seen in some cases.

Type I MPGN accounts for 90% of cases and is mostly seen in adolescents and young adults. There is accentuated lobularity of glomerular segments (*Figs 17.19a* and *17. 20*), which is caused by proliferation of mesangial cells. Capillaries are greatly thickened due to subendothelial deposits of immune complex containing IgG or IgM and C3. Thickening is also due to ingrowth of mesangial cell cytoplasm between the endothelium and basement membrane, with the formation of a double-contour or tram-track basement membrane (*Figs 17.19a* and *17.20*). A very rare variant of type I MPGN (sometimes called **type III**) has deposits in other parts of the basement membrane.

Typically there is progressive deterioration in renal function over a period of about 10 years, resulting in chronic renal failure.

Type II MPGN accounts for 10% of cases and is also seen in children and young adults. There is marked thickening of the GBM, but mesangial proliferation is usually not as prominent as in type I. The characteristic feature is large, continuous, dense ribbon-like deposits within the basement membrane, giving rise to the alternative name of **dense deposit disease** (Figs *17.19b* and 17.21). By immunohistochemistry these deposits contain no immune complexes and are composed of complement factor C3. The pathogenesis of this disease has been related to activation of the alternative complement pathway (see pink box, page 373). Some cases are associated with partial lipodystrophy.

Type II MPGN also has a poor prognosis, with gradual development of chronic renal failure over 10–15 years.

In both types there is a high incidence of recurrence of the disease in transplanted kidneys, particularly in type II MPGN, with linear dense deposits accumulating in the glomeruli of the transplant.

type I membranoproliferative
glomerulonephritis

type II membranoproliferative
glomerulonephritis

a

b

Fig. 17.19
Membranoproliferative glomerulonephritis. There are two main patterns, type I (a) and type II (b). In both, there is apparent exaggeration of the lobularity of the glomerulus because of increase in mesangial cells and matrix (1). The basement membrane is markedly thickened by a combination of mesangial cytoplasm intrusion into membrane (2) and large immune complex deposits (3) which are subendothelial and discontinuous in type I, but form a continuous linear dense deposit in type II.

Fig. 17.20 Type I membranoproliferative glomerulonephritis. Methenamine silver stain. This photograph shows an early stage of type I disease. The basement membrane is thickened (arrows), and the glomerular segments are variably expanded by proliferation of the mesangium (**M**).

Fig. 17.21 Type II membranoproliferative glomerulonephritis (EM). This electron micrograph shows the continuous electron dense immune complexes in the basement membranes of two adjacent capillary loops (**DD**). Proliferating mesangial cells (**MC**) have largely occluded the capillary lumina.

Pathogenesis of MPGN

Membranoproliferative glomerulonephritis is basically the result of abnormalities of complement deposition and handling in the glomerulus. In type I MPGN, complement deposition in the GBM is supplemented by an immune complex disease component, circulating complexes being present in up to 50% of cases. The main complement found in glomerular deposits is C3, and immunoglobulins include IgG, IgM and occasionally IgA. The presence of C1q and C4 in deposits supports the contention that activation of the classic complement pathway plays a part in the pathogenesis. Complement activation causes consumption of serum complement, and serum levels of C3 are reduced in 60% of cases. In type II MPGN there are no immune complexes and the

dense deposits of C3 in the basement membrane are caused by abnormal activation of the complement system. This is mediated by a circulating autoantibody to C3 convertase, which prevents its normal breakdown. Normally, C3 convertase activates C3, but has a very short half-life. The autoantibody, termed C3 nephritic factor, stabilizes C3 convertase, allowing continued activation of C3. The absence of C1q and C4, the early components of the classic pathway, is explained by direct action of C3 convertase. The complement activation may cause consumption of serum complement, and serum levels of C3 are markedly reduced in most cases. There is a familial predisposition to the development of this condition in some cases.

Rapidly progressive glomerulonephritis is characterized by the presence of numerous crescents

An epithelial crescent is the result of breaks in the glomerular basement membrane permitting the leak of fibrin, blood proteins and white blood cells (particularly monocyte/macrophages) into the urinary space. These stimulate active proliferation of the epithelial cells lining Bowman's capsule, forming a crescent which enlarges relentlessly to compress

the glomerular tuft, which shrivels and becomes nonfunctional. Large numbers of glomeruli showing crescents indicates a poor prognosis, with rapid progression to renal failure. Rapidly progressive glomerulonephritis is not a distinct etiological disease, but can occur in many of the other forms of glomerulonephritis when glomerular damage is particularly severe and associated with breaks in the basement membrane; it is therefore particularly associated with tuft necrosis lesions. Important causes of crescentic glomerulonephritis are given on page 378.

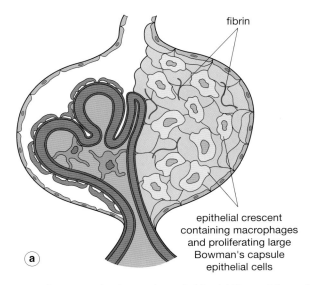

fibrin

epithelial crescent containing macrophages and proliferating large Bowman's capsule epithelial cells

(a)

(b)

Fig. 17.22 a&b Crescentic glomerulonephritis. (a) The rapidly proliferating epithelial crescent crushes the glomerular tuft, which may show a range of changes including focal proliferative glomerulonephritis, segmental tuft necrosis, mesangiocapillary glomerulonephritis, or acute proliferative glomerulonephritis. (b) This photomicrograph shows a glomerulus (**G**) being compressed by a proliferating crescent (**C**); the crescent is squashing the damaged glomerular tuft out of existence.

Focal segmental proliferative glomerulonephritis can be either primary or secondary

In almost every case focal glomerulonephritis is also 'segmental,' only occasional lobules of the glomerular tuft being involved in disease. A range of histological appearances can be seen:

- **Focal mesangial cell proliferation** with increased matrix production, with immune complex deposits visible on electron microscopy, the nature and location of the deposits depending on the disease.
- In addition to the proliferative changes, there may be segmental **tuft necrosis.**
- When tuft necrosis is present, some affected glomerular segments may show crescent formation. When many segments of many glomeruli show crescent formation the prognosis is poor.
- In old lesions the affected segment may show hyalinization, i.e. replacement of glomerular structures

by a large mass of acellular mesangial matrix material, and the changes are indistinguishable from those of **focal glomerulosclerosis** (see page 376).

In the evaluation of focal segmental glomerulonephritis, electron microscopy and immunohistochemistry of a renal biopsy sample are essential to establish the location and nature of the immune complexes characteristic of the many different types, as this pattern of glomerular disease can be caused by several different diseases, divisible into two groups:

Primary types, which include IgA nephropathy (Berger disease), and some patterns of Goodpasture syndrome.

Secondary types, in which focal segmental glomerulonephritis occurs as a component of other systemic diseases, particularly:

- Infective endocarditis, mainly SBE.
- Small vessel vasculitis syndromes, e.g. Henoch–Schönlein nephritis (see page 375).
- Some patterns of systemic connective tissue disorders, particularly SLE (see pages 561–3).

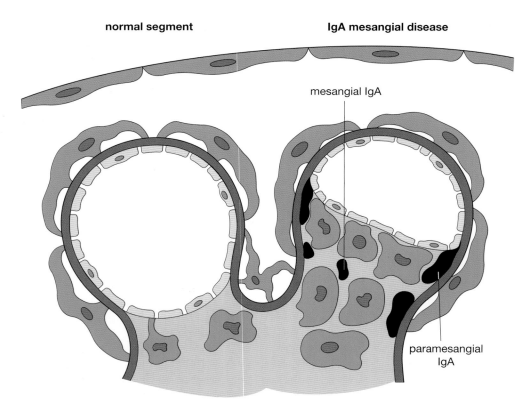

normal segment   IgA mesangial disease

mesangial IgA

paramesangial IgA

Fig. 17.23 Focal segmental proliferative glomerulonephritis (IgA nephropathy). This diagram shows a typical appearance in early focal segmental disease. One glomerular capillary loop is structurally normal, but its neighbor shows proliferation of mesangial cells in association with immune complex deposition; in this case of IgA nephropathy, the deposits are of IgA which is deposited in mesangium and in a paramesangial location. Eventually, the affected segment will be obliterated by mesangial matrix produced in excess by the proliferated mesangial cells.

Fig. 17.24 a&b IgA Nephropathy (a) 1 μm resin section, Toluidine blue stain. (b) Immunoperoxidase method for IgA. In (a) the bottom half of the glomerulus is normal by light microscopy but the upper half shows segmental increase in mesangial matrix and cells within which are paramesangial and mesangial deposits of IgA, just detectable here as darker blue blobs (arrows). In (b) the IgA is seen to be fairly widespread within the mesangium, but with more in the proliferated segments (arrows) on the left than in the structurally normal segments on the extreme right.

IgA (Berger) nephropathy is the most common cause of glomerulonephritis in adults

As its name implies, this is associated with deposits of IgA in the glomerulus. It usually presents with recurrent hematuria or persistent proteinuria, more rarely with nephritic syndrome or rapidly progressive renal failure.

The glomerulus usually shows a focal and segmental glomerulonephritis, due largely to mesangial cell proliferation in response to the presence of deposits of IgA in the mesangium and at the junction between the mesangium and the basement membrane (paramesangial) (*Figs 17.23* and *17.24*). Tuft proliferation is followed by mesangial matrix deposition and eventual sclerosis of the segment.

In the early stages the disease may be asymptomatic except for persistent microscopic hematuria with mild proteinuria, but as more segments of more glomeruli become involved, more severe hematuria, and proteinuria sufficient to cause nephrotic syndrome, may develop.

Around 25% of patients progress to eventual chronic renal failure over a period of many years, when sufficient segments of sufficient glomeruli have been damaged to lead to glomerular sclerosis and death of nephrons.

In some cases the mesangial changes are not focal and segmental, but more extensive ('mesangioproliferative glomerulonephritis'), and rarely there may be crescentic glomerulonephritis, in which case progression to renal failure may be rapid.

The pathogenesis of the disease is uncertain. The IgA that is deposited in the mesangium almost certainly comes from bone marrow rather than from mucosal sites. Consequently, previous suggestions that chronic mucosal allergies predispose to the condition are unlikely to be correct.

Goodpasture's syndrome is a rare cause of glomerulonephritis

This is characterized by the presence of autoantibodies to type IV collagen in the glomerular basement membrane (anti-GBM, see page 365), seen on immunohistochemistry as linear deposition of IgG and C3. The histological pattern may be either a focal segmental glomerulonephritis or a diffuse glomerulonephritis, often with crescents. As the autoantibody also reacts with alveolar basement membrane, there is also pulmonary hemorrhage.

Secondary types of focal segmental glomerulonephritis are particularly associated with systemic vasculitis and connective tissue diseases

Focal segmental glomerulonephritis is a feature of many types of small vessel vasculitis when they affect the kidney (e.g. microscopic polyarteritis, Wegener arteritis, Henoch–Schönlein disease). Henoch–Schönlein nephritis is usually seen in childhood in association with other manifestations such as skin purpura, arthralgia and abdominal pain, all thought to be due to small vessel vasculitis. The glomeruli and small vessels elsewhere contain IgA, so the renal appearances overlap with those of IgA nephropathy. About 20% of cases of infective endocarditis show focal segmental glomerulonephritis, with immune complex deposits. It is also a feature of some of the so-called connective tissue diseases, particularly systemic lupus erythematosus (SLE) and progressive systemic sclerosis (see pages 561–4). In many of the secondary causes, fibrinoid tuft necrosis, often with consequent crescent formation, is a frequent feature (*Fig. 17.27*).

Focal segmental glomerulosclerosis accounts for many cases of nephrotic syndrome

Focal segmental glomerulosclerosis may occur:

- as a primary idiopathic disease.
- in association with HIV infection.
- as an end-stage of the various types of focal segmental proliferative glomerulonephritis.

It is a common cause of persistent proteinuria and nephrotic syndrome, and accounts for 10% of cases of nephrotic syndrome in children and 20% of cases in adults. There is focal and segmental hyalinization due to increased mesangial matrix synthesis, which eventually obliterates the glomerular capillaries. Granular IgM and C3 are seen with immunochemistry.

In children and young adults focal glomerulosclerosis is seen as an idiopathic disease, accounting for most cases of nephrotic syndrome that fail to respond to steroid therapy.

In later adult life it is seen secondary to other disorders. Increasingly this pattern of glomerular damage is being seen in association with HIV infection as part of HIV nephropathy.

Focal glomerulosclerosis has a poor prognosis. There is progression of disease over many years, with hyalinization of glomeruli and loss of functioning nephrons leading to chronic renal failure.

Minimal change disease is a common cause of nephrotic syndrome in childhood

Minimal change disease is mainly seen in children under the age of 6 years, in whom it causes proteinuria and nephrotic syndrome. In adults the condition is less common, but still accounts for 10–15% of cases of nephrotic syndrome.

The characteristic feature, and the reason for the name, is that by light microscopy there is nothing abnormal to see in the glomeruli. By electron microscopy there is fusion of the foot processes of podocytes (see *Fig. 17.12*). Immune complexes and deposits are not seen. Tubules may show accumulation of lipid in lining cells, giving rise to the old-fashioned alternative name of **lipoid nephrosis**, which is sometimes still used.

Treatment with steroids usually brings about remission of disease within 2 weeks, although relapse is frequent when steroids are stopped.

An immune pathogenesis is suggested by the response of the disease to steroid therapy, and it has been proposed that minimal change disease is caused by non-complement-fixing antibodies to antigens on the glomerular epithelial cell membrane. Detailed study of the basement membrane has shown that it becomes depleted of polyanionic charges, leading to failure of retention of proteins. In adults, disease has been associated with the presence of tumors such as lymphomas and renal cell carcinomas.

Fig. 17.25 a&b Minimal change glomerulonephritis. Shown diagrammatically (a), normal foot processes are regularly spaced, but in this pattern of disease they become fused. In (b), which is a biopsy from the kidney of a child with the nephrotic syndrome, the complex secondary foot process arrangement is lost and the primary foot processes (**Pl**) lie directly on the basement membrane (**BM**).

The glomerulus is affected in several ways in SLE

In the kidney in SLE, immune complex deposition can give various patterns of glomerulonephritis. These are:

- **Mesangial pattern (WHO Class II)** in which there is only mild mesangial cellular and matrix increase, with largely normal basement membranes. Immune complexes are present in the mesangium. Mild proteinuria and intermittent microscopic hematuria are the usual clinical manifestations.
- **Focal segmental pattern (WHO Class III)** in which there is a focal and segmental glomerulonephritis with immune complexes in mesangium and basement membranes. Sometimes there is tuft necrosis, and crescents may form in affected glomeruli. Proteinuria and hematuria are the usual clinical features. This pattern may progress to:

Fig. 17.26 Lupus nephropathy. This pattern of lupus glomerular involvement is similar to that in membranous nephropathy, forming wire-loop lesions (arrows).

Fig. 17.27 Segmental tuft necrosis. This glomerulus shows one segment where the normal structure has been completely destroyed by red-staining fibrinoid tuft necrosis. This is an important glomerular feature in a range of diseases in which there is acute damage to small blood vessels.

- **Diffuse proliferative pattern (WHO Class IV)** in which there is diffuse and global proliferation of mesangial and endothelial cells with variable basement membrane thickening. Immune complexes are in mesangium and basement membrane; in the basement membrane the deposits may be in subepithelial, intramembranous or subendothelial locations, often all three. Very large subendothelial deposits produce 'wire-loop' thickening of the membrane, visible on light microscopy. In severe lesions tuft necrosis (see *Fig. 17.27*) and crescents may develop. Hematuria and severe proteinuria, often sufficient to produce the nephrotic syndrome, are almost invariable.
- **Membranous pattern (WHO Class V)** in which the lesions resemble those in membranous nephropathy, with immune complexes in the usual subepithelial position, but in addition they are present in the mesangium and in a subendothelial location. When the latter are large, 'wire loops' may form (see *Fig. 17.26*). The nephrotic syndrome is the usual presenting symptom.

The immune complexes found vary in composition, but the 'full house' pattern of three immunoglobulins (IgG, IgM and IgA) and two complement factors (C3 and C1q) is particularly common, particularly in the membranous pattern. The focal and diffuse proliferative patterns are more common than the mesangial and membranous patterns. The **Class I pattern** (histologically normal glomeruli) is very rare.

In addition to the glomerular lesions, tubulointerstitial inflammation is frequent, and the same sort of immune complexes seen in the glomerular lesions can also be found in the basement membranes of the tubules.

Renal lesions occur in other systemic connective tissue disorders

The kidney is vulnerable in other connective tissue diseases, particularly when those diseases have a vasculitic component.

Polyarteritis nodosa affecting large and medium-sized arteries produces multiple medium or small infarcts in the kidney. The variant in which only small vessels are involved, **microscopic polyarteritis**, affects arterioles and the small vessels of the glomerular tuft, producing infarction of entire glomeruli or segments, visible as fibrinoid tuft necrosis, similar to that illustrated in *Fig.17.27*. Crescent formation often develops in response to the tuft necrosis.

Wegener granulomatosis (see page 166) is a necrotizing vasculitis affecting the lung, upper respiratory tract and kidney. In the kidney there is extensive focal segmental glomerular involvement, with tuft necrosis and extensive crescent formation. In 90% of cases the kidney is involved at some time in the natural history of the disease, presenting initially with hematuria, but rapidly progressive renal failure develops if crescent formation is extensive.

Rheumatoid arthritis occasionally involves the kidney in a similar way to the small vessel vasculitic syndromes above, but acute rheumatoid vasculitis is rare, and kidney damage due to rheumatoid-associated amyloid, or tubular damage by anti-rheumatoid drugs (e.g. gold therapy, penicillamine) are much more common.

Systemic scleroderma (progressive systemic sclerosis) involves the kidney in two main ways:

- Concentric lamellar thickening of the tunica intima of interlobular arteries and some arterioles. Although this is the result of proliferation of intimal cells, a substantial component of the thickening is amorphous acellular matrix rich in glycosaminoglycans (*Fig. 17.28*)
- Fibrinoid tuft necrosis affecting segments of many glomeruli.

The vascular changes produce systemic hypertension which is frequently of the severe accelerated ('malignant') type, and it is in this group that tuft necrosis is seen to be most severe and extensive; it is not known whether this is the cause or effect of the accelerated hypertension. These changes lead to rapidly progressive renal failure.

Fig. 17.28 Progressive systemic sclerosis. This small renal artery is from a patient who died of rapidly progressive renal failure, with extensive tuft necrosis of glomeruli and these widespread arterial changes. The vessel lumen is almost obliterated by concentric intimal proliferation.

Key Facts
Nephrotic syndrome

Nephrotic syndrome comprises:

- Severe proteinuria
- Hypoalbuminemia
- Generalized edema
- Hypercholesterolemia and hyperlipidemia

Key Facts
Rapidly progressive glomerulonephritis

- Not a distinct etiological entity, but develops as a consequence of severe glomerular damage in other glomerular lesions
- Characterized by the presence of epithelial crescents
- Crescents result from leakage of blood components into urinary space
- Crescents cause compression destruction of glomeruli
- Causes rapidly progressive renal failure
- The causes of crescent formation are given in the adjacent Key Facts list.

Key Facts
Nephritic syndrome

Nephritic syndrome comprises:

- Overt hematuria
- Oliguria
- Azotemia and uremia
- Edema (often facial)
- Mild hypertension

Key Facts
Causes of crescent formation

Diffuse glomerulonephritis types

- Acute diffuse proliferative glomerulonephritis (occasional)
- Membranoproliferative glomerulonephritis (rare)
- Diffuse pattern of Goodpasture's glomerulonephritis

Focal segmental glomerulonephritis types

- Segmental lupus nephritis
- Small vessel vasculitis (microscopic polyarteritis, Wegener's arteritis, Henoch–Schönlein nephritis etc.)
- Acute scleroderma of kidney

Clinical presentation of glomerular diseases

Presenting condition	Possible glomerular pathology	Non-glomerular causes
Asymptomatic proteinuria or hematuria	Focal segmental GN (early) (particularly IgA disease) Membranous nephropathy Early diabetic nephropathy Early glomerular amyloid	Postural proteinuria
Macroscopic hematuria	Focal segmental GN (early) Acute proliferative GN (early) Membranoproliferative GN (early) Crescenteric GN with tuft necrosis (see key facts)	Kidney, ureteric or bladder tumor Bladder infection Kidney trauma or infarction
Nephritic syndrome	Acute proliferative GN Focal segmental GN (advanced – all causes) SLE nephritis (some patterns; see page 563)	None
Nephrotic syndrome without red cell casts	Minimal change nephropathy Focal segmental glomerulosclerosis Membranous nephropathy Diabetic glomerulonephropathy Amyloid nephropathy	None
Nephrotic syndrome with red cell casts (mixed nephritic/ nephrotic)	Membranoproliferative GN Mesangioproliferative GN Crescenteric GN (early) SLE nephritis (some patterns; see page 563)	None
Acute renal failure	Crescenteric GN (rapidly progressive) Diseases with extensive tuft necrosis (e.g. SLE vasculitis syndromes etc.)	Hypoperfusion (pre-renal) Toxic tubular necrosis Extensive renal infarction Extensive renal infection Septicemia Disseminated intravascular coagulation in multi-organ failure (all causes)
Chronic renal failure	End stages of all of the above glomerular lesions in this column	Congenital diseases (see page 389) Hypertensive renal disease Tubulointerstitial disease (e.g. chronic renal infection, nephrotoxic drugs)

The kidney is frequently affected in diabetes mellitus

Diabetes is now one of the most common causes of end-stage kidney disease. The kidney lesions can be divided into three main forms:

- Lesions of the arterial and arteriolar supply to the glomeruli.
- Lesions of the glomerulus.
- Lesions of the tubules and interstitium.

Glomerular lesions are particularly frequent in long-standing juvenile (type I) diabetes (see page 569), whereas the vascular and tubulointerstitial lesions occur in both type I and type II (maturity onset diabetes).

Vascular disease in diabetes reduces blood flow through the glomeruli

Diabetics have particularly severe atheromatous disease which not only involves large and medium arteries but also extends into smaller branch arteries than is the case in non-diabetics. The intimal thickening associated with atheroma leads to a reduction of the vessel lumen, particularly marked in the small arteries. The arterioles undergo hyaline thickening of their walls, similar to that seen in benign hypertensive nephrosclerosis (see *Fig. 17.11*). The reduction in luminal size of arteries and arterioles leads initially to poor glomerular perfusion by blood, with reduced glomerular filtration rates (see page 359), and ultimately to glomerular ischemia.

Diabetic glomerular disease involves three main changes

The three main features are:

- **Diffuse thickening of the glomerular capillary basement membranes.** The membranes show homogeneous thickening, and can be up to three to five times normal thickness late in the illness

(*Fig. 17.29a*). Although thick, these basement membranes leak protein, and the patient initially develops proteinuria, eventually leading to the nephrotic syndrome.
- **Diffuse mesangial sclerosis ('diffuse diabetic glomerulosclerosis')** is due to increased mesangial matrix production throughout all glomeruli, and leads to enlarged glomeruli with a prominent mesangium. Exudative lesions due to a combination of thick permeable basement membrane and abnormal mesangium may be visible as masses of red-staining coagulated protein (fibrin caps) on the surface of some segments of the glomerulus (*Fig. 17.29b*).
- **Nodular diabetic glomerulosclerosis** is localized pattern of mesangial sclerosis, confined to occasional segments, formed when the mesangial cells deposit matrix in a concentrically laminated pattern, so that the sclerotic mass is spherical (*Fig. 17.29c*). These lesions are called Kimmelstiel–Wilson nodules, and are virtually only seen in advanced diabetic kidney disease.

Although the basement membrane thickening produces proteinuria and the nephrotic syndrome, the other two features lead to expansion of the mesangial matrix, crushing the glomerular capillaries, which are usually already poorly perfused because of the arterial and arteriolar disease. When blood ceases to flow through a glomerulus, the nephron dies. As more nephrons die, the patient develops chronic renal failure.

There are probably many factors involved in the pathogenesis of the glomerular lesions in diabetic nephropathy. The metabolic disorders in diabetes mellitus (hyperglycemia, insulin deficiency) may be responsible for the alteration in capillary basement membrane thickness and in its biochemical structure and integrity, particularly in the amount and nature of the protein and proteoglycan present. Such factors may also be responsible for the increase in mesangial matrix which occurs, culminating in progressive glomerular sclerosis.

Fig. 17.29 Diabetic renal disease. (a) Basement-membrane thickening. (b) Exudative lesions. (c) Nodular glomerulosclerosis.
Diabetes causes basement-membrane thickening, seen on electron microscopy (a). Exudative lesions (b) are seen as fibrin-like material (**F**) over the tips of glomerular capillary loops. In nodular glomerulosclerosis (c), rounded hyaline areas develop in glomeruli, termed 'Kimmelstiel–Wilson nodules' (**K**).

Diabetes affects tubulointerstitial tissues in three main ways

Diabetes can affect the tubules and interstitium in the following ways:

- The combination of diabetic vascular and glomerular disease (page 569) leads to reduced glomerular blood flow, with consequent poor flow through afferent arterioles and peritubular capillaries. This leads to **chronic ischemic injury** to tubules and interstitium. The tubules atrophy, and the interstitium shows fibrosis.
- In diabetics, the kidney is particularly prone to acute bacterial infection (**acute pyelonephritis**, page 382), which particularly affects tubules and interstitium. Many collecting tubules and ducts contain pus, with the naked-eye cut surface appearance of linear yellow streaks in the medulla and small abscesses in the cortical tubules and interstitium (*Fig. 17.32*).
- The combination of chronic renal tubular and interstitial ischemia, with superimposed bacterial infection, predisposes to **renal papillary necrosis** (*Fig.17.30*) in which the papillae and variable amounts of the medullary pyramids undergo acute necrosis, possibly due to inflammatory thromboses in the vasa recta in the medulla. This acute phenomenon is not confined to diabetics, but may also occur when there is obstructive uropathy, with or without associated infection, in analgesic nephropathy (see page 384), and in patients with sickle cell disease, which particularly affects tubules and interstitium.

Whereas chronic ischemic injury plays a role in the slow relentless progression into chronic renal failure, both acute pyelonephritis and papillary necrosis usually precipitate acute renal failure, particularly in diabetics in whom renal functional impairment is already established.

Key Facts
Diabetic renal disease

- Severe atheroma of the aorta, main and branch renal arteries, with hyaline arteriolosclerosis, causes glomerular and tubular ischemia.
- Three patterns of glomerular abnormality (diffuse basement membrane thickening, diffuse and focal nodular glomerulosclerosis) lead to progressive glomerular hyalinization, with nephrotic syndrome and eventual chronic renal failure.
- Increased risk of pyelonephritis and papillary necrosis, both of which can precipitate acute renal failure.

Fig. 17.30 Renal papillary necrosis (a) macro (b) LP H&E. (a) & (b) Renal papillae (**P**) are pale and necrotic, with a line of demarcation from the adjacent viable kidney. The necrotic papillae are later shed.

Deposition of amyloid in glomeruli causes nephrotic syndrome and chronic renal failure

The kidney is a target organ in amyloidosis, a condition in which extracellular fibrillar protein is deposited in a variety of tissues. For a more detailed discussion, see Chapter 25. The amyloid is deposited as fibrils in the GBM and in the mesangium. As amyloid is deposited in the basement membrane, the membrane thickens and its permeability is increased, so that the first manifestation is **proteinuria**. With heavy deposition of amyloid, the protein loss increases until the patient develops features of the **nephrotic syndrome**.

Amyloid is an important cause of the nephrotic syndrome in adults. Heavy amyloid deposition in the mesangium, in combination with increased mesangial matrix formation, can eventually lead to expansion of the mesangium, ultimately leading to compression of the glomerular capillary system, and transition into **chronic renal failure**. Amyloid is also deposited in the walls of intrarenal vessels, particularly afferent arterioles.

Fig. 17.31 Amyloid in glomerulus TEM. The central capillary loop **C** is so far unaffected, but the two loops on either side are obliterated by the deposition of amyloid **A**.

> ## Key Facts
> ### Nephrotic syndrome in adults
>
> - Diabetes, SLE, amyloidosis, and other systemic disorders (40%).
> - Membranous nephropathy (20%).
> - At stages in natural history of most forms of glomerulonephritis (10–15%).
> - Focal glomerulosclerosis (10–20%, depending on local incidence of HIV).
> - Minimal change nephropathy (10%).
> - Membranoproliferative glomerulonephritis (5%).

> ## Key Facts
> ### Nephrotic syndrome in childhood
>
> - Minimal change glomerulonephritis (60%).
> - Focal glomerulosclerosis (10%).
> - At stages in natural history of some forms of glomerulonephritis (10%).
> - Membranoproliferative glomerulonephritis (10%).
> - Membranous glomerulonephritis (5%).
> - Secondary to systemic disorder (5%).

DISEASE OF RENAL TUBULES AND INTERSTITIUM

Disease of the renal tubules and interstitium accounts for a large number of cases of renal failure. The main causes of disease are infections, ischemia, and toxic and metabolic disorders. The main types of disease are **pyelonephritis** (acute and chronic), **acute tubular necrosis**, and **interstitial nephritis** (acute and chronic).

The most important and common type of tubulointerstitial inflammation is acute pyelonephritis due to bacterial infection

Acute pyelonephritis is caused by bacterial infection, with organisms entering the kidney by two routes:

- **Ascending infection from the lower urinary tract** (most common). Predisposing factors that lead to ascending urinary tract infection are pregnancy, diabetes mellitus, stasis of urine, e.g. due to lower urinary tract destruction by a calculus, enlarged prostate, or malignant invasive tumor in the pelvis, structural defects of the urinary tract, and reflux of urine from bladder into ureters (vesicoureteric reflux).
- **Bloodstream spread in bacteremic or septicemic states** (unusual). Although less common, this seems to be the most likely cause in elderly patients who develop pyrexia of unknown origin, often with rigors, and acute renal failure.

Clinically patients develop fever, rigors and pain in the back, often associated with signs of a lower urinary tract infection. Diagnosis is made by examination of urine, especially culture to demonstrate the organism responsible.

Most cases of infection are caused by *E. coli*, other enteric organisms being seen less frequently.

Macroscopically the kidneys show variable numbers of small, yellowish white cortical abscesses, which are usually spherical, under 2 mm in diameter, and sometimes surrounded by a zone of hyperemia; the cortical abscesses are often most prominent on the subcapsular surface, after the capsule has been stripped away (see *Fig. 17.32a*). In the medulla the abscesses tend to be in the form of yellowish-white linear streaks that converge on the papilla. The pelvicalyceal mucosa may be hyperemic or covered with a fibrinopurulent exudate.

Histologically the kidney shows neutrophilic purulent infiltrate throughout the cortex and medulla. In the medulla there is pus in the lumina of the collecting tubules and ducts, and in the cortex, pus lies within tubules and as small spherical abscesses within which bacterial colonies can sometimes be seen (see *Fig. 17.32b*).

If untreated, acute pyelonephritis may give rise to the following complications:

- **Acute renal failure** – particularly if the infection is bilateral, or renal function is already impaired by some other disease, e.g. diabetes.
- **Gram-negative septicemia** – with severe shock, and often multiorgan failure.
- **Papillary necrosis** – often with shedding of necrotic papillae into urine, and almost invariably followed by acute renal failure (see pages 381, 571).
- **Perinephric abscess** – if infection spreads out of the kidney into perinephric fat. This is particularly likely to occur when there is pyelonephritis (see below), associated with the presence of large calculi in the pelvicalyceal system (see page 392).
- **Pyonephrosis** – in which the pelvicalyceal system becomes distended with pus; this tends to occur when there is obstruction at the pelviureteric junction or lower (e.g. by a calculus – see page 392).

Fig. 17.32 Acute pyelonephritis. Macroscopically, small microabscesses are visible as white spots beneath the renal capsule (a). Histologically (b), the kidney is infiltrated with neutrophils (**N**) with occasional bacterial colonies (**B**) visible.

Fig. 17.33 Tuberculous pyelonephritis. Caseous material fills the renal pelvis and calyces.

Chronic pyelonephritis is characterized by chronic interstitial inflammation associated with large scars of the kidney

Chronic pyelonephritis is a common cause of end-stage chronic renal failure, accounting for about 15% of all cases. The disease is characterized by interstitial chronic inflammation and scarring, which destroys nephrons. The areas of scarring are associated with distortion of the pelvicalyceal system of the kidney. Renal-induced hypertension may develop, and hypertension-induced vascular damage (page 164) can increase renal damage.

There are two forms of chronic pyelonephritis: reflux-associated and obstructive.

In the most common form, **reflux-associated chronic pyelonephritis**, reflux of urine from the bladder up the ureters predisposes to recurrent bouts of inflammation, leading to scarring. This occurs in childhood, and disease becomes manifest in early adult life, with progressive impairment of renal function.

In **obstructive chronic pyelonephritis**, recurrent episodes of infection occur in a kidney in which there is obstruction to the pelvicalyceal drainage. The obstruction, which can be at any level in the lower urinary tract, may be due either to anatomical abnormality or to renal tract stone.

Kidneys have irregular areas of scarring, seen as depressed areas 0.5–2 cm in size. The scars are sited over a club-shaped distorted renal calyx and are associated with fibrous scarring of the renal papilla. The most common site for these areas of scarring is the renal calyces at the poles of the kidney.

Histologically the kidney has irregular areas of interstitial fibrosis with chronic inflammatory cell infiltration. Tubules are atrophic or may be dilated and contain proteinaceous material. Glomeruli show periglomerular fibrosis and many demonstrate complete hyalinization.

Tuberculous pyelonephritis may lead to destruction of the whole kidney

Tuberculous pyelonephritis is characterized by white caseous material filling the pelvicalyceal system, which may be unilaterally or bilaterally affected (*Fig. 17.33*). Infection is initially renal, but over a period of months or years enlarges and ruptures into the pelvicalyceal system, releasing tubercle bacilli into the lower urinary tract. This can lead to the development of tuberculous ureteritis, cystitis and, in the male, prostatitis and epididymo-orchitis.

With time, extension of caseous granulomatous inflammation leads to destruction of cortex and medulla, so that at the end stage of the disease the kidneys are reduced to cystic masses of partially calcified caseous material; if both kidneys are affected, chronic renal failure results.

This pattern of renal involvement in TB is distinct from renal involvement in rapidly progressive **miliary TB**, in which the kidney is just one of many organs that receive large numbers of tubercle bacilli, spread from a fulminating lung infection. In miliary TB there are very large numbers of small tuberculous granulomas scattered throughout both kidneys. The patient usually dies before the individual granulomas can enlarge and show much caseation.

Acute tubular necrosis is a common and important cause of reversible acute renal failure

In acute tubular necrosis (ATN), metabolic or toxic disturbances cause necrosis of renal tubular epithelial cells. Although the tubular epithelial cells die and are shed, regeneration is possible if the damaging stimulus is corrected, as residual viable tubular epithelial cells can proliferate to repopulate the tubules. It is this regenerative capacity of the tubular epithelial cells that permits adequate tubular functioning after renal transplantation following a prolonged period of hypoxia of the graft.

There are two main groups of causative factors: ischemic and toxic. **Ischemic tubular necrosis** is caused by failure of renal perfusion. This is usually the result of hypotension and hypovolemia in shock, or may occur after extensive acute blood loss. Clinical situations that carry a high risk of developing ischemic ATN are major surgery, severe burns, hemorrhage, and causes of severe hypotension and shock.

Toxic causes of ATN are rarer and include:

- **Endogenous products**, including hemoglobinuria and myoglobinuria.
- **Heavy metals**, including lead and mercury.
- **Organic solvents**, including chloroform and ethylene glycol.
- **Drugs,** including NSAIDs, some antibiotics, and cyclosporine.
- **Other toxins**, including paraquat, phenol, and products of some poisonous fungi.

There are three phases to ATN:

1. **Oliguric phase**. A damaging stimulus causes necrosis of renal tubular epithelium. There is blockage of renal tubules by necrotic cells, and a secondary reduction in glomerular blood flow (caused by arteriolar constriction) reduces glomerular filtration. Macroscopically, the kidneys are diffusely swollen and edematous (*Fig. 17.34a*). Patients develop acute renal failure and oliguria. Supportive measures are required to prevent hyperkalemia and fluid overload.
2. **Polyuric phase**. Over 1–3 weeks, regeneration of renal tubular epithelium takes place, with removal of dead material by phagocytic cells, as well as in the form of casts in urine. As tubules open up and glomerular blood flow increases, patients develop polyuria. This is because the regenerated tubular cells are undifferentiated and have not developed the specializations necessary for resorption of electrolytes and water. Replacement of fluid and electrolytes is needed to compensate for excessive loss from urine.
3. **Recovery phase**. Tubular cells re-establish differentiation and there is restoration of homeostatic renal function.

Fig. 17.34 Acute tubular necrosis. (a) Shows the kidney to be pale and swollen, with loss of corticomedullary demarcation. (b) Histology of the cortex shows degeneration and necrosis of tubular epithelium, with swelling of cytoplasm and pyknosis of nuclei.

Interstitial nephritis is an inflammatory disease of renal interstitium and tubules

Interstitial nephritis is characterized by inflammation in the interstitium, associated with tubular atrophy or damage. There are many causes, the main one of which is exposure to drugs, particularly certain analgesics and antibiotics. Less commonly, physical agents such as irradiation cause a similar pattern of tubulointerstitial damage. Many cases of diagnosed chronic interstitial nephritis have no determinable cause and are regarded as idiopathic.

Drug-induced acute interstitial nephritis presents 2–3 weeks after exposure to a causative agent, with fever, hematuria, proteinuria and elevated blood urea. In some cases acute renal failure develops. There is edema of the interstitium, associated with lymphocytic and eosinophil inflammatory infiltration. Tubules may show epithelial degeneration or necrosis. It is thought that an immune reaction to drugs is the underlying mechanism. Recovery usually takes place on withdrawal of the causative agent.

Drug-induced chronic interstitial nephritis is characterized by the development of chronic renal failure after exposure to a causative agent. There is interstitial fibrosis, chronic inflammation, and atrophy of tubules.

Analgesic nephropathy is a form of tubulointerstitial disease caused by the administration of analgesic agents, particularly phenacetin and NSAIDs. It is also associated with renal papillary necrosis. After long-term exposure to the causative agent, patients develop renal tubular failure with polyuria, metabolic acidosis and, ultimately, chronic renal failure. Analgesic nephropathy is associated with an increased risk of development of carcinoma of the urothelium (see page 393).

Radiation nephritis is seen after the kidneys are included in the field of radiation used to treat malignancy. There is hyalinization of glomeruli and small vessels, with later ischemic tubular atrophy and interstitial fibrosis.

Metabolic abnormalities may cause secondary tubular damage

Urate nephropathy is seen in a small proportion of patients with hyperuricemia. Precipitation of urate crystals occurs in the renal collecting ducts, causing tubular damage, inflammation and later scarring.

Nephrocalcinosis is caused by persistent hypercalcemia. Calcification occurs in the renal parenchyma, particularly the tubular basement membrane, with tubular damage and later fibrosis. During the development of this condition there is failure of tubular function and the development of polyuria.

Myeloma (see page 314) causes casts of secreted Bence Jones protein to precipitate out in renal tubules, causing physical obstruction of tubules. Amyloid may develop in glomeruli (see Chapter 25) and, if the myeloma is associated with hypercalcemia due to bone destruction, there may be superimposed nephrocalcinosis. Urography with certain contrast agents may precipitate acute tubular blockage and acute renal failure.

Oxalate is an end-product of sugar and amino acid metabolism, and is usually efficiently excreted by the kidney. However, when in excess, it reacts with calcium ions to form crystalline calcium oxalate which can be the basis of some renal calculi (see page 392). In the rare autosomal recessive disorders primary hyperoxaluria types 1 and 2, very high blood levels of oxalate lead to extensive calcium oxalate deposition in the tubules and interstitium of the kidney, leading to chronic renal failure (*Fig. 17.35*) as the deposition eventually destroys all the nephrons. The disease recurs in transplanted kidneys unless the underlying liver enzyme defects are addressed by simultaneous liver transplantation.

RENAL TRANSPLANTATION

Renal transplantation is increasingly being performed as a treatment for end-stage renal failure. After transplantation, several complications may occur, including thrombosis of the surgical vascular anastomosis leading to ischemia in the graft, transplant rejection, or recurrence of disease in transplanted kidney, e.g. membranoproliferative glomerulonephritis.

Four patterns of renal transplant rejection are recognized

The four patterns of rejection seen after renal transplantation are hyperacute rejection, acute rejection, accelerated acute rejection, and chronic rejection.

Hyperacute rejection occurs within a very short time of the organ being perfused by the host's blood. It takes the form of widespread intravascular thrombosis in small vessels, with focal necrosis and neutrophil infiltration. It is the result of preformed host antibodies reacting instantly with antigens in the graft, and in the past was almost entirely due to host antibody against donor blood group substances; it was therefore nearly always the result of blood-group incompatibility. More recently, it is due to preformed anti-HLA antibodies in recipient blood, formed by prior exposure to blood transfusions, or from previous grafts. Although a problem in early renal transplants, since testing recipients for the presence of antibodies to donor lymphocytes became routine practice, hyperacute rejection is now almost never seen.

Acute rejection occurs within a week or so of the graft being inserted, but may also appear after cessation of immunosuppressive therapy. It is termed 'acute' because it typically progresses rapidly, being mediated by both humoral and cell-mediated mechanisms.

- The cellular component of acute rejection is mediated by T-cells reacting against donor HLA antigens, particularly class II. The graft becomes infiltrated by lymphocytes, most of which are T cells, and the lymphocytes destroy various components of the graft, including tubules (**acute cellular rejection**).
- The humoral component of acute rejection is characterized by vasculitis with endothelial necrosis, neutrophil infiltration of vessel walls, and damage to the intima and elastic lamina of the larger arteries in the graft (**acute vascular rejection**).

Fig. 17.35 Oxalate deposits in kidney: 2 μm resin section. (Toluidine blue). Postmortem histology from a patient who died in chronic renal failure due to primary hyperoxaluria. The kidneys were small, hard and gritty due to massive oxalate deposits (clear crystals, arrowed). The inset shows the crystals by polarising microscopy.

Parenchymal damage caused by the cellular acute rejection usually responds rapidly to immunosuppressive therapy, whereas damage caused by vascular pathology associated with the humoral component may be permanent. A typical case of acute rejection has a mixture of both components.

Accelerated acute rejection can occur in a patient who has had a previous unsuccessful graft and is therefore already sensitized to donor antigens.

Chronic rejection occurs slowly and progressively over some months. The result of slow breakdown of the host's tolerance to the graft, it may be due to inadequate immune suppression. Histologically, there is intimal fibrosis in arteries in the graft, leading to secondary ischemic damage to the parenchyma. The interstitium is infiltrated by plasma cells and lymphocytes.

TUMORS OF THE KIDNEY

Benign tumors of the kidney are commonly seen as an incidental finding and are of little clinical significance. The main tumors of the kidney in adults are renal adenocarcinomas; metastatic tumors are seen, but they are uncommon. Transitional cell carcinomas of the renal pelvis are considered in the section on disease of the lower urinary tract. The only other important renal tumor is nephroblastoma (Wilms' tumor), which is seen almost exclusively in early childhood.

Benign tumors of the kidney are frequent incidental findings

Benign tumors of the kidney are common incidental findings at postmortem examination and may also be encountered as incidental findings on imaging.

Renal cortical adenomas are benign tumors derived from renal tubular epithelium. They are spherical, well circumscribed, and pale yellow in color. The histological appearances are varied, but with a papillary pattern predominating, hence they are often called renal papillary adenomas. They share macroscopic and microscopic features with the papillary pattern of renal adenocarcinoma (see below), but are generally smaller. In order to separate them from adenocarcinomas, an arbitrary cut-off point of 3 cm was once adopted, but proven metastases from tumors less than 3 cm has spoilt the story, and these tumors are regarded as being of low-grade malignancy or of having malignant potential.

Renal medullary fibromas are very common small spherical white benign tumors found in the renal medulla. They are typically 3–10 mm in diameter, and discovered incidentally at necropsy. They are composed of spindle cells, and may be hamartomas rather than true neoplasms

Renal oncocytomas are benign epithelial tumors composed of large cells with granular eosinophilic cytoplasm containing many mitochondria.

Angiomyolipomas are tumors composed of smooth muscle, adipose tissue and large blood vessels. Sometimes they are associated with tuberous sclerosis (see page 479).

Renal adenocarcinoma is the most common malignant tumor of the kidney

Usually seen after the age of 50 years, renal adenocarcinoma classically presents with hematuria and loin pain. In the early stages, the hematuria (due to tumor infiltrating into the pelvicalyceal system) may be intermittent and insignificant, hence easily missed or ignored. Loin pain, and later an awareness of a mass in the loin, is suggestive of a large tumor stretching or invading the renal capsule. Renal adenocarcinoma is one of the tumors that occasionally presents as a result of bloodborne metastases, such as bone pain or pathological fracture due to bone secondaries, or brain symptoms due to a cerebral metastasis. Multiple rounded lung metastases ('cannonball secondaries') are usually associated with a primary renal tumor invading a main renal vein (see below). Renal carcinomas are often also associated with paraneoplastic syndromes of hypercalcemia, hypertension, polycythemia, or Cushing's syndrome caused by ectopic or inappropriate hormone secretion. Renal adenocarcinomas account for around 3% of all carcinomas in adults.

Macroscopically these tumors are usually rounded masses, with a yellowish cut face marked with areas of hemorrhage and necrosis (*Fig. 17.36*). There are three main histological patterns:

- **Clear cell carcinoma** is the most common (over 70%), and is composed of tumor cells with clear cytoplasm due to the high content of glycogen and lipid (*Fig. 17.37*)
- **Papillary renal carcinoma** is the second most common (10–20%) and may be multiple. The overlap with apparently benign papillary tumors has already been mentioned.
- **Chromophobe carcinoma** is the rarest pattern, and has cytological similarities with the benign oncocytoma.

Fig. 17.36 Adenocarcinoma of the kidney. A renal carcinoma appears as a yellow mass (**M**), with areas of necrosis and hemorrhage.

Fig. 17.37 Renal adenocarcinoma. Clear-cell carcinoma of the kidney is composed of uniform vacuolated cells.

The tumor spreads by local expansion (breaking through the renal capsule into perinephric fat), by lymphatics to regional lymph nodes, and by bloodborne metastasis (involving lungs, bone, brain and other sites as a result of tumor invasion of the renal vein). A characteristic behavioral feature is that large tumors may grow as a solid core along the main renal vein, even entering the inferior vena cava. Prognosis depends on the stage at presentation: if tumor is confined within the renal capsule, there is a 70% 5-year survival; however, prognosis is very poor if the tumor has broken through the capsule into perinephric fat, if there is renal vein invasion, or if metastases are present at diagnosis.

Etiology and molecular pathology of renal cell carcinoma

Recent work has revealed common cytogenetic abnormalities that relate to specific histological subtypes of tumor.

- **Clear cell carcinoma** is associated with inactivation of the tumor suppressor gene VHL located on chromosome 3p25. Clear cell carcinoma is increased in von Hippel–Lindau syndrome (see page 479) as a consequence of inherited somatic mutations in the VHL gene. However, in the more common sporadic cases of clear cell carcinoma, inactivation of the VHL gene is due to gene deletion resulting from allelic loss of entire segments of chromosome 3p, containing the VHL gene, followed by somatic mutation or hypermethylation of the remaining copy.
- **Papillary renal cell tumors** can also be divided into familial and sporadic forms. In contrast to clear cell carcinomas, papillary renal cell carcinomas are associated with amplification of the MET proto-oncogene on chromosome 7q31. Familial cases are associated with trisomy of chromosome 7 linked to mutations in MET that result in overexpression. Sporadic cases also show trisomy of chromosome 7 but, in contrast, mutations in MET are absent. Sporadic cases can also show trisomies of other chromosomes. The genes associated with these chromosomes have not been identified.
- **Chromophobe renal cell carcinomas** show multiple combinations of chromosome loss. The cytogenetic patterns in these tumors are so diverse that the underlying genetic mutation has not been identified. Although these different cytogenetic findings do not appear to correlate with the stage, grade or biological behavior of tumors, they are opening the way for a molecular, rather than a histological, classification of this type of carcinoma.

Nephroblastoma is one of the common malignant tumors of childhood

Nephroblastoma (Wilms' tumor) is an embryonal tumor derived from the primitive metanephros. Although it does occasionally occur in adults, it is predominantly a tumor of young children, with a peak incidence between the ages of 1 and 4 years.

The tumor presents as an abdominal mass or, less frequently, with hematuria. Macroscopically, tumors are rounded masses that replace large amounts of the kidney, appearing as solid, fleshy, white lesions with frequent areas of necrosis (see *Fig. 17.38*). Histologically, there are various combinations of four elements, these being primitive small-cell blastomatous tissue resembling the developing meta-nephric blastema, immature-looking glomerular structures, epithelial tubules, and stroma composed of spindle cells and striated muscle. Other heterologous components, such as cartilage and osteoid, neural tissue, and even mucinous and squamous epithelium, are occasionally seen.

Prognosis is related to spread of tumor at diagnosis, lung metastases often being present. The presence of histological features of anaplasia (cells with large pleomorphic and hyperchromatic nuclei and frequent abnormal mitoses) in tumors is associated with a poor prognosis. Although these tumors grow rapidly and there is often evidence of spread at the time of diagnosis, treatment with a combination of nephrectomy, radiotherapy and intensive chemotherapy achieves a high cure rate. Even with metastases, current therapy produces a 90–95% 2-year survival rate, provided there is no extensive anaplasia in the original tumor at diagnosis. A 2-year survival can be regarded as cure.

Fig. 17.38 Nephroblastoma. The kidney is extensively replaced by fleshy, white tumor.

Molecular pathology of Wilms' tumor

Wilms' tumor appears to represent more than one genetic entity. At least three different genes seem to be important in the origin of Wilms' tumor, the best characterized being WT1, a tumor-suppressor gene on chromosome 11. Mutations in this gene may be associated with congenital loss of iris (aniridia), and it is likely that the development of Wilms' tumor follows a 'two-hit' model for tumor suppressor genes (see Chapter 6), in that there are cases in which both copies of the gene are defective or lost.

CONGENITAL DISEASES OF THE KIDNEY AND LOWER URINARY TRACT

DEVELOPMENTAL DISEASES OF THE URINARY TRACT

Developmental diseases of the kidneys are often seen associated with other abnormalities of development

Developmental renal disease is a common clinical problem, often found in association with other congenital abnormalities. The main developmental abnormalities of the kidney can be classified as: agenesis, failure of differentiation (renal dysplasia), abnormal anatomic development, abnormalities of renal tubular transport, and developmental abnormalities of structural elements.

Bilateral renal agenesis occurs as part of Potter's syndrome. Affected infants have abnormal facies and, frequently, abnormalities of the lower urinary tract, lungs and nervous system. Characteristically, because the kidneys are not present to contribute to amniotic fluid, there is oligohydramnios in pregnancy.

During development, there may be failure of differentiation of metanephric tissues, leading to **renal dysplasia**. This may affect a whole kidney or just one segment, and may be unilateral or bilateral. The affected areas are replaced by solid and cystic masses in which cartilage is usually prominent (see *Fig. 5.4* and page 57).

Renal development may be anatomically abnormal, leading to **horseshoe kidney** (see *Fig. 17.34*), in which the two kidneys are fused across the midline, and **pelvic kidney** in which the kidney is sited low in the pelvis.

Fig. 17.39 Horseshoe kidney. The kidneys are fused across the midline in front of the aorta (**A**). The ureters are kinked over the joining segment, and this may be an unusual cause of hydronephrosis.

Genetic defects in type IV collagen production lead to inherited kidney disease

There are two main divisions, **Alport syndrome** and **thin basement membrane disease** (also called benign familial hematuria), which have different clinical manifestations, although both usually initially present with microscopic persistent or recurrent hematuria. Both are associated with mutations in the genes coding for the A3, A4 and A5 components of type IV collagen.

Alport syndrome may be X-linked, autosomal recessive or autosomal dominant, but most cases are X-linked (>80%). In the early stages the hematuria is associated with diminished hearing, and with the passage of time these progress to chronic renal failure and sensorineural deafness, often with visual impairment due to a range of eye abnormalities, particularly anterior lenticonus (an abnormality in lens shape). The renal lesion is due to an abnormally thin and irregular glomerular basement membrane, followed by progressive mesangial sclerosis leading to slow destruction of the glomeruli and progressive loss of nephrons. Most males with the X-linked pattern develop end-stage renal disease between the ages of 20 and 40, often having passed through a phase of heavy proteinuria and the nephrotic syndrome. Women with X-linked disease also have hematuria, but a much smaller percentage progress to renal failure, and more slowly.

Thin basement membrane disease is also due to abnormalities in the genes for A3 and A4 components of type IV collagen, but the disease shows autosomal dominant inheritance, is not associated with extrarenal disease, and the renal lesion does not progress to end-stage renal failure, although renal biopsies late in the disease show increased focal and segmental mesangial sclerosis, and there is an increased incidence of hypertension. The underlying renal abnormality is again diffuse thinning of the glomerular basement membrane (see *Fig. 17.40*).

CYSTIC DISEASE OF THE KIDNEY

Cysts in the kidney are common, but few lead to renal impairment

Cysts in the kidney are a common finding at postmortem and have many causes, but only a few types cause impairment of renal function. This forms a useful basis for memorizing the types.

Cystic diseases that do not cause renal failure

- **Simple benign renal cyst** is the most common type and may be single or multiple. They are thin-walled and filled with clear yellow fluid. They have no impact on renal function, but may cause confusion with renal carcinoma on some radiological investigations.
- **Medullary sponge kidney** occurs in adults and is usually asymptomatic. All the papillae contain cystically dilated collecting ducts (*Fig.17.41*). It may be complicated by calcification and calculus formation in the cysts, with occasional symptoms due to the calculi or secondary infection.
- **Dialysis-associated cystic disease** occurs in the kidneys of patients who already have end-stage renal failure and have been treated by dialysis for many years. The cysts occur in both cortex and medulla, and may contain oxalate crystals.

Cystic diseases that cause renal failure

- **Autosomal dominant polycystic kidney disease (ADPKD)** is the most common of this group. Both kidneys gradually become entirely replaced by large numbers of enlarging fluid-filled cysts which are sometimes hemorrhagic. The functioning renal parenchyma is gradually compressed out of existence by the enlarging cysts over a period of years, so that renal failure usually only develops in adult life,

Fig. 17.40 Thin basement membrane disease (EM). At first sight, these glomerular basement membranes appear normal, but multiple measurements show thicknesses range between 170 and 280 nm (normal range 300–400 nm). The diagnosis can easily be missed.

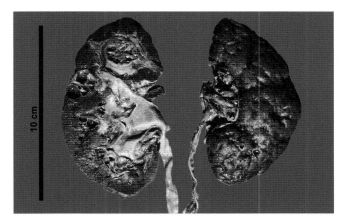

Fig. 17.41 Medullary sponge kidney. The cut surface of the left kidney shows clusters of small cysts confined to the medullae. The other specimen shows the surface of the right kidney from the same patient; the surface scarring is due to repeated attacks of secondary pyelonephritis.

Fig. 17.42 Adult polycystic disease. The kidney is converted into a mass of large cysts. Hemorrhage into cysts is common, leading to bloodstained contents.

unfortunately often after the patient has passed on the gene mutation. The vast majority (90%) of cases result from mutations in the *PDK1* gene that encodes the cell matrix protein polycystin 1. The remaining 10% are the result of mutations in the *PDK2* gene encoding polycystin 2. Polycystins 1 and 2 form heterodimers, and loss of either protein results in cyst formation following the classic 'second-hit' hypothesis. By the time chronic renal failure develops, the patient usually has systemic hypertension and the kidneys are often enormously enlarged, so that the patient may also complain of abdominal swelling. This type is illustrated in *Fig. 17.42*. Cysts also occur in the liver, lungs and pancreas, but cause no symptoms in these sites.

There is also an association with berry aneurysms of the cerebral arteries (page 456) which, with the often associated hypertension, predispose to subarachnoid hemorrhage (page 460).

- **Autosomal recessive polycystic kidney disease (ARPKD)** is rare, and both kidneys are always involved. There are perinatal, neonatal, infantile and juvenile types, of which the perinatal type is the most severe (with renal failure before or at birth) and the juvenile type the least severe. The kidneys are larger than normal and show an unusual radial pattern of elongated cysts replacing cortex and medulla. Cystic

changes are also present in the liver, associated with periportal fibrosis and bile ductule proliferation; these changes are particularly prominent in the rare juvenile type, and may produce portal hypertension. A wide range of gene mutations has been described in this condition, all associated with chromosome 6p.

- **Nephronophthisis (uremic medullary disease)** is the term applied to a group of diseases that begin mainly in childhood and are associated with multiple small cysts concentrated mainly at the corticomedullary junction. It is likely that these are secondary changes to the primary abnormality, which is interstitial fibrosis associated with progressive destruction of cortical and medullary tubules. There are three patterns of this disease complex, with both autosomal dominant and recessive types having differing clinical features, but all tend to present in childhood with polyuria and polydipsia (due to early failure of concentrating capacity of the renal tubules) and to progress to renal failure by the age of 10 years. A fourth rare type presents in adult life. The autosomal recessive type (familial juvenile nephronophthisis) is the most common pattern.

Cystic change also occurs in renal dysplasia (see page 57) which, when bilateral, leads to renal failure.

DISEASES OF THE LOWER URINARY TRACT

The lower urinary tract extends from the calyces in the kidney to the distal end of the urethra, and is structurally adapted to transmit urine from the kidney to the exterior, the bladder being modified to act as a reservoir. The lower urinary tract is lined by urothelium (**transitional-cell epithelium**), which is capable of resisting the osmotic stresses of contact with urine.

There are five main groups of disorders in the lower urinary tract: **infection**, which is often secondary to stasis of urine, following obstruction to flow; **obstruction** by intrinsic occlusion or extrinsic pressure; **stone formation**, which is often secondary to stasis of urine combined with infection; **tumor formation**, i.e. neoplasia of transitional-cell epithelium; and **developmental abnormalities**.

INFECTION

Infections in the lower urinary tract are predisposed to by obstruction and stasis

Lower urinary tract infection is usually due to Gram-negative coliform bacilli, e.g. *E. coli* and *Proteus* spp., which are normally commensals in the large bowel; because they have a short urethra, women are particularly prone to developing ascending infections. In men, lower urinary tract infection is usually associated with structural abnormalities of the lower urinary tract and stasis due to obstruction.

Diabetes mellitus also predisposes to infection. In most cases the lower urinary tract infection remains localized to the urethra and bladder, but organisms may ascend the ureter and enter the pelvicalyceal system, particularly when there is an obstructive lesion. An **acute bacterial urethritis** and **cystitis** may lead to an ascending **ureteritis** and **pyelitis** (inflammation of the renal pelvis and calyces). In this way, organisms may gain access to the renal parenchyma to produce **acute pyelonephritis**, with the formation of abscesses in the renal medulla and cortex (see page 382).

The main complications of lower urinary tract infection are acute and chronic pyelonephritis (see page 382–3), pyonephrosis (distension of the pelvicalyceal system with pus, usually the result of infection superimposed on obstruction, often at the pelviureteric junction), and papillary necrosis in severe infections, particularly in diabetics.

OBSTRUCTION

Obstruction of the drainage of urine from the kidney causes hydronephrosis

Obstruction, one of the most important consequences of disease of the lower urinary tract, may occur at any place in the tract:

- **Renal pelvis** – calculi, tumors.
- **Pelviureteric junction** – stricture, calculi, extrinsic compression.
- **Ureter** – calculi, extrinsic compression (pregnancy, tumor, fibrosis).
- **Bladder** – tumor, calculi.
- **Urethra** – prostatic hyperplasia or carcinoma, urethral valves, urethral stricture.

If obstruction occurs in the urethra, the bladder develops dilatation and secondary hypertrophy of muscle in its wall. This predisposes to development of outpouching of the bladder mucosa (diverticula).

If obstruction occurs in a ureter, there is dilatation of the ureter (**megaureter**), with progressive dilatation of the renal pelvicalyceal system, termed **hydronephrosis** (*Fig. 17.43*). Fluid entering the collecting ducts cannot empty into the renal pelvis and there is intrarenal resorption of fluid. At this stage, if the obstruction is relieved, renal function returns to normal. However, if obstruction persists, there is atrophy of renal tubules, glomerular hyalinization, and fibrosis. As an end-stage, the renal parenchyma becomes severely atrophic and renal function is permanently impaired (*Fig. 17.43b*). Usually, the end-stage of hydronephrosis develops only with unilateral obstruction of a ureter, as renal function is maintained by the non-obstructed kidney. With bilateral obstruction, most usual with lesions in the bladder base or retroperitoneal tissues, renal failure develops before severe atrophy of both kidneys does. The causes of hydronephrosis are shown in the clinical box below. Urinary tract obstruction also predisposes to infection and stone formation.

Hydronephrosis

Causes of hydronephrosis
Hydronephrosis can be caused by obstruction to the drainage of the kidney at many levels:

Idiopathic obstruction at the pelviureteric junction
Extrinsic compression of ureter (tumor or
   retroperitoneal fibrosis)
Tumor in renal pelvis or ureter (transitional cell
   carcinoma)
Calculus in ureter
Congenital ureteric abnormality (ureterocele)
Disease at base of bladder (carcinoma)
Compression of prostatic urethra (hyperplasia or
   carcinoma)
Urethral obstruction (urethral stricture of valves)

Fig. 17.43
Hydronephrosis.
(a) External. (b) Cut surface. In hydronephrosis (a) there is dilatation of the renal pelvis (**P**). In advanced disease (b) there is severe loss of renal parenchyma around a grossly dilated renal pelvicalyceal system.

URINARY CALCULI

Most renal calculi are composed of calcium oxalate and phosphate

Urinary calculi may form anywhere in the lower urinary tract (**urolithiasis**), the most common sites being the pelvicalyceal system and bladder. The two main predisposing factors for stone formation are increased concentration of solute in urine (low fluid throughput or primary increase in metabolite), and reduced solubility of solute in urine (due to persistently abnormal urinary pH). Conditions that cause these factors to operate are low fluid intake, urine stasis, persistent urinary tract infection, and primary metabolic disturbances.

Renal calculi are of four main types by chemical composition; in order of commonness they are:

- Calcium oxalate and phosphate calculi.
- Magnesium ammonium phosphate calculi (also called struvite stones).
- Uric acid calculi.
- Cystine calculi.

The most common urinary stones, accounting for 80% of cases, are composed of calcium oxalate or phosphate. Half of these cases are associated with idiopathic hypercalciuria, with only about 10% being caused by hypercalcemia. Other cases may be caused by hyperoxaluria, which has several associations, e.g. inflammatory bowel disease. The second most common type of calculi, accounting for 15% of cases, are those composed of magnesium, ammonium, and calcium phosphates (**struvite**). They are associated with infection in the lower urinary tract as a result of urea-splitting organisms, which make urine permanently alkaline.

Uric acid stones account for about 5% of cases and are predisposed to by conditions causing hyperuricemia, e.g. gout. However, 50% of patients with uric acid stones do not have hyperuricemia, and it is suggested that the production of persistently acid urine is the predisposing factor.

Cystine stones are rare, accounting for less than 1% of cases. They are seen in heritable tubular transport defects causing cystinuria.

Stones at different sites in the urinary tract have different appearances

Stones formed at different sites in the urinary tract have different morphological appearances. For example, calculi in the pelvicalyceal system are often multiple and may be small, taking the form of gravel. However, large, branching **staghorn calculi** occasionally form due to the constant accretion of calcium salts, conforming to the contours of the pelvicalyceal system (*Fig. 17.44*).

The presence of calculi in the pelvicalyceal system predisposes to persistent pelvicalyceal infection, pyonephrosis and perinephric abscess, and development of squamous metaplasia in the urothelium. Squamous cell carcinoma may occasionally occur in the metaplastic areas.

Most stones in the ureter have developed in the renal pelvis, secondarily passing down the urinary tract. Often this is associated with intense loin pain, termed **ureteric colic**, which may be associated with ureteric obstruction and hydronephrosis. In the bladder the stones are usually spherical and laminated, and may reach a large size. The main predisposition for stone formation in the bladder is stasis and chronic infection. The presence of bladder calculi causes squamous metaplasia in the urinary bladder and may be associated with development of squamous carcinoma.

> ### Key Facts
> #### Urinary calculi
>
> - Due to increased concentration of solute in urine or reduced solubility of product in urine.
> - Infection, stasis, and metabolic abnormalities are the main underlying causes.
> - Most commonly composed of calcium oxalate and phosphate, some being caused by hypercalciuria or hyperoxaluria.
> - The second most common are triple-phosphate stones caused by chronic infections.
> - Uncommon types are urate and cystine stones.

Fig. 17.44 Renal staghorn calculus. The renal pelvis is filled with a large calculus that is shaped to its contours, resembling the horn of a stag (**S**). The calyceal system at the lower pole contains separate rounded calculi.

TUMORS OF THE LOWER URINARY TRACT

Tumors of the lower urinary tract are derived from the transitional cells of the urothelium

Most tumors of the lower urinary tract, from renal calyces down to urethra, arise from urothelium, and are mainly caused by environmental agents excreted in high concentration in the urine (see pink box on page 394). A field change takes place throughout the urothelium, such that all areas are at risk of developing urothelial neoplasia; for this reason, multiple tumors are common.

The bladder is the most common site for the development of these tumors (*Fig. 17.45*), but they also occur in the renal pelvis (*Fig. 17.46*), the ureters and, rarely, the urethra. Most urothelial tumors have a papillary pattern, with delicate fronds protruding into the lumen of the lower urinary tract, covered by urothelial transitional type epithelium. Hence these are frequently called **transitional cell tumors** or **urothelial neoplasms**.

All urothelial tumors present with painless hematuria, sometimes accompanied by dysuria and frequency of micturition. When the tumor blocks a ureteric orifice there may be symptoms secondary to the obstruction, e.g. pyelonephritis.

Transitional cell urothelial tumors show a wide range of behaviors, from the almost completely benign, with little predilection for invasion, to the highly malignant with a high chance of invasion and metastasis.

Some indication of the likely behavior of a urothelial tumor is given by **histological grading** (WHO) into the following types:

- **Urothelial papilloma.**
- **Urothelial neoplasm of low malignant potential.**
- **Papillary urothelial carcinoma-low grade.**
- **Papillary urothelial carcinoma-high grade.**

This grading is based on the degree of cytological atypia exhibited by the urothelial cells of the tumor.

In urothelial papilloma they are virtually normal urothelial cells that form a covering of normal thickness, whereas in a urothelial tumor of low malignant potential the cell layer is thicker and the urothelial cells have large nuclei. The other two grades show increasing degrees of cytological atypia and nuclear pleomorphism, so that the high-grade lesion shows severely dysplastic cells with numerous cells in mitosis.

In these high-grade lesions the tumors are less papillary and may have little papillary element remaining at diagnosis, assuming the pattern of a flat raised or ulcerated plaque, by which time they are already showing invasive behavior.

True urothelial papilloma is rare. About 80% of tumors are low grade or of low malignant potential when first encountered, and 20% are high grade, of which a high proportion already show evidence of invasion at first diagnosis.

Fig. 17.45 Transitional-cell carcinoma. (a) A papillary urothelial carcinoma arises from the dome of the bladder as a fronded papillary lesion (T). (b) Histologically, lesions are composed of papillae covered with transitional epithelium. This is a low-grade tumor.

A further important pattern is **urothelial carcinoma in situ,** in which the urothelium shows patches of dysplastic epithelium with severe cytoplasmic and nuclear pleomorphism, and mitotic figures, but without any papillary pattern. These patches are often multiple and appear on cystoscopy as patches of red thickening of the normally pale bladder lining. This pattern is important because of the frequency of invasion, often forming a flat ulcerated lesion as described above.

Once invasion is present the prognosis depends not on the grading but on the staging based on the TNM classification (see pages 79–81). For urothelial tumors this is:

Tis – carcinoma in situ, no invasion.
T1 – tumor invades lamina propria only.
T2 – tumor invades muscularis propria.
T3 – tumor invades outside bladder.
T4 – tumor invades adjacent structures (e.g. colon).

Fig. 17.46 Transitional-cell carcinoma of the renal pelvis. Papillary transitional cell carcinoma (**T**) fills the renal pelvis with dilatation of the renal calyces caused by urinary obstruction.

Fig. 17.47 Urothelial carcinoma in situ. Urothelial carcinoma in situ is a flat lesion characterized by severe epithelial dysplasia but with no invasion across the basement membrane.

Fig. 17.48 Invasive urothelial carcinoma. This photomicrograph shows high-grade (poorly differentiated) urothelial carcinoma (**C**) invading into the muscle layers (**M**) of the bladder (stage T2).

Carcinogenesis in transitional-cell carcinoma

Transitional-cell carcinomas of the lower urinary tract can develop as a result of exposure to environmental agents excreted in high concentration in the urine. This is sometimes the result of occupational exposure to a carcinogen, and some cases of transitional-cell carcinoma are regarded as industrial diseases that are liable for compensation. The main carcinogens responsible are associated with cigarette smoking, aniline dyes, and the rubber industry (car-tire plants). Half of the population inherit two deleted genes for glutathione S transferase M1 (GSTM1), the enzyme that normally acts to detoxify many carcinogens. Studies have shown that the deleted 0/0 genotype for GSTM1 increases the risk of development of transitional-cell carcinoma in patients exposed to the carcinogenic effects of cigarette smoke; it has been estimated that this common genetic predisposition underlies about 25% of cases of transitional-cell carcinoma. Molecular genetic studies have shown several abnormalities in transitional-cell carcinoma. Monosomy and loss of heterozygosity for chromosome 9 suggest that a specific tumor suppressor gene is missing in a high proportion of tumors, and the hunt is on to characterize the gene responsible. Mutation of the p53 gene is seen in many tumors and is associated with tumor progression and invasion. Abnormal expression of several other oncogenes has been documented, and these are also associated with tumor progression.

Squamous cell carcinoma and adenocarcinoma of the bladder are uncommon lesions with special etiology

Non-transitional-cell carcinomas of the bladder, which account for about 15% of all tumors, can be broken down into squamous cell carcinomas, pure adenocarcinomas, mixed tumors (transitional-cell and adenocarcinomas), undifferentiated carcinomas, and spindle-cell carcinomas.

Squamous cell carcinomas of the lower urinary tract are most often seen in the bladder and renal pelvis. They are derived from metaplastic epithelium, most commonly associated with chronic irritation from a calculus. In endemic areas an important cause of squamous metaplasia and subsequent carcinoma is **schistosomiasis.**

Adenocarcinomas of the bladder are uncommon but are usually seen in the dome region, where they are believed to derive from persistent glandular tissue in urachal remnants. In some cases these tumors spread along a remnant track to the umbilicus. The rare congenital condition of exstrophy of the bladder, which is due to failure of closure, predisposes to the later development of adenocarcinoma.

Developmental abnormalities of the lower urinary tract

Developmental abnormalities in the lower urinary tract often accompany complex congenital malformation syndromes. They may also occur as isolated abnormalities, the most clinically significant being:

- **Ureteric defects** forming bifid or double ureters. These may be associated with vesicoureteric reflux, and predispose to recurrent infections.
- **Ureterocele** is a cyst of the lower ureter, sited at its passage through the bladder wall. The cyst bulges into the bladder and causes obstruction of the ureter, leading to hydroureter and hydronephrosis. The majority of cases (90%) are unilateral.
- **Persistent urachus** leads to a vesicoumbilical fistula, urachal cysts, and urachal sinuses.
- **Exstrophy of the bladder** (ectopia vesicae) is uncommon and is caused by failure of closure of the bladder, associated with a defect in the pelvis and abdominal wall. The bladder lining is exposed and the infant develops recurrent infections, leading to metaplasia of the transitional-cell epithelium to a glandular type. This condition predisposes to the development of adenocarcinoma of the bladder.
- **Posterior urethral valves** are folds of lining mucosa in the urethra that cause obstruction leading to hydronephrosis. They are more common in males than in females, and predispose to ascending pyelonephritis in children.

Case-based questions

Cases 1 and 2 Two boys with hematuria

Two boys, JB aged 7 and PD aged 9, are admitted to the Pediatric Nephrology Unit in the same week with almost identical symptoms of hematuria and limb edema. JB also had facial edema, and his mother thought that her son had been passing reduced quantities of urine for a few days; the mother of PD was not sure whether her son also had this symptom. Examination confirmed that both boys had edema, and also showed that both had hypertension, slightly worse in PD. Simple urine testing in the unit confirmed that they had hematuria, and laboratory testing showed that both had a raised blood urea and creatinine. According to the parents, both boys had suffered from a sore throat in the preceding couple of weeks.

1. What syndrome are these boys suffering from?

It is decided to treat them conservatively, with a mild diuretic to reduce edema and limit hypertension, but with regular monitoring of blood pressure, urine output and blood urea. JB showed reduction of edema, and his blood pressure and blood urea and creatinine began to reduce after 4 days. However, PD showed no improvement, and his blood pressure slowly increased as did his blood urea and creatinine. After 5 days of slow deterioration, it was decided to perform a renal biopsy on patient PD.

2. What do you think the biopsy in PD might show?
3. If JB had been subjected to biopsy on admission, what do you think the biopsy would have shown?

JB was discharged symptom free 2 weeks after admission, with a normal blood urea and normal blood pressure, the only residual abnormality being mild proteinuria, whereas PD's blood urea and creatinine continued to rise despite treatment, and he remained hypertensive. Over the following few weeks PD developed end-stage chronic renal failure and required regular dialysis until a renal transplant was performed. ▶

▶ **4. Describe the sequence of events that led to the destruction of almost all of PD's nephrons.**

JB made a complete recovery, with eventual disappearance of his mild proteinuria. In a small percentage of cases the proteinuria persists and slowly worsens over many years, sometimes leading to the nephrotic syndrome and eventual chronic renal failure.

5. What is happening at glomerular level in such cases?

Cases 3 and 4 Two girls with limb edema

Two girls, AW aged 6 and JL aged 9, are admitted to the Pediatric Nephrology Unit in the same week. Both have been referred by their family practitioners because of swelling of the lower legs and hands. The parents of both had noted that their urine had appeared 'thick' and frothy over the previous couple of weeks. The family practitioners had tested the urine of both girls and found severe proteinuria. On admission, examination confirmed the presence of edema, and laboratory investigations confirmed severe proteinuria and hypoalbuminemia.

1. What syndrome are these girls suffering from, and what is the most likely cause at this age?

Both girls were treated with prednisolone, and over the next couple of weeks AW showed improvement, with a reduction in proteinuria and gradual improvement in her blood albumin level and edema. JL, however, showed little or no improvement, and renal biopsy was performed.

2. If renal biopsy had been performed on AW on admission, what glomerular and tubular changes would you expect to see?
3. When renal biopsy was performed on JL after 5 weeks of non-response to steroids, what changes might you see?
4. If JL had been aged 43, what would have been the most likely causes of her syndrome?

Case 5 A routine urine analysis

During a routine medical examination for life insurance purposes a 23-year-old man is discovered to have microscopic hematuria and is referred to his family practitioner, who repeats the test on three further occasions, finding microscopic hematuria on each occasion. Although the patient feels well and has no symptoms, he is referred to the Nephrology Unit for assessment. Full examination reveals no abnormality, and there are no features in the clinical history to suggest a cause. Renal function is normal. Renal biopsy is performed, and the pathologist reports that preliminary H&E-stained paraffin sections show a focal segmental proliferative glomerulonephritis affecting three of the 12 glomeruli present in the first section of the biopsy.

1. What further investigative techniques would the pathologist apply to the biopsy sample?
2. What do you think these further investigations are most likely to reveal in this case?

The patient is discharged and followed up in the Nephrology Clinic at regular intervals. The microscopic hematuria never disappears, and he is noted to have slowly increasing proteinuria.

3. What is happening to the glomeruli in this case, and what is the likely long-term outcome without treatment?

Case 6 An accident victim

A 57-year-old man is admitted as an emergency with multiple injuries following a road traffic accident in which he sustained compound fractures of the tibia and fibula on both sides. On admission he is pale and shocked, with a blood pressure of 80 systolic and 40 diastolic despite intravenous fluid and plasma expanders given by paramedics at the site of the accident. It quickly becomes apparent that there is continuous intra-abdominal bleeding, and emergency laparotomy shows a ruptured spleen, which is removed, and a tear in the liver which is sutured with a hemostatic sponge in place. Despite blood transfusion he remains hypotensive throughout the subsequent orthopedic procedures to pin and plate his leg fractures. After all surgical procedures it is noted that he is not passing urine.

1. What has happened to his kidneys to prevent the formation of urine?
2. What is the most likely mechanism in this case?
3. What is the outlook for his renal function?

Brief answers to these case-based questions are given on pages 591–2. More detailed answers and other study resources are available online at www.studentconsult.com.

Male genital system   18

REVISION OF MALE GENITAL SYSTEM STRUCTURE

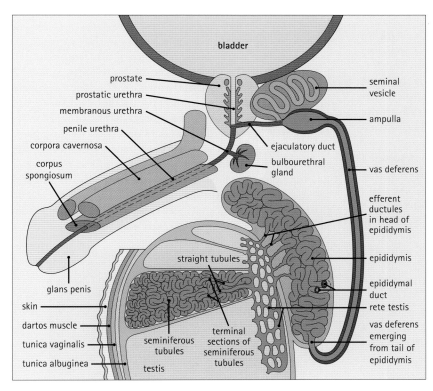

Fig. 18.1 Diagram of the male reproductive system. Spermatozoa production (spermatogenesis and spermiogenesis) occurs in the seminiferous tubules of the testis, and the spermatozoa pass along the lumina of the tubules to the rete testis at the hilum of the testis. From there they pass through several efferent ductules which fuse to form a single epididymal duct, which is highly coiled to form the structure called the epididymis. Within this duct they acquire their motility. The spermatozoa then pass into a long straight tube, the vas deferens, which carries them from within the scrotal sac to the ejaculatory ducts in the pelvis, on the way receiving the thick nutrient-rich secretions from the seminal vesicles. The right and left ejaculatory ducts pass through the prostate gland, receiving more secretions, and open into the prostatic urethra. The spermatozoa, suspended in the mixed secretions from seminal vesicles, prostate gland and bulbo-urethral glands (semen), pass along the penile urethra into the vagina during sexual intercourse.

Fig. 18.2 Histology of normal testis. The mature testis is largely composed of seminiferous tubules **T**, shown here in transverse and oblique section. Each tubule is highly convoluted so those shown here probably represent a single tubule, cut at many levels as it is folded back and forth. Each tubule has a distinct basement membrane sitting on a fibrocollagenous layer in which are located scattered contractile myoid cells, the whole being called the tunica propria (**arrows**). The seminiferous tubules are lined by the germinal epithelium which is responsible for producing spermatozoa. For details, refer to a histology textbook. In the interstices between tubules are blood vessels and clumps of Leydig (interstitial) cells (**L**), responsible for the synthesis of testosterone.

Maldescent of the testis (cryptorchidism) leads to increased risk of development of testicular tumors

In the embryo the testis develops high on the posterior abdominal wall from the genital ridge, and the germ cells migrate to the genital ridge from the yolk sac. At about the seventh month of gestation the testes descend from the posterior abdominal wall, through the inguinal canal and ring into the scrotum, guided by a cord, the gubernaculum. Occasionally, this descent fails to occur and the testis becomes arrested somewhere along its route, most commonly at or near the external inguinal ring or in the inguinal canal. Premature infant boys are particularly likely to be born with at least one undescended testis (about 30%), but it is also seen in a small proportion of term infants (3–5%).

Most undescended testes will descend into the scrotum spontaneously within the first 4 months of life, possibly stimulated by the rapid increase in gonadotropin and testosterone secretion that occurs in that period. If the testis has failed to descend by about 1 year of age, surgical correction by orchidopexy is usually undertaken, in which the testis is pulled down into the scrotum from the inguinal canal, and tethered to prevent its return.

The rationale for orchidopexy is that an undescended testis in the inguinal canal will not develop normally, in that germ cell maturation into spermatozoa will not take place and the testis remains small, with the seminiferous tubules being lined by Sertoli cells only. This may be because the body temperature in the inguinal canal is higher than in the scrotum, and this may be the factor that inhibits germ cell maturation. Orchidopexy within the first year of life increases the chances of normal or near-normal function in the affected testis.

One further reason for surgical intervention is that an undescended testis has a far greater chance of developing a malignant germ cell tumor later in life. This risk can be minimized if the testis is relocated into the scrotum. For this reason, undescended testes that have not even got as far as the inguinal canal and are still located in the abdomen are removed as a precaution. Sometimes no testis can be found (**anorchia**), or only an undeveloped remnant (**hypoplasia**).

Infections of the testis commonly also involve the epididymis

Infection of the testis (orchitis) is often associated with an infection that enters through the epididymis (epididymitis), resulting in **epididymo-orchitis**. The most important infections of the testis and epididymis are acute bacterial epididymo-orchitis, viral orchitis, and tuberculous epididymo-orchitis.

Acute infection is usually due to gonococci and *Chlamydia* (sexually transmitted) or *Escherichia coli* and other Gram-negative bacilli. Infection spreads from the urethra and lower urinary tract. Clinically the testis and epididymis are greatly enlarged and very tender. Histologically there is extensive infiltration of the seminiferous tubules and interstitium by neutrophils, later followed by lymphocytes and plasma cells; interstitial edema is considerable, and there is often patchy hemorrhage. Successful treatment with antibiotics is followed by healing and scarring, but there may be permanent damage to seminiferous tubules and epididymis, with consequent impairment of fertility.

Viral orchitis is usually the result of infection by the mumps virus after puberty. The disease is usually unilateral, and is associated with tender enlargement of the testis. The inflammatory infiltrate is mainly composed of lymphocytes and plasma cells. In a small proportion of cases bilateral disease after puberty can result in reduced fertility.

Tuberculosis may affect the testis and epididymis (**tuberculous epididymo-orchitis**) at a late stage of disease. Albeit currently rare, its incidence can be expected to increase with the increasing incidence of tuberculosis anticipated with the emergence of antibiotic-resistant strains of *Mycobacterium tuberculosis* (see page 117). The organisms may gain access to the epididymis by bloodstream spread during a phase of active pulmonary TB. The organisms are sequestered in the epididymis, and produce caseating granulomas over a period of many years, often continuing long after the initial pulmonary tuberculous lesion has healed. Eventually the epididymis is destroyed by caseating necrosis, and the infection spills over into the testis (*Fig. 18.3*). Epididymal infection may also arise by spread of infection from the kidney and lower urinary tract (see page 383).

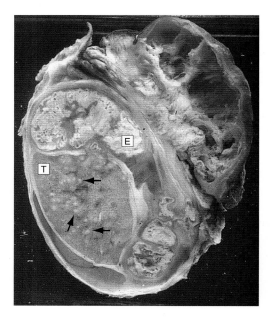

Fig. 18.3 Tuberculous epididymitis. The epididymis (**E**) is converted into a mass of caseous necrosis, and there is often associated tuberculous prostatitis and cystitis. The testis **T** contains tiny whitish specks (**arrows**) which are small early caseating granulomas, direct spread from the extensive epididymal involvement.

Granulomatous orchitis may mimic a testicular tumor clinically

Granulomatous orchitis is a disease of unknown etiology which presents with a painless, or only slightly tender, testicular enlargement; this is the common presenting symptom of most malignant germ-cell tumors of the testis (see page 402), so granulomatous orchitis is important in the differential diagnosis.

There is usually diffuse enlargement of the testis which has a pale cut surface appearance, resembling that of the most common germ cell tumor, seminoma (see page 404). Histologically, the seminiferous tubules show destruction of most of the germ cells, and replacement by an infiltrate of macrophages, plasma cells and lymphocytes, within which are numerous Langhans'-type multinucleate giant cells (*Fig. 18.4*).

The disease is most common in middle-aged men, the same age group in which seminoma occurs. Although the cause is not known, an autoimmune basis has been postulated. In the UK, a flurry of cases occurred when vasectomy first became fashionable, but the incidence has fallen in recent years. In the USA it is most common in African-Americans. Some cases apparently follow accidental trauma, groin surgery (e.g. hernia repair), prostatic surgery, or lower urinary tract infections.

Torsion of the testis causes venous infarction

Torsion of the testis, which is mainly seen in children and adolescents, occurs when the testis twists on its pedicle, obstructing the venous return. Blood continues to enter the testis and, with venous return mechanically obstructed, venous infarction occurs.

After torsion, the affected testis is swollen and excruciatingly painful, and there may be associated scrotal swelling, abdominal pain, nausea and vomiting. Thus the symptoms may simulate those of an acute bacterial orchitis. With advanced torsion, the testis is swollen and almost black as a result of being engorged with venous blood, which cannot escape because of the blocked venous drainage. As the pressure in the testis rises, arterial blood is unable to enter, and the testis becomes ischemic and eventually undergoes irreparable infarction (*Fig. 18.5*).

If the patient presents early, manual detorsion can be attempted (twisting the testis outwards and laterally through 180°) through the scrotum under analgesia, and may be temporarily successful in some cases, with great relief of pain. Open surgery, with untwisting and tethering of the testis, may enable the testis to be conserved with some function. A salvage rate of over 80% is achievable in patients who are operated on within 6 hours of the onset of the torsion, but the chances of any useful testicular function is virtually non-existent after 12 hours, and the infarcted testis might as well be removed.

The same clinical features may be exhibited by torsion of the tiny hydatid of Morgagni (a cystic remnant of the

Fig. 18.4 Granulomatous orchitis. The seminiferous tubules show destruction of their normal germ cell component, which is replaced by a chronic inflammatory infiltrate of lymphocytes, plasma cells and macrophages, with numerous Langhans' giant cells, forming granuloma-like structures.

Fig. 18.5 Torsion of testis. This testis and epididymis was removed surgically from a 7-year-old boy who had had a swollen and painful testis for 8 hours. Attempts at manual detorsion before scrotal exploration had been unsuccessful, and untwisting the torsion during the operation brought about no change in colour or evidence of resumed blood flow, so the testis was excised. The epididymis **E** is deeply congested by venous infarction, and the testis **T** shows complete infarction with much loss of tubular architecture.

Müllerian duct situated on the top of the testis), but the pain and swelling are less severe.

Other benign intrascrotal lesions are common, but not life-threatening

The most important are:

- **Hydrocele** – see later.
- **Epididymal cysts** – also known as spermatoceles, are cystic dilatations of the head of the epididymis, forming a spherical or ovoid thin-walled translucent mass distended with clear or slightly milky fluid.

- **Varicoceles** – are abnormally enlarged and thick-walled veins of the pampiniform plexus, forming an irregular mass in the scrotum.

Much less common are:

- **Sperm granuloma** – a very tender indurated nodule, usually found somewhere along the length of the vas deferens. Histologically it shows a chronic inflammatory reaction to remnants of spermatozoa, particularly the heads, and is thought to represent a reaction to spermatozoa that have leaked out of the ductular system. It may also be found in the region of the head of the epididymis. Sometimes there is a history of preceding trauma or surgery, e.g. vasectomy.
- **Adenomatoid tumor** – a benign neoplastic growth of mesothelial origin. It occurs as a small well-circumscribed, firm white nodule in, or near, the epididymis. They are most common in middle-aged men.

Hydrocele is the commonest cause of scrotal enlargement

The inner lining of the scrotal wall is a dense collagenous layer, the **parietal tunica vaginalis**, which has a smooth inner layer of flat mesothelial cells. This tunica is reflected over the external surface of the testis and epididymis, the **visceral tunica vaginalis**, which is also covered by mesothelial cells. Normally the mesothelial layers of the two tunica are in close contact, with only a thin layer of fluid (secreted by the mesothelial cells) separating them.

Hydrocoele is the result of fluid accumulating in the cavity bounded by the tunica vaginalis (*Fig. 18.6*a), producing a scrotal enlargement characterized clinically by being a fluctuant swelling which transilluminates when a lighted torch is viewed through the enlarged scrotum, as the fluid

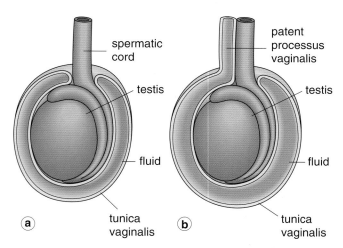

Fig. 18.6 Hydrocele. (a) In a **hydrocele** the tunica vaginalis surrounding the testis is distended by fluid. (b) In **congenital hydrocele** there is associated patency of the processus vaginalis, with continuity with the peritoneal cavity.

is usually crystal clear. Although most hydroceles arise as a primary phenomenon, they sometimes occur secondary to the development of a testicular tumor. Treatment of a hydrocele by aspirating the fluid is sometimes complicated by bleeding into the cavity; if severe, there may be sufficient blood to form a firm, dark clotted mass within the cavity, a **hematocele**.

Congenital patency of the processus vaginalis may be a cause of hydrocele in childhood (*Fig. 18.6*b).

TESTICULAR TUMORS

Tumors of the testis are important, for they account for a high proportion of malignant tumors seen in men in early and mid-adult life, particularly between the ages of 15 and 45 years. In the second half of the 20th century the incidence of testicular tumors increased in western countries, particularly in some parts of Europe; the rising incidence has given cause for concern that one or more unidentified environmental agents may be responsible.

The two main groups of testicular tumors are:

- **Germ cell tumors** (95%) – derived from the multipotential germ cells lining the seminiferous tubules.
- **Sex cord stromal tumors** (5%) – derived from the specialized and non-specialized support cells of the testis.

Testicular germ cell tumors are predisposed by maldescent and a chromosomal abnormality

Maldescent of the testis (cryptorchidism; see page 398) is an important predisposing factor in the development of some types of testicular germ cell tumor. The incidence of tumor development is 20–40 times higher than in normally descended testes. The highest risk is in testes that remain within the abdominal cavity.

An abnormality of chromosome 12 (an isochromosome of the short arm called I(12p) is found in 90% of testicular germ cell tumors, and other abnormalities of 12p are found in the other 10%. An abnormality at this locus is present in all testicular germ cell tumors, and is also seen in the ovarian germ cell-equivalent tumors.

The nomenclature and classification of testicular tumors are difficult because so many have mixed elements

About 95% of the tumors are **germ cell tumors**, derived from the germinal epithelium lining the seminiferous tubules, and the germ cells are multipotent, being capable of differentiating along a number of cell lines.

Some tumors (about 40%) are entirely composed of one single cell line, but the rest are mixtures of two or usually more histological types derived from the totipotent germ cells. The various cell lines are:

- Seminoma
- Spermatocytic seminoma.
- Embryonal carcinoma.
- Teratoma.
- Yolk sac tumor.
- Choriocarcinoma.

The derivation of these cell lines from the totipotent testicular germ cells is discussed in the blue box below, and illustrated diagrammatically in *Fig. 18.7*. The most important types of single-pattern and mixed pattern tumors are discussed in some detail on pages 402–5.

Classification and nomenclature of germ-cell tumors

The UK Testicular Tumor Panel classification of testicular tumors is no longer used, and the WHO classification and associated nomenclature is widely accepted.

Testicular totipotent germ cells can form different types of tumor, depending on which line of differentiation occurs:

- Totipotent germ cells which differentiate to spermatocytic cell lines form tumors called **seminomas**.
- Primitive totipotent cells which differentiate to various somatic embryonal tissues such as epithelium, cartilage, smooth muscle, neural tissues etc. form tumors called **teratomas**.
- Primitive totipotent germ cells which differentiate into extraembryonic tissues such as trophoblast and yolk sac form two types of tumor, **yolk sac tumor** and **choriocarcinoma** (trophoblastic tumor).

- Primitive totipotent germ cells which show no specific differentiation produce a primitive undifferentiared tumor, but with some epithelial pattern characteristics, called **embryonal carcinoma**.

All of the tumors can occur as single-pattern types (about 40% of all testicular tumors), but mixed-pattern tumors are more common (about 60%).

Some of the types are rare as single-pattern tumors, but are an important and common component of mixed-pattern tumors. There is also a great variation in tumor type with age. For example, yolk sac tumor is the most common testicular tumor in infants and very young children as a single-pattern tumor, but is extremely rare as a single-pattern tumor in adults; it is an important component of mixed-pattern tumors, usually combined with embryonal carcinoma (see page 405). Seminoma is the most common single-pattern tumor in adults.

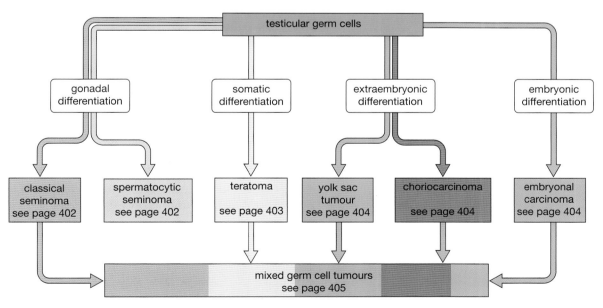

Fig. 18.7 Germ cell tumors of the testis (WHO).

SINGLE-PATTERN GERM CELL TUMORS

Seminoma is the most common single-pattern tumor of the testis

Seminoma occurs both as a single-pattern tumor and as a component of some mixed-pattern tumors. As a single-pattern tumor it is most common in those aged between 30 and 45 years, characteristically presenting with a painless, progressive enlargement of one testis; bilateral involvement is rare.

Macroscopically the normal, pale-brown testicular tissue is replaced by a homogeneous creamy-white tumor mass (*Fig. 18.8*a). In contrast to other types of germ-cell tumor, there is no evidence of cyst formation or hemorrhage; necrosis occurs only in the largest, neglected tumors.

The most common histological type of seminoma is termed **classic** (or typical) **seminoma.** Histologically these tumors are composed of sheets of regular, tightly packed cells that have central nuclei and clear cytoplasm.

A characteristic feature is the presence of fibrous septa, in which numerous lymphocytes are found (*Fig. 18.8*b). Seminoma shows immunoreactivity for placental alkaline phosphatase (PLAP).

In some tumors there is increased pleomorphism and mitotic activity, often with tumor giant cells, and this group was formerly called 'anaplastic' seminoma. However, despite these cytological indicators of more malignant behaviour, these tumors behave in exactly the same way as classic seminomas, have the same prognosis, and are not treated any differently. The distinction is therefore of no prognostic or management value.

Seminomas with trophoblastic (human chorionic gonadotropin-containing) giant cells are encountered in 10% of cases, but the biological relevance of the trophoblastic tissue is uncertain. Such tumors may be associated with increased blood levels of human chorionic gonadotropin (hCG) secreted by trophoblasts.

Seminoma may be found in association with other germ-cell elements, forming mixed germ-cell tumors.

Seminoma is the most common tumor type complicating cryptorchid testis (see page 398), and may therefore occur as a primary tumor in the inguinal canal or high on the posterior wall of the abdomen.

Spermatocytic seminoma is distinct from classic seminoma

Spermatocytic seminoma is a rare tumor which occurs in elderly men (60+). Like the classic seminoma it presents as progressive enlargement of a testis and may reach a large size; it may be bilateral in a small proportion of cases. The cut surface of the tumor is pale yellow and mainly homogeneous, but with occasional areas of mucoid cystic change. Histologically it is composed of a mixture of

Fig. 18.8 Seminoma. Macroscopically (a) the testis is replaced by firm, white tumor (T). Histologically (b) neoplastic cells are polygonal, with clear cytoplasm and large nuclei. Septa containing lymphoid cells (L) are a prominent feature.

three cell types; some are large mononuclear or multinucleated cells with abundant pale-staining or eosinophilic cytoplasm, and others are small cells with hyperchromatic nuclei and only a narrow rim of eosinophilic cytoplasm, but the majority are intermediate cells which often show a characteristic filamentous chromatin pattern in the nuclei. Unlike classic seminoma, there is no lymphocytic infiltrate in the scanty supporting stroma, but the stroma may be edematous, with droplets of pale pink proteinaceous material.

Although this tumor may show increased mitotic activity histologically, it behaves in a benign manner and does not metastasize.

Teratomas contain derivatives of all three embryonic germ cell layers

By definition, teratomas are tumors that contain elements derived from ectoderm, mesoderm and endoderm. True testicular teratomas can be shown to contain elements from all three, commonly including squamous epithelium (ectoderm), cartilage (mesoderm) and respiratory and intestinal-type epithelium (endoderm). The tissues may be **mature**, closely resembling the adult type, or **immature**, resembling the forming tissues as seen in the embryo.

Some descriptions of testicular teratomas include a variant called monodermal teratoma, in which derivatives of only one germ cell layer is present; this is an oxymoron, as by definition all three germ cell layers should be represented.

Testicular teratomas composed entirely of mature somatic elements are seen in young children

All three germ cell layers are represented, and occur in a well-differentiated and mature form, so that a wide range of tissues (e.g. skin, cartilage, bone, respiratory or intestinal epithelium) can be identified. They usually appear cystic (see *Fig. 18.9*a) and have a good prognosis, as they behave in a benign manner.

Teratomas composed solely of immature somatic elements are rare as a single-pattern tumor

The immature somatic elements are recognizable but resemble the immature tissues seen in the developing embryo (*Fig. 18.10*), rather than the well-formed mature elements seen in the childhood tumor. Tumors composed entirely of such teratomatous elements are rare and occur in an older age group than the mature teratomas, most commonly in the post-pubertal male (15–25 years) Unlike the childhood tumors these teratomas are malignant, and metastatic spread can occur in up to 30% of cases. Some more mature elements may also be present.

Although rare as a single-pattern tumor, immature teratoma is an important and common component of **mixed-pattern tumors** (see page 405).

In this post-pubertal group, the chromosomal abnormality I(12p) is present in almost all cases, but it is important to note that the chromosomal abnormality is not seen in the mature teratoma of early childhood.

The tumors have a heterogeneous cut surface appearance with frequent cystic areas. Extensive sampling of the tumor must always be undertaken to exclude the presence of elements of other germ cell tumors.

Fig. 18.9 Teratoma composed of mature elements. Macroscopically, differentiated teratomas are usually cystic (a). Histologically (b), a variety of differentiated elements such as epithelium (**E**) and cartilage (**C**) are seen.

Fig. 18.10 Teratoma composed of immature elements. This field of teratoma shows immature cartilage **C** and primitive columnar, focally mucus-secreting, epithelium **E**.

Yolk sac tumor occurs as a single-pattern tumor in infants, but as a component of mixed-pattern tumors in adults

Yolk sac tumor (also called endodermal sinus tumor) is the most common testicular tumor in children under 3 years of age. On cut surface the tumor is homogeneous and creamy in color, often with a glistening or slightly mucoid appearance. Histologically it shows many different patterns of arrangement of the small cuboidal cells of which it is mainly composed; there are solid, glandular, alveolar, reticular and microcystic patterns. A characteristic feature is the presence of papillary structures covered externally by a layer of the cuboidal cells, with a central fibrovascular core; these are called **Schiller–Duval bodies**.

Some cells in yolk sac tumors are positive for α-fetoprotein (AFP), as are small hyaline droplets which are invariably present.

In young children, yolk sac tumors have a good prognosis because of their response to chemotherapy regimens.

Fig. 18.11 a & b Yolk sac tumor. (a) shows a selected field from a yolk sac tumor showing Schiller-Duval bodies (arrowed). (b) is an immunochemical method showing the focal presence of AFP (alpha fetoprotein)

In adults, yolk sac components are found in many of the mixed-pattern germ cell tumors, particularly when AFP immunocytochemistry is used to search for them.

α-fetoprotein is also secreted into the blood and can be detected as a tumor marker.

Trophoblastic tumors are rare as single-pattern tumors but more common as mixed-pattern tumors

The most common type of trophoblastic tumor is **choriocarcinoma**, composed of cytotrophoblasts and syncytiotrophoblasts, and identical to the tumor seen in placenta (see Chapter 19, page 436). This tumor is highly malignant, growing rapidly and with a predisposition to erode blood vessels, which makes bloodborne metastasis very common. They appear as small hemorrhagic tumors, usually less than 3 cm in diameter, and often smaller. The ability to invade blood vessels from the outset means that these tumors may present with bloodborne metastases (e.g. in the lungs) before the patient is aware of any testicular enlargement.

They are much more common as a component of a mixed-pattern tumor, their presence often indicated by foci of hemorrhage and necrosis within an otherwise pale tumor mass. This element can be identified by immunohistochemical detection of HcG, which may also be detected in the blood as a tumor marker.

Embryonal carcinomas are composed of immature cells resembling those of the early embryo

Embryonal carcinoma comprises about 5% of single-pattern germ cell tumors, but is an important component of about 40–50% of mixed-pattern tumors (see page 405). On cut surface the tumors have a variegated appearance, with both solid fleshy and cystic or necrotic areas (see *Fig. 18.12*a).

Histologically they are composed of large undifferentiated cells of embryonic appearance, with pale-staining vesicular nuclei in which nucleoli are prominent and mitoses frequent. The cytoplasm is pale or slightly eosinophilic.

Although the cells are primitive and immature, they are often arranged in patterns shown by epithelial cells, namely papillary, tubular or acinar forms (see *Fig. 18.12*b), as well as in solid masses.

Embryonal carcinoma behaves in a highly malignant fashion, with early invasion of lymphatics and thin-walled blood vessels, so lymph node and bloodborne metastasis is common. Nevertheless, the tumor responds well to cytotoxic chemotherapy.

Both single-pattern embryonal carcinomas and mixed-pattern tumors containing a significant component of embryonal carcinoma occur most commonly in the 20–30-year age group, and less commonly in adolescents (15–20 years).

The mixed-pattern tumors that contain that contain seminoma tend to occur at a later age than those without a seminomatous component, but overall the main age range for mixed-pattern tumors is 20–35 years.

Accurate identification of the various components of mixed tumors is important, so thorough histological sampling must be undertaken, with the application of histochemical tumor marker methods such as AFP and hCG (see page 406).

Over 80% of adults with germ cell tumor of the testis also show in situ germ cell neoplasia

In the testicular tissue around established germ cell tumors can be found areas of non-invasive, in situ germ cell neoplasia in the form of cytologically malignant germ cells still contained within seminiferous tubules by the tubule basement membrane. The abnormal cells are large, with abundant pale cytoplasm and large irregular nuclei containing nucleoli. Immunocytochemically these cells show positivity

Fig. 18.12 Embryonal carcinoma. (a) The typical cut surface appearance of an embryonal carcinoma. The tumor is pale and has a variegated appearance, with a mixture of solid and cystic areas. (b) The histological appearance, mainly solid clumps of undifferentiated cells but with some focal tubular and acinar epithelial arrangement.

Fig. 18.13 Examples of germ cell tumors of mixed pattern. (a) A mixed embryonal carcinoma/seminoma. The seminoma **S** shows the typical appearance of classic seminoma (see also *Fig. 18.8b*), although the lymphocytic infiltrate of the stroma is not apparent in this field. *Fig. 18.13b* shows a field from a mixed germ cell tumor, containing immature teratoma **T** (mainly immature cartilage) and a column of embryonal carcinoma **E**.

About 60% of all germ cell tumors of the testis are mixed-pattern

The most common combinations are:

- Embryonal carcinoma + yolk sac tumor + teratoma + trophoblastic tissue.
- Embryonal carcinoma + yolk sac tumor + teratoma + seminoma.
- Embryonal carcinoma + yolk sac tumor + teratoma.
- Teratoma + seminoma.

It can be seen that almost all combinations occur, but spermatocytic seminoma never occurs as a component of mixed-pattern germ cell tumors.

with placental alkaline phosphatase (PLAP), and are also positive for OCT3/4, which is a marker for pluripotent stem cells. These in situ neoplastic cells have the same appearance irrespective of the nature of the malignant germ cell tumor involving the testis; they do not show the abnormality of chromosome 12 (see page 400) until they become invasive.

Testicular germ cell tumors can metastasize via lymphatic or blood vessels

Local invasion of neglected or rapidly growing tumors can involve the rete testis, epididymis and spermatic cord, but prognostically the most significant spread is by way of lymphatic and blood vessels.

The pattern of lymphatic spread is characteristic, with involvement of retroperitoneal para-aortic lymph nodes in the first instance, and subsequent spread to lymph node groups above the diaphragm, usually mediastinal and supraclavicular nodes.

Bloodstream spread is usually to the lungs, but brain, liver and bone are other common sites of bloodborne metastasis.

This pattern of spread can be shown by all types of germ cell tumor except spermatocytic seminoma, which does not metastasize; tumors that contain trophoblastic elements are particularly likely to spread by the bloodstream at an early stage, sometimes before the patient is aware of a testicular mass.

The staging of testicular tumors is based on the extent of spread at first diagnosis

Successful treatment of germ cell tumors is based on a combination of surgery (orchidectomy, sometimes with retroperitoneal lymph node dissection), radiotherapy, and appropriate and timely chemotherapy. The precise regimen is based on the nature of the tumor and the stage at first diagnosis. The commonly used staging is:

- **Stage I** – tumor confined to the testis, epididymis or spermatic cord
- **Stage II** – metastases confined to the retroperitoneal lymph nodes below the diaphragm.
- **Stage III** – metastases in lymph nodes above the diaphragm, or in other organs.

Stage II is sometimes further subdivided into IIA (nodes <2 cm in diameter), IIB (nodes 2–5 cm in diameter) and IIC (nodes >5 cm in diameter), the size of the nodes being assessed by imaging.

An important component of treatment is regular surveillance after the initial treatment, with regular chest X-rays and measurement of tumor markers (see later), and abdominal scans if appropriate.

Use of tumor cell markers in testicular germ cell tumors

Tumor cell markers play an important role in both the accurate diagnosis of germ cell tumors and the surveillance of the patient.

In **histological diagnosis** of an excised tumor, the use of immunohistochemical methods for various tumor cell markers facilitates the identification of some components of mixed-pattern germ cell tumors. For example, AFP (α-fetoprotein) is used to identify yolk sac tumor elements, and hCG (human chorionic gonadotrophin) identifies trophoblastic elements. hCG can also be used to identify trophoblastic giant cells within a seminoma (see page 402).

Assay of blood levels of tumor markers is important in the **surveillance** of patients with germ cell tumors. The serum levels of AFP and the β unit of hCG are measured before and after removal of any testicular tumor, as these proteins are produced by many testicular germ cell tumors.

- Trophoblastic germ cell tumors have elevated levels of hCG.
- Yolk sac tumors have elevated levels of AFP.
- 80% of germ cell tumors except seminoma have elevated AFP/hCG or both.
- About 10% of seminomas have a slightly elevated levels of hCG because of the presence of occasional trophoblastic giant cells.

If tumor is confined to the testis (stage 1), levels of marker will drop after orchidectomy. If levels do not fall to normal, it indicates that there is metastatic disease (i.e. not stage 1). In follow-up after treatment, increasing levels of a marker protein are an indication of tumor recurrence, usually before recurrence is manifest clinically or detectable by imaging.

Lactic dehydrogenase (LDH) is also usually measured before and after treatment. This enzyme is ubiquitous and not specific for testicular germ cell tumors, but is a useful marker of tumor bulk. Serial LDH measurements therefore allow the monitoring of the effects of therapy on tumor bulk.

Sex-cord and stromal tumors of the testis are less common than germ-cell tumors

Tumors may be derived from the non-germ-cell components of the testis (the interstitial Leydig cells and the Sertoli cells), but these are much less common than germ-cell tumors and account for about 5% of all cases. The testis may also be a site for development of primary lymphoma.

Leydig-cell tumors (also termed **interstitial cell tumors**) may occur at any age from childhood to late adult life. In childhood, tumors may cause precocious development of secondary sexual characteristics; in adults they often cause loss of libido and gynecomastia, reflecting secretion of either testosterone or estrogen, or both. Macroscopically, tumors appear circumscribed and are yellow (*Fig. 18.14*). They are composed of cells that resemble normal Leydig cells. Although the majority of tumors are benign, those over 5 cm in diameter and those with mitoses may behave in a malignant fashion.

Sertoli-cell tumors (also called **androblastoma**) may arise at all ages, including infancy, but have a peak incidence in the fourth decade. Typically, they are well circumscribed and composed of cells resembling the normal Sertoli cells of the tubules. Most lesions are benign, but tumors with many mitoses may behave in a malignant fashion.

Testicular disease may result in male infertility

Male infertility is the result of failure of the production of mature motile spermatozoa. Initial tests involve the analysis of a sample of semen for the presence of spermatozoa.

In some cases no spermatozoa are seen in the ejaculate. Several conditions are recognized as being responsible, the most common being: destruction of testicular tissue or scarring in ducts as a result of inflammatory disease, e.g. following infection; congenital absence of the vas deferens or seminal vesicles; or the presence of cryptorchid testes. The chromosomal disorder **Klinefelter's syndrome** (XXY) is associated with severe atrophy of testicular tubules and absent germ cells. Serum levels of FSH are elevated in cases

of failure of the testis, in which case no function can be expected.

Other disorders are associated with abnormally small numbers of spermatozoa. Endocrine causes, particularly disease of the hypothalamopituitary axis and estrogen excess (endogenous or exogenous), must always be suspected. Germ cells are very sensitive to abnormal environments and are easily damaged; they are particularly sensitive to the effects of systemic chemotherapy and irradiation. For normal germ-cell development and maturation to take place, the testicular temperature should be lower than core temperature. Exposure to high temperature, due either to maldescent or an environmental cause, may result in infertility.

In some cases the cause of reduced spermatozoa production is uncertain after investigation, and testicular biopsy may be performed for diagnosis. Sometimes the seminiferous tubules show a complete absence of germ cells, being lined only by Sertoli cells. Alternatively, early stages of spermatogenesis may be normal, but the late stages leading to the formation of mature spermatozoa are defective (so-called **maturation arrest**).

PROSTATE GLAND

The main diseases of the prostate are inflammatory disorders, hyperplasia and carcinoma

There are three important conditions of the prostate: **prostatitis** (which may be acute or chronic), **benign prostatic hyperplasia**, and **prostatic adenocarcinoma**. In younger men, disease of the prostate is mainly due to infections, some of which are sexually transmitted diseases. In older men enlargement of the prostate is an almost universal phenomenon, most commonly due to prostatic hyperplasia, and leads to obstruction of the urinary outflow through the prostatic part of the urethra. Occasionally, clinically apparent prostatic urethral obstruction may be caused by the development of carcinoma.

Prostatitis is caused mainly by infections that gain access from the urethra

Acute inflammation of the prostate usually follows acute infection in the bladder or urethra, and is particularly common following surgical instrumentation of the urethra. The usual causative organisms in older males are those that infect the bladder and urethra, particularly *E. coli* and *Proteus* spp. Sexually transmitted diseases may also cause prostatitis, particularly gonococcus and *Chlamydia* (a cause of non-gonococcal urethritis). Acute infections are characterized by the presence of a heavy neutrophilic infiltrate, often with abscess formation.

Fig. 18.14 Leydig-cell tumor of the testis. A Leydig-cell tumor is seen as a well-circumscribed tumor (T), with a yellow cut surface.

Chronic infective prostatitis is also associated with lower urinary tract infection, and results from inadequately treated acute prostatitis. A further cause of chronic prostatitis is TB, cases usually being associated with renal or epididymal TB. Chronic prostatitis usually shows an admixture of neutrophils with lymphocytes and plasma cells; in tuberculous cases there is a giant-cell histiocytic reaction, with focal caseation.

Benign prostatic hyperplasia affects most men over the age of 70 years

Benign prostatic hyperplasia is the most common disorder of the prostate. It affects almost all men over the age of 70, but is found with increasing frequency and severity from about the age of 45 onwards. Clinically it presents with difficulty with micturition, due to compression of the prostatic urethra by the enlarging prostate gland. In most cases it is the two lateral lobes that are markedly enlarged. However, in some cases the posterior lobe shows the greatest enlargement, which may obstruct the urinary outflow tract at the internal urinary meatus at the bladder neck. Prolonged prostatic obstruction is the most common cause of chronic obstructive uropathy, and may lead to marked hypertrophy of the bladder wall, with trabeculation of bladder muscle, and acute or chronic retention of urine in the bladder. In such cases the failure to empty the bladder may lead to reflux of urine into the pelvicalyceal system, producing mega-ureter and hydronephrosis and predisposing to infection.

The pathogenesis of benign prostatic hyperplasia is not known, but it is believed to be due to androgen–estrogen

Fig. 18.15 Benign prostatic hyperplasia. In prostatic hyperplasia, the prostate is enlarged by hyperplastic nodules in the periurethral gland zone (PUG), compressing and distorting the urethra (U). The peripheral zone glands (PZG) are not involved, but this is the zone in which carcinoma arises.

imbalance (see pink box below). The area that is hormone sensitive, and which undergoes this pattern of hyperplasia, is the periurethral group of prostatic glands, not the true prostatic glands at the periphery. Continuing enlargement of the periurethral glands compresses the peripheral true prostatic glands, leading to their collapse, leaving only their fibrous supporting stroma behind.

Macroscopically the hyperplastic component of the prostate shows a nodular pattern of hyperplastic glandular acini separated by fibrous stroma (*Fig. 18.15*). Some of the nodules are cystically dilated and contain a milky fluid. Others contain numerous calcified concretions (corpora

Pathogenetic factors in prostatic hyperplasia

A metabolite of testosterone called **dehydrotestosterone (DHT)** is produced in the stroma of the prostate by the action of an enzyme called 5α-reductase, which is located in the stromal cells, on circulating testosterone. DHT promotes proliferation of both stromal and epithelial cells by binding to androgen receptors on the nuclei of both cell types, leading to the production of growth factors that stimulate the proliferation of epithelial and stromal cells.

Clinical studies with 5α-reductase inhibitors (e.g. finasteride and episteride) have shown a reduction in prostatic size, with relief of symptoms of obstruction.

However, there are other factors involved in prostatic enlargement, including the rise in estradiol levels in old age, the estrogens possibly rendering the prostatic glandular epithelium and stroma more sensitive to the effect of DHT.

One further factor involved in prostatic obstruction is contraction of smooth muscle fibers within the prostate, particularly at the bladder neck, mediated by α-adrenergic receptors in the prostate stroma. This is the basis of the use of α-adrenergic blocker drugs such as prazosin and doxazosin to relax the smooth muscle in the prostate and help relieve obstruction.

amylacea). Histologically the acini are hyperplastic and tightly packed, lined by tall columnar epithelial cells with small basal nuclei, and the epithelium is sometimes thrown up into irregular papillary folds. Another component of the prostatic enlargement is muscular hypertrophy, particularly in the region of the bladder neck.

Carcinoma of the prostate is the second most common type of cancer in men

Carcinoma of the prostate is an important and common malignant tumor in men, occurring with increasing frequency over the age of 55.

Carcinoma of the prostate is an adenocarcinoma which arises in the true prostatic glands at the periphery of the prostate, unlike benign prostatic hyperplasia which originates in the glands in the transition zone in the inner part of the gland around the urethra (*Fig. 18.15*). Because the tumor arises in the peripheral glands, local invasion outwards through the prostatic capsule is most likely before the tumor infiltrates medially towards the urethra. For this reason, attempts to obtain biopsy samples of the prostate to establish a diagnosis of malignancy by using the transurethral route may give false negative results; a needle biopsy of the outer prostate using a transrectal approach is more likely to be successful.

The pathogenesis of the tumor is uncertain, although some etiological factors are recognized, and some possibly relevant genetic factors have been identified in cases where there is a strong family history. In the absence of any firm and consistent causative factors, no primary preventive strategies offer themselves for carcinoma of the prostate; efforts are therefore directed towards screening to detect early-stage disease using blood testing for prostate specific antigen (PSA).

Because of its peripheral origin, prostatic cancer is often well established before the patient develops symptoms of difficulty with micturition due to urethral obstruction, and some tumors may remain locally silent, even in the presence of widespread metastases.

Prostatic cancer can be divided clinically into three groups on the basis of their behaviour:

- **Invasive prostatic carcinomas** Clinically important, as they invade locally and metastasize.
- **Latent prostatic carcinomas.** These are small foci of well-differentiated carcinoma, frequently an incidental finding in the prostatic glands of elderly men. They appear to remain confined to the prostate for a long time.
- **Occult carcinomas** are not clinically apparent at the primary site, but present as metastatic disease.

Macroscopically, carcinomas of the prostate appear as diffuse areas of firm, white tissue which merge into the fibromuscular prostatic stromal tissues. Distortion and extension outside the capsule of the prostate is common,

producing a hard, irregular, craggy mass that can be palpated on rectal examination.

Grading of prostatic carcinoma uses the Gleason system

The most widely used histological grading scheme is that proposed by Gleason, based on the architectural differentiation of the tumor. This scheme recognizes that different patterns may occur within the same tumor. There are five grades, numbered 1 to 5, with grade 1 being the best differentiated and grade 5 the least differentiated. Tumors are given two grades based on the most common and second most common architectural pattern. The two grades are added together to give a final **Gleason score**, which will lie somewhere between 2 and 10. For example, a well-differentiated tumor may have a Gleason score of 3, and a poorly differentiated one may have a score of 9.

The prognosis of prostatic cancer varies greatly with Gleason score and also stage; in general, tumors with a Gleason score of less than 6 are low-grade and not aggressive. The main limitation of the Gleason (or any other) histological grading system is that the only tissue usually available for histological assessment is one or more small needle biopsy cores, so the sampling may not be representative.

Fig. 18.16 Prostatic adenocarcinoma. (a) A Gleason grade 1 tumor, closely resembling normal prostate, with well-formed separate glands with lumina, pale cytoplasm and predominantly basal nuclei. (b) A Gleason grade 4 tumor, with incomplete gland formation and scanty lumina. This is the most common pattern; these two patterns rarely appear together.

PSA and prostate cancer diagnosis

Prostate-specific antigen (PSA) is a glycoprotein synthesized almost exclusively in the epithelial cells of the prostate gland, and blood measurement of PSA can be used in the diagnosis of prostatic carcinoma and in the assessment of response to therapy.

The normal PSA level is <5 ng/L, and levels >10 ng/L are strongly suggestive of tumor. However, many factors influence PSA levels and in most cases (unless grossly elevated) they are not reliable as a screening method.

The main value is in sequential measurements of PSA to determine whether metastatic spread has occurred and to monitor the success or otherwise of treatment.

Staging is based on the extent of the tumor, i.e. whether it is confined to the prostate gland (T1 and T2), has spread outside the prostatic capsule (T3) or invades adjacent organs (T3). Accurate staging is difficult unless sophisticated imaging methods are used.

Carcinoma of the prostate metastasizes to bone and nodes and invades the bladder base

Prostatic carcinomas spread by three main routes:

- **Direct spread** to base of bladder and adjacent tissues. This causes obstruction of the urethra (difficulty in micturition) and may block the ureters, causing hydronephrosis (see page 391).
- **Lymphatic spread** to pelvic and para-aortic nodes.
- **Vascular spread** to bone. Bone metastases from prostatic carcinoma may be sclerotic with bone production (dense on radiograph), rather than lytic with bone destruction.

Occasionally, the first manifestation of disease is from metastatic spread, for example compressing the spinal cord after vertebral metastasis. The pathological diagnosis of metastatic prostatic carcinoma is assisted by immunohistochemical detection of PSA and prostate-specific antigen in biopsy material. This may also be used as a serum marker for disease, levels being particularly raised when there is metastatic disease.

As many prostatic carcinomas are dependent on testosterone for growth, orchidectomy, or treatment with estrogenic drugs or agonists of luteinizing hormone-releasing hormone, may induce tumor regression.

PENIS

Hypospadias and epispadias are congenital abnormalities of the penile urethra

Normally the penile urethra opens to the exterior through the tip of the glans at the end of the penis. Occasionally, maldevelopment of the urethral canal may lead to the urethra opening further back on the penile shaft, on to either the ventral (underside) surface (**hypospadias**) or the dorsal (upperside) surface (**epispadias**).

Hypospadias is the more common of the two, and the opening may be near the corona, in midshaft, or situated much further back at the root of the penis in a scrotal or perineal location. An opening at or near the corona is the commonest site (about 85%) and the easiest to deal with surgically; the scrotal/perineal location is rarest (about 5%) and is more difficult to treat.

In epispadias, the urethral opening can again be located in the glans/corona region, in midshaft, or close to the root of the penis (peno-pubic). The latter are associated with separation of the pubic bone and abnormalities of the bladder neck such that urinary incontinence is common.

In both hypospadias and epispadias, a location close to the root of the penis may interfere with normal ejaculation.

Phimosis is an abnormality of the foreskin

In the uncircumcised male the foreskin can normally be retracted to behind the corona. When the prepuce is too small or rigid to permit this, the condition is called phimosis; it may be the result of abnormal development of the foreskin leading to a tight prepuce, but it more commonly occurs as a result of undue rigidity of the preputial ring due to fibrous scarring from trauma, repeated infection, or balanitis xerotica obliterans (see below).

Forcible retraction of a tight prepuce may result in **paraphimosis**, in which the tight preputial ring leads to constriction at the corona and swelling of the glans penis to such an extent that the foreskin cannot be returned to its normal position. Paraphimosis causes severe pain and swelling of the glans, and may constrict the penile urethra leading to acute urinary obstruction.

Infections of the penis include infections of the penile urethra (urethritis) and infections of the glans and foreskin (balanitis)

Gonococcal urethritis is caused by *Neisseria gonorrhoeae*, acquired as a sexually transmitted disease. It presents with urethral pain and a purulent discharge. If untreated, scarring of the urethra may lead to a urethral stricture.

Non-gonococcal urethritis is mainly caused by *Chlamydia trachomatis*. It causes a purulent urethral discharge and, in rare cases, may lead to the development of **Reiter's syndrome** (arthritis, urethritis and conjunctivitis).

Balanitis may be caused by a wide variety of organisms, including the fungus *Candida albicans*, and by both pyogenic and anaerobic bacteria. In uncircumcised men poor hygiene and phimosis are predisposing factors.

The penile mucosa is the site of original infection in **sexually transmitted diseases** such as syphilis (the syphilitic chancre (see *Fig. 8.3*) and herpes genitalis. In the latter, typical herpetic blisters form on the glans penis. A particular type of viral infection seen on the penis and around the perineum is **condyloma acuminatum**, caused by one of the human papilloma viruses (see page 511); the warts have a cauliflower-like appearance. Although uncommon in western countries, ulcerated lesions on the penis may be caused by *Haemophilus ducreyi* (chancroid), *Calymmato-bacterium granulomatis* (granuloma inguinale) and *Chlamydis trachomatis* (lymphogranuloma venereum).

The penis is prone to develop a number of skin diseases

The most important of these is **balanitis xerotica obliterans (BXO)**, in which the foreskin, particularly around the prepuce, becomes abnormally thickened and scarred, predisposing to phimosis. It is a fibrosing condition of the dermis, identical in pathology to the vulval and skin disease **lichen sclerosus** (see page 414).

Other skin diseases such as lichen planus, psoriasis, viral warts and molluscum contagiosum also affect the penis; they are discussed in more detail in Chapter 23.

The most common tumor of the penis is squamous carcinoma

Invasive squamous carcinoma of the penis usually occurs in uncircumcised elderly men (70+) and presents as a warty, cauliflower-like growth on the glans which occasionally bleeds, but grows slowly. These tumors are often neglected because of patient embarrassment, so tend to present to clinician when already fairly advanced, necessitating amputation of the distal penis; the most common site of metastatic spread is to the inguinal lymph nodes via lymphatics.

Carcinoma in situ may occur in the skin of the penile shaft, where clinically and histologically it resembles intraepidermal carcinoma elsewhere in the skin (see page 522). On the glans penis, penile intraepithelial neoplasia (PIN) appears as persistent and expanding red patches, eventually becoming raised and indurated (Queyrat's erythroplasia); many cases are associated with human papilloma virus infection.

Peyronie's disease leads to distortion of the erect penis

Peyronie's disease is a distressing condition of the penis affecting 1–3% of all men; it most commonly occurs between the ages of 40 and 60, but can also occur in young and elderly men. A proliferation of cellular fibrous tissue occurs in the fibrous tunica albuginea which surrounds the erectile corpora of the penis. This most commonly occurs on the dorsal aspect of the penile shaft, and progressive collagenization of the proliferated fibroblastic tissue leads to a dense, rigid collagenous plaque. When the penis becomes erect, this plaque produces an upward curvature and can also make the erect penis painful. The plaque less commonly arises on the undersurface, in which case the curvature is downwards, or on one lateral surface, producing lateral curvature.

The cause is unknown; fibrous scarring following trauma has been postulated, even though few patients give a history of significant trauma. Furthermore, the histological appearances of both the early cellular and the late collagenous lesions are identical to those seen in another proliferative fibrosis disease, Dupuytren's contracture of the hand (see page 559). The probable link between these two diseases is reinforced by the observation that about 30% of patients with Peyronie's disease also have, or eventually develop, Dupuytren's contracture.

The scrotum is covered by hair-bearing skin

The scrotal skin can be affected by almost any of the common skin diseases discussed in Chapter 23. Eczema, contact dermatitis, psoriasis, fungal infections, epidermal cysts and nevi are particularly common.

Case-based questions

Case 1 A boy with a painful swollen testis

A 6-year-old boy was seen in the hospital Emergency Room screaming with pain. According to his mother he had been miserable that evening and had been unable to settle when he went to bed; she heard him crying during the night and found him apparently in great pain, holding his scrotum. She saw that his left testis was swollen and extremely tender, and brought him to the Emergency Room. She thought it had been about 2 hours since he began crying with the pain.

1. What is the most likely diagnosis?
2. Why is the time interval since onset important?

After unsuccessful initial treatment in the Emergency Room, he was taken to surgery where his condition was successfully treated without recourse to excision of the testis.

► 3. **What treatment was attempted in the ER?**
4. **What treatment was successful in surgery, and what fact in the history suggested that orchidectomy might be avoided?**

Case 2 A boy with a painless swollen testis

While bathing her 2-year-old son, a mother noticed that the right side of his scrotum seemed larger than the left, and on careful palpation thought that the right testis was much larger than the left. She had not noticed this a few days before when she had last given him a long and playful bath. She took him to the family practitioner, who confirmed that the testis was enlarged and referred the child to a pediatrician as a matter of urgency.

1. **What is your differential diagnosis?**
2. **Which on your list is the most likely diagnosis, given the history as above?**

The pediatrician ordered some blood tests and imaging investigations before orchidectomy.

3. **What investigations did he undertake, and for what purpose?**

The imaging investigations showed no abnormality, but the blood tests showed a raised level of AFP (α-fetoprotein).

4. **What do these investigations suggest?**

The enlarged right testis, with epididymis and spermatic cord, were removed surgically and the child was followed up with repeated blood AFP measurements which were fortunately never elevated again.

Cases 3 and 4 Two adults with painless enlargement of the testis

Two men were seen in the Genitourinary Surgery Unit on the same day, both complaining of an enlarged testis. Patient 3, aged 42, had noticed a dragging discomfort in his left testis about 6 weeks previously, and had realized over the following 3 or 4 weeks that the testis was becoming slowly enlarged. On examination the testis was enlarged to about two or three times normal size, uniformly firm but non-tender.

Patient 4, aged 21, had become aware that his right testis was enlarged while showering after a tennis game. He had no other symptoms, and felt well.

Examination by the surgeon confirmed testicular enlargement in both cases.

1. **What is the most likely diagnosis in each case, and why?**
2. **What tumor cell markers would be of value in preoperative diagnosis, and what results might you expect in the two cases?**

Case 5 An old man with low back pain

A 68-year-old man, previously fit and well, developed persistent pain in his lower back. Despite bed rest and analgesics, the pain was unremitting and he eventually saw his family practitioner, who noted that the patient had tenderness on pressure to the fourth and fifth lumbar vertebrae.

The family practitioner performed a rectal examination and felt the prostate gland to be enlarged, hard and irregular, with loss of the median sulcus. He referred the patient to a genitourinary surgeon for further investigation.

1. **What is the most likely pathology of the prostate gland in this case?**
2. **What is the most likely cause of the back pain?**

The genitourinary surgeon confirmed the clinical findings of the family practitioner and ordered blood tests and imaging. He later performed a transrectal biopsy of the prostate gland.

3. **What blood and imaging investigations do you think the surgeon requested, and what do you think they would reveal?**
4. **Why was a transrectal biopsy performed rather than a transurethral biopsy?**

Brief answers to these case-based questions are given on page 592. More detailed answers and other study resources are available online at www.studentconsult.com.

Gynecologic and obstetric pathology

19

GYNECOLOGIC AND OBSTETRIC PATHOLOGY

FEMALE GENITAL TRACT

Diseases of the female genital tract form a large component of clinical practice

Abnormalities of the female genital tract which are not directly related to conception, pregnancy or childbirth are called **gynecologic pathology**, and form the bulk of this chapter. A large part of a gynecologist's clinical practice is associated with bleeding from the genital tract and pain, usually due to disorders of menstruation, which can have many causes (e.g. benign abnormalities of endometrium or myometrium), but sometimes due to the important tumors **carcinoma of the endometrium** (in postmenopausal women) and **carcinoma of the uterine cervix** (mainly in premenopausal women). Early detection of carcinoma of the uterine cervix before it becomes invasive is based on regular microscopic examination of smears taken from the surface epithelium of the cervix (**cervical cytology**). There are, however, many other simple benign causes of non-menstrual bleeding from the female genital tract, particularly benign **polyps** of the endometrium and uterine cervix. The main pathological conditions affecting the ovaries are benign and malignant cysts and solid tumors. Hormonal dysfunction of the ovaries is usually manifest as disorders of menstruation or problems with conception and pregnancy. The vulva is composed of skin, and is heir to many of the diseases of skin at other sites, including allergic and contact dermatitis, psoriasis, epidermal cysts, benign nevi, viral warts, and the malignant tumor **squamous cell carcinoma**. Three skin conditions which are particularly common in the vulva are **lichen sclerosus**, **lichen planus** and **lichen simplex chronicus**. Most inflammatory skin diseases of the vulva present clinically with itching, soreness and irritation. The vagina is relatively free of pathology, with the exception of infections including sexually transmitted diseases.

Abnormalities related to conception, pregnancy or childbirth are described in **obstetric pathology** (see pages 433–7). This section of the chapter outlines the main clinical problems and their underlying pathology.

DISEASES OF THE VULVA

The vulva is frequently affected by skin diseases, often not recognized or diagnosed by gynecologists

The labia majora and minora are skin, and subject to a wide range of skin diseases, particularly inflammatory skin disease, causing pruritus and soreness. One of the most frequent, and often misdiagnosed, is **acute contact dermatitis** (**allergic dermatitis**, *Fig. 19.1*) following the use of topical applications such as deodorants, creams and ointments used for the treatment of vulval irritation and soreness (particularly antiseptic or disinfectant solutions and creams).

There is an enormous range of materials that can cause contact dermatitis in the vulva, including soap, detergents in shower gels and bubble baths, detergents used in washing underwear, and constituents of various cosmetics, including perfumes etc. Even rubber and chemicals in contraceptives and nail varnish may produce an allergic type of dermatitis as, ironically, may local anesthetic creams and topical steroids given as treatment.

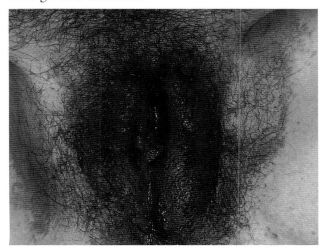

Fig. 19.1 Acute contact dermatitis. The labia majora and minora are red, swollen and sore-looking, and the redness also involves the groin. This is due to a local contact dermatitis to a disinfectant solution.

Other types of inflammatory skin disease can also affect the vulva, e.g. psoriasis, (see page 510), seborrheic dermatitis (see page 508), drug rashes of various types (see page 519) and blistering diseases (see pages 515–8). Careful history taking, combined with examination of the rest of the skin, will often enable a diagnosis to be made. Unfortunately, gynecologists rarely examine the rest of the patient, and often miss the diagnosis.

Lichen simplex chronicus is a pattern of chronic dermatitis which produces thickening of the vulval skin

Constant repeated frictional trauma, almost always due to the repeated scratching of a chronically itching vulva, causes thickening of the epidermis by proliferation of squamous keratinocytes (acanthosis), thickening of the overlying keratin layer (hyperkeratosis), and fibrosis of the underlying dermis; for clinical and histological details see page 502 and *Fig. 23.3*. This condition is erroneously called 'hypertrophic vulval dystrophy' by gynecologists and gynecologic pathologists, a term that should be abandoned as should the specious and imprecise acronym NNED (non-neoplastic epithelial disorder), loosely used to describe any vulval disorder which is NOT vulval intraepithelial neoplasia (VIN) or invasive carcinoma. Proper management is based on the investigation and treatment of the underlying cause of the original itching, often a contact or allergic dermatitis, or one of the specific inflammatory skin diseases that particularly affect the vulva, lichen sclerosus or lichen planus.

Lichen sclerosus et atrophicus is an important skin disease and commonly affects the vulva

Lichen sclerosus et atrophicus, (another example of a so-called NNED!), results in epidermal atrophy and densely collagenous upper dermal fibrosis of unknown etiology. The condition has a particular predilection for the skin in the genital area, occurring frequently in the vulva, and less commonly in the penis (balanitis xerotica obliterans, see page 411). It presents as white papules or confluent patches, which are covered by atrophic epidermis in which telangiectatic blood vessels are prominent (*Fig. 19.2*). The histology is identical to that seen in affected skin elsewhere, with compact hyalinization of the upper dermis with an underlying lymphocytic infiltrate.

Long-standing inadequately treated lichen sclerosus may lead to severe scarring and narrowing of the introitus, and is a predisposing factor to the eventual development of squamous carcinoma. Chronic scratching of lichen sclerosus lesions may produce coexistent lichen simplex chronicus, a combination inaccurately called 'mixed vulval dystrophy,' another term that should be dispatched to oblivion.

Lichen planus is a common inflammatory condition of the skin which frequently affects the vulva; the diagnosis is often missed

In the vulva, the lesions may resemble those seen in the skin at other sites: raised purplish plaques and patches, particularly on the labia majora. However, on the labia

Fig. 19.2 Lichen sclerosus of vulva. This vulva shows extensive, thick, white patches due to collagenous thickening, overlaid by an atrophic epithelium.

Fig. 19.3 Erosive lichen planus. The labia show reddening and there is an area of red denudation of mucosa, producing an erosion. This is typical of the erosive pattern of lichen planus.

minora it is frequently clinically different, producing very sore, superficial red weeping erosions (*Fig. 19.3*). This pattern can also be seen in the other common orificial site of lichen planus, the mouth. The disease may be confined to the vulva, but careful history taking and examination of the skin elsewhere will usually reveal current lesions or evidence of past skin or oral involvement with lichen planus.

Like lichen sclerosus, lichen planus is curable with strong topical steroids if diagnosed clinically and histopathologically; hence vulval biopsy to establish or confirm an accurate diagnosis is an important part of the management of such cases. Also like lichen sclerosus, some cases of vulval lichen planus are clinically and histologically modified by lichen simplex chronicus due to repeated scratching. Long-standing under-treated lichen planus may also predispose to the development of squamous carcinoma.

Most infections of the vulva are caused by viruses or fungi

The vulval skin is frequently involved with infective disease, usually due to viruses and fungi. Viral infections of the vulval skin are due either to herpes virus or to the human papillomavirus (HPV). Fungal infections are usually caused by superficial dermatophytes or *Candida*.

Herpes vulvitis produces initially painless blisters, which subsequently break down to form a painful, sore, eroded area. The herpes virus is acquired through sexual contact, and the disease is therefore mainly seen in young women.

HPV (human papillomavirus) is also sexually transmitted and may be associated with thickening of vulval skin and mucosa in the labia minora (**flat condyloma**), or may present as multiple protuberant warts (**condylomata acuminata**), which are either sessile or pedunculated. HPV strains 6 and 11 are responsible for most vulval lesions. There is a strong link between HPV infections of the vulva and intraepithelial neoplastic change in the vulva (see page 416) and cervix (see page 418).

Fungal infections of the vulva are mainly due to *Candida albicans.* There is usually associated fungal vaginitis, presenting with a copious vaginal discharge and vulval reddening and soreness. The infection and its manifestations are often severe in diabetics. Infection of vulval skin with dermatophytic fungi also produces similar superficial inflammation and soreness.

Sexually transmitted disease affecting the vulva can be caused by a number of different types of organism

In addition to sexually transmitted herpes virus and HPV, a number of other organisms can produce vulval lesions as a result of sexually transmitted infection, although many of them are confined to tropical countries. Among the most important are *Calymmatobacterium granulomatis*, which causes **granuloma inguinale** and produces ulcerating nodules on the vulva, and *Chlamydia trachomatis*, which

causes **lymphogranuloma venereum** with ulcerating vulval papules and enlarged inguinal lymph nodes.

Hemophilus ducreyi causes **chancroid**, with multiple tender papules and ulcerating nodules on the vulva, associated with tender enlargement of the inguinal lymph nodes.

Treponema pallidum is the causative organism of **syphilis**. The lesions are small, indurated vulval or vaginal papules (chancre) in the first stage (representing the site of entry of the organism), and multiple moist, warty, vulvovaginal and perineal lesions (condylomata lata) in the second stage.

Benign cysts on the vulva are common and may be derived from skin or Bartholin's glands

The hair-bearing skin component of the vulva may be the site of formation of benign keratin-filled epidermal cysts similar to those seen elsewhere in the skin. Bartholin's glands are mucus-secreting glands in the posterior part of the labia majora. They discharge their secretions into the vestibule through short ducts that are normally lined by transitional-cell epithelium, although squamous-cell metaplasia is common. Cystic dilatation of the ducts and glands may result from duct obstruction, the cysts being lined by mucus-secreting columnar epithelium, transitional or squamous epithelium, or a mixture.

The most important malignant tumor of the vulva is squamous-cell carcinoma

Squamous carcinoma of the vulva, which usually occurs in elderly women, may show extensive local invasion and metastases in inguinal lymph nodes. One variant in very old women, **verrucous carcinoma**, produces a large, warty, cauliflower-like growth that grows slowly, invading local tissues, but almost never metastasizes (*Fig. 19.4*). Well-differentiated squamous carcinomas of the vulva have a good prognosis provided they are confined to the vulva and inguinal nodes; the prognosis is worse if there is local invasion to other pelvic organs (e.g. bladder, rectum), metastatic tumor in iliac lymph nodes, or evidence of bloodborne metastasis.

Although most invasive squamous carcinomas of the vulva appear to arise de novo, some arise in epithelium in which there is severe dysplasia amounting to carcinoma in situ (*Fig. 19.5*). This phenomenon, **vulval intraepithelial neoplasia** (**VIN**), is generally seen in patients younger than those with invasive tumors, and there may be coexisting evidence of HPV warty change in the affected and adjacent epithelium. Furthermore, HPV16 can be demonstrated in many cases (70–90%) of vulval carcinoma arising in VIN. There is also an increased risk of cancer progression in young women who smoke cigarettes, suggesting a possible interaction between cigarette smoking and HPV infection in the etiology of invasive vulval carcinoma in younger women.

Other neoplastic lesions of the vulva are mainly melanocytic lesions or skin appendage tumors

Apart from squamous-cell carcinomas, other tumors arising in the vulva are derived from melanocytes or skin appendages. **Benign intradermal** and **compound nevi** are common on the vulval skin, and the labia majora are an important site for the development of malignant melanoma. The features of both benign nevi and **malignant melanoma** are identical to those occurring in the skin (see Chapter 23). Although any of the skin-appendage tumors described in Chapter 23 can occur in the skin of the vulva, only **papillary hidradenoma** (derived from the eccrine ducts) is frequently seen.

Fig. 19.4 Verrucous carcinoma of the vulva. This radical vulvectomy specimen shows a verrucous carcinoma that has invaded the right labium majus.

Rarely, Paget's disease of the vulva may occur, representing intraepidermal spread of a carcinoma derived from an adenocarcinoma of skin appendages. It is histologically similar to the disease of the nipple.

DISEASES OF THE VAGINA

The most important diseases of the vagina are infections (vaginitis)

The vagina can become infected by the same agents that cause vulvitis, e.g. herpes simplex virus, HPV, *Candida albicans, Gardnerella vaginalis.* The vagina has an abundant natural bacterial flora, the principal organism in which is *Lactobacillus acidophilus.* This produces lactic acid by the breakdown of glycogen in the surface vaginal epithelium, thereby creating an acid environment in which most other organisms cannot proliferate. However, this barrier only works effectively against bacteria. Infective vaginitis is usually sexually transmitted, presenting with vulvovaginal soreness and discharge.

Trichomonas vaginalis is a common cause of vaginitis in young women and is usually sexually transmitted. The vaginal mucosa becomes red and inflamed, with a frothy white discharge on its surface.

Gardnerella vaginalis is a very common cause of non-specific vaginitis, commonly associated with a thin, milky white vaginal discharge.

Herpes simplex produces erosive vaginal lesions, and the organism may be transmitted to the fetus during passage through the birth canal. Usually, there are associated vulval herpetic lesions.

Candida albicans is a normal commensal in the vagina, but its proliferation is usually suppressed by the normal vaginal flora. Clinical infection can occur when the vaginal flora is destroyed, e.g. by antibiotics. White plaques of fungal hyphae develop on an inflamed vaginal mucosa, and there is

Fig. 19.5 Vulval intraepithelial neoplasia (VIN). In (a) there is very extensive red thickening of the vulva, extending onto the perineum and perianal region. This is due to extensive VIN. In the micrograph (b) the full thickness of the vulval epithelium shows dysplastic squamous cells, with many mitoses (VIN III).

vaginal discharge associated with severe vulval irritation. Infection may be severe in patients with diabetes mellitus.

Less common causes of vaginal infection include the gonococcus (usually secondary to gonococcal cervicitis), *Mycoplasma*, and HPV (usually associated with extensive vulval and perineal condylomata which extend up the vagina at a late stage), and some forms of staphylococci. Staphylococci are usually introduced into the vagina with a tampon, and proliferation of bacteria in a neglected or retained tampon may lead to production of bacterial exotoxins, giving rise to the **toxic shock syndrome**.

Primary tumors of the vagina are very rare

Primary tumors of the vagina in adults are exceptionally rare, but the vagina is frequently the site of metastases, particularly from malignant tumors of the cervix, endometrium and ovary. Vaginal bleeding after hysterectomy for uterine or ovarian malignancy should always be investigated and biopsied because of the frequency of metastatic tumor in the residual vaginal vault.

The main primary vaginal tumors are **squamous-cell carcinomas** and, even more rarely, adenocarcinomas. Clear-cell carcinoma of the vagina is seen in women exposed in utero to the synthetic estrogen diethylstilboestrol, preceded by replacement of normal vaginal epithelium by glandular epithelium, termed **vaginal adenosis**.

In childhood the vagina may be the site of development of **rhabdomyosarcoma**, which macroscopically appears as a polypoid, gelatinous mass protruding into the vagina.

DISEASES OF THE CERVIX

The cervix is an important site of pathology, particularly in women of reproductive age. The ectocervix is covered by squamous epithelium, and the endocervical canal by mucus-secreting columnar epithelium, which shows glandular downgrowths. At various stages in a woman's reproductive life the junction between the squamous and columnar epithelium migrates onto the convexity of the ectocervix, then back into the endocervical canal. This **squamocolumnar junction** is the seat of most of the epithelial diseases that occur in the cervix.

The original squamocolumnar junction is usually located in the region of the external os, but its precise location at birth is influenced by exposure to maternal hormones in utero.

Around puberty, hormonal influences cause extension of the columnar epithelium onto the ectocervix, forming an **ectropion** or **cervical erosion** (*Fig. 19.6*). This process is augmented by a first pregnancy, particularly when it occurs shortly after menarche.

Before puberty, the pH of the vagina and cervix is alkaline, but afterwards bacterial breakdown of glycogen in the vaginal and cervical squamous epithelium renders it an acidic environment, the pH being about 3.

Exposure of the sensitive columnar epithelium of the ectropion to the postpubertal acidic environment of the vagina induces squamous metaplasia and a transformation zone between the endocervical columnar epithelium and

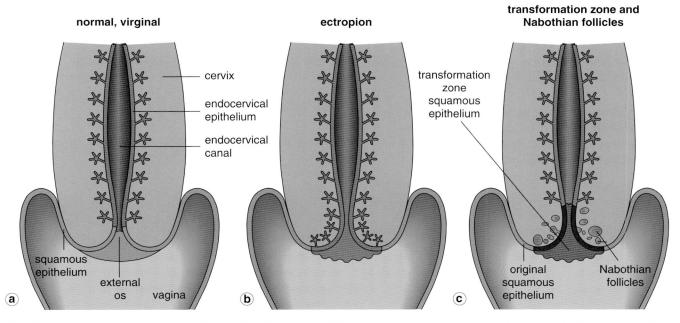

Fig. 19.6 Squamocolumnar junction of the cervix. The mobility of the squamocolumnar junction, the development of ectropion, and the formation of the transformation zone are illustrated. (a) The squamocolumnar junction is originally situated in the region of the external os. (b) At puberty the endocervical epithelium extends distally into the acid environment of the vagina, forming an ectropion. (c) A transformation zone forms as squamous epithelium regrows over the ectropion. The openings of the crypts may be obliterated in the process, which leads to the formation of mucus-filled Nabothian follicles.

the ectocervical squamous epithelium. This zone is composed of new squamous epithelium in an area previously occupied by columnar epithelium.

Thus the squamocolumnar junction is of variable size, but its site always approximates to the external os. In older women it may retreat into the endocervical canal.

The most important diseases of the cervix are listed in *Fig. 19.7*.

Chronic cervicitis is produced by the same organisms responsible for infective vaginitis

The term 'chronic cervicitis' is sometimes applied inaccurately by clinicians when the area of ectocervix around the external os is red and irregular; in most cases this is not inflammation, but represents the extension of columnar epithelium onto the external os, sometimes called **ectropion** or, inaccurately, a 'cervical erosion'.

Acute cervicitis with erosion may be seen in herpes simplex infection, and there is usually herpetic disease of the vulva and vagina. Genuine chronic endocervicitis, with a heavy lymphocytic and plasma cell infiltrate, may be found in association with infections of the vagina by *Trichomonas*, *Candida*, *Gardnerella* and gonococcus.

Microglandular endocervical hyperplasia is mainly seen in pregnancy and in women taking oral contraceptives with a progestogen component

Microglandular endocervical hyperplasia is a common cervical change, induced by hormonal changes. It is a pattern of endocervical proliferation in which the cervical crypts multiply and become architecturally disordered, sometimes associated with decidual change in the stroma. This change is seen particularly during pregnancy, and is the result of progestogen stimulation of the endocervix; however, the changes may persist after the removal of the causative stimulus. It is also seen in women taking oral contraceptives containing progestogen.

The lesion may be asymptomatic, but there is often a complaint of an excessive mucous vaginal discharge, and in severe cases the cervix looks to be the seat of numerous small endocervical polyps.

Cervical polyps are a common cause of intermenstrual bleeding

Cervical polyps are common abnormalities which, through erosion and ulceration, may cause intermenstrual bleeding. They are seen in about 5% of women. Macroscopically they appear smooth, rounded or pear-shaped, and are typically 1–2 cm in diameter. The polyps derive from the endocervix, protruding from the cervix through the external os. They are composed of endocervical stroma and glands, the latter often being distended with mucus. The surface of the polyp may show ulceration and inflammation and, if long-standing, there may be surface squamous metaplasia.

Benign tumors of the cervix are uncommon, the most frequent being leiomyomas

True benign neoplasms of the cervix are uncommon, most nodules associated with the cervix being endocervical polyps. Leiomyomas may occur in the cervix, but are less common at this site than in the uterus (see page 427, *Fig. 19.19*). Derived from the smooth muscle of the cervix wall, they expand the cervix asymmetrically, producing distortion and compression of the endocervical canal.

HPV infection is common in the ectocervical epithelium and is an important etiological agent in cervical cancer

HPV infection of the cervix is sexually acquired. Over 70 subtypes of HPV have been defined, each of which has been allocated a number.

Occasionally, HPV infection may produce papillary lesions of cervical squamous epithelium (**condyloma acuminatum**), which are similar to those seen on the vulva (see page 415). They are usually located on the ectocervical squamous epithelium or on the squamous epithelium of the transformation zone, and may be multiple.

Fig. 19.8 Wart-virus change in the cervix. The cervical epithelium shows the characteristic features of wart-virus change in a 'flat condyloma' from the transformation zone; the epithelium is atypical, with koilocytes in the upper layers of the epithelium.

More often, HPV infection causes **flat condylomas**. These cannot normally be seen with the naked eye, but may be recognizable on colposcopic examination after painting the cervix with dilute acetic acid, which turns them white.

Histologically the epithelium in flat condylomas is abnormal, with binucleate cells (particularly in the upper layers of the epithelium), and so-called 'koilocytic change' in the most abnormal epithelial cells (*Fig. 19.8*). These viral changes can be recognized on cervical-smear cytology. Both patterns of wart-virus involvement of the cervical squamous epithelium are most frequent in the transformation zone epithelium, and may coexist with changes of intraepithelial neoplasia.

Different types of HPV are differently associated with invasive carcinoma of the cervix: HPV 16 and 18 are frequently associated, whereas HPV 6 and 11 are rarely associated with malignant transformation.

HPV types 16 and 18 contain gene segments that integrate into the cellular genome, resulting in the expression of proteins that inhibit the action of tumor suppressor genes (such as *TP53*) and that activate cyclin E. These defects in cell cycle regulation result in uncontrolled cellular proliferation (page 85). HPV types 6 and 11, in contrast, do not integrate into the host genome.

Despite the frequent association of HPV 16 and 18 with the development of carcinoma, it must be emphasized that of all women harboring these infections, only a small minority go on to develop carcinoma.

Cervical intraepithelial neoplasia is an important precursor of invasive malignancy

The metaplastic epithelium of the transformation zone is susceptible to change during reproductive life. Mild degrees of nuclear enlargement can be seen in response to chronic inflammation, in reparative epithelium, and in association with HPV infection. However, more severe atypia is now regarded as a preneoplastic proliferation and is called **cervical intraepithelial neoplasia** (CIN) (*Fig. 19.9*). This change takes place in the metaplastic epithelium of the transformation zone of the cervix and is usually associated with infection by HPV.

Three grades of severity are recognized, depending on the proportion of the thickness of the cervical epithelium that is replaced by atypical cells.

CIN I corresponds to mild dysplasia. Atypical cells are confined to the lower third of the epithelium, the upper two-thirds showing normal differentiation and maturation with flattening of cells.

CIN II corresponds to moderate dysplasia. Atypical cells occupy the lower half of the epithelium, but evidence of differentiation and maturation with flattening of cells is seen in the upper half. Nuclear abnormalities may extend through the full thickness of the epithelium, but are most marked in the lower half, where there may be increased mitoses with some abnormal forms.

CIN III corresponds to severe dysplasia and carcinoma in situ. Atypical cells extend throughout the full thickness

Fig. 19.9 Cervical intraepithelial neoplasia. (a) The junction between normal ectocervical epithelium and severe full-thickness CIN. Note the ease with which the abnormal epithelial cells from the atypical epithelium can desquamate (arrows); this forms the basis of diagnostic exfoliative cytology. (b) Mild/moderate atypia of cervical epithelium (CIN I–CIN II). The atypical cells are confined to the deeper parts of the epithelium but cells at the surface show maturation with flattening. (c) Moderate/severe atypia of cervical epithelium (CIN II–CIN III). Atypical cells with pleomorphism and mitotic activity extend through the full thickness of the epithelium. (d) Foci of early microinvasion (arrow) arising in an area of CIN III.

of the epithelium, with minimal differentiation and maturation on the surface. Mitotic figures and abnormal mitoses are present through all layers, and there may be extension of the change along endocervical crypt necks, and foci of true microinvasion.

Histological appearances of typical CIN patterns are shown in *Figs 19.9b* and *c*.

These abnormal epithelial changes occur in the transformation zone, but may extend over the ectocervical surface and up the endocervical canal. In about 10% of cases, atypia termed **cervical glandular intraepithelial neoplasia** (CGIN) is also seen in endocervical epithelium.

The presence of abnormal epithelial cells can be detected by cytological examination of a smear of surface epithelial cells removed from cervix; this is the basis of screening for disease (see blue box below).

CIN I is associated with a small risk of progression to carcinoma, CIN II and CIN III being associated with a higher risk of development of carcinoma. The natural history of CIN is important, as it determines how often screening is required to detect progression of disease.

- 50% of patients with CIN I have spontaneous regression of disease.
- 30% of patients with CIN I have persistent low-grade atypia.
- 20% of patients with CIN I progress through CIN II to CIN III over a period of about 10 years.

- 20% of patients with CIN III progress to develop invasive carcinoma of the cervix within 10 years.

It has been suggested that smears repeated every 3 years are adequate for the purposes of population screening. Despite this frequency, it is still possible for some individuals to progress from CIN I to invasive carcinoma in a short space of time.

Invasive carcinoma of the cervix is most commonly squamous-cell carcinoma

Invasive carcinoma of the cervix may occur at any time during the reproductive and postmenopausal years, but the average age of development is about 50 years. It accounts for 3–5% of cases of carcinoma in females.

Macroscopically, early lesions appear as areas of granular irregularity of the cervical epithelium, progressive invasion of the stroma causing abnormal hardness of the cervix. Late lesions appear as fungating, ulcerated areas, which destroy the cervix (*Fig. 19.11*).

The vast majority of carcinomas of the cervix are **squamous-cell carcinomas**, arising from the transformation zone or ectocervix. Lesions fall into three histological patterns: keratinizing squamous-cell carcinoma, non-keratinizing large-cell squamous carcinoma, and non-keratinizing small-cell squamous carcinoma.

Although squamous-cell carcinoma of the cervix is predisposed by a variety of factors, the common denominator

---

Diagnostic cervical cytology

The development of abnormalities in the cervical epithelium is an important factor in the prevention of subsequent invasive carcinoma of the cervix. Detection of abnormal cells is based on the presence of abnormal cytology. Using a specially shaped spatula, cells are scraped from the ectocervix and lower cervical canal and smeared onto a slide. They are fixed in a preservative solution and sent to a pathology laboratory for cytological examination after the addition of Papanicolaou stain (the origin of the term 'Pap smear'). In CIN, the exfoliated cells have an increased nuclear: cytoplasmic ratio and a clumped, irregular chromatin pattern, being termed **dyskaryotic** (*Fig. 19.10*).

If atypical epithelial cells are detected in a cervical smear, patients are recalled. The site of abnormal epithelium is identified by colposcopy, and the diagnosis confirmed by biopsy of the abnormal area. If the lesion is non-invasive and completely visible, not extending high up into the endocervical canal, ablation of the atypical area can be performed using laser or cryotherapy. If the

topmost edge of the lesion cannot be seen in the endocervical canal, the lesion has to be removed as part of an excision biopsy.

Fig. 19.10 Cervical cytology smear in CIN. This cytology preparation shows a clump of cervical epithelial cells demonstrating moderate and severe dyskaryosis.

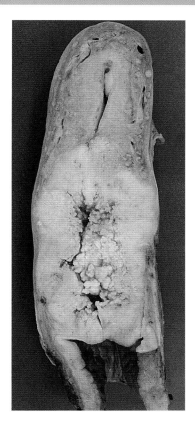

Fig. 19.11 Invasive squamous carcinoma of the cervix. In this hemisection through the uterus, cervix and upper vagina, a fungating lesion has completely destroyed the cervix and is invading the lower part of the body of the uterus.

is sexual activity, suggesting that exposure to environmental agents (particularly infection) is most important.

Adenocarcinoma of the cervix is less common than squamous carcinoma, but may be increasing in incidence

Adenocarcinoma of the cervix is almost always derived from the mucus-secreting columnar epithelium lining the endocervical canal, and may be preceded by adenocarcinoma in situ. Both invasive and in-situ carcinoma can be detected by cervical smear cytology. Invasive adenocarcinomas comprise 5–10% of all primary malignant tumors of the cervix; there is evidence of an apparent increase in incidence, but this may be largely explained by a reduction in the incidence of invasive squamous carcinomas. Compared with invasive squamous carcinoma, adenocarcinoma tends to metastasize to lymph nodes earlier and to be less radiosensitive; it is generally regarded as having a worse prognosis.

Prognosis of squamous cell carcinoma of the cervix is related to stage at diagnosis

The common presenting symptom is vaginal bleeding in the early stages, but advanced neglected tumors may cause urinary obstruction due to bladder involvement.

The histological type of the tumor is less important for prognosis than is the staging at diagnosis. Microinvasive

---

Risk factors in cervical squamous-cell carcinoma

Sexual intercourse: very low incidence in virgins.

Age at first intercourse: higher incidence in women who have intercourse before the age of 17, and in those who marry early (presumably also a reflection of earlier intercourse).

Sexually transmitted diseases: higher incidence in women with a history of sexually transmitted disease, and also in prostitutes (see HPV below).

Socioeconomic status: incidence higher in the lower social groups, but this may be related to lifestyle and sexual habits rather than any other factor.

Smoking: epidemiological studies suggest a link between heavy smoking and cervical carcinoma, particularly CIN. Although it is difficult to rule out other factors, such as different social and sexual lifestyles in smoking and non-smoking women, depression of local immune surveillance by Langerhans' cells has been suggested as important.

Male factors: to explain the importance of sexual intercourse, carcinogenic agents have been sought in

smegma, spermatozoa and other components of the semen, but no definite evidence of a chemical carcinogen has been found.

HPV: the coexistence of HPV with CIN and invasive carcinoma, seen frequently in cone biopsy and colposcopy specimens, suggests a link. Furthermore, the identification of DNA from HPV types 16, 18 and 33 in more than 60% of cervical carcinomas strongly suggests a link and possible causative factor. This is currently an area of intense research. Proteins produced by HPV inactivate products of tumor suppressor genes, thereby facilitating tumor development.

HIV infection: carcinoma of the cervix is predisposed by immunosuppression and has increased in incidence as a consequence of AIDS.

Other infective agents: attempts to prove a role for infective agents such as *Chlamydia* and herpes simplex have been inconclusive, the link usually being no stronger than the fact that both diseases are the result of sexual intercourse.

Fig. 19.12 Stage and 5-year survival for carcinoma of the cervix

Stage	5-year survival (%)	Degree of local invasion
I	90	Confined to cervix
II	82	Invasion of upper part of vagina or adjacent parametrial tissues
III	35	Spread to pelvic side wall, lower vagina or ureters
IV	10	Invasion of rectum, bladder wall or outside pelvis

carcinomas show minute foci of very superficial invasion, only detected histologically, and have a very good prognosis after local excision. Invasive carcinomas are staged according to the degree of local invasion, and survival is related to stage (*Fig. 19.12*). Invasion of paracervical and external iliac nodes occurs early.

DISEASES OF THE ENDOMETRIUM

The endometrium lines the uterus, responding to cyclical hormonal stimulation during the menstrual cycle. The histology of the endometrium can be used as a reliable index of the phase of the menstrual cycle. The main diseases of the endometrium include histological changes in response to endocrine effects, inflammatory diseases causing endometritis, polyps, hyperplasia (divided into several types and important in predisposing to neoplasia), tumors (epithelial tumors, mostly carcinomas and rarer tumors of endometrial stroma), endometriosis (a condition in which endometrium grows outside the uterus), and adenomyosis (a condition in which endometrium grows down into the muscle of the uterine wall).

Histological changes reflecting endocrine defects are commonly seen in the endometrium

Histological examination of the endometrium is frequently undertaken as part of the investigation of disordered menstruation or infertility. The histological pattern of endometrium is correlated with the stated last date of menstrual period and with any relevant drug therapy.

Among the most common abnormalities encountered in clinical practice is **senile atrophy**, seen after the menopause. Glands are simple, lined by inactive cuboidal cells and may form large cystic spaces. There is no evidence of mitotic activity, reflecting lack of estrogenic stimulation.

Anovulatory cycles are common at the start and end of reproductive life. They are associated with irregular men-

struation. The effects of excessive estrogen stimulation are manifest in the endometrium as proliferation of glands.

Luteal-phase defect or irregular ripening is associated with infertility. This may be caused by failure of production of progesterone by the corpus luteum, or by defective receptors for progesterone within endometrium. Examination of the endometrium in the second half of the menstrual cycle shows inadequate or absent development of secretory changes in the endometrium.

Persistence of the corpus luteum at the end of the normal menstrual cycle causes failure of normal endometrial shedding, leading to abnormal uterine bleeding. Examination of the endometrium reveals a mixed pattern of menstrual-phase, secretory-phase and proliferative-phase patterns.

Oral contraceptive pills cause changes in the structure of the endometrium, which is greatly reduced in bulk. Glands become small and inactive, with poor development of the stroma.

Intrauterine contraceptive devices (IUCDs) are sometimes associated with chronic endometritis and *Actinomyces* infection.

Metaplasia of the endometrium is usually seen in postmenopausal women, arising less commonly in normal cycling endometrium. The main types are squamous metaplasia and metaplasia to epithelial patterns resembling tubal or endocervical epithelium.

Acute endometritis is usually encountered as a complication of pregnancy

Acute endometritis is characterized by infiltration of endometrial glands by neutrophils. Caused by bacterial infection, it is usually seen as a complication of parturition or miscarriage. The organisms most commonly responsible are streptococci, staphylococci and clostridia, which are often associated with anaerobic organisms when there is retained dead tissue within the uterine cavity postpartum.

In severe cases of acute inflammation a **pyometra** may develop, when the uterine cavity is filled with pus. This is the consequence of obstruction of the cervical os, complicated by infection of the uterine cavity. The main reasons for obstruction of the cervix are tumors, and scarring as a result of previous surgical intervention.

Chronic endometritis is usually associated with recent gestation, pelvic inflammatory disease, or IUCD use

Chronic endometritis may be associated with menstrual irregularities, but is also found in women who are being investigated for infertility. Histologically the endometrium shows lymphoid infiltration, with the formation of plasma cells. The majority of cases are associated with a definite clinical risk factor for developing inflammation. The condition occurs after recent pregnancy, miscarriage or instrumentation in 50% of cases, in association with pelvic inflammatory disease (e.g. salpingitis) in 25% of cases, and in association with previous use of IUCDs in about 20% of cases. In the remaining 5% of cases without a defined risk factor, chronic endometritis may be caused by gonococcal or chlamydial infection, or TB.

In tuberculous endometritis, because granulomas form only in secretory endometrium, they may not be seen in samples taken from early in the cycle. The condition is commonly part of more widespread infection involving fallopian tubes.

In adenomyosis, endometrium burrows deep within the wall of the uterus

Adenomyosis is a condition in which endometrium grows down to develop deep within the myometrium. The condition may cause enlargement of the uterus and is sometimes associated with menstrual abnormalities and dysmenorrhea.

Macroscopically, small irregular pink areas, some with small cysts, are seen in the affected myometrium (*Fig. 19.13a*). Histologically, islands of endometrium are seen deep within muscle (*Fig. 19.13b*). If traced, these deep islands are found to be in continuity with surface endometrium. This process may affect the myometrium diffusely or may occur focally, producing apparently circumscribed nodules of hypertrophied muscle and deep endometrium (**nodular adenomyosis**).

Ectopic growth of endometrium outside the uterus is termed 'endometriosis'

Endometriosis is a condition in which ectopic endometrium develops outside the uterine cavity. It affects 1 in 15 (7%) women of reproductive age, with associated infertility in about 30% of cases. The pathogenesis is discussed in the pink box on page 424.

The common sites for ectopic endometrial growth are the ovaries, fallopian tubes, round ligaments, and pelvic peritoneum. Less common sites are the intestinal wall, bladder, umbilicus, and laparotomy scars. Rarely, involvement of lymph nodes, lung and pleura is seen.

The ectopic endometrium still responds to cyclical hormonal stimulation, with phases of proliferation and breakdown with bleeding. The bleeding and breakdown stimulate the formation of fibrous adhesions and accumulation of hemosiderin pigment.

Macroscopically, foci of endometriosis appear as cystic and solid masses, which are characteristically dark brown from iron pigment accumulated as a result of repeated bleeding. Histologically, endometrial glands and stroma are seen, together with fibrosis and macrophages containing iron pigment.

Endometrial tissue growing in abnormal sites stimulates fibrosis and may cause fibrous adhesions between adjacent organs. When peritoneum is involved, adhesions may cause bowel obstruction. The condition usually presents with cyclical pelvic pain, dysmenorrhea, and infertility. When it affects the fallopian tubes and ovaries the whole of the fallopian tube and ovary may be converted to a cystic mass containing brown, semi-liquid material (chocolate cyst).

Treatment by endocrine manipulation of endometrial growth is usually effective.

Endometrial polyps are localized overgrowths of endometrial glands and stroma

Endometrial polyps are very common and are usually seen in the perimenopausal age range. They are thought to be caused by over-proliferation of glands in response to estrogenic stimuli. Macroscopically they vary in size, but are usually 1–3 cm in diameter and are usually sited in the uterine fundus. They appear as firm smooth nodules within

Fig. 19.13 Adenomyosis of the uterus. (a) In this uterus, removed because of heavy, irregular and painful periods, the myometrium is expanded as a result of severe adenomyosis, particularly posteriorly. The islands of endometrium can be seen as yellowish brown areas surrounded by hypertrophied smooth muscle (nodular adenomyosis). (b) Histology of an area of endometrial glands and stroma within hypertrophied myometrium, taken from the specimen in (a).

Pathogenesis of endometriosis

The reason for the development of endometriosis remains uncertain, but there are three main theories:

1. **Retrograde menstruation.** In normal women it is well documented that fragments of endometrium migrate into the peritoneal cavity along the fallopian tube at the time of menstruation. It has been proposed that this material implants in some cases, causing endometriosis, and that although in normal women the immune system destroys such implanted endometrium, in women susceptible to endometriosis the immune surveillance is absent.

2. **Metaplasia of peritoneal epithelium** may cause it to differentiate to form endometrium. Metaplasia may also cause the development of tubal-pattern epithelium, causing the related condition of endosalpingosis. The stimulus for such metaplasia remains uncertain.

3. **Metastatic spread of endometrium.** This theory suggests that endometrium found in nodes, pleura, lung and umbilicus has been spread by lymphatics or blood vessels.

None of these hypotheses alone explains endometriosis in all of its manifestations, and it is likely that all three mechanisms are operative to differing degrees.

It is well established that endometriosis is dependent on estrogen for continued growth and proliferation, with disease becoming inactive after oophorectomy or onset of the menopause. This is the rationale for treatment that induces a hypoestrogenic state by suppression of the hypothalamopituitary–ovarian axis with analog of gonadotrophin-releasing hormone (GnRH).

---

the endometrial cavity (*Fig. 19.14*), occasionally prolapsing through the cervical os.

Histologically they are made up of cystically dilated endometrial glands in a vascular stroma. They are clinically associated with menstrual abnormalities and dysmenorrhea, but may develop ulceration or undergo torsion.

Endometrial hyperplasia is caused by estrogenic stimulation and may be preneoplastic

Endometrial hyperplasia is seen in response to estrogenic stimulation. An endogenous response may be seen with successive anovulatory cycles or estrogen-secreting tumors, and an exogenous response with estrogen-containing drugs.

The importance of endometrial hyperplasia is that it is associated with an increased risk of developing adenocarcinoma of the endometrium. It is divided into non-atypical and atypical types by the WHO classification.

Of the non-atypical hyperplasias, **simple hyperplasia** is the most common pattern, diffusely affecting the whole endometrium. Proliferation of glands can be seen, with evident mitoses and stratification of cells. Glands grow in a regular tubular pattern, but are often dilated (*Fig. 19.15a*); however, there is no cytological atypia of the nuclei. This type is associated with a very slightly increased risk of malignancy after a long period of time, typically over 10 years. **Complex hyperplasia** is almost always seen focally within the endometrium. There is obvious proliferation of epithelium, evident by mitotic figures, but the glands grow in an irregular pattern, with branched irregular contours and little intervening stroma. The cells forming the glands do not show cytological atypia. This type is associated with a slightly increased risk of developing malignancy.

Fig. 19.14 Benign endometrial polyp. The microcystic appearance is due to cystically dilated endometrial glands within the polyp.

Atypical hyperplasia is commonly seen only focally within the endometrium and, like non-atypical hyperplasia, is divided into simple and complex types; however, most show a complex pattern. There is proliferation of epithelium, evident by mitotic figures, and the glands grow in an irregular pattern, with branched irregular contours (*Fig. 19.15b*). However, the cells forming the glands show cytological atypia, with pleomorphism and hyperchromatism. About 30% of cases with this pattern of hyperplasia will develop a carcinoma of the endometrium, usually within 5 years of diagnosis.

Endometrial carcinoma is the most common cancer of the female genital tract

Carcinomas of the endometrium are nearly all adenocarcinomas, with several histological subtypes. This type of carcinoma is the most frequent invasive malignancy in the

Fig. 19.17 Surgical stage of endometrial carcinoma, and outcome after treatment with surgery and radiotherapy

Stage	Proportion of cases (%)		5-year survival (%)
I	80	Corpus of uterus only	90
II	5	Corpus and cervix	50
III	5	Invasion confined to pelvis	30
IV	10	Invasion outside pelvis or involves bladder or rectal mucosa	10

Fig. 19.15 Endometrial hyperplasia. (a) This endometrium shows simple hyperplasia, with cystic dilatation of glands showing no other architectural or cytological atypia. (b) This endometrium shows complex atypical hyperplasia, with irregular branching glands and dark-staining epithelium due to cytological atypia.

female genital tract, accounting for about 7% of all tumors in women. Endometrial carcinoma can be divided into two main groups:

- Tumors that occur at a time close to menopause, associated with endometrial hyperplasia and abnormal estrogenic stimulation of the endometrium. This is the largest group and is associated with a generally good prognosis.
- Tumors that occur in older, postmenopausal women, not associated with estrogenic stimulation or endometrial hyperplasia. Tumors in this group are more often associated with a poor prognosis.

Macroscopically, small tumors appear as diffuse, solid areas or polypoid lesions in the endometrium, whereas larger tumors fill and distend the endometrial cavity with soft, white, friable tissue (*Fig. 19.16a*). Necrosis of tumor is common and leads to a frequent presenting feature of postmenopausal bleeding.

Fig. 19.16 Endometrial adenocarcinoma. (a) The endometrial cavity is distended by soft, friable endometrial adenocarcinoma, showing necrosis and hemorrhage. There is considerable depth of invasion, the tumor being close to penetrating the serosal surface at the fundus of the uterus. (b) Histology of the tumor in (a) shows a moderately differentiated endometrioid type of adenocarcinoma (the most common type) extensively invading the smooth muscle of the myometrium.

Most tumors associated with estrogenic excess are **endometrioid adenocarcinomas** (60% of all cases). These can be graded (I–III) according to the amount of glandular and solid pattern with tumor (*Fig. 19.16b*). A high grade is associated with a worse prognosis. In some cases, areas of squamous metaplasia or true squamous carcinoma (**adenosquamous carcinoma**) are also present.

Two other main types of tumor are seen, mostly in the non-estrogen-related postmenopausal group. **Uterine papillary serous carcinoma** is a highly aggressive tumor. Even in the absence of significant myometrial or vascular invasion, recurrence, widespread metastasis and death may occur. **Uterine clear-cell carcinoma** also behaves in a highly malignant fashion. Papillary serous and clear cell carcinomas are not graded.

Spread of carcinoma of the uterus is mainly by local invasion and is divided into four stages (I–IV). Stage I tumors are confined to the corpus uteri, stage II tumors involve extension into the cervix, stage III have spread beyond the uterus but are confined to the true pelvis and stage IV tumors show distant metastasis or involvement of other viscera. Survival figures for each stage are given in *Fig. 19.17*.

Spread along the lumina of the fallopian tubes leads to frequent involvement of ovaries, and with **venous and lymphatic invasion** there may be involvement of the vagina and para-aortic nodes. Widespread hematogenous metastasis is uncommon, except with papillary serous carcinomas and clear-cell carcinomas. The prognosis of carcinoma of the uterus is related to stage, as outlined in *Fig. 19.17*.

Tumors of endometrial stroma may be pure or seen as part of mixed tumors

Less than 2% of all uterine tumors involve neoplastic proliferation of the stromal element of the endometrium. These tumors are thought to be derived from primitive Müllerian cells that can variably differentiate into endometrial stroma, epithelium, or support tissues. Tumors present as expansile masses within the uterine cavity, causing postmenopausal bleeding; with the more malignant tumors there is evidence of dissemination.

Endometrial stromal sarcoma is composed of malignant stromal spindle cells and can be graded from low to high.

Adenosarcoma contains malignant stroma and a histologically benign epithelial component. Tumors commonly recur after hysterectomy.

Carcinosarcoma (malignant mixed Müllerian tumor) has both malignant stromal and epithelial components. Often the stromal component contains tissues not normally seen in the uterus, e.g. cartilage, fat and skeletal muscle. This typically occurs in elderly women and has an extremely poor prognosis (*Fig. 19.18*).

DISEASES OF THE MYOMETRIUM

The myometrium is composed of smooth muscle. Apart from changes in pregnancy, the myometrium is affected in adenomyosis (see page 423) and by tumors (either leiomyomas or, rarely, leiomyosarcomas and adenomatoid tumors).

Pathogenesis of endometrial carcinoma

In the perimenopausal age group, the majority of endometrial adenocarcinomas are associated with hyperestrogenism and endometrial hyperplasia. Hyperestrogenism may be exogenous or endogenous in origin.

Clinical associations carrying a higher risk of development of adenocarcinomas are obesity (due to endogenous production of estrogen in adipose tissue), diabetes mellitus, nulliparity, and hypertension.

An increased incidence of endometrial carcinoma is also seen in some families, in which it is associated with an increased risk of breast cancer, and the occurrence of dominant-acting oncogenes seems likely in this group. Mutation of K-*ras* oncogene is a common event in the development of about 10% of sporadic endometrial cancers. Abnormality in p53 is also a common event, particularly in papillary serous carcinomas which have a poor prognosis.

Fig. 19.18 Malignant mixed Müllerian tumor of the endometrium. The endometrial cavity is greatly distended by a soft, fleshy, partly necrotic and hemorrhagic tumor. This old lady presented with postmenopausal bleeding, abdominal distension and pain, and had pulmonary and peritoneal metastases at the time of diagnosis.

Diagnosis of endometrial disease

The diagnosis of endometrial disease is aided by several imaging and histological techniques.

- **Transvaginal ultrasonography** can indicate lesions within the uterus, and establish the thickness of the endometrium.
- **Hysteroscopy** may identify endometrial polyps or submucosal myomas.
- **Endometrial biopsy** is frequently performed, for example to distinguish anovulatory from ovulatory bleeding, and to exclude a hyperplastic condition or a carcinoma.

Endometrial biopsy by pipette aspiration removes a small sample. This procedure may be performed as a clinic or office procedure without anesthetic.

Cervical dilatation and curettage (D and C) of endometrium is a means of obtaining a large sample of endometrium, but requires a general anesthetic. Material may be sent for culture (to establish the cause of endometritis) or histology.

In the evaluation and staging of tumors, **MR imaging** is increasingly being used to establish the extent of tumor spread preoperatively.

Fig. 19.19 Leiomyomas of the myometrium. This patient presented with heavy, irregular, painful periods. The uterus is distorted by multiple well-circumscribed benign leiomyomas in intramural, subserosal and submucosal sites.

Leiomyomas (fibroids) are the most common tumors of the uterus

Leiomyomas, also called fibroids, are the most common benign tumors of the female genital tract. They affect over half of all women over the age of 30, usually becoming symptomatic in the decade before the menopause.

Macroscopically, leiomyomas appear as rounded, rubbery, pale nodules, which have a whorled appearance on cut surface. They may arise in several locations within the uterus (e.g. intramural, submucosal and subserosal) and are very commonly multiple (*Fig. 19.19*).

Leiomyomas vary in size, ranging from under 1 cm in diameter to giant lesions 20–30 cm in size. The typical diameter for lesions responsible for clinical problems is 2–4 cm.

Histologically, tumors are composed of smooth-muscle cells and intervening collagenous stroma. Importantly, there is no cellular atypia and very few mitoses are seen. Several uncommon histological variants of leiomyoma are also described, characterized by unusual cellular or stromal patterns, e.g. myxoid change.

Degenerative changes and complications occur in these tumors. For example, tumors may outgrow their blood supply, becoming replaced by hyaline material, as well as undergoing calcification. In pregnancy, and less commonly at other times, tumors may develop ischemic degeneration in which lesions become soft and uniformly dark red (so-called 'red degeneration'). Pedunculated tumors may undergo torsion, developing venous infarction.

Clinically these tumors are associated with abnormal menstrual bleeding, dysmenorrhea, or infertility. Occasionally they cause problems because of their effects as a large abdominal mass, e.g. compressing the bladder. During pregnancy, leiomyomas may cause complications such as spontaneous abortion, premature labor, and obstruction of labor.

Uterine leiomyomas depend on the trophic action of estrogen for maintenance of size, and usually shrink after the menopause. Treatment with GnRH agonists, which induce hypoestrogenism, is being used to cause shrinkage of the uterus and fibroids to allow easier surgical removal by myomectomy. For most women who no longer wish to conceive, the treatment is to have a hysterectomy.

Leiomyosarcomas of the uterus are a tumor of the postmenopausal age group

Overall, leiomyosarcomas of the uterus are uncommon, accounting for about 2% of all tumors in the female genital tract. They arise most frequently in the postmenopausal age group.

Macroscopically tumors are typically large, fleshy masses within the myometrium, which may be necrotic. They are usually around 10–15 cm in diameter. Histologically tumors are composed of smooth-muscle cells but, unlike a benign tumor, there is greater cellularity, with mitoses and nuclear hyperchromatism. The single most useful assessment in deciding whether a smooth-muscle tumor is benign or malignant is to perform a mitotic count. Lesions with high mitotic counts are regarded as biologically malignant. In between those lesions with very high or very low counts are borderline lesions termed '**smooth-muscle tumors of uncertain malignant potential**'.

As with most sarcomas, leiomyosarcomas of the uterus tend to metastasize preferentially by vascular spread, particularly causing pulmonary metastases.

DISEASES OF THE FALLOPIAN TUBES

The fallopian tubes run from the endometrial cavity, through the wall of the uterus, forming the fimbriated end applied to the ovaries, which is responsible for guiding released ova into the uterus.

The main diseases of the fallopian tubes are inflammatory diseases (e.g. salpingitis), uncommon tumors of the epithelium and smooth-muscle wall, and ectopic pregnancy (see page 435). Postinflammatory scarring and obliteration of the fallopian tube is an important and common cause of infertility.

Salpingitis is an important cause of late tubal obstruction and infertility

Salpingitis is nearly always caused by infection that has gained access by ascending from the uterine cavity. Most cases result in acute salpingitis with acute inflammation, but others result in a chronic inflammatory reaction. The main associations for salpingitis are following pregnancy and endometritis, IUCD use, sexually transmitted disease (*Mycoplasma*, *Chlamydia* and gonococcus), TB and *Actinomyces*.

In cases of acute salpingitis the tubes are macroscopically swollen and congested, with a red, granular appearance to the serosal surface, due to vascular dilatation. Histologically the lumen may contain pus, and there is infiltration of the tubal epithelium by neutrophils. With resolution, chronic inflammation may supervene, associated with distortion of mucosal plicae, fibrosis and occlusion of the tubal lumen. A **pyosalpinx** occurs when there is massive distension of the tubal lumen by pus.

Chlamydial colonization of the tubal mucosa is increasingly being recognized as a cause of impaired tubal function in infertile women and a common cause of ectopic pregnancy. This is usually in the absence of symptoms and laparoscopic signs of active infection. The histological correlates of such infection are uncertain.

Tuberculous salpingitis is acquired by hematogenous spread from a site outside the genital tract. The tubes develop multiple granulomas in the mucosa and wall, causing adhesions to adjacent tissues (especially ovary). In advanced cases the tube may be converted to a cavity filled with caseous necrotic material.

Infection by *Actinomyces* is predisposed by colonization of the female genital tract in association with IUCD use. The pus in the tubal lumen contains colonies of *Actinomyces*, visible macroscopically as 'sulfur granules.'

In many cases of infection of the fallopian tube, adhesions form between the tube and the ovary, and infection involves the tube, ovary and adjacent parametrial tissues. This situation gives rise to a matted clump of tissue and fibrosis, referred to as a **tubo-ovarian mass**, in which individual components are hard to discern.

Hydrosalpinx is dilatation of the fallopian tube, with flattening of the mucosa, the lumen being distended by clear, watery fluid. This is believed to be a sequel to previous inflammatory damage to the tube, acquired with healing of previous inflammation (*Fig. 19.20*).

Tumors of the fallopian tube are very uncommon

Neoplastic lesions of the fallopian tube are rare, but among those that do occur are benign adenomatoid tumors, encountered in the mesosalpinx, and primary adenocarcinomas, seen in postmenopausal women. As the latter are usually seen at an advanced stage, they generally have a poor prognosis.

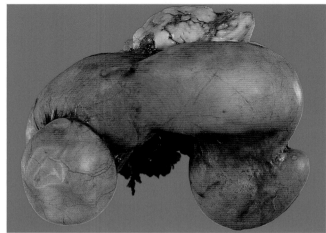

Fig. 19.20 Fallopian tube showing hydrosalpinx. The fallopian tube is distended, very thin-walled, and contains clear fluid. It is convoluted and distorted by fibrous scarring, the result of healing of previous inflammation (salpingitis).

In addition, tumors of the endometrium may spread up the tubal lumen, and metastatic disease in the pelvic peritoneum may involve the tubal serosa. Small cysts at the fimbrial end of the fallopian tube are common and, generally, clinically silent.

DISEASES OF THE OVARIES

The ovaries are paired organs attached to the back of the broad ligament. The important components of the ovary are surface 'germinal' epithelium, stroma responsible for production of many steroid hormones, and follicles containing the germ cells.

The main diseases of the ovary are non-neoplastic cysts, stromal hyperplasia, and tumors (there is a wide variety of benign and malignant lesions derived from epithelium, stroma, or germ cells).

Non-neoplastic cysts of the ovaries are common

Non-neoplastic cystic lesions in ovaries are extremely common, the majority arising from the development of Graafian follicles, others being derived from surface epithelium. Among the main types are **mesothelial-lined inclusion cysts**, which are small lesions ranging from microscopic up to 3–4 cm in diameter. They are lined by cells that are the same as those of the ovarian surface epithelium, and are filled with clear fluid.

Follicular cysts are derived from ovarian follicles and are lined by granulosa cells, with an outer coat of thecal cells (*Fig. 19.21*). Cysts are, by definition, over 2 cm in diameter. In some cysts the thecal coat becomes luteinized. Although most cysts are clinically insignificant, some may be a cause of hyperestrogenism.

Corpus luteum cysts are caused by failure of involution of the corpus luteum. Cysts are typically 2–3 cm in diameter, with a thick, yellow lining of luteinized granulosa cells. There is continued production of progesterone, resulting in menstrual irregularity.

Fig. 19.21 Follicular ovarian cyst. This micrograph shows part of the wall of a small follicular cyst, in which follicle granulosa cells can be seen lining the wall.

 Polycystic ovary syndrome (Stein–Leventhal syndrome) is a common cause of infertility

The polycystic ovary syndrome is an important and common cause of infertility. Patients are often obese, hirsute, and have acne and menstrual abnormalities (amenorrhea or irregular periods). The ovaries show thickening of the capsule, and multiple follicular cysts with stromal hyperplasia (*Fig. 19.22*).

The pathogenesis of this syndrome is still uncertain, but there are three possible theories. Defects in the hypothalamopituitary–gonadal axis may cause abnormal secretion, release or interference with the pulse frequency of gonadotropin-releasing hormone and/or luteinizing hormone, resulting in increased ovarian androgen production.

A defect in ovarian steroidogenesis may favour androgen production.

Finally, insulin resistance in peripheral tissues, often detected in obese patients, may divert metabolic pathways towards androgen synthesis.

The syndrome now has specific diagnostic features, as defined by the Rotterdam criteria.

Fig. 19.22 Polycystic ovary syndrome (Stein–Leventhal syndrome). These ovaries from a patient with Stein–Leventhal syndrome show enlargement by multiple follicular cysts, which are particularly arranged around the periphery, together with thickening of the ovarian stroma.

Theca–lutein cysts are usually seen as multiple bilateral cysts, up to 1 cm in diameter, filled with clear fluid. They are caused by high levels of gonadotropin, which precipitates follicle development (e.g. in hydatidiform mole and drug treatment).

Endometriosis may be the cause of cystic ovarian lesions filled with dark brown, iron-containing fluid (see page 423).

Stromal hyperplasia is a cause of virilization in postmenopausal women

Hyperplasia of the ovarian stroma associated with luteinization is commonly seen in the ovaries of postmenopausal women. Ovaries are usually enlarged and have a firm texture, being replaced by proliferated stromal cells. Clinically, affected women often show virilization, as the stromal cells produce androgens.

Hyperplasia of the stroma is also seen in association with a variety of neoplastic and non-neoplastic growths within the ovary, and may be associated with endocrine effects.

NEOPLASTIC DISEASE OF THE OVARIES

Primary tumors of the ovary may be derived from any of the normal cellular constituents of the ovary. They are divided into those derived from surface epithelium (70%), those from sex-cord and stromal cells (10%), and those from germ cells (20%).

In addition to primary tumors, the ovary is frequently involved in metastatic disease from other sites. Malignant tumors of ovary spread locally and particularly seed to peritoneum, when ascites is an important complication.

Epithelial tumors of the ovary can differentiate into several types

The epithelial tumors of the ovary are derived from the surface epithelium which in turn is derived from embryonic celomic epithelium. Tumors with this origin differentiate into a variety of tissues.

- **Endocervical differentiation**: mucinous ovarian tumors.
- **Tubal differentiation**: serous ovarian tumors.
- **Endometrial differentiation**: endometrioid and clear-cell ovarian tumors.
- **Transitional differentiation**: Brenner tumors.

In the histological assessment of epithelial tumors of the ovary it can be difficult to decide which lesions are benign and which are malignant. In between those tumors that are obviously benign or malignant are some cases in which there are histological features of atypical cells and abnormal tissue architecture, but no evidence of invasion. Such lesions are termed '**tumors of borderline malignant potential.**' Most borderline tumors behave in a benign fashion, the remainder behaving as low-grade malignant tumors.

Serous tumors of the ovary contain watery fluid and are often bilateral

Benign serous tumors of the ovary (70%) are termed **serous cystadenomas** (*Fig. 19.23a*). These thin-walled, unilocular cysts contain watery fluid and are bilateral in about 10% of cases. Histologically they are lined by a cuboidal, regular epithelium in which small papillary projections may be seen. A related tumor, termed an **adenofibroma**, is a benign, sometimes solid and sometimes cystic (cystadenofibroma) tumor, composed of benign serous epithelium and spindle-cell stroma.

Malignant serous tumors of the ovary are termed 'serous cystadenocarcinomas' (*Fig. 19.23b, c*). These are the most common form of ovarian carcinoma and are bilateral in about half of all cases. Macroscopically, tumors may be cystic, mixed solid and cystic, or largely solid in appearance. Histologically they are composed of cystic cavities lined by columnar and cuboidal cells, with papillary proliferations of cells and solid areas. Cells are pleomorphic and mitoses are seen. Importantly, invasion of the ovarian stroma does occur, confirming the malignant character. These lesions are associated with an overall 20% 5-year survival. If the tumor has penetrated the ovarian capsule, the survival rate falls dramatically.

Borderline serous tumors of the ovary are bilateral in about 30% of cases. Macroscopically, tumors may be cystic, or mixed solid and cystic. Histologically they are composed of cystic cavities lined by columnar and cuboidal cells, with papillary proliferations of cells and solid areas. Cells are pleomorphic and mitoses are seen. However, invasion of the ovarian stroma does not occur, despite the presence of cellular atypia. These lesions are associated with an overall 75% 10-year survival.

Mucinous tumors of the ovary are usually multilocular and contain gelatinous material

Benign mucinous tumors of the ovary are multilocular cystic lesions that contain glutinous viscid mucoid material (*Fig. 19.24a,b*). They are bilateral in only 5% of cases. Histologically the cysts are lined by a single layer of columnar, mucin-secreting cells with regular nuclei and no atypical features or mitoses.

Malignant mucinous tumors of the ovary, termed **mucinous cystadenocarcinomas** (*Fig. 19.24c, d*) are bilateral in 25% of cases. These tumors may occur in young women, and the median age at diagnosis is 35 years. Macroscopically they are multilocular cystic lesions that contain viscid or gelatinous mucoid material. They may grow to a very large size. Solid areas may be seen in the walls of some cysts. Histologically the tumors are composed of columnar, mucin-secreting cells, which show heaping of nuclei, solid areas, pleomorphism and mitoses. Importantly, invasion of ovarian stroma is seen, confirming the malignant nature of the lesion. Overall survival is 34% at 10 years, which is better than that for the equivalent malignant serous tumors;

Fig. 19.23 Serous tumors of the ovary. Benign serous cystadenomas are thin-walled, unilocular cysts bearing small papillary projections (a). The malignant counterpart of (a) is the serous cystadenocarcinoma (b), showing a mixed solid and cystic pattern. Note that the tumors are bilateral, a frequent feature. Histology of the tumor in (b) shows the papillary pattern of adenocarcinoma (c), with papillary fronds covered by pleomorphic atypical epithelium.

Fig. 19.24 Mucinous tumors of the ovary. In (a) a fresh, unfixed, benign mucinous tumor of the ovary has a characteristic multilocular cystic appearance and a shiny mucoid content. Histology of a cyst wall shows well-differentiated, tall columnar epithelium (b), with basal nuclei, and luminal cytoplasm distended with mucin, which is also present in the cyst cavity space. Like the benign tumor in (a), the malignant mucinous cystadenocarcinoma in (c) is multilocular, but the solid areas in the walls of some cysts are malignant. Histology from one of the solid areas in (c) shows that the epithelium is much more pleomorphic and less well differentiated (d) than that seen in the benign tumor (b).

however, with modern chemotherapy the stage of the tumor is assuming greater importance in predicting survival.

Borderline mucinous tumors of the ovary are bilateral in 10% of cases. Apart from the fact that there is no evidence of invasion of ovarian stroma, they resemble mucinous cystadenocarcinomas both macroscopically and histologically. Overall survival is 90% at 10 years.

Endometrioid tumors of the ovary are usually malignant and often bilateral

Benign and borderline endometrioid tumors are uncommon, the vast majority of cases being malignant (**endometrioid carcinomas**). These account for 20% of ovarian carcinomas and are bilateral in about 40% of cases. Clear-cell carcinomas of the ovary are a variant of endometrioid

carcinoma, characterized by cells that have clear cytoplasm and contain abundant glycogen. Overall, endometrioid carcinomas have a 40% 5-year survival.

Mixed Müllerian tumors are composed of both epithelial and stromal elements, including cartilage and skeletal muscle. These lesions are also considered a variant of endometrioid carcinoma and have an extremely poor prognosis.

Brenner tumors of the ovary contain transitional-type epithelium, as well as a spindle-cell stroma

Brenner tumors are composed of nests of epithelium resembling transitional cell epithelium of the urinary tract, associated with a spindle-cell stroma. Macroscopically, lesions are solid and have a firm, yellowish white cut surface and range in size from a few centimeters up to 20 cm in diameter. Histologically, nests of transitional cell epithelium are separated by a spindle-cell stroma. The epithelial component may vary from histologically benign to highly atypical, allowing pathological classification into benign, borderline, and malignant Brenner tumors.

There are several forms of sex-cord stromal tumors of the ovary

About 10% of ovarian tumors are derived from the stromal cells and sex-cord cells of the ovary. As several of this group secrete estrogen, patients may develop endometrial hyperplasia and a predisposition to endometrial neoplasia.

Fibromas are benign tumors, usually seen in postmenopausal women. They are tough, whorled, white lesions composed of spindle cells and collagen. This type of tumor may be accompanied by ascites and pleural effusion in under 1% of cases (**Meigs' syndrome**).

Thecomas are solid tumors composed of the spindle cells of the ovarian stroma. These stromal cells are commonly functional, producing estrogen. Macroscopically, tumors are yellow due to the cellular content of lipid (*Fig. 19.25*). The vast majority of lesions are benign.

Some lesions show features of fibroma with focal areas developing features of thecoma (**fibrothecoma**). This reflects a common origin of both fibroma and thecoma from the spindle cells of the ovarian stroma.

Granulosa-cell tumors are composed of the granulosa cells derived from follicles. Around 75% secrete estrogen and present with signs of hyperestrogenism. Macroscopically, tumors are soft and yellow, and can vary in size from

Molecular pathology of ovarian carcinoma

Like many carcinomas, ovarian carcinomas are associated with several oncogene abnormalities, which increase in number with high-grade tumors. For example, p53 and *Ki-ras* mutations are not seen in benign epithelial tumors, but are seen in high-grade carcinomas. Overexpression of *c-erb-B2* oncogene is associated with greater biological aggressiveness and an unfavorable disease course.

Some cases of carcinoma of the ovary are associated with a penetrant dominant genetic predisposition. Clinical suspicion should be aroused by the presence of several affected members in a family, patients with both ovarian and breast cancer, and families in which there are multiple cancers in both males and females. Many families with this pattern of disease have an abnormality in a gene termed '*BRCA1*' (on chromosome 17), which is also an important cause of familial breast cancer.

a few centimeters to large masses. If confined to the ovary, they are associated with an excellent prognosis. If tumors are large or extend outside the ovary, they are more likely to behave in an aggressive manner, with local recurrence or metastasis.

Sertoli–Leydig cell tumors (androblastomas) are very uncommon and most are small benign lesions confined to the ovary. They may cause masculinizing effects from secreted hormones.

Fig. 19.25 Fibrothecoma of the ovary. A large, well-circumscribed, spherical tumor with a whorled cut-surface appearance replaces one ovary. The slightly yellow tinge is a reflection of accumulated lipid within the plump spindle cells of the thecoma component. On the left is the cut surface of the attached uterus.

Fig. 19.26 Benign cystic teratoma of the ovary (dermoid cyst). The ovarian cyst cavity contains a partly gelatinous and partly 'buttery' material in which some hairs can be seen. The cyst is lined largely by skin epithelium with skin appendages, including hair follicles.

Germ-cell tumors of the ovary may be benign or malignant, histologically resembling those seen in the testis

Germ-cell tumors account for 20% of ovarian neoplasms, occurring from childhood onwards. The classification of these lesions closely follows that for germ-cell tumors of the testis (see pages 400–6).

Benign cystic teratomas (dermoid cyst of ovary) are the most common ovarian germ-cell tumors, accounting for about 10% of all neoplasms of the ovary. Macroscopically the affected ovary is replaced by a cyst lined by skin with skin appendage structures, particularly hair (*Fig. 19.26*). Teeth, bone, respiratory tract tissue, mature neural tissue and smooth muscle are other common elements. Lesions can vary in size from 2–3 cm up to masses 10–20 cm in diameter. These lesions are benign, but are bilateral in 10% of cases. A small number of cases develop secondary malignant change in one of the elements of the teratoma, commonly squamous-cell carcinoma of the epidermal component.

Solid teratomas are very uncommon and are seen mainly in adolescents. These large, solid lesions are composed of a variety of tissue components such as squamous epithelium, cartilage, smooth muscle, respiratory mucosa, and neural tissue. In most cases small areas of primitive embryonal tissue are also seen, or other types of germ-cell tumor are encountered (classifying the lesions as 'malignant immature teratoma' or 'mixed malignant germ-cell tumor with a propensity for metastasis', respectively). In cases in which only mature tissues are seen, there is a good prognosis after removal.

Struma ovarii is composed of mature thyroid tissue. Considered by many to be a teratoma with only one line of maturation, it may cause hyperthyroidism.

Dysgerminomas of the ovary are similar to seminomas of the testis. Affected ovaries are enlarged and replaced by soft, white tumor with histological appearances like those seen in seminoma.

Yolk-sac tumor is a rare, highly malignant form of germ-cell tumor, usually seen in women under the age of 30. Lesions are typically large and necrotic, secreting α-fetoprotein, detectable in the blood as a tumor marker.

Choriocarcinoma is a rare form of germ-cell tumor composed of trophoblastic cells. It is highly malignant, with a propensity for vascular spread. Tumors secrete hCG, which can be used as a tumor marker.

Metastatic tumors of the ovary are usually from the breast and gastrointestinal tract

Tumors often metastasize to the ovary, the most common sites of origin being breast, stomach, and colon. A so-called **Krukenberg tumor** is an ovary enlarged by metastatic signet ring-cell adenocarcinoma (commonly from the stomach), which stimulates stromal hyperplasia. Such tumors are usually bilateral.

OBSTETRIC PATHOLOGY

It is not our purpose to provide a detailed text on obstetric pathology, but rather to offer an outline of the important pathology related to common or significant conditions likely to be encountered in community obstetric practice, and some pathology relating to conditions met in hospital obstetric practice.

Pregnancy is associated with a number of important abnormalities, among which is **hyperemesis gravidarum**. Although nausea and occasional vomiting are common in early pregnancy, true hyperemesis gravidarum, with uncontrollable persistent vomiting leading to hemoconcentration and electrolyte abnormalities, is rare. Its cause is not known, but the rapid rise in estrogens and progesterone in early pregnancy is thought to be important.

Anemia of two types may occur, namely iron deficiency and folate deficiency. In both cases the most common cause is an increased requirement due to the additional burden of the growing fetus, particularly in multiple pregnancies. Occasionally, reduced intake may be a factor. This is usually as a result of inadequate diet due to poverty or to poor food intake, or the consequence of the repeated vomiting associated with hyperemesis.

Pregnant women are prone to develop **urinary tract infection** because of stasis in the bladder and urinary tract, possibly associated with dilatation and kinking due to relaxation of smooth muscle under the influence of increased progesterone levels. This may be augmented by an obstructive element due to the enlarging uterus compressing the bladder and ureters in late pregnancy. About 2% of women develop clinically manifest acute urinary tract infection, a further 5% having asymptomatic bacterial colonization of urine.

Skin rashes in pregnancy are usually the result of drugs taken for anemia or urinary tract infection. Specific pregnancy-related skin rashes include a blistering skin eruption of unknown cause, and **herpes gestationis**. The latter occurs in the second and third trimesters, presenting as urticated spots that then blister, usually on the abdomen and trunk.

Hypertension in pregnancy is usually due to mild pre-eclamptic syndrome. However, pregnancy may unmask a latent tendency to develop benign essential hypertension. Rarer causes include underlying glomerular disease and a previously asymptomatic pheochromocytoma of the adrenal medulla. The dangers of hypertension in pregnancy are cardiac failure and predisposition to cerebral hemorrhage.

Pre-eclamptic toxemia syndrome comprises raised blood pressure, proteinuria and peripheral edema

Pre-eclamptic toxemia is common in the UK, occurring in about 10% of all pregnant women. Seen particularly in association with multiple pregnancies, primigravidae and

Pathogenesis of pre-eclampsia

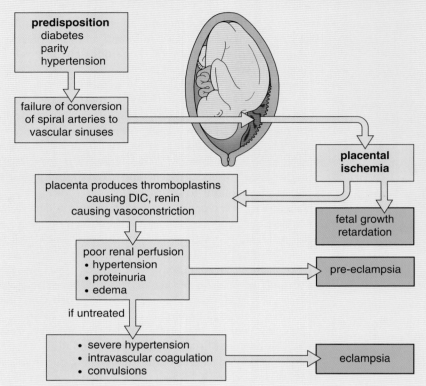

predisposition
diabetes
parity
hypertension

failure of conversion of spiral arteries to vascular sinuses

placental ischemia

placenta produces thromboplastins causing DIC, renin causing vasoconstriction

fetal growth retardation

poor renal perfusion
• hypertension
• proteinuria
• edema

pre-eclampsia

if untreated

• severe hypertension
• intravascular coagulation
• convulsions

eclampsia

Fig. 19.27 Pathogenesis of pre-eclampsia.
Pre-eclampsia is predisposed to by maternal factors of parity, diabetes and hypertension. First pregnancy carries most risk. A main factor in development is failure of conversion of narrow spiral arteries to low-resistance vascular sinuses in the placenta. Placental ischemia results in poor fetal growth and liberation of substances which cause vasoconstriction and promote hypertension. In the kidney, endothelial cells become swollen, with deposition of fibrin in glomeruli, leading to proteinuria. If untreated severe hypertension and intravascular coagulation occur with development of cerebral ischemia and fits.

women over the age of 35 years, it is a syndrome characterized by increased blood pressure, proteinuria and peripheral edema.

Most cases are mild, with the blood pressure under 100 mmHg diastolic and no proteinuria; in severe cases the diastolic pressure is consistently above 100 mmHg, and there is proteinuria and severe peripheral edema.

The pre-eclamptic syndrome has hazards for both mother and fetus, but maternal problems are rare, being largely confined to severe pre-eclampsia, which may progress into full-blown eclampsia (see below). A feature of pre-eclampsia is reduced placental blood flow; this may lead to fetal hypoxia in late pregnancy, particularly during labor, with increased risk of perinatal mortality. The fetus may also suffer intrauterine growth retardation and have low birth-weight. The mechanisms thought to be involved in the genesis of hypertension, proteinuria and edema in the pre-eclamptic syndrome are outlined in *Fig. 19.27*.

Eclampsia is now a rare complication of pregnancy

Rarely, a small proportion of patients with severe pre-eclampsia develop eclampsia. Patients develop severe systemic disturbance, experiencing frontal headaches, rapid and sustained rise in blood pressure, shock, anuria and fits. They develop disseminated intravascular coagulation, with widespread occlusion of blood vessels, fibrinoid necrosis of vessel walls, and, in fatal cases, widespread microinfarcts in the brain, liver, kidney and other organs. Fatal eclampsia is now rare owing to treatment of the pre-eclamptic syndrome.

Spontaneous abortion is very common, often occurring before a woman is aware of her pregnancy

Many fertilized ova fail to implant successfully, and it has been estimated that more than 40% of conceptions fail to convert into recognizable pregnancies; of those that do, 15% terminate as clinically recognized spontaneous abortion. There are many causes of spontaneous abortion throughout the gestation period, the causes differing at different stages:

• **First trimester causes.** The majority are associated with abnormal fetuses, most being linked to abnormal chromosome karyotypes, particularly X0 (Turner's syndrome). Structural developmental abnormalities, such as neural tube defects, are also important.

Maternal systemic lupus erythematosus (SLE) and the presence of circulating antiphospholipid antibodies are a recognized cause of repeated spontaneous abortion in the first trimester, and the disease may be clinically undiagnosed. Transplacental infection, e.g. *Brucella*, *Listeria*, rubella, *Toxoplasma*, cytomegalovirus and herpes, may lead to spontaneous abortion early in pregnancy.

- **Second trimester causes** include chorioamnionitis, rupture of membranes, placental hemorrhages and structural abnormalities of the uterus (e.g. congenital uterine malformations), large submucosal leiomyomas, and incompetence of the cervix. Abortions due to abnormal placentation may occur in this period, but are more common in the third trimester.
- **Third trimester causes** are mainly the result of maternal abnormality such as uncontrolled hypertension or eclampsia. The various types of placental abnormality, e.g. placental hemorrhage, abruption and infarction, are important causes in this trimester.

In ectopic pregnancy the fertilized ovum implants in an abnormal site

Ectopic gestation occurs when a fertilized ovum implants outside the uterine cavity. The most common site is the fallopian tube. A common cause is infection by chlamydial organisms. Tubal ectopic pregnancy is also likely when there is some structural abnormality of the fallopian tube, usually scarring resulting from previous episodes of salpingitis, although an increasingly common predisposing factor is previous tubal surgery for contraceptive purposes.

The fertilized embryo implants in the tubal mucosa and submucosa, and proliferation of trophoblast erodes submucosal blood vessels, precipitating severe bleeding into the tubal lumen (*Fig. 19.28*). Many tubal ectopic pregnancies present as an acute abdominal emergency, with severe lower abdominal pain that is usually localized to the side of the ectopic pregnancy; however, some tubal ectopics rupture, leading to bleeding into the peritoneal cavity, in which case the pain is less well localized. Rupture usually occurs in the early stages of pregnancy, and the patient may not be aware that she is pregnant; occasionally, ectopic pregnancies do not cause early hemorrhage and may be sustained for some weeks, during which the endometrium develops decidual changes.

Other sites of abnormal implantation are very rare but include peritoneal cavity, ovary and cervix.

Abnormal development of gestational trophoblast may lead to hydatidiform mole

Several disorders of abnormal trophoblast development are recognized, ranging from abnormal proliferative conditions through to highly malignant tumors. These are grouped under the term **trophoblastic diseases**. Many of these disorders follow a preceding abnormal gestation and are associated with cytogenetic abnormalities.

Hydatidiform mole is a benign abnormal mass of cystic vesicles derived from the chorionic villi (*Fig. 19.29a,b*). Hydatidiform moles may be partial or complete:

Fig. 19.29 Hydatidiform mole. The uterine contents in a hydatidiform mole are entirely composed of abnormal cystic vesicles (a). No normal placenta or fetal parts are identified. This is a complete mole. (b) Histology shows the cystic vesicles to be enormously enlarged chorionic villi (**V**) with hyperplasia of the surface trophoblast (**T**) cells.

Fig. 19.28 Ectopic pregnancy in fallopian tube. The distal fallopian tube is distended by a blood clot in which there are chorionic villi eroding the tubal wall; fetal parts are rarely seen.

- In **partial mole** the vesicular degeneration of the chorionic villi affects only part of the placenta. Fetal parts and some normal placental villi are present, along with the abnormal trophoblastic tissue. This has a low risk of subsequent development of malignancy.
- In **complete mole** no normal placenta is identified and the mole forms a bulky mass, which can fill the uterine cavity. No fetal parts or normal placental villi are present. This has a low risk of subsequent development of malignancy.

In both cases a characteristic feature of the mole is atypical hyperplasia of the syncytiotrophoblast and cytotrophoblast cells on the surface of the distended villi. The incidence of both types of mole is about 1 in 2000 in the UK and USA. However, they occur far more frequently in some parts of Asia, South America and Africa, the incidence in Taiwan, for example, being 1 in 400 pregnancies.

A small proportion (probably about 10%) of both partial and complete moles show invasion of the myometrium by the molar component, but this is not evidence of the development of malignant neoplasm.

Cytogenetics of hydatidiform mole

In some cases it is difficult to be certain of the nature of hydropic villi with abnormal trophoblastic proliferation. Cytogenetic analysis of molar tissue has offered an insight into the possible origin of these diseases, as well as a means of assisting diagnosis.

The majority (80%) of complete hydatidiform moles are 46XX, both X chromosomes being derived from paternal spermatozoa. The implication is that a single haploid spermatozoon has penetrated an 'empty' ovum (i.e. monospermic or homozygous) or, alternatively, two single haploid sperms, both bearing the X chromosome, have penetrated (i.e. dispermic or heterozygous). It is claimed that dispermic moles are more likely to lead to persistent trophoblastic disease than monospermic moles.

A small percentage of complete moles have a chromosome constitution 46XY, both the X and Y chromosomes being derived from paternal spermatozoa; this is probably the result of penetration of an empty ovum by two haploid spermatozoa, one bearing an X chromosome, the other a Y chromosome.

Most partial moles have a chromosome constitution 69XXY, i.e. they are triploid.

Evacuation of both complete and partial moles from the uterus may not be complete; some residual trophoblastic tissue is frequently left behind, particularly where there is deep invasion of the myometrium. Detection of such cases is by ultrasound imaging, as well as by demonstrating continued elevated levels of hCG secreted by trophoblast. These cases should be regarded as having **persistent trophoblastic disease**, and require chemotherapy to eradicate the residual trophoblastic tissue.

In some cases of persistent trophoblastic disease, there is a risk of subsequent development of malignant tumor of trophoblast, choriocarcinoma.

Choriocarcinoma is a malignant tumor of trophoblastic tissue

Around 50% of choriocarcinomas develop from a hydatidiform mole, only 20% arising after a normal pregnancy. The time-lag between pregnancy and the development of choriocarcinoma is very variable: it is usually a matter of a few months, but may occasionally take many years. It is rare in the UK and USA (approximately 1 in 50 000 pregnancies) but, like mole, is more common in Asia, South America and Africa.

The tumor forms hemorrhagic masses in the endometrial cavity, with a peripheral rim of viable tumor surrounding extensively necrotic and hemorrhagic debris. Histologically (*Fig. 19.30*) it is composed of masses of cytotrophoblastic cells, often covered by a rim of pleomorphic syncytiotrophoblast; there is no evidence of structured villus formation. Trophoblastic tissue has a propensity for invading vessel walls, and bloodborne metastases occur early to many sites, particularly lung and brain. Formerly rapidly fatal, this tumor responds to cytotoxic chemotherapy, and the prognosis with correct treatment is now excellent (particularly if post-treatment monitoring of hCG levels is carried out).

Fig. 19.30 Choriocarcinoma of uterus. In choriocarcinoma the uterine cavity contains masses of pleomorphic trophoblast, which invades myometrium (**M**). To the naked eye this appears as a hemorrhagic and necrotic mass resembling a blood clot.

There are two main causes of antepartum hemorrhage

Antepartum hemorrhage is bleeding from or into the female genital tract after the 28th week of pregnancy and before delivery. The main causes are **placental abruption** and **placenta previa**. The above account for two-thirds of all cases and have a roughly equal incidence. In the remaining one-third the cause is not apparent, but some trivial cause in the lower genital tract, e.g. a cervical polyp, may occasionally be responsible.

Placental abruption is due to abnormal premature separation of a normally located placenta

Premature separation of the placenta is termed **placental abruption** and is an important cause of antepartum hemorrhage (see below), which may lead to stillbirth and even maternal death. The mechanisms of premature separation are not known, but it is particularly likely to occur in women who have a history of abruption, a history of many previous pregnancies, hypertension, or polyhydramnios and premature rupture of membranes.

In most cases placental separation is manifest as abdominal pain with vaginal bleeding. However, the hemorrhage may occasionally be concealed, the blood being contained within the placental bed. In such cases the patient develops lower abdominal pain, followed rapidly by hypotension and clinical manifestations of shock.

Placenta previa is implantation of the placenta low in the uterus so that it encroaches on the lower segment

The lower segment of the uterus does not contract during labor, but becomes passively stretched as the uterus enlarges. In placenta previa the fact that the placenta overlies the lower segment may lead to antepartum hemorrhage or an obstructed labor, depending on the precise location of the placenta. Four grades of placenta previa are recognized (*Fig. 19.31*):

- **Grade I.** The edge of the placenta encroaches on the lower segment, but does not reach the internal os.
- **Grade II.** The placenta occupies the lower segment, with its edge reaching the internal os but not covering it.
- **Grades III/IV.** The placenta is implanted in the lower segment and either partly (Grade III) or completely (Grade IV) covers the internal os.

All grades are likely to present with antepartum hemorrhage, as the lower segment stretches before delivery. Grades III and IV are particularly likely to lead to an obstructed labor, the placenta preventing the passage of the presenting fetal part into the os, thereby necessitating cesarean section.

In addition to leading to antepartum hemorrhage, placenta previa is particularly likely to lead to postpartum hemorrhage because the stretched lower segment of the uterus contracts less than the rest of the uterus after delivery, allowing continued seepage of blood from the placental bed.

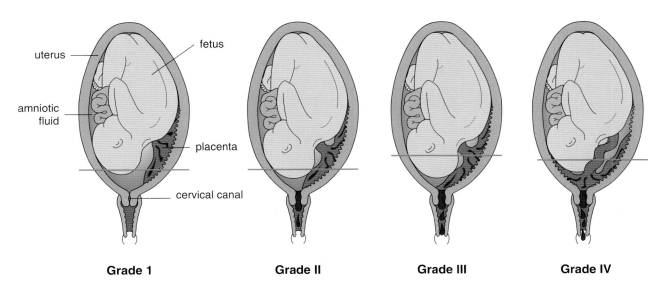

Grade 1   Grade II   Grade III   Grade IV

Fig. 19.31 Grades of placenta previa. Normally the placenta does not extend into the lower uterine segment (below the blue line in diagram). In placenta previa, different grades of severity are associated with increasing encroachment of placenta on the lower segment and cervical os.

Case-based questions

Case 1 A young teacher with infertility

A 32-year-old school teacher presents to her gynecologist with a 4-year history of infertility. Her husband has been investigated and has a normal sperm count and normal sperm motility. On further questioning, she gives a history of lower abdominal pain premenstrually, as well as dysmenorrhea, particularly in her sacral region, and also dyspareunia.

On examination she appears to be mildly tender in the region of the right ovary, and small nodules (approximately 1 cm in diameter) are palpable posterior to the uterus on vaginal examination. No other abnormality is found. Investigations show a normal hemoglobin, platelet and white cell count.

Laparoscopy is performed. The right ovary is enlarged and is fixed by adhesions to the fallopian tube and broad ligament, with ill-defined dark-brown cystic areas. The posterior aspect of the uterus and the pouch of Douglas show similar cystic dark brown lesions up to 5 mm in maximum extent.

The right ovary and fallopian tube are excised and sent for histology. They show scattered cystic areas 3–5 cm in maximum dimension, containing thick brown fluid. Within the fibrous walls surrounding the cysts, endometrial glands and stroma are seen. Abundant macrophages containing hemosiderin pigment are present.

The appearances are those of pelvic and ovarian endometriosis.

1. What is the colloquial name often given to the ovarian cysts caused by endometriosis, and why?
2. What are the possible theories with regard to the pathogenesis of endometriosis?
3. What therapies may be used to treat the disease?
4. What are the major complications of the disease?

Case 2 A woman with post-menopausal bleeding

A 65-year-old retired accountant presents to her doctor with a 5-month history of irregular postmenopausal bleeding. She has not been taking hormone replacement therapy. On examination, she appears pale. Vaginal examination shows no obvious local source for the bleeding. Full blood count shows a hemoglobin of 9.5 g/dL, with a normal white cell and platelet count.

She undergoes dilatation and curettage, which produces bulky uterine curettings. An enlarged right

ovary can be felt under anesthetic but is not biopsied. Histological examination shows severe cytological and architectural atypia of the endometrium and a diagnosis of endometrial adenocarcinoma is made.

She has a hysterectomy with a cuff of vagina excised, and a bilateral salpingo-oophorectomy. The operative specimen is sent for pathological examination. The uterine cavity is filled with a focally necrotic, pale, friable tumor measuring approximately 7 cm in maximum dimension. This extends into the myometrium, up to – but not through – the serosal surface. The cervix is not infiltrated by carcinoma/tumor which does not extend into the fallopian tubes. The right ovary is enlarged with a well-defined yellow tumor 4 cm in diameter, with a firm cut surface. Histological examination confirms that the uterine tumor is a moderately differentiated (grade 2) endometrial adenocarcinoma of the endometrioid type. The right ovarian tumor is a benign thecoma.

1. What is the association between endometrial carcinoma and the ovarian thecoma?
2. How do endometrial carcinomas spread?
3. How are endometrial carcinomas staged and what is the prognosis, based on stage, for this patient?

Case 3 A student with an unpleasant vaginal discharge

A 23-year-old drama student presents to her family doctor because she has developed a foul-smelling vaginal discharge. She complains of some associated vulval and vaginal itching and soreness. She is otherwise well. On examination, the vaginal and cervical mucosa are reddened, and a frothy, white, fishy-smelling discharge is noted. A high vaginal swab is taken. Microscopic examination showed motile flagellated protozoa approximately 30 μm in diameter. The appearances are those of *Trichomonas vaginalis*.

1. What other organisms may cause vulval and vaginal infections?
2. How is *Trichomonas* usually transmitted?
3. What is the treatment?

Case 4 A woman with heavy menstrual bleeding

A 41-year-old woman who runs her own home-made pie and farm shop business, presents to her doctor complaining of heavy periods. She is otherwise well, and her menstrual cycle is regular. She has one child and does not want more. On examination, she is pale and

▶ has a bulky irregularly shaped uterus. Her ovaries are both palpable and bulky.

Her hemoglobin is 9.9 g/dL, her white cell and platelet counts are normal.

She is admitted to hospital for routine hysterectomy, which reveals a grossly enlarged irregular uterus. Macroscopic examination shows multiple, well-defined, rubbery, pale tumors of the myometrium, with a whorled cut surface. The largest measures 12 cm in maximum dimension. Histological examination confirms that these are leiomyomas (fibroids).

1. **What are the possible presentations and complications of leiomyomas?**
2. **How is a leiomyoma distinguished from a leiomyosarcoma?**

Case 5 A nurse with an 'acute abdomen'

A 29-year old intensive care nurse, presents as an emergency to hospital with acute abdominal pain. Her menstrual cycle has been regular and she has had a period nine days earlier. She is tender in the right iliac fossa and, on bimanual examination, a mass thought to be ovarian in origin can be palpated. Her full blood count is normal and a pregnancy test is negative.

She has a laparotomy and a haemorrhagic right ovarian mass is removed. In addition, her left ovary contains a smaller tumour and this was also resected. She makes an uneventful recovery. The removed ovarian tissue is sent for pathological examination.

Macroscopic examination reveals bilateral cystic ovarian tumours: the larger right tumour measuring 8 cm in maximum extent. This has a purple, haemorrhagic appearance and, on opening, is unilocular, containing greasy material, teeth and hair. Histology confirms that both are benign cystic teratomas (dermoid cysts) with mature bone, muscle, neural, respiratory and skin elements.

1. **How common are mature cystic teratomas of the ovary?**
2. **Why did the patient present with acute abdominal pain?**
3. **What are the complications of ovarian mature cystic teratomas?**
4. **What are the other four types of germ-cell tumour and what is their behaviour?**

Case 6 A veterinary surgeon presents with a history of recurrent, spontaneous abortions

A 29-year old veterinarian develops bleeding *per vaginam* in the ninth week of pregnancy. She has abdominal cramps and, by the time she reaches hospital, has passed several large, haemorrhagic tissue fragments. She continues to bleed PV. On examination, the cervical os is dilated. Intravenous fluids are given and a dilatation and curettage are performed. Scanty material only is recovered and sent for histology.

Histological examination confirms that features of products of conception are present, including decidua and trophoblastic tissue. There is no evidence of an infective agent histologically.

1. **What proportion of fertilized ova fail to implant successfully?**
2. **What are the causes of first-trimester spontaneous abortions?**
3. **Are there any occupational hazards to be considered?**

Brief answers to these case-based questions are given on pages 592–3. More detailed answers and other study resources are available online at www.studentconsult.com.

Breast disease 20

THE NORMAL BREAST

Tissues contain endocrine-responsive epithelium and stroma

The normal adult female breast is composed of lobules of glandular epithelial tissue (small ducts terminating in terminal ductules or acini). These link by branching to larger ducts that eventually converge and drain at the nipple (*Fig. 20.1*). Surrounding the lobular epithelial components is a cellular, specialized hormone-responsive stroma (intralobular stroma). Surrounding the lobules, the breast contains non-specialized fibrocollagenous support tissue and prominent adipose tissue (extralobular stroma).

INFLAMMATORY DISORDERS OF THE BREAST

Mastitis and breast abscess are seen as a complication of lactation

Infections of the breast are usually associated with lactation, the organisms (commonly *Staphylococcus aureus* and *Streptococcus*) gaining access through cracks and fissures in the nipple and areola. The initial infection causes an **acute mastitis**, with painful tender enlargement of the breast, which generally resolves after treatment with appropriate antibiotics.

Without antibiotic therapy, bacterial mastitis is often followed by the development of a **breast abscess**, which may require surgical drainage.

Chronic inflammation of the breast is rare, but may develop after incomplete resolution of an acute mastitis. Tuberculous mastitis may occur, but is uncommon in western countries.

Fat necrosis follows trauma and can clinically mimic neoplastic disease

Following episodes of trauma, localized areas of inflammation of the breast may occur as a result of fat necrosis.

The trauma causes necrosis of adipose tissue, which stimulates a localized inflammatory and reparative response to the dead fat cells Macrophages which have phagocytosed lipid material are generally prominent (*Fig. 20.2*).

Organization with fibrous repair takes place, producing a hard, irregular lump in the breast. The main clinical significance of this condition is that patients may not be able to recall a history of trauma, and these lesions may clinically resemble a breast carcinoma with the presence of tethering of the overlying skin.

Fig. 20.2 Fat necrosis. In the response to fat necrosis (**N**) there is an initial acute inflammatory reaction, followed by a chronic inflammatory response in which numerous plasma cells are seen (**P**). Macrophages phagocytose lipid released from adipocytes, forming multinucleate giant cells, as well as foam cells (**F**), also termed 'lipophages.'

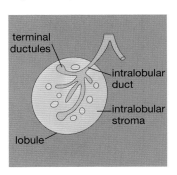

Fig. 20.1 Lobule. The normal breast lobule contains epithelial elements in the form of ducts and terminal ductules. These are surrounded by a cellular specialised intralobular stroma. Each lobule drains by a small terminal duct.

Duct ectasia is caused by inflammatory destruction of support tissues around ducts

Mammary duct ectasia is a disease of uncertain pathogenesis. There is abnormal progressive dilatation of large breast ducts, which accumulate retained secretory products and shed epithelium. The disease is mainly seen in parous women in the perimenopausal age range.

Although the precise cause is uncertain, it is thought that an important abnormality is inflammatory destruction of the normal elastic-containing support tissues around ducts, which then allows dilatation. The inflammatory component has led to the alternative term 'periductal mastitis' for this condition.

Clinically, patients develop a firm breast lump, which may resemble a carcinoma, or there may be a nipple discharge. Macroscopically, affected areas of breast show distended ducts, up to 1 cm in diameter, filled with inspissated creamy material.

Histology shows dilated ducts containing proteinaceous material and phagocytic macrophages distended with lipid. There is fibrosis around ducts, associated with non-specific chronic inflammation.

BENIGN DISEASES OF THE BREAST

Fibrocystic change is common with increasing age

The term fibrocystic change describes alterations in structure seen in both the epithelial and connective tissue components of the breast. It is common in the breasts of mature women, with an increasing incidence towards the menopause. This condition has also been known by a variety of other terms including 'fibroadenosis,' 'cystic mammary dysplasia,' 'cystic hyperplasia,' 'cystic mastopathy' and 'chronic mastitis,' but these terms are now no longer preferred.

The cause of fibrocystic disease is uncertain. Most believe that it is due to disturbances of cyclical ovarian estrogen and progesterone levels, accompanied by altered responsiveness of breast tissues in women approaching the menopause.

There are two components to fibrocystic change, divided into non-proliferative and proliferative.

Cysts and fibrosis represent non-proliferative fibrocystic changes

Macroscopically, areas of fibrocystic disease appear as firm, rubbery replacement of breast tissue, in which cysts may be visible.

Cysts are a prominent component, increasing in incidence with the approach of the menopause. They range in size from those detectable only by histology to palpable lesions 1–2 cm in diameter. Cysts are lined by flattened epithelium derived from the lobular–ductal unit and are filled with watery fluid. The epithelium lining cystic ducts may become transformed from the normal low cuboidal to a columnar pattern (**columnar transformation**). In many cases the epithelium lining cystic ducts undergoes metaplasia to a form similar to that of normal apocrine glands (**apocrine metaplasia**) (*Fig. 20.3*).

Fibrosis is noted as increased collagen deposition around cystically dilated ducts within the breast tissue. Fibrocystic disease may be manifest as replacement of breast tissue by dense fibrous tissue, termed **mammary fibrosis**, particularly in women after the menopause.

Proliferative epithelial changes may be seen in fibrocystic change

Epithelial hyperplasia in ducts and lobules may be seen in about 30% of cases of fibrocystic disease; this is important, as this type of change is associated with an increased risk of the later development of carcinoma (*Fig. 20.4*).

In most cases the cytology and architecture of the proliferated epithelium show no atypia, and lesions are classified as **hyperplasia of usual type**. In other cases, abnormalities in cell cytology or architecture are noted in which instances the term **atypical hyperplasia** is used (*Fig. 20.5d*).

For patients who have hyperplasia of usual type (about 25% of all cases of fibrocystic disease) the risk of subsequent development of carcinoma is increased twofold. For those who have atypical epithelial hyperplasia (about 5% of cases), the risk of subsequently developing a carcinoma increases fourfold.

Fig. 20.3 Fibrocystic change. In fibrocystic change there is proliferation of ducts, lobular tissue and stromal support tissues to form a mass of cystic spaces (**C**) and fibrous tissue (**F**). The epithelium of some ducts is replaced by bright, pink-staining epithelium (**P**) resembling normal apocrine glands.

(a)

(b)

(c)

Fig. 20.4 Fibrocystic change.
(a) In fibrocystic change intralobular stroma is replaced by collagenous tissue and there is frequent cystic dilatation of small ducts lined by cytologically bland epithelium. Apocrine metaplasia is commonly seen as bright-pink-stained lining to cysts.
(b) In a proportion of patients there are proliferative epithelial changes within lobules (**epithelial hyperplasia**). This results in expansion of the cellularity within lobules. Histological examination can distinguish between **hyperplasia of usual type**, in which there is no architectural or cytological atypia, and **atypical hyperplasia,** in which architecture or cytology raise concerns.
(c) Sclerosing adenosis is characterized by proliferation of both stromal and epithelial elements within the lobule. Superficially this pattern can resemble the histological pattern seen in some types of carcinoma.

Histology in the lobule

Fig. 20.5 Histology in the lobule.

(a) In the normal lobule, epithelium lining ductules are cuboidal with small, regular nuclei.

(b) Columnar cells may replace cuboidal epithelium in ductules in some patterns of ductal hyperplasia (columnar transformation).

(c) Hyperplasia of usual type is characterized by heaped-up epithelial growth, with cytologically bland but overlapping, stratified nuclei

(d) In atypical hyperplasia, cells are regularly distributed, appear monotonous, with punched-out gland space.

Fig. 20.6 Sclerosing adenosis. The breast lobule is distorted by overgrowth of intralobular stroma and proliferated small ductules, which become compressed into narrow ribbons and slits.

Sclerosing lesions of the breast are commonly seen in radiographic screening

Several lesions of the breast are characterized by a predominant fibrous component that forms a localized area of irregular, stellate, collagenous sclerosis in which epithelial elements are also present. These lesions have become significant in modern clinical practice, as they can be confused with a carcinoma on mammographic screening. The main types are:

• **Sclerosing adenosis.** This may present as a solitary, palpable lesion in young women, in addition to being seen in areas of fibrocystic change in older women. There is proliferation of specialized hormone-responsive stromal tissue and myoepithelial cells, separating and compressing proliferated acinar and ductal structures into narrow ribbons of cells (*Figs 20.4c* and *20.6*).

- **Radial scars and complex sclerosing lesions** are composed of collagenous and elastic tissue enclosing distorted ductules. Careful histological examination of these lesions is required, as some forms of carcinoma (tubular carcinoma) can adopt this pattern of growth.

Fibroadenoma presents as a mobile lump in the breast of young women

One of the lesions most commonly responsible for causing a lump in the breast is the **fibroadenoma**, a benign, localized proliferation of branching duct-like structures and abundant stroma. There is debate as to whether this lesion is a true neoplasm or actually represents a nodular form of hyperplasia. Fibroadenomas are seen most frequently in women aged 25–35 years as solitary discrete lesions, but small foci of histologically similar areas may also be a component of fibrocystic change. Clinically these are typically highly mobile, firm, smooth lumps that evade easy clinical evaluation by slipping between the finger and thumb of the palpating hand. This mobile, elusive property gave rise to the colloquial description of a 'breast mouse'.

Macroscopically, fibroadenomas are typically 1–4 cm in diameter, appearing as firm, rubbery, well-circumscribed white lesions. They have a glistening cut surface and a tough texture.

There are two histological components (*Fig. 20.7*): the **epithelial component**, which forms complex, branching gland-like structures lined by duct-type epithelium, and the **stromal component**, which is a loose, cellular fibrous tissue around the epithelial areas.

NEOPLASTIC BREAST DISEASES

BENIGN BREAST TUMORS

Benign tumors of the breast are less common than malignant tumors

There are several benign tumors of the breast. The breast may also be the site of development of benign tumors of support tissues, e.g. lipomas and leiomyomas. The main benign tumors of the breast are breast hamartomas, adenomas, duct papillomas, and phyllodes tumors.

Hamartomas of the breast are seen on mammographic screening

Mammographic screening is currently revealing a number of asymptomatic benign lesions of the breast. These are coming to the attention of pathologists as they are now being excised or biopsied. Macroscopically hamartomas resemble fibroadenomas. They are composed of a mass of fibrous stroma, which encloses lobular and ductal structures.

Duct papillomas are a common cause of a bloodstained nipple discharge

Papillomas of mammary duct epithelium may arise as solitary or multiple lesions. **Solitary papillomas** are usually located in the larger lactiferous ducts near the nipple. They are most common in middle-aged women and are a common

Fig. 20.7 Fibroadenoma. The fibroadenoma is composed of both epithelial (**E**) and stromal (**S**) components. Although lesions form localized, circumscribed lumps, they are believed to be hyperplastic rather than neoplastic.

Fig. 20.8 Papilloma of the breast. A breast papilloma is shown within a dilated duct. It is composed of fronds of tissue, with a vascular stroma covered by a two-layered ductal epithelium.

cause of a bloody nipple discharge (*Fig. 20.8*). Lesions are usually 1–2 cm in size and consist of a delicate supporting stroma covered by a double layer of cuboidal or low columnar epithelial cells, resembling the lining of a duct; with larger lesions, the duct is often dilated. Malignant change is rare.

Multiple papillomas are far less common than solitary lesions and are usually located in smaller ducts deeper in the breast in young women. This type is associated with increased risk of later development of breast carcinoma.

True adenomas of the breast are uncommon primary tumors

Compared to nodular proliferative lesions such as fibroadenomas and sclerosing lesions, true adenomas of the breast are uncommon.

Tubular adenomas occur in young women and are composed of regular tubular-shaped glands and a minimal stroma. There is no associated risk of developing carcinoma.

Adenoma of the nipple commonly presents as ulceration and reddening of the nipple, clinically confused with Paget's disease of the nipple (see page 446). These lesions are composed of duct-like structures associated with a collagenous stroma.

Phyllodes tumors are composed of both epithelial and stromal elements

A phyllodes tumor is composed of epithelial-lined, cleft-like spaces surrounded by a cellular spindle-cell stroma (*Fig. 20.9*). These lesions were previously called 'cystosarcoma phyllodes' or 'giant fibroadenomas,' names that are no longer recommended.

Clinically, tumors present as a breast lump and can be seen at any age after puberty, although most are encoun-

tered after the age of 40 years. Macroscopically they are rubbery, white lesions in which a whorled pattern of slit-like spaces and solid areas can be seen.

The histological appearance of these lesions is variable and it is possible to classify phyllodes tumors as benign, of borderline malignant potential, or definitely malignant.

In 90% of cases both epithelial and stromal elements are bland and give no cause for concern. However, in the remaining 10% there are atypical features to the stromal element, with pleomorphism and mitoses, leading to a borderline or malignant classification.

Biologically the majority of phyllodes tumors are benign, but about 10% recur locally. Tumors with atypical histological features are particularly prone to recur, and the very small minority with marked atypical histological features (classified as malignant) may spread, with the development of metastases.

MALIGNANT TUMORS OF THE BREAST

Carcinoma of the breast affects up to 1 in 10 women

Malignant tumors of the female breast are extremely common, accounting for 20% of all malignancies in women.

About 1 in 10 women will develop carcinoma of the breast at some time in their life. The incidence increases steeply through the reproductive ages, and then less steeply from the age of the menopause at around 50. The main risk factor for breast cancer relates to estrogen exposure, and this relates to several epidemiological risk factors associated with increased risk of disease.

Most tumors are **invasive adenocarcinomas**, which arise from the terminal ducts and lobular units, forming **invasive lobular carcinomas** or **invasive ductal carcinomas**. Carcinoma of the breast may also be encountered at a stage prior to invasion, in the form of carcinoma in situ of mammary ducts or lobules (**ductal carcinoma in situ** and **lobular carcinoma in situ**), and this is a risk factor for the later development of invasive breast carcinoma.

In addition to the two main groups of ductal and lobular carcinoma, there are less common, special types of breast carcinoma, which are often associated with a better prognosis, e.g. tubular carcinoma and mucinous carcinoma.

Breast carcinoma presents in four main ways:

- A palpable lump in the breast, increasingly being detected by patients themselves as a result of health education.
- Abnormality detected on mammography as a result of developing breast-screening programs.
- Incidental histological finding in breast tissue removed for another reason.
- First manifest as metastatic disease (see page 449).

Fig. 20.9 Phyllodes tumor. Phyllodes tumors are composed of a spindle-celled stroma (**S**), containing clefts lined by epithelium.

Intraductal carcinoma of the breast is a form of carcinoma in situ

Non-invasive ductal carcinoma in situ (DCIS) may present as a breast lump (about 5% of such cases) or be detected as a mammographic abnormality (about 20% of such cases). It is most common in women between the ages of 40 and 60 years.

Histologically, atypical cells fill and distend small and medium-sized ducts (*Fig. 20.10*). There are two main histological types: low grade and high grade. In high-grade DCIS, ducts are dilated by solid or centrally necrotic masses of atypical epithelium with significant nuclear pleomorphism. In low-grade DCIS cells are monotonous and form complex micropapillary or cribriform (sieve-like) architectural patterns within expanded ducts.

It has been estimated that, if left untreated, about 30% of cases would progress to invasive carcinoma. If treated by mastectomy, intraductal carcinoma has an excellent prognosis.

Lobular carcinoma in situ increases the risk of invasive breast cancer in both breasts

Lobular carcinoma in situ accounts for about 6% of all cases of breast cancer. It does not usually present as a palpable mass, often being encountered as a histological finding in breast tissue removed because of a suspicious mammographic appearance. Histologically, abnormal cells fill the mammary lobules (*Fig. 20.11*).

The importance of this disease is that it carries a high risk of subsequent development of invasive carcinoma. It has been estimated that about 20% of patients with lobular carcinoma in situ will develop invasive carcinoma after 20 years. The risk of neoplasia is present for both breasts, not just the breast carrying the in situ disease, and either lobular or ductal invasive carcinoma may develop.

Paget's disease of the nipple is a pattern of spread of in-situ tumor to the skin

Paget's disease of the nipple is a pattern of spread of intraductal carcinoma of the breast.

Patients develop reddening, thickening and scaling of the skin of the nipple and areola, resembling eczema (*Fig. 20.12a*), sometimes followed by ulceration. Any eczema-like rash involving the nipple should prompt consideration of this diagnosis

Histologically the epidermis of the nipple and areola is infiltrated by large pale pleomorphic neoplastic epithelial cells, termed 'Paget's cells' which are typically spread along the basal layer (*Fig. 20.12b*).

Eczematous or inflammatory conditions of the nipple must always be regarded with suspicion, and biopsy should be performed to exclude Paget's disease.

Fig. 20.10 Ductal carcinoma in situ of the breast. (a) High grade DCIS shows pleomorphism, often with central necrosis in ducts containing calcium. (b) Low-grade DCIS is characterized by complex architectural patterns with monotonous cells. (c) Histology of high-grade DCIS showing calcification in a necrotic region. Stroma (S) is not invaded.

Fig. 20.11 Lobular carcinoma in situ of the breast. In non-invasive lobular carcinoma the normal lobular architecture is maintained, but lobules (**L**) are increased in size, being packed with atypical cells that fill and expand them. The basement membrane remains intact and there is no evidence of invasion of the stroma (**S**).

Fig. 20.13 **Invasive breast cancer with abundant stroma.** On cut surface an area of invasive carcinoma of the breast is seen as an irregular yellowish white area (**T**). Because of the stromal response, these are sometimes termed 'scirrhous carcinomas.' The stromal fibrous response has caused dimpling of the overlying skin with retraction of the nipple (**N**), sometimes an important physical sign.

Fig. 20.12 **Paget's disease of the nipple.** Macroscopically (a) Paget's disease appears as a red, scaling rash around the nipple. Histologically (b) the lower part of the epidermis is replaced by large, pale cells with pleomorphic nuclei (**P**). These are breast carcinoma cells that have spread along the mammary and nipple ducts to invade the epidermis. In the underlying breast there is either intraductal or invasive ductal carcinoma.

The macroscopic appearance of invasive carcinoma is determined mainly by the non-neoplastic stromal component

An invasive carcinoma of the breast can vary in size from less than 1 cm in diameter to masses occupying the whole of a breast; however, the majority are 1–3 cm in diameter at the time of diagnosis. In recent years the size of treated tumors has become smaller as an increasing proportion are detected at an early stage by public health self-screening promotion or active mammographic screening programs.

Macroscopically, the appearance of a carcinoma of the breast is determined mainly by the quality and quantity of its induced stromal component. Stromal responses are important in the biology of most tumors, and a supporting stroma is an essential requirement for tumor growth.

Invasive carcinoma of the breast is divided into six main histological types, only two of which are common

There are six main types of invasive breast carcinoma, each named according to its histological pattern and occurring with varying frequency.

- invasive ductal carcinoma, no special type (55%)
- mixed ductal and lobular carcinoma (30%)
- pure invasive lobular carcinoma (10%)
- special types (see page 448) (5%)

In contrast to in situ neoplasia, there is invasion into local tissues, with the possibility of metastatic spread.

- Most carcinomas of the breast excite a fibrous stromal reaction (desmoplastic response) and appear as irregular areas of gritty, firm yellowish white tissue with the consistency of an unripe apple (*Fig. 20.13*).
- Tumors which have little in the way of a desmoplastic response are mainly composed of neoplastic cells with scant fibrous stroma, appearing soft and fleshy.
- Some carcinomas secrete large amounts of mucin into the stroma, and appear white with a gelatinous consistency (mucoid or colloid carcinoma).

The most common types of invasive carcinoma of the breast are ductal and lobular

Invasive ductal carcinoma is the most common type of breast cancer. It may occur as a pure form or may be mixed with another pattern of carcinoma, most commonly lobular carcinoma. Tumor cells invade breast tissue and there is usually a desmoplastic response, creating a dense fibrous stroma (*Fig. 20.14*). A minority of tumors are low-grade lesions, the majority being either intermediate or high-grade poorly differentiated types. When ductal carcinoma is mixed with specialized tumors that have a good prognosis (e.g. tubular or colloid carcinoma), the prognosis is slightly better than for the pure ductal tumor.

Invasive lobular carcinoma is the second most common type of breast cancer. Importantly, the tumor is often multifocal within the breast, and this type is associated with a high frequency of bilateral breast involvement relative to other subtypes. Tumor cells invade breast tissue, with a desmoplastic response. Characteristically, tumor cells are compressed into narrow cords, described as an 'Indian file' pattern of invasion (*Fig. 20.15*).

Although uncommon, some specialized carcinomas of the breast are associated with a better prognosis

Although they account for about 5% of all invasive breast cancers, certain specialized histological types of invasive carcinoma are associated with a better prognosis than the ductal and lobular types.

Tubular carcinomas are composed of well-differentiated cells that form regular tubular structures resembling small ducts. Although they represent 2% of all invasive carcinomas, they account for about 20% of cases detected by mammography. There is usually a desmoplastic response, with fibrous stroma forming a stellate pattern. Cells are well differentiated in this form of carcinoma, and this pattern is associated with a very good survival compared to standard ductal carcinoma.

Mucoid carcinoma (also termed 'colloid carcinoma') is most commonly seen in postmenopausal women. Cells in the lesion secrete mucin into the stroma, giving tumors a soft, slimy texture. This pattern of tumor is associated with a very good survival compared to ductal carcinomas of a similar size.

Fig. 20.14 Invasive ductal adenocarcinoma of the breast. Moderately differentiated invasive ductal adenocarcinoma of the breast show diagrammatically (a) and on histology (b). Tumor islands invade adjacent stroma (**S**). The tumor still forms tubule-like structures (**T**).

Fig. 20.15 Invasive lobular carcinoma of the breast. Lobular carcinoma shown diagrammatically (a) and on histology (b) is characterized by invasion in narrow cords of cells, termed 'Indian file' invasion. Cells are smaller than those seen in typical ductal carcinomas.

Medullary carcinomas of the breast are most commonly seen in postmenopausal women. They form apparently well-circumscribed masses and, lacking much of a desmoplastic response, are soft and fleshy. The neoplastic cells are generally large and highly pleomorphic, with numerous mitoses. A characteristic feature is a dense infiltrate of reactive lymphoid cells at the tumor periphery, representing a host response to tumor. These lesions are associated with only a slightly better survival than similarly sized ductal carcinomas.

Carcinoma of the breast spreads in a characteristic fashion

Carcinoma of the breast spreads in a characteristic fashion, which explains several of the common clinical manifestations of disease. Metastatic disease and recurrence of tumor may be a late event, occurring many years after local treatment of disease.

Local spread is into adjacent breast, into overlying skin (skin tethering), and deeply into pectoral muscles (deep fixation of tumor).

Lymphatic spread is into local lymphatics in the breast. When lymphatic drainage of the skin is involved, this gives rise to a *peau d'orange* appearance. Spread to axillary lymph nodes and nodes in the internal mammary chain is caused by embolization of tumor to nodes.

Vascular spread leads to dissemination of tumor to distant sites. The preferred sites for metastasis are **bone** (pathological fractures, hypercalcemia, leukoerythroblastic anemia, spinal-cord compression), **lung** (breathlessness), **pleura** (effusion and breathlessness), and **ovary** (Krukenberg tumor, see pages 255 and 433). Other sites are commonly involved but with less consistency.

Prognostic factors can be used to predict survival in breast cancer

Breast cancer is not one disease and there is great variation in survival following treatment. The factors related to prognosis in breast cancer are clinically important as they allow informed counseling of patients.

Stage of tumor is widely regarded as the most powerful prognostic factor. Several staging systems are in use including the TNM classification (see pages 79–81).

- Large primary tumor size (>2 cm) or fixation to local tissues is associated with poor prognosis.
- Spread to nodes is associated with significant reduction in 5-year survival from around 80% to 60%.
- Vascular spread is associated with a poor prognosis and a 5-year survival of about 10%.

The link between early stage and good clinical outcome is one of the main reasons for promoting breast-screening programs.

Grade of tumor assessed by looking at the degree of gland formation, pleomorphism and numbers of mitoses, provides additional prognostic data. Carcinomas can be assigned to three groups, which are related to survival at 10 years:

- Grade I (85%).
- Grade II (60%).
- Grade III (45%).

Histological type of tumor is another prognostic factor, some specialized types of carcinoma of the breast (tubular, mucoid) being associated with better prognosis than the common ductal and lobular types, as they have a low propensity for metastasis.

Prognosis can also be related to **hormone receptor status.** Patients with breast tumors that express receptors for estrogen and progesterones have a longer disease-free survival than those that do not. This is a reflection of tumor differentiation and likely response to anti-hormone therapy. Recent molecular profiling has identified subtypes of tumor with prognostic significance (*Fig. 20.16*).

The cause of breast cancer is uncertain, but there are several defined risk factors

Epidemiological studies have shown that breast cancer is related to several risk factors. Environmental factors contribute 75% risk and genetic factors about 25%.

Geographical The incidence of disease is five times greater in developed western countries than in less developed areas.

Familial breast cancer There is an increased genetic risk of developing breast cancer in about 5% of all cases (see pink box, page 451).

Proliferative breast disease Usual epithelial hyperplasia is associated with an approximately twofold increased risk of the development of carcinoma. Atypical hyperplasia is associated with a fourfold increased risk in women with no family history of breast cancer, but the risk increases 11-fold in women with a family history of breast cancer.

Early onset of menarche A 5% risk reduction is associated with each year of delay.

Childbirth One child reduces the risk by 25%, five children by 50% compared to nulliparous women.

Late menopause There is a 3% increase in risk for each year of delay in reaching the menopause.

Exogenous hormones There is an increased risk in patients on hormone-replacement therapy after the menopause. There is an increase in risk for women taking combined oral contraceptives.

Dietary factors A 50% increased risk of developing breast cancer has been linked to obesity in the premenopausal period, and also to a high alcohol intake, estimated at 10% increase per 10 g of ethanol consumed per day.

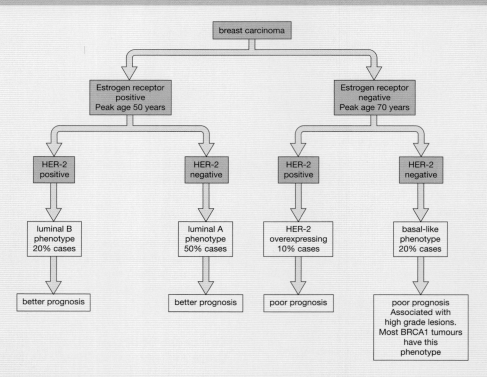

Fig. 20.16 Molecular classification of breast cancer. The application of gene profiling has allowed the identification of subtypes of carcinoma related to prognosis based on expression of ER and HER-2 (also called ErbB2 or Neu, a tyrosine kinase, and members of ErbB receptor family). The poor prognosis basal phenotype can be confirmed by demonstrating expression of specific keratins. The drug herceptin can be used to treat HER2-expressing tumors.

Diagnosis of breast cancer

The diagnosis of breast cancer is made using a 'triple approach.'

Clinical No woman should be allowed to have a lump in the breast without a firm diagnosis. More women practice self-examination, and all lumps discovered should be investigated clinically.

Imaging Some types of breast cancer do not produce palpable lumps. Mammographic screening may detect lesions by microcalcification or altered patterns of soft-tissue shadowing.

Fine-needle aspiration with cytology Diagnostic information can be obtained by aspirating cells using a fine needle followed by cytology (*Fig. 20.17*).

Fig. 20.17 Fine-needle aspiration cytology. Aspiration of breast tumors by needle can produce cytological preparations that are reliable in diagnosis of the nature of the lesion. In this case, large nuclei with an abnormal chromatin pattern indicate a carcinoma.

Familial breast cancer

Approximately 5% of cases of carcinoma of the breast are associated with a penetrant dominant genetic predisposition. Clinical suspicion is warranted in the presence of several affected members in a family, patients with early onset of disease, patients with bilateral breast cancers, patients with both ovarian and breast cancer, and families in which there are breast, ovarian, endometrial and colon cancers, or sarcomas in both males and females.

Germline mutations have been noted in several genes, all involved in maintaining genetic integrity, leading to an increased risk of breast cancer.

- Of all families with a strong familial history of breast cancer, many have an abnormality in the *BRCA1* or the *BRCA2* gene, also associated with development of carcinoma of the ovary. The breast cancer risk by age 70 years is 35% for *BRCA1* and 50% for *BRCA2*.
- About 5% of families have a mutation of the p53 gene (Li–Fraumeni syndrome). Family members develop a wide range of other tumors in addition to breast cancer.
- Cowden's disease associated with PTEN mutations involves breast cancer as part of the syndrome.
- Mutations in CHEK2, ATM, NBS1, RAD50, BRIP1, and PALB2 are associated with doubling of the breast cancer risk.
- In 2007 50% of familial cases had no identified gene.

Carcinoma of the breast in men is uncommon

Adenocarcinoma of the breast in men accounts for only 1% of all cases of breast cancer. Lesions fall into the same spectrum as those seen in the female breast, with the exception of lobular carcinoma in situ (as the male breast contains no lobular tissue). Paget's disease (see pages 446–7) may also be seen in males, and any rash of the nipple should be viewed with the same suspicion as in females.

Invasion of the chest wall is seen more often in males, possibly because of the small size of the breast, and lesions are more often locally advanced at diagnosis. A high proportion of tumors are ER positive, making anti-estrogen therapy possible in most cases.

In the breast, malignant tumors other than carcinomas are uncommon

Malignant tumors other than carcinomas are uncommon in the breast. Mention has already been made that **phyllodes tumors** may be malignant (see page 447) and can result in local invasion and metastatic disease.

Primary sarcomas in the breast are uncommon. The main types are angiosarcomas, malignant fibrous histiocytomas, and fibrosarcomas.

Lymphomas may occur in the breast as primary disease or as part of a systemic lymphoma.

Gynecomastia of the male breast is most commonly idiopathic

The male breast is normally undeveloped and inactive, consisting of fibroadipose tissue containing rudimentary mammary ducts. Enlargement of the male breast, termed **gynecomastia**, may be unilateral (70% of cases) or bilateral. In most cases it is idiopathic and presents shortly after puberty. Other causes include:

- Klinefelter's syndrome (see page 407).
- Estrogen excess (cirrhosis, puberty, adrenal tumor, exogenous estrogens).
- Gonadotrophin excess (testicular tumor).
- Prolactin excess (hypothalamic or pituitary disease).
- Drug-related (spironolactone, chlorpromazine, digitalis).

There is enlargement of the breast as a firm, raised, rubbery mass beneath the nipple (*Fig. 20.18*).

Fig. 20.18 Gynecomastia. In gynecomastia the simple mammary ducts (**D**) become enlarged, often with thickening of the epithelial layer, and there is an increase in periductal fibrous tissue (**T**), which may be markedly collagenous.

Case-based questions

Case 1 – A woman with a carcinoma of the breast

A 67-year-old retired shopkeeper presents to her doctor with a 1-month history of a lump in the right breast. On examination, this is firm, ill-defined with skin tethering, and is adherent to the underlying pectoralis muscle. It measures approximately 4 cm in maximum extent. Enlarged lymph nodes are palpable in the right axilla.

Fine-needle aspiration cytology (FNAC) confirms that carcinoma cells are present. The patient undergoes simple mastectomy with axillary clearance. The operative specimens are sent for pathological examination.

Histological examination reveals a grade 3 invasive ductal adenocarcinoma/no special type. Four out of eight axillary lymph nodes contained metastatic carcinoma.

1. What is the incidence of breast cancer?
2. What are the benefits of FNAC, and what are the features of malignancy in a cytology preparation?
3. How, and to where, does breast carcinoma spread?
4. When you see the patient to discuss prognosis, how will your understanding of the natural history of disease be used to inform your discussion?
5. What other pathological investigation results would you be interested in knowing about in relation to the tumor before you see the patient?

Case 2 A suspicious mammogram

A 60-year-old woman attends for breast screening. She is in good health. A spiculate lesion is noted on her mammogram and she is recalled for assessment. No mass is palpable clinically. The radiological appearances are considered suspicious of carcinoma, and she undergoes stereotactic fine-needle aspiration cytology which reveals carcinoma cells. The lesion is localized by a marker wire and she has a therapeutic excision and lymph-node sampling. The operative samples are sent to pathology for analysis.

Histology reveals a small (0.9 cm maximum extent) grade 1 tubular carcinoma of the breast. The five axillary lymph nodes are free of tumor.

1. What histological features are assessed to determine histological grade of a breast carcinoma?
2. Apart from grade, what other features can be useful in predicting prognosis in a woman with breast carcinoma?
3. What is the prognosis?

Case 3 – Breast lumps and axillary tenderness

A 44-year-old woman presents to her doctor with an ill-defined area of lumpiness and pain in the right upper outer quadrant of her breast. This has been causing her discomfort ever since she began a parachute jumping course about 3 months ago. She is otherwise well. A full history reveals that she had always had menstrual irregularities, has taken the oral contraceptive pill, and has also recently noted right axillary tenderness. In the past she has had breast pain, particularly premenstrually. On examination she has multiple lumps in both breasts, several of which appear to be cystic. Fine-needle aspiration cytology is performed and cyst fluid is drained. This reveals sheets of benign cells showing apocrine metaplasia. A diagnosis of fibrocystic change (FCC) is made.

1. How common is fibrocystic change and what is the etiology?
2. What are the histological components of fibrocystic change?
3. Which of these features is important with respect to increased risk of developing breast carcinoma, and how high is this risk?
4. What is the likely cause of the axillary tenderness?

Brief answers to these case-based questions are given on page 593. More detailed answers and other study resources are available online at www.studentconsult.com.

Nervous system and muscle 21

INTRODUCTION

The nervous system is affected by general pathological processes, such as inflammation and infarction, but it is also the site of specific diseases of the specialized tissues of the nervous system, such as neurodegenerative diseases and demyelinating disorders.

The main cell types of pathological significance in the nervous system are: **neurons**; **astrocytes**, which act as specialized support cells; **oligodendrocytes**, which form myelin; and **microglia**, which are resident cells of the monocyte/macrophage type.

The compact anatomy of the nervous system means that even small lesions may produce severe functional disturbances. Importantly, any neurons that are lost cannot be replaced, as they lack the capacity for cell division.

RESPONSES OF THE NERVOUS SYSTEM TO INJURY

The nervous system has several pathological responses to injury that are not seen in other tissues.

Neuronal chromatolysis is a reparative response of neurons following damage to the axon (*Fig. 21.1*). The neuronal cell body swells due to the accumulation of neurofilaments and there is peripheral migration of the Nissl substance, associated with nuclear swelling. Chromatolysis is part of the regenerative response whereby neurons can regrow a severed axon (see page 485).

Phagocytosis. Following cell death, damaged tissues are removed by phagocytic resident microglial cells, which are supplemented by recruitment of monocytes from the blood. These phagocytic cells become vacuolated by accumulated lipid from dead cells, forming foam cells.

Gliosis. Astrocytes become activated, proliferating to fulfill a metabolic role in protecting neurons. Following cell death and their removal by phagocytes, damaged areas are replaced by proliferation of astrocytes, which form a **glial scar**. In large areas of damage, astrocytic gliosis may not entirely replace a defect, and an area remains that is partly cystic and partly gliotic.

Cerebral edema is accumulation of tissue fluid in between the cells of the nervous system. Seen after damage from many different causes, it is the result of breakdown of the blood–brain barrier due to ischemia, trauma, inflammation, and metabolic disorders. This breakdown also occurs around tumors.

Severe cerebral swelling is associated with a rise in the pressure within the skull (**raised intracranial pressure**).

Expanding intracranial lesions cause raised intracranial pressure

Raised intracranial pressure is an important consequence of several disorders affecting the brain. The commonest causes include the effects of bleeding in or around the brain, swelling associated with cerebral infarction and the growth of brain tumors.

The cranial cavity is divided simplistically into three spaces by the falx and tentorium cerebelli. If a lesion expands within the skull, there is only a limited amount of room to accommodate it. Initially, reduction in the size of the ventricles and subarachnoid space occurs as limited compensatory shifts in volume. Once this volume is used, further

Fig. 21.1 Neuronal chromatolysis. This neuron shows central chromatolysis. The neuron is swollen with no visible Nissl substance. The nucleus is large, centrally placed with an open chromatin pattern.

increase in the size of a lesion is associated with increase in intracranial pressure. There are two main consequences of raised pressure: first, brain structures shift and can become compressed or compromised; second, the pressure within the skull can be so high that it exceeds the arterial perfusion pressure, leading to brain death.

Swellings within the brain are particularly dangerous when they lead to rapid local expansion of one part, causing it to shift from one brain compartment to another, a process termed **cerebral herniation**. There are four types of cerebral herniation.

Transtentorial herniation (*Fig. 21.2a* and *b*) is caused by lesions expanding in one cerebral hemisphere. There is herniation of the medial part of the temporal lobe down over the tentorium cerebelli to compress the upper brain stem (*Fig. 21.2b*). The third cranial nerve becomes first stretched, then compressed on the side of the lesion, giving rise to a fixed dilated pupil. Branches of the posterior cerebral artery are also compressed as the brain herniates, causing secondary infarction of the occipital lobe. As the midbrain is distorted by compression, small vessels are torn and secondary hemorrhage into the brain stem occurs, leading to death.

Cerebellar tonsillar herniation (*Fig. 21.2a*) is caused by expanding lesions in the posterior fossa. There is herniation of the lower part of the cerebellum (cerebellar tonsils), which pushes down into the foramen magnum and compresses the medulla; this process is also known as **coning**. As the medulla is compressed, it causes cessation of respiration and death. This may be precipitated by performing a lumbar puncture in a person with a mass in the brain. Withdrawal of CSF allows a pressure gradient to develop and there is rapid coning with death. Lumbar puncture should never be performed until the possibility of a mass lesion in the cranial cavity has been excluded.

Cingulate gyrus (subfalcial) herniation (*Fig. 21.2a* and *c*) is caused by a lesion in one of the cerebral hemispheres, resulting in movement of the cingulate gyrus beneath the falx cerebri. This is often associated with compression of the adjacent anterior cerebral artery, leading to secondary cerebral infarction.

Diencephalic herniation is caused by generalized swelling of both cerebral hemispheres. There is compression of the ventricles, with descent of the thalamus and midbrain through the tentorial hiatus.

Fig. 21.2 Cerebral herniation. (a) If there is expansion of a lesion on one side of the brain, for example a tumor or a hematoma, a pressure gradient develops. The cingulate gyrus may move beneath the falx cerebri and the parahippocampal gyrus may herniate through the tentorial hiatus. If pressure increases in the posterior fossa, herniation of the cerebellar tonsils into the foramen magnum may occur. (b) Herniation of the parahippocampal gyrus through the tentorial hiatus. The free edge of the tentorium cerebelli has indented the cerebrum (arrows) along the margin of the herniated brain tissue. (c) Herniation contusions (arrow) may be visible where the uncus or parahippocampal gyrus has been pressed against the edge of the tentorium, in this case by a subdural hematoma (not visible in figure). Histologic examination of the contusions reveals focal necrosis and small hemorrhages. The subdural hematoma has also displaced midline structures and caused subfalcine herniation of the cingulate gyrus (arrowhead).

CEREBROVASCULAR DISEASE

Cerebrovascular diseases are the third most common cause of death in western countries. The most frequent manifestation of disease is a sudden episode of neurological deficit termed a **stroke**, which is the result of cerebral hemorrhage or cerebral infarction in the majority of cases.

Arteriovenous malformations predispose to intracranial hemorrhage

Arteriovenous malformations (AVMs) are developmental abnormalities of blood vessels (both arteries and veins) in which leashes of unusually fragile vessels are formed. They occur most commonly in relation to the cerebral hemispheres, but other sites (including the spinal cord) are also affected.

Macroscopically, lesions may involve the meninges, extend deep into the brain, or be mixed in pattern. They vary in size, but are typically 3–4 cm in diameter. Lesions have several feeding arterial vessels and several draining channels, making surgical removal very difficult. Increasingly interventional transvascular approaches are allowing therapeutic embolization of lesions

Histologically they are composed of abnormal blood vessels surrounded by areas of gliotic brain tissue (*Fig. 21.3*) Evidence of previous bleeding may be inferred by the presence of iron-containing hemosiderin pigment within the gliotic brain tissue.

Clinically, AVMs are a cause of epilepsy and of other focal neurological signs. The major problem is that the fragile vessels bleed, causing life-threatening intracranial hemorrhage.

Fig. 21.3 Arteriovenous malformation. An arteriovenous malformation is composed of abnormal blood vessels, some with thick walls, lying within gliotic cerebral tissues.

Clinical features of raised intracranial pressure

Patients with raised intracranial pressure may develop symptoms and signs due to an expanding cerebral lesion. In slowly expanding lesions, compensation takes place and signs develop slowly. In rapidly expanding lesions, signs and symptoms can develop within minutes.

There may be **vomiting** due to movement of the medulla and stimulation of vomiting centers, **headache** due to stimulation of pain-sensitive nerve endings associated with stretched vessels, and **papilledema** due to impaired flow of axonal cytoplasm in the optic nerves, caused by increased pressure of the CSF in the optic nerve sheath.

If a lesion expands rapidly, there is danger of cerebral herniation. It is usual to observe patients carefully on a regular basis to detect the earliest signs of an enlarging brain lesion. This is usually done after head trauma to detect any developing cerebral pathology.

- The pupils are observed. A sluggish pupillary reaction to light is seen when there is stretching of the third cranial nerve in early transtentorial herniation. A fixed dilated pupil indicates crushing of the nerve and is seen in more advanced herniation.
- Conscious level is assessed. As the brain stem is compressed, there is a progressive reduction in conscious level.

In the late advanced stages of raised intracranial pressure, **bradycardia**, **hypertension** and **neurogenic pulmonary edema** develop. These are usually seen only in patients who are close to death from a cerebral mass lesion.

Cerebral blood vessels are prone to atheroma, arteriolosclerosis and amyloid deposition

The cerebral arteries are prone to the general pathological processes that affect systemic arteries.

Atheroma principally affects the main named cerebral arteries. It is generally more severe in the basilar artery than in the anterior and middle cerebral vessels. The main complications of atheroma are thrombosis and aneurysm formation (*Fig. 21.4*). Atheroma is particularly important in the extracranial cerebral arteries, the carotid and vertebral vessels in the neck. It is now appreciated that the majority of cerebral ischemic events are caused by disease in the extracranial vessels, especially in the region of the carotid bifurcation.

Arteriolosclerosis affects the small vessels that penetrate the brain and is caused by long-standing hypertension or diabetes. Vessels show replacement of the muscular media by hyaline material, which weakens the walls and predisposes to intracerebral hemorrhage. Reduction in

Fig. 21.4 Fusiform atherosclerotic aneurysm. The basilar artery is replaced by a large fusiform aneurysm (**A**) caused by atherosclerosis.

Fig. 21.5 Berry aneurysm. This is the circle of Willis, with anterior (**A**), middle (**M**) and posterior (**P**) cerebral arteries linked by communicating vessels. Berry aneurysms (**B**) are seen arising where the internal carotid bifurcates into middle and anterior cerebral vessels.

the size of the lumen of small vessels also predisposes to very small cerebral infarcts (**lacunar infarcts**) see page 459).

Amyloid (see Chapter 25), especially that derived from Aβ peptide (as seen in Alzheimer's disease), is frequently deposited in the cerebral vessels of the elderly, causing **amyloid angiopathy**. This predisposes to intracerebral hemorrhage in a peripheral distribution in the cerebral hemispheres termed lobar cerebral hemorrhage; it is the cause of cerebral hemorrhage in about 10% of cases in patients over the age of 70.

Berry aneurysms are the most common type of aneurysm of cerebral arteries

Berry aneurysms are small saccular aneurysms that occur in about 2% of the population. Macroscopically they appear as rounded swellings arising from the cerebral arteries (*Fig. 21.5*). Although they can be 0.2–3 cm in diameter, most are under 1 cm. Occurring particularly at the branch points of vessels around the circle of Willis, they are frequently multiple.

- 45% arise in the region of the anterior communicating cerebral artery.
- 30% arise from the middle cerebral artery as it divides deep in the sylvian fissure.
- 20% arise in the region of the internal carotid arteries, usually at the origin of the posterior communicating artery.
- 5% arise elsewhere in the cerebral circulation.
- Aneurysms are prone to rupture, with consequent subarachnoid hemorrhage (see pages 460–1).

Berry aneurysms arise because of developmental defects in the internal elastic lamina of vessels. The stress of the systolic waves causes herniation of the intima, with the formation of saccular aneurysms. This is accentuated by hypertension, and aneurysms are commonly seen in association with coarctation of the aorta and adult polycystic renal disease.

Less common are **atherosclerotic** and **infective (mycotic) aneurysms**. Atherosclerotic aneurysms are most common in the basilar artery, where they tend to be fusiform (*Fig. 21.4*). Infective (mycotic) aneurysms arise in cases of infective endocarditis, when a small segment of arterial wall is acutely inflamed and dilates due to local bacterial infection from a small septic embolus.

Stroke is common in the general population

Stroke occurs in 2 per 1000 of the general population. A clinical diagnosis, defined as the sudden onset of non-traumatic focal neurological deficit, it has several pathological causes, and is mainly seen in the elderly population. The causes of stroke can be divided into two main groups: **ischemic** (85%), caused by cerebral infarction; and **hemor-**

rhagic (15%), caused by intracerebral and subarachnoid hemorrhage. Routine early imaging plays a key role in distinguishing between hemorrhage and ischemia in patients who present with clinical stroke.

The **clinical diagnosis of ischemic stroke** is defined as a sudden onset of non-traumatic focal neurological deficit that causes death or lasts for over 7 days.

Transient ischemic attacks (TIA) are defined as brief episodes of non-traumatic neurologic dysfunction caused by focal brain or retinal ischemia, with clinical symptoms typically lasting less than 1 hour, and without evidence of acute infarction.

The terms **minor stroke** and **reversible ischemic neurological deficit** (RIND) has been used when an episode lasts over 24 hours with recovery of clinical features occurring after a period of time, usually defined as 7 days. Imaging investigation commonly reveals small areas of permanent structural ischemic damage in such cases.

Episodes of TIA or RIND carry an increased risk of the patient developing a completed stroke, which is 2–4% at 1 month for example, those with severe carotid atheroma.

Diffusion-weighted magnetic resonance imaging (DWI), which is sensitive to detecting ischemic changes in the brain, has highlighted overlap in findings between these clinical groups. It has been proposed that the term **acute ischemic cerebrovascular syndrome (AICS)** be used as a collective term to incorporate clinical groups such as TIA, RIND and ischemic stroke.

Hemorrhages and ischemic lesions caused by trauma are discussed later in this chapter (see page 461 et seq.).

BRAIN ISCHEMIA AND INFARCTION

There are four types of ischemic brain damage: large vessel, small vessel, venous and global

The four main types of ischemic brain damage are classified according to the pathogenesis of reduced blood flow to the brain.

Large vessel disease causes regional infarction, the main mechanisms being embolism and thrombosis in the large, named cerebral arteries. Resulting areas of infarction correspond to territories of supply of named cerebral arteries and their main branches.

Small vessel disease causes microinfarcts known as lacunar infarcts. These are caused by arteriolosclerosis predisposed to by hypertension and diabetes. The main sites for this type of infarction are the pons and the basal ganglia/internal capsule region.

Venous infarction causes hemorrhagic necrosis in affected areas. These are caused by thrombosis in a main cerebral venous sinus and are usually associated with an identifiable abnormal predisposition to thrombosis, e.g. dehydration or one of the recognized thrombophilia syndromes.

Global ischemia causes widespread neuronal necrosis and can lead to laminar cortical necrosis in which the majority of large neurons in the cerebral cortex die. It is seen when there is global reduction in cerebral blood flow as, for example, with sustained cardiorespiratory arrest. When blood flow is reduced but not completely absent (as in severe hypotension), infarction at arterial boundary zones occurs, sometimes termed 'watershed infarction'.

Mechanisms of hypoxic and ischemic damage

Hypoxic and ischemic damage to the brain results in failure of supply of energy sources. Neurons have small metabolic reserves and are extremely sensitive to energy deprivation. This situation is seen in: **failure of blood oxygenation**, which occurs in severe respiratory disease, asphyxiation and carbon monoxide poisoning; **failure of blood flow**, which may be either focal (as occurs in occlusion of a cerebral artery) or generalized (as occurs with a cardiac arrest); and **severe hypoglycemia**, which causes energy deprivation to the brain despite an adequate supply of blood and oxygen.

Failure of supply of energy substrates to the brain causes death of neurons, with sparing of vessels and support cells, which are more robust. The neurons that are most vulnerable are the large cells in the hippocampus and those in the cerebellar cortex (Purkinje cells).

Total irreversible cessation of blood flow leads to cerebral infarction in the territory supplied by the artery involved. This affects all cell types, including glial cells and vessels.

An important event in ischemic damage is **activation of glutamate receptors**, which causes uncontrolled entry of calcium into neurons, leading to cell death. This concept, termed excitotoxicity, is believed to be a common factor in many types of neuronal death, including that seen in severe epilepsy. Use of drugs that block certain types of glutamate receptor can prevent neuronal death following ischemia.

Regional cerebral infarction is caused by occlusion of named cerebral arteries

Regional cerebral infarcts are caused by the occlusion of main named arteries supplying the brain. The most common causes originate outside the cranial cavity, e.g. emboli from the heart, aorta or carotid vessels, and thrombosis in the carotid or vertebral arteries (see *Fig. 21.6*), predisposed to by atheroma. Less common causes of infarction are seen in younger stroke patients (see blue box). There are three zones conceptually considered in relation to an area of cerebral ischemic damage: tissue that are certain to die (infarct core), tissue that will generally survive by collateral perfusion (oligemic periphery), and tissues in between that may either die or survive (the ischemic penumbra). Some strategies of treatment in stroke are concerned with preventing neuronal death in the penumbra.

Cerebral infarcts correspond to the territory of supply of the occluded arteries. It is difficult to see an infarct in the first 24 hours, as changes are limited to focal swelling and blurring of the normal demarcation between gray and white matter, termed a **pale or anemic infarct**. If there is lysis of an occlusive thrombus, the infarcted area may be reperfused with blood, resulting in a hemorrhagic infarct (*Fig. 21.7*).

Fig. 21.6 Carotid artery thrombosis. This is the carotid artery dissected from the neck of a patient who died of cerebral infarction. There is complete occlusion by thrombus complicating an established atheromatous plaque at the level of the bifurcation.

Fig. 21.7 Recent hemorrhagic cerebral infarct. This is a slice through a brain, in the same plane as seen in routine CT scans. A large infarct, corresponding to the territory of the middle cerebral artery is seen as an area of swollen hemorrhagic brain (**I**). The hemorrhage was caused by reperfusion after lysis of an occluding thrombus.

Fig. 21.8 Old healed cerebral infarct. This is a transverse axial brain slice. With time, a regional cerebral infarct is replaced by a cystic gliotic cavity (**C**).

Stroke in younger patients

The causes of strokes in younger patients are different from those seen in the elderly.

- 40% are the result of **non-traumatic intracerebral hemorrhage**, the main causes being hypertension, berry aneurysms, AVMs, and bleeding into tumors. Cocaine and heroin abuse also predisposes to hemorrhage.
- 20% of cases have **subarachnoid hemorrhage**, the majority being due to ruptured berry aneurysms or vascular malformations.

- 40% of cases have **cerebral infarction**. In 30% of these cases no cause is ascertained. In the other 70% there are diverse and sometimes unusual causes including **vascular occlusion** (cardiogenic emboli, premature atherosclerosis, vasculitis, arterial dissection), **vascular spasm** (migraine-associated, recreational drugs), **increased thromboembolic tendency** (oral contraceptives and pregnancy, alcohol and smoking, antiphospholipid antibodies), and **heritable conditions** (congenital lack of inhibitors of coagulation).

By about 1 week the infarcted area becomes macroscopically soft and is infiltrated by macrophages, which remove dead tissue. Proliferation of astrocytes occurs around the margins of the infarct, and these partly replace the dead tissue, usually being well established by about 2 weeks. Larger regional areas of infarction invariably heal as fluid-filled cystic spaces bounded by gliosis (*Fig. 21.8*).

Although a number of clinical syndromes related to occlusion of individual arteries are described, the most important practical distinction is between those affecting the **carotid territory** (frontal, temporal, parietal lobes or basal ganglia/internal capsule) and those affecting the **vertebrobasilar territory** (occipital lobe, cerebellum or brain stem).

Large cerebral infarcts may cause death by associated cerebral swelling, leading to herniation, and brainstem compression. Infarcts in critical sites, particularly brain stem infarcts, may interfere with vital functions and lead to death. Immobility and difficulty in swallowing lead to the development of pneumonia in many patients.

Lacunar infarction is caused by arteriolosclerosis of small vessels

Lacunar infarcts are small, often slit-shaped, areas of infarction less than 1 cm in maximum diameter. They are an important form of cerebral infarct, particularly in patients with hypertension and diabetes, being caused by **hyaline arteriolosclerosis**.

Macroscopically, lesions are usually multiple and are seen in the sites normally supplied by fine perforating branches, such as the basal ganglia, internal capsule, thalamus and pons (*Fig. 21.9*).

Clinically, lacunar infarcts can be asymptomatic or may cause very restricted neurological deficits such as monoparesis. Multiple lacunar infarcts in the basal ganglia cause a syndrome of rigidity and abnormal gait termed vascular pseudo-parkinsonism, which superficially resembles Parkinson's disease. Lacunar infarction is also associated with ischemic white-matter degeneration, an important cause of dementia. Because hypertension and diabetes are risk factors for ischemic heart disease and atheroma, lacunar infarcts are often seen in association with regional infarcts caused by large vessel disease.

Cortical laminar necrosis is caused by generalized failure of perfusion

Diffuse necrosis of cerebral cortical neurons is the pattern of infarction seen in generalized failure of blood flow or oxygenation as seen, for example, following cardiac arrest, with severe hypoglycemia, and after carbon monoxide poisoning.

Changes develop 24 hours after resuscitation from the damaging episode. There is widespread damage to the cerebral cortex, with death of the majority of cortical neurons. With time, there is phagocytosis of dead neurons with astrocytic gliosis.

Macroscopically the cerebral cortex is shrunken and there is extensive loss of axons from the brain, causing secondary white matter loss (*Fig. 21.10*).

Patients who survive global laminar necrosis generally have severe brain damage, existing in a vegetative state devoid of higher cortical functions. Lesser degrees of hypoxia or cerebral perfusion failure result in similar damage, limited to the particularly vulnerable areas of the hippocampus and cerebellar cortex.

Fig. 21.9 Lacunar infarcts of brain. Lacunar infarcts are seen as small slit-shaped cavities (**S**), a few millimeters in size, in the basal ganglia on both sides. They are caused by disease of small perforating vessels.

Fig. 21.10 Cortical laminar necrosis. The cortex is replaced by a band of yellow gliotic tissue, most evident in the superior part of the brain compared to the temporal lobes.

Fig. 21.11 Sagittal sinus thrombosis. This shows the inside of the dura from the skull. The sagittal sinus is thrombosed with propagation of thrombus down cortical veins that have been stripped off with the dura.

Venous infarction is caused by venous sinus thrombosis

Venous infarction is the least common pattern of cerebral infarction. It occurs when there is occlusion of the venous sinuses and cerebral cortical veins by local thrombosis (*Fig. 21.11*).

Predisposing factors include dehydration in children, spread of infection from adjacent foci in the head (nasal sinus and middle ear) and disorders that cause hypercoagulability of blood, particularly polycythemia, oral contraceptive therapy and pregnancy.

Macroscopically the affected brain shows severe hemorrhagic infarction caused by vascular congestion.

SPONTANEOUS INTRACRANIAL HEMORRHAGE

Spontaneous intracranial hemorrhage accounts for about 15% of all strokes and is caused by intracerebral hematoma and subarachnoid hemorrhage. Petechial hemorrhage is a less common pattern. Hemorrhage caused by trauma is considered in a later section (see page 462).

Cerebral hematomas are most commonly caused by hypertensive vascular damage

The most common cause of cerebral hemorrhage is hypertensive vascular damage. Prolonged hypertension results in arterio- and arteriolosclerosis and in the development of small microaneurysms (Charcot–Bouchard aneurysms) that

Fig. 21.12 Intracerebral hematoma. A large hematoma effaces the basal ganglia, with compression of adjacent brain. Blood has ruptured into the ventricles.

predispose to vessel rupture, resulting in a hematoma. The common sites for hypertensive intracerebral hematoma are those supplied by fine perforating vessels (basal ganglia, internal capsule, thalamus, cerebellum and pons).

In patients over the age of 70 years, 10% of cerebral hemorrhages are caused by the presence of cerebral artery amyloid, which is composed of Aβ peptide (see page 574). This causes hematomas, seen in the periphery of cerebral hemispheres (lobar hemorrhages).

Less common causes of a cerebral hematoma are bleeding into a tumor, rupture of vascular malformations, cerebral vasculitis, bleeding associated with disordered coagulation, and bleeding occurring in association with leukemias.

Macroscopically, hematomas appear as a large blood clot, causing compression and damage to adjacent brain (*Fig. 21.12*). Large hematomas in the basal ganglia or thalamus often rupture into the ventricular system. If the patient survives a bleed, the hematoma is removed by phagocytic cells; astrocytic gliosis takes place, leaving a cavity stained yellow-brown with hemosiderin. Large bleeds that cause raised intracranial pressure, and those that rupture into the ventricular system, are commonly fatal.

Subarachnoid hemorrhage is most often caused by a ruptured berry aneurysm

Bleeding into the subarachnoid space (between the arachnoid and the pia) is termed **subarachnoid hemorrhage**. A cause of stroke from adolescence to old age, it accounts for about 5% of all cases. In most cases, the cause of subarachnoid bleeding is rupture of a berry aneurysm; less common causes are rupture of an intracerebral hematoma into the subarachnoid space, or rupture of a vascular malformation.

Macroscopically, a layer of blood is present over the brain surface in the subarachnoid space (*Fig. 21.13*). Blood is therefore present in the cerebrospinal fluid (CSF) and can

Fig. 21.13 Subarachnoid hemorrhage. Owing to rupture of a berry aneurysm just visible in the sylvian fissure (arrow), blood is present in the subarachnoid space over the cerebral hemispheres.

be detected on lumbar puncture. There are two effects of subarachnoid hemorrhage:

- Blood around vessels causes vascular spasm and leads to widespread cerebral ischemia and brain swelling.
- There may be blockage of CSF resorption, causing acute hydrocephalus.

About 30% of patients die immediately; others who present with headache and signs of meningeal irritation may have intervention and occlusion of the aneurysm. Intervention is commonly a transvascular coiling of the aneurysm, or alternatively craniotomy and clipping of the aneurysm neck. In the absence of intervention, 30% of patients have a re-bleed within 1 year, most within 1 month of the first. A long-term complication is development of hydrocephalus caused by blockage and fibrosis in the CSF pathways.

Diffuse petechial hemorrhage in the brain is caused by damage to small vessels

The least common form of cerebral hemorrhage is multiple petechial hemorrhages scattered throughout the brain. These are 1–2 mm in size and are concentrated in the white matter. They are caused by disease that disrupts the walls of small cerebral blood vessels, allowing extravasation of red cells. Patients with this pattern of disease tend to present with confusion and reduced conscious level, rather than with focal neurological signs. The main causes are acute hypertensive encephalopathy, fat embolism, vasculitis of small cerebral vessels (e.g. polyarteritis), cerebral malaria and acute hemorrhagic leukoencephalitis (allergic vasculitis of cerebral vessels).

TRAUMA TO THE CENTRAL NERVOUS SYSTEM

Head injury is one of the most common causes of disability and death in young men, mainly sustained during road traffic accidents and falls. Injury is divided into two types:

- **Non-missile trauma** (closed head injury) is the result of acceleration/deceleration forces to the head and the resultant rotational and shearing forces on the brain, which cause movement of the brain within the skull. This happens when the head is thrown violently forward, or when a head travelling at speed is suddenly brought to a halt (motor cyclist's head in contact with road). This is the most common pattern of head trauma encountered clinically.
- **Missile trauma** (open head injury) is caused by penetration of the skull or brain by an external object such as a bullet.

Brain pathology from head injury may be divided into two groups: primary and secondary

Brain pathology from head injury may be divided into two broad categories, primary (i.e. the immediate consequence of impact damage) and secondary (i.e. occurring as a delayed consequence of brain swelling, bleeding, hypoxia or secondary infection) (*Fig. 21.14*).

There are two main patterns of primary brain damage in closed head injury.

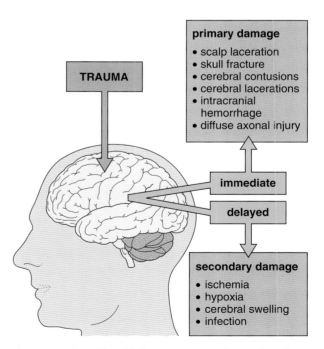

Fig. 21.14 Closed head injury. Primary and secondary damage related to non-missile head injury.

1. **Cerebral contusions** occur when the brain moves within the cranial cavity, causing parts of the brain to be crushed by violent contact with the skull or dural membranes. For the most part, these occur adjacent to the site of impact (*coup* lesions) and diagonally opposite (*contrecoup* lesions). The most common sites for this pattern of damage are the underside of the frontal lobes, the tips and inferior aspects of the temporal lobes, the occipital poles, and the cerebellum. Early contusions appear as petechial hemorrhage into cortical gray matter and underlying white matter. Over a period of several hours there is oozing of blood, and contusions become hemorrhagic, with severe swelling of the brain (*Fig. 21.15*).

   Severe contusions may be associated with extensive intracerebral, subarachnoid and subdural hemorrhage. Contusions heal by gliosis, which is often associated with brown hemosiderin deposition (caused by the associated hemorrhage).

2. **Diffuse traumatic axonal injury** is the result of shearing of axons due to acceleration, deceleration, and torsional forces, leading to severe damage to white matter tracts. Patients with this pattern of damage who survive are generally severely disabled. Most of the changes are only seen histologically, consisting of axonal tearing visible as swellings of the torn ends of nerve fibers (axonal retraction balls) (*Fig. 21.16*). Petechial hemorrhages may also occur in the corpus callosum and brain stem, and their detection at these sites, either by imaging or at autopsy, is a useful indicator of this type of severe head injury.

Secondary brain damage occurs after the immediate impact. Head injury is often associated with widespread trauma, which leads to problems maintaining blood oxygenation and blood pressure. As a consequence, head injury is often complicated by the development of secondary hypoxic brain damage and cerebral edema.

Tearing of blood vessels with trauma leads to four main types of cerebral hemorrhage: **intracerebral hematoma**, caused by tearing of vessels within the brain parenchyma; **subarachnoid hemorrhage**, caused by tearing of vessels adjacent to the subarachnoid space; **subdural hemorrhage**, caused by tearing of veins (discussed below); and **extradural hemorrhage**, caused by tearing of vessels in the skull (discussed below).

Fig. 21.15 Cerebral contusions. Primary impact damage has caused severe hemorrhagic contusion of the left frontal lobe (**C**) – coup lesion, with smaller contusions on the right parietal lobe (**P**) – contrecoup lesion. Swelling of the left side of the brain has caused cerebral herniation with compression of the midbrain (**M**).

Fig. 21.16 Diffuse axonal injury. If silver stains are used on white matter normal axons are seen as long thin black-stained structures. Axonal swellings can be seen as oval-shaped structures caused by axonal damage in head injury.

Extradural hemorrhage is caused by tearing of vessels that run outside the dura

Extradural hemorrhage causes a hematoma in the potential extradural space between the skull and the dura (*Fig. 21.17*) and is almost always the result of skull fracture, which tears an artery or a main venous sinus running outside the dura. A vessel commonly involved is the **middle meningeal artery** (associated with fracture of the temporal bone).

The extradural hematoma appears as a gelatinous layer of blood clot outside the dura. This accumulation causes compression of the brain and development of transtentorial herniation. In many cases, high-pressure arterial blood accumulates rapidly, leading to an acute decline in conscious level with raised intracranial pressure. In other cases blood accumulates over a period of hours in which trauma is followed by gradually progressive coma.

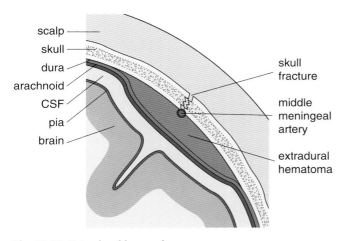

Fig. 21.17 Extradural hemorrhage.

scalp
skull
dura
arachnoid
CSF
pia
brain

skull
fracture

middle
meningeal
artery

extradural
hematoma

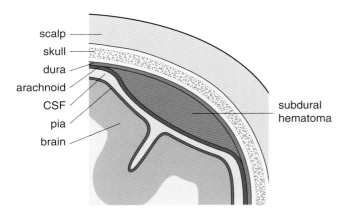

Fig. 21.18 Subdural hemorrhage.

scalp
skull
dura
arachnoid
CSF
pia
brain

subdural
hematoma

Some subdural hematomas are caused by minor head trauma and have a chronic pattern of evolution

Subdural hemorrhage results in a hematoma developing in the subdural space between the dura and the arachnoid (*Fig. 21.18*). It is caused by traumatic tearing of venous vessels that traverse the subdural space. There are two patterns.

Acute subdural hematomas are usually seen after a severe head injury and are associated with other types of brain injury. They cause rapid accumulation of blood, leading to acute neurological deterioration as a result of raised intracranial pressure.

Chronic subdural hematomas usually occur as a result of minimal trauma and are mainly seen in the very young (including childhood non-accidental injury) and the elderly. Blood typically accumulates slowly over a period of days or weeks, becoming localized by a membrane of fibrovascular granulation tissue. In addition to the osmotic effects of degenerating blood clot drawing in fluid from the CSF, increase in the size of the hematoma occurs with further

bleeding. Clinical symptoms and signs may only become obvious weeks after an apparently trivial injury, as a result of raised intracranial pressure.

Macroscopically a subdural hematoma is seen as a layer of gelatinous blood clot (acute type) or as an organized layer of dark liquefied clot surrounded by membranes (chronic type), which flattens and compresses the underlying brain, staining the outside of the arachnoid with hemosiderin.

Trauma to the spinal cord is a common cause of disability in young men

Most spinal cord injuries occur in young males as a result of road traffic accidents, falls and sport, and in young females in horse-riding accidents.

Injury is mainly caused by fracture and dislocation of the vertebral column, causing compression of the spinal cord by distortion of the spinal canal (*Fig. 21.19*). Minor contusions of the cord result in transient recoverable neurological abnormality. Severe contusions cause damage to ascending and descending tracts, as well as necrosis of neurons at the segments damaged.

The consequence of cord damage depends on the spinal level of the injury; cervical lesions cause tetraplegia, whereas lower thoracic lesions cause paraplegia. Denervated muscles undergo atrophy, with secondary contractures and deformities in limbs. Denervation of the bladder leads to problems with micturition, urinary stasis and recurrent infections.

Penetrating injuries of the spinal cord are uncommon, but may be seen after stabbings or shootings. Complete

Fig. 21.19 Spinal cord trauma. Fracture of a vertebra (**F**) is associated with narrowing of the spinal canal and compression of the cord, which appears slightly yellowed and swollen at the site of injury.

Fig. 21.20 Causes of spinal cord compression

Prolapse of intervertebral disc

Osteophytes caused by spondylosis

Bone disease (rheumatoid or Paget's)

Extradural tumor or abscess, or meningeal fibrosis

Intradural tumor (schwannoma, arteriovenous malformation,

meningioma)

transection of the cord may occur, hemisection giving rise to a Brown–Séquard syndrome.

In addition to trauma, the spinal cord and nerve roots are vulnerable to damage by non-traumatic compression, the main causes of which are summarized in *Fig. 21.20*.

Fig. 21.21 Hydrocephalus. The lateral ventricles (**L**) including the temporal horns (**H**) are dilated. In this case the cause was obstruction of CSF flow through the cerebral aqueduct.

HYDROCEPHALUS

Excess CSF in the intracranial cavity is termed 'hydrocephalus' and most cases are caused by obstruction of the flow of CSF

The term hydrocephalus is used to describe conditions in which there is increase in the volume of CSF within the brain, with expansion of the cerebral ventricles. The most common type, which is termed **non-communicating hydrocephalus** or **obstructive hydrocephalus**, is caused by blockage of the CSF pathway from the ventricles to the subarachnoid space. A less common type is communicating hydrocephalus, in which there is impairment of resorption of CSF at the arachnoid villi along the dural venous sinuses, usually precipitated by previous infection or bleeding into the subarachnoid space.

Among the main causes of obstructive hydrocephalus is **congenital hydrocephalus**, seen in about 1 in 1000 births. Some cases have stenosis of the aqueduct of Sylvius, some have an associated Arnold–Chiari malformation (see page 477), and some are inherited as an X-linked trait.

Tumors may obstruct the ventricular system, particularly those located in the brain stem, cerebellum, or pineal region which block the cerebral aqueduct or fourth ventricle.

Scarring and **blockage of the CSF exit foramina** at the base of the brain are common complications of meningitis or subarachnoid hemorrhage.

Hemorrhage in the brain or subarachnoid space may obstruct CSF drainage pathways.

Macroscopically, there is dilatation of the ventricular cavities of the brain proximal to the site of obstruction (*Fig. 21.21*). The effects of hydrocephalus depend on the speed of development of disease and age of the patient.

In **acute hydrocephalus**, swelling of the brain may be rapid and may cause death from cerebral herniation.

In **chronic hydrocephalus**, signs and symptoms develop slowly and there are clinical features of raised intracranial pressure. When hydrocephalus develops in children, before the skull bones have fused, there is progressive enlargement of the head circumference. In adults, where the skull is rigidly fused, prolonged disease causes thinning of the skull vault. In the absence of treatment, long-standing disease causes axonal damage and gliosis in the white matter. In children this leads to mental subnormality and in adults can lead to the development of a dementia syndrome, with early gait disturbance and incontinence as prominent features.

Treatment of hydrocephalus involves the placement of a permanent shunt to drain CSF into the peritoneal cavity. This leads to other pathological complications because shunts become periodically blocked, leading to acute attacks of hydrocephalus. Shunts also become infected with low-virulence organisms, producing signs and symptoms of infection, as well as immune-mediated glomerular disease.

SYRINGOMYELIA

A syrinx is a fluid-filled cavity in the cord or brain stem

A syrinx is a fluid-filled slit-like cavity that develops in the spinal cord (**syringomyelia**) or brain stem (**syringobulbia**), causing compression of the white matter tracts and resulting in neurological disability. Most syringeal cavities are secondary to trauma or ischemia, or are associated with tumors of the spinal cord. Less commonly, a syrinx may be a primary developmental phenomenon. Syringeal cavities are most frequent in the cervical spinal cord and may extend over many segments.

Clinical manifestations of syringomyelia are due to compression of the spinal cord tracts and include wasting of the intrinsic muscles of the hand, spastic weakness in the legs, and loss of pain and temperature sensation, with preservation of touch.

INFECTION OF THE CENTRAL NERVOUS SYSTEM

Infection of the central nervous system (CNS) is an extremely common clinical problem that can be caused by most classes of infecting organism. There are four main patterns of associated inflammation, corresponding to the primary seat of the infective process:

1. **Meningitis** (inflammation of the meninges) is divided into leptomeningitis (inflammation centered on the subarachnoid space) and pachymeningitis (inflammation centered on the dura).
2. **Cerebritis** and **cerebral abscess** (focal inflammation of the brain).
3. **Encephalitis** (diffuse inflammation of the brain) or **myelitis** (diffuse inflammation of the cord).
4. **Meningoencephalitis** (combination of diffuse inflammation of the brain and inflammation of leptomeninges).

There are three main types of leptomeningitis

Leptomeningitis is a form of inflammation centered on the subarachnoid space. Infecting organisms circulate and spread by the CSF route. Initial infection is nearly always the result of bloodborne spread of the infecting organism, but may also be caused by direct spread from infection in the middle ear, mastoid, nasal sinuses, and dural venous sinuses. Penetrating wounds, including fracture of skull, can also predispose to leptomeningitis.

Leptomeningitis can be divided into three main groups: **acute purulent meningitis**, which is mainly caused by bacterial infection; **lymphocytic meningitis**, which is mainly caused by viral infection; and **chronic** and **granulomatous meningitides**, which are caused by TB and unusual organisms (see Chapter 8).

Acute purulent meningitis is almost always caused by bacterial infection

Acute purulent meningitis is a severe infection that is nearly always caused by bacterial infection. Patients are severely unwell and have signs of infection, neck stiffness and photophobia. CSF examination shows turbid fluid with many neutrophil polymorphs and a low sugar; bacteria may be seen on special staining.

Macroscopically, the subarachnoid space contains a cream-colored acute inflammatory exudate rich in neutrophils (*Fig. 21.22*). The severe inflammation causes second-

Fig. 21.22 Acute purulent leptomeningitis. The subarachnoid space contains a creamy purulent exudate caused by bacterial meningitis. This is an acute inflammatory exudate that is rich in neutrophils.

ary thrombosis of superficial vessels and cerebral ischemic damage. If treated early, there may be resolution of disease. However, complications caused by organization of the inflammatory exudate may lead to obstruction of the CSF drainage pathways and the development of hydrocephalus.

The main causes of acute purulent meningitis vary according to age. In neonates *Escherichia coli*, streptococci and *Listeria monocytogenes* are responsible, and in children *Haemophilus influenzae* and *Neisseria meningitidis* are the principal causes. *Neisseria meningitidis* and *Streptococcus pneumoniae* type 3 are involved in adults, and in the elderly the main causative organisms are *Streptococcus pneumoniae* type 3 and *Listeria monocytogenes*.

Lymphocytic meningitis is usually caused by viruses and is a benign self-limited disease

Lymphocytic meningitis is a self-limited disease caused by several viral infections. In most cases patients have clinical malaise and meningism, and require investigation to exclude the presence of bacterial meningitis. Typically the CSF is clear and has a normal glucose level, but has a mild elevation of protein and contains an increase in lymphoid cells.

The cause of infection is ascertained by virological or serological examination of CSF and blood. The most common causes are infection by the mumps, Coxsackie, echo, Epstein–Barr, lymphocytic choriomeningitis and polio viruses. In many cases no organism is detected.

Chronic and granulomatous meningitides are severe inflammatory diseases that lead to meningeal fibrosis and cranial nerve lesions

Chronic and granulomatous meningitides are forms of severe productive chronic inflammation and fibrosis. The

CSF is typically opalescent, with a raised protein level, reduced glucose level, and an increased lymphocyte count with the presence of plasma cells. The important causative organisms are *Mycobacterium tuberculosis*, *Treponema pallidum* (syphilis), *Cryptococcus neoformans*, and *Borrelia burgdorferi* (Lyme disease).

Macroscopically there is thickening and opacity of the leptomeninges, with marked thickening and fibrosis in advanced disease. Histologically, there is lymphocytic and plasma-cell infiltration of the meninges with fibrosis. The cause of chronic meningitis may be apparent on examination. In tuberculous meningitis caseating granulomas are seen, and mycobacteria may be visible on Ziehl–Neelsen (ZN) staining. In cryptococcal infection, fungi are usually clearly visible, with the use of special stains (see *Fig. 8.25*).

Meningeal fibrosis and inflammation have two main effects: they lead to obstruction of the drainage pathways for CSF, causing hydrocephalus (see page 464), and vascular lesions cause infarction and cranial nerve and spinal root palsies.

Pachymeningitis is caused mainly by direct spread of infection from bone

Pachymeningitis is a pattern of inflammation caused by infection centered on the dura. In the vast majority of cases it is the result of direct spread from a focus of infection in the adjacent bone, e.g. penetrating wounds with fracture of the skull, osteomyelitis of vertebra or skull, or infection in the middle ear, mastoid, or nasal sinuses.

The main causative organisms are streptococci and *Staphylococcus aureus*; Gram-negative organisms are also involved, as well as anaerobic organisms.

One of the main complications of pachymeningitis is epidural abscess. This may cause septicemia, spread to cause leptomeningitis, or act as a mass compressing nervous tissue. Another complication is subdural empyema with spread of infection in the subdural space.

Cerebritis and cerebral abscess are examples of severe focal infection of the brain

Focal inflammation of the parenchyma of the brain, termed cerebritis, frequently leads to the formation of a cerebral abscess. These patterns of inflammation develop in four main ways:

1. Secondary to meningitis and caused by the same types of organism.
2. Local extension from sepsis in the middle ear or mastoid cavities (see Fig. 21.23).
3. Hematogenous, particularly associated with bacterial endocarditis, cyanotic congenital heart disease, and pulmonary bronchiectasis.
4. Trauma following open injuries to the CNS.

Areas of brain affected by cerebritis appear as ill-defined areas of swelling which are congested and soft on cut surface, being composed of necrotic brain infiltrated by neutrophils. An abscess is a rounded cavity, typically 1–2 cm in diameter, filled with pus and walled off both by gliosis and by fibroblasts derived from tissue adjacent to blood vessels (*Fig. 21.23*). Certain brain areas are preferred sites for abscess formation, according to etiology. For example, infection of the middle ear causes abscesses in the temporal lobe or cerebellum; nasal sinus infection causes abscesses in the frontal lobes; chronic lung sepsis tends to cause abscesses in frontal lobes; and septic emboli tend to cause abscesses in parietal lobes.

Microbiology usually reveals mixed bacterial organisms in cerebral abscesses, including a high frequency of anaerobic bacteria. TB may form a localized caseous abscess termed a '**tuberculoma.**' Cerebral abscesses may also be caused by fungal infection, e.g. *Candida*, *Aspergillus* and amebas, and some cases of cerebritis and abscess are due to *Toxoplasma*, predisposed to by immunosuppression. If they are not excised or drained surgically, abscesses may rupture to cause meningitis or ventriculitis.

Encephalitis and myelitis are diffuse inflammatory processes leading to neuronal death and brain swelling

Diffuse inflammation of the brain (**encephalitis**) and cord (**myelitis**) is caused by viral, rickettsial and certain bacterial organisms (mainly *Listeria*, *Treponema*, and *Borrelia*). The main viral organisms responsible for this pattern of infection are herpes simplex, polio and rabies. Clinically, inflammation causes neurological dysfunction manifest by myelopathy (motor and sensory signs) or encephalopathy (confusion and reduced level of consciousness).

Fig. 21.23 Cerebral abscess. An abscess (**A**) containing yellow pus is seen in the temporal lobe. This was caused by spread of infection from the middle ear.

Macroscopically, there is hyperemia of the meninges, petechial hemorrhages in the brain, and brain swelling due to edema. In some types, e.g. encephalitis due to herpes simplex, there is extensive brain necrosis. The results of encephalitis or myelitis are death of neurons, cuffing of cerebral blood vessels by lymphoid cells, and astrocytic gliosis. Depending on the cause, viral cellular inclusion bodies may be seen. For example, cytoplasmic Negri bodies are seen in rabies, and nuclear viral inclusion bodies are seen in herpes encephalitis.

VIRAL DISEASES OF THE NERVOUS SYSTEM

Viral diseases of the nervous system are seen in four main patterns:

- **Viral meningitis**, characterized by the development of lymphocytic meningitis (see page 465).
- **Cytolytic**, in which there is cell destruction producing encephalitis or myelitis. This is the most clinically severe pattern of involvement and is most commonly seen with herpes simplex (*Fig. 21.24*).
- **Latent**, in which virus is integrated into the host cells, with the potential for reactivation as a cytolytic infection. This is extremely common with herpes zoster, causing shingles.
- **Persistent**, in which there is slow, smoldering degeneration of neuronal tissues caused by viral infection in the absence of elimination by immune responses, e.g. measles virus infection causing subacute sclerosing panencephalitis.

The main viral infections of the CNS are summarized in *Fig. 21.25*. Diffuse infections lead to headache, drowsiness, and coma. Systemic viral infections can also predispose to immune-mediated demyelinization or vasculitis in the nervous system.

AIDS commonly affects the nervous system

One of the most common causes of viral infection of the nervous system is HIV. Not only does HIV directly affect the brain and spinal cord, AIDS also predisposes to several complications as a result of immunosuppression. HIV appears to gain entry to the CNS via infection of macrophages. Productive infection is seen within microglia in the brain.

Lymphocytic meningitis is seen in patients around the time of seroconversion.

HIV-associated dementia (HIV-D) is a clinical syndrome that has elements of intellectual impairment, and behavioral and motor changes. Several pathologically defined changes underlie this clinical syndrome.

HIV encephalitis is a multifocal process characterized by inflammatory foci, including multinucleate giant cells, mainly seen in white matter, basal ganglia and brain stem.

HIV leukoencephalopathy is characterized by loss of myelin, gliosis, phagocytic macrophages and scattered multinucleate giant cells in white matter.

Vacuolar myelopathy is the term used to describe vacuolation in myelin sheaths, with myelin loss in the spinal cord. This leads to a spastic paraparesis and ataxia.

Cerebral vasculitis is seen most prominently in childhood HIV disease of the brain.

Painful sensory neuropathy (HIV-SN) is increasingly recognized and may be potentiated by antiviral therapy.

Cerebral atrophy with neuronal loss is seen in some patients, especially affecting frontal and temporal regions.

The immunosuppression induced by AIDS predisposes to several opportunistic infections of the CNS, particularly atypical mycobacteria, cryptococcal meningitis, cytomegalovirus (CMV), herpes zoster encephalitis, toxoplasmosis, progressive multifocal leukoencephalopathy due to papovavirus, and *Candida* and *Aspergillus* infection.

AIDS patients are at risk of developing primary cerebral lymphomas (see page 484).

Fig. 21.24 Herpes encephalitis. In herpes simplex encephalitis (a) necrosis of the temporal lobes (**T**) is a typical development. Brain biopsy is useful in diagnosis when the virus can be seen by electron microscopy (b) as rounded particles with a dense core. Virus can also be identified by immunostaining or culture. In early cases, PCR can be used to identify viral DNA in CSF samples.

Fig. 21.25 Main viral infections of the CNS

Virus	Notes
Herpes zoster	Causes shingles in peripheral nerve dermatomes from latent infection of CNS dorsal root ganglion cells. Causes a vasculitis of the CNS
Herpes simplex	(HSV)HSV-1 causes necrotizing encephalitis affecting temporal lobes (*Fig. 21.24*). HSV-2 causes meningitis and neonatal necrotizing encephalitis
HIV-1	The causative virus of AIDS causes HIV encephalitis and myelopathy of spinal cord
Poliovirus	This is a picorna enterovirus. Most infections are subclinical. May cause lymphocytic meningitis or paralytic poliomyelitis with motor neuron death
Cytomegalovirus	Causes encephalitis in immunosuppressed patients, e.g. AIDS. Also causes congenital infection of the CNS in utero, resulting in microcephaly and cerebral calcification
Rubella	Causes infection of the brain in utero and leads to microcephaly
HTLV-1	Causes tropical spastic paraparesis, a form of demyelination of the spinal cord
Rabies virus	Rhabdovirus, transmitted by animal bite, travels in peripheral nerves to CNS, causing severe meningoencephalitis with a high fatality rate. Negri bodies are viral inclusions seen in nerve cells
Measles	Causes subacute sclerosing panencephalitis in childhood, characterized by neuronal death and gliosis
JC virus	A papovavirus causing progressive multifocal leukoencephalopathy (multiple foci of demyelination in immunosuppressed patients)
Arbovirus infections	Vertebrate hosts and mosquito vectors, causing epidemic encephalitis with a high mortality (eastern and western equine encephalitis, Venezuelan encephalitis, Japanese B and Murray Valley encephalitis)

Spongiform encephalopathies are caused by an unconventional protein-only agent

Creutzfeldt–Jakob disease (CJD) is an uncommon nervous system disorder. It is characterized by the accumulation of a modified normal cell-membrane protein, termed **prion protein** (PrP). The precise way in which the protein is modified is debatable (see Ch. 8, page 128).

The disease is associated with a rapidly progressive dementia in humans, with histological vacuolation in the brain known as **spongiform encephalopathy** (*Fig. 21.26*). It is similar to kuru in humans, scrapie in sheep, and bovine spongiform encephalopathy (BSE) in cattle, which are also characterized by the accumulation of PrP. It is now recognized that this is a protein-only infective disorder, a biologically unique phenomenon.

Variant CJD has been caused by transmission to humans of the agent that causes BSE in cattle, by ingestion of contaminated meat in the diet. This disease is characterized by early psychiatric symptoms followed by sensory symptoms, cerebellar ataxia, and only late dementia. The brain shows prominent accumulation of PrP amyloid plaques (*Fig. 21.27a*). Importantly in this condition PrP also accumulates in the lymphoid tissues in affected patients, allowing diagnosis by tonsil biopsy in life (*Fig. 21.27b*).

Although most human CJD is sporadic, cases have resulted from transplantation of tissue from an affected

Fig. 21.26 Spongiform encephalopathy. This shows cerebral cortex with large areas of coarse as well as fine vacuolation, characteristic of spongiform encephalopathy. In affected areas, neuronal loss and astrocytic gliosis develop. Special techniques can be used to detect abnormal accumulations of prion protein in the brain.

person, as well as from administration of growth hormone derived from cadavers. Identical and transmissible disease can result from hereditary mutations in the gene coding for the prion protein in man (hereditary CJD and Gerstmann–Straussler syndrome, causing familial cases of ataxia and dementia).

Fig. 21.27 Variant CJD. (a) An amyloid plaque composed of PrP in the brain from a patient with new variant CJD. (b) Tonsillar tissue stained with an antibody that detects PrP. This has accumulated in the follicle center in the lymphoid tissue. Similar PrP accumulates in other lymphoid sites such as spleen, nodes and appendix. This does not happen in sporadic CJD.

FUNGAL INFECTIONS OF THE CNS

Fungal infection of the nervous system is usually seen in patients who are immunosuppressed

Infection of the nervous system by fungi is frequently seen in patients who are immunosuppressed (most commonly following organ transplantation or anticancer chemotherapy, or with HIV infection and AIDS).

Candidiasis causes multiple small cerebral abscesses in the CNS, usually secondary to septicemia caused by primary *Candida* infection elsewhere. *Aspergillus* is another organism that affects the brain by hematogenous spread, usually from primary lung involvement, leading to formation of fungal abscesses.

Phycomycoses (mucormycosis, zygomycosis) infect the brain by local spread from primary infection of the paranasal sinuses. Fungi typically invade along vessels, causing vascular thrombosis and cerebral infarction.

Cryptococcosis is due to a yeast-like organism that most commonly causes a fungal meningitis in immunosuppressed

patients, but may also affect patients with normal immune function (see page 123 and *Fig. 8.25*).

PARASITIC INFECTION OF THE NERVOUS SYSTEM

Parasitic infection of the nervous system by protozoa and metazoa is increasing in western countries

Infection of the nervous system by protozoa was formerly uncommon in western countries, but is being increasingly seen because of international travel and the increased risk of infection in patients with immunosuppression.

Toxoplasma can cause a congenital infection resulting in hydrocephalus and cerebral calcifications. It is also now frequently seen in patients with AIDS, causing cerebritis and brain abscesses (see page 133 and *Fig. 8.40*).

Worldwide, **malaria** is the most common protozoan disease to involve the brain (particularly infection with *Plasmodium falciparum*), causing vascular thromboses with petechial hemorrhages (cerebral malaria) (see pages 129–31). In acute disease **trypanosomiasis** may be associated with an encephalomyelitis.

Entamoeba histolytica can cause an amebic abscess by spread from the gut, whereas meningitis is caused by free-living amebas such as *Naegleria*, usually acquired by swimming in contaminated pools in warm climates.

The two main metazoan parasites to infect the brain are *Echinococcus granulosus* (causing hydatid disease) and the larval form of the pork tapeworm, *Taenia solium* (causing cysticercosis) (see page 136).

TUBERCULOSIS OF THE BRAIN

Infection of the nervous system with TB may cause meningitis or abscess

Infection of the CNS by *Mycobacterium tuberculosis* is by bloodborne spread from a site of primary infection, most commonly the lung. There are two main types of infection.

Meningitis is characterized by numerous granulomas in the leptomeninges, with features of a chronic meningitis (see pages 465–6). Infection is most marked around the base of the brain, and even when infection is treated there is often the development of meningeal fibrosis to cause hydrocephalus.

Tuberculous abscess (tuberculoma) forms with infection of the brain parenchyma. A tuberculoma is typically a firm, lobulated mass of granulomatous inflammation with central caseous necrosis, up to several centimeters in diameter, and walled off by fibrous tissue. Lesions occur within the cerebral hemispheres, but are most common in the cerebellum. Treatment with antibiotics is usually ineffective and surgical excision is required.

DEMYELINATING DISEASES

The demyelinating disorders are diseases in which the main abnormality is damage to CNS myelin. Myelin loss is seen in many disease processes after axonal loss, but this type of secondary myelin loss is not considered as part of the group of demyelinating diseases. The most important condition causing demyelination is **multiple sclerosis**.

Multiple sclerosis is an immune-mediated disease of uncertain cause

Multiple sclerosis (MS) is a disease in which there are relapsing episodes of immunologically mediated demyelination in the CNS. Loss of myelin leads to failure of axonal function and neurological dysfunction.

The lesions of MS are confined to the brain and spinal cord. Areas of demyelination are termed plaques, best seen at the angles of the lateral ventricles, in the cerebellar peduncles, in the optic nerves and in the brain stem, although they can occur at any site in the CNS, including the spinal cord.

Areas of active recent demyelination appear as salmon-pink granular patches of softening in white matter. Histologically, there is myelin loss associated with lymphocytic cuffing of small vessels. Macrophages enter the lesion and phagocytose damaged myelin, accumulating lipid and forming foam cells. Astrocytes around plaque margins become enlarged. Remyelination may then take place in plaques, which may then be subject to further episodes of demyelination.

Areas of complete myelin loss appear as sharply demarcated patches of firm, gelatinous, grayish-pink discoloration (*Fig. 21.28*). These inactive plaques, sometimes called burnt-out plaques, show loss of myelin, very few inflammatory cells, and are largely occupied by astrocytes.

Although the axons that span a plaque are mostly preserved, there is clear evidence of loss of axons from plaque areas, and this feature of MS may be related to clinically progressing disability.

There is great variation in outcome. Some patients have a relatively benign form of disease, experiencing only minor disability and few episodes of demyelination. Others have frequent repeated episodes of myelin loss, progressing such that in the late stages of disease they are rendered blind, paraplegic and incontinent, with cognitive dysfunction caused by loss of hemispheric white matter (progressive relapsing–remitting MS). The least common form is characterized by unremitting rapid progression from onset (primary progressive MS).

Etiology and pathogenesis of multiple sclerosis

MS has a peak incidence between the ages of 20 and 40 years, with a slight female preponderance. Many theories have been advanced to explain the disease, but the etiology of the condition is uncertain.

Although viral infection has been postulated, none has been consistently detected or directly implicated in disease. Immunological mechanisms are central to disease pathogenesis, and an active immunological response is present in areas of demyelination. The cause of the immune response remains uncertain. An association with certain HLA antigens (HLA-DR2) has also been demonstrated. It is likely that the disease is the result of a genetic susceptibility, predisposing to the mounting of an inappropriate immune response to viral infections.

In the region of active plaques, microglial cells show enhanced expression of class II major histocompatibility antigens, suggestive of immune activation. Lesions are infiltrated by T cells, B cells and macrophages, again emphasizing immune activation. Trials with cytokine agents that modulate the immune response are under evaluation.

Fig. 21.28 Multiple sclerosis. A large plaque (**P**) is seen adjacent to the lateral ventricle (**V**). Histologically, areas of myelin loss are revealed on myelin stains.

The diagnosis of MS is based on clinical evaluation and the exclusion of other causes of focal neurological disease. Several diagnostic procedures are particularly helpful.

Electrophysiology shows increased time for conduction in CNS tracts, measured by showing increased latency for visual and auditory evoked responses.

Magnetic resonance imaging can show even small areas of demyelination within the brain and spinal cord, particularly if gadolinium enhancement is used.

CSF examination usually shows a mild increase in lymphoid cells, and a mild increase in protein with a normal glucose level. Activation of the immune system in the CNS can be identified by demonstrating oligoclonal bands of immunoglobulin in the CSF by electrophoresis.

Myelin loss is seen in several diseases as a secondary process

Demyelination is a prominent component of several diseases.

Leukodystrophies are inborn errors of metabolism in which there is abnormal formation or metabolism of myelin, sometimes termed **dysmyelination**. The main types are metachromatic leukodystrophy due to aryl sulfatase A deficiency, and adrenoleukodystrophy caused by metabolic defects in peroxisomal metabolism of long-chain fatty acids.

Binswanger's disease is caused by ischemic damage to myelin as a result of widespread cerebral arteriolosclerosis. There is loss of myelin from the cerebral hemispheres, leading to cognitive decline.

Progressive multifocal leukoencephalopathy is caused by infection with papovavirus, usually seen in patients who are immunosuppressed (see page 125).

NEURODEGENERATIVE DISEASES

The neurodegenerative diseases are common disorders in which there is degeneration of specific groups of neurons or brain areas, causing characteristic clinical syndromes. The incidence of these diseases rises with age, particularly after the age of 65 years, and many are increasingly being recognized as familial. The main clinical syndromes caused by neurodegenerative disease are dementia syndromes with

Fig. 21.29 Motor neuron disease. The crossed (**C**) and uncrossed (**U**) corticospinal tracts in the cervical spinal cord show pallor due to loss of axons (Luxol fast blue/cresyl violet).

cognitive decline, movement disorders (particularly defects of cerebellar and extrapyramidal systems), motor weakness, and autonomic failure.

An increasingly accepted concept in the majority of these diseases is that they are the result of abnormal accumulation of protein within neurons, glial cells, or both. Different diseases are characterized by the accumulation of distinct proteins. Protein accumulation may then form histologically recognizable inclusions bodies. This has given rise to the idea that the neurodegenerative diseases are 'proteinopathies.' In rare diseases mutation in the gene coding for a protein leads to its accumulation. In most instances disease is regarded as sporadic.

Motor neuron disease (amyotrophic lateral sclerosis) causes paralysis due to death of motor neurons

Motor neuron disease is mainly seen in old age, a small number of patients presenting in middle age. Disease typically begins as mild weakness in one limb. There is then progression to severe paralysis, with loss of swallowing and respiration leading to death in 2–3 years. The cause of the disease is unknown. Different subtypes relate to the loss of different groups of motor neurons:

- **Amyotrophic lateral sclerosis** is the most common pattern, showing loss of both cortical motor neurons and lower motor neurons in the spinal cord and brain stem.
- **Progressive bulbar palsy** is common and shows loss of brain stem motor neurons.
- **Progressive muscular atrophy** is uncommon and shows loss restricted to spinal lower motor neurons.
- **Primary lateral sclerosis** is rare and shows loss of neurons restricted to the motor cortex.

There is loss of motor neurons from cortex, brain stem and spinal cord, and gliosis with secondary degeneration of motor tracts (*Fig. 21.29*). Inclusion bodies containing the proteins TDP-43 and ubiquitin are found in surviving neurons.

Parkinson's disease results from loss of neurons from the substantia nigra

Parkinson's disease is a movement disorder that mainly affects patients over the age of 45 years. It is characterized clinically by disturbance of movement, with rigidity, slowness of voluntary movement (bradykinesis), and rest tremor. Severity of disease is related to loss of the neuromelanin-containing nerve cells from the substantia nigra in the midbrain; these cells normally produce dopamine, their loss reducing the amount of dopamine in the basal ganglia.

Macroscopically, there is loss of pigment from the substantia nigra, which is the result of death of the melanin-containing dopaminergic cells (*Fig. 21.30*). The surviving cells in the substantia nigra contain spherical inclusions termed **Lewy bodies** (*Fig. 21.31*), which contain the protein alpha synuclein.

Rare cases of Parkinson's disease are familial. The cause of sporadic disease is related to abnormal aggregation of α-synuclein in the brain, defective elimination of aggregated protein, and impairment of mitochondrial function. The natural history of the disease is for patients to develop failure of response to treatment, with death eventually occurring from wasting and poor nutritional intake. A significant proportion of patients develop dementia (Parkinson's disease dementia).

Molecular genetics of Huntington's disease

The gene for Huntington's disease is located on chromosome 4. The cause of the disease is an abnormally long, tandemly repeated trinucleotide (CAG). In normal individuals this gene has between 9 and 34 repeats, whereas in Huntington's disease patients have around 70 repeats. The protein produced by the gene, which has been named **huntingtin**, is expressed in many tissues but has no homology with other proteins; its function is currently unknown. Protein accumulates inside neuronal nuclei, forming inclusions as well as accumulating inside some nerve cell processes.

The age of onset of disease is related to the length of the repeat sequence: patients with large repeat sequences have early onset. With passage of the gene through generations, the repeat sequence increases in length, resulting in progressively earlier ages at presentation, a phenomenon termed **anticipation**.

Now that the gene has been identified, confident genetic testing for the disease is possible, with all its attendant ethical and social implications.

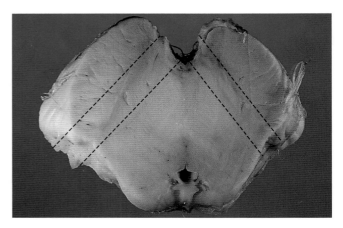

Fig. 21.30 Parkinson's disease. In this section through the midbrain, pigmented neurons have been lost from the substantia nigra (between lines), which is abnormally pale.

Fig. 21.31 Lewy body in Parkinson's disease. Lewy bodies (**L**) are spherical inclusions seen in the melanin-containing neurons in Parkinson's disease. Typically they have a hyaline core and a pale halo. They are based on aggregated neurofilaments and α–synuclein.

Fig. 21.32 Huntington's disease. This shows slices from two brains. On the right is a normal brain with normal caudate (**C**); on the left the brain from a patient with Huntington's disease shows severe atrophy of the caudate (**A**).

Huntington's disease is an autosomal dominant disease causing chorea and dementia

Huntington's disease is a neurodegenerative disease that causes choreiform movements and dementia, with onset in middle life. The disease is an autosomal dominant disorder with a prevalence of approximately 1 in 20 000; the gene has been characterized at its location in the short arm of chromosome 4 (see pink box).

Macroscopically the brain shows atrophy of the caudate and putamen due to cell loss and gliosis (*Fig. 21.32*), and more subtle loss of neurons from the cerebral cortex.

The natural history of this disease is for affected individuals to develop progressive cognitive decline, with an increase in severity of the movement disorder. Patients die as a result of their severe mental and physical incapacity.

Alzheimer's disease is the most common cause of dementia

Alzheimer's disease is the most common neurodegenerative disease and the most common cause of dementia. Clinically, patients develop progressive failure of memory, degeneration of temporal and parietal association cortex (causing dyspraxia and dysphasia) and, frequently, disturbances in emotion. With progression of disease over many years patients become immobile and emaciated, death commonly being due to the development of a pneumonia.

The cause of the disease is unknown, but there are well-defined genetic predispositions (see pink box on page 474).

The brain in Alzheimer's disease is smaller than normal and its weight is reduced, evident as shrinkage of gyri and widening of sulci of the cerebral hemispheres (*Fig. 21.33*).

Atrophy is most evident in the temporal lobe, particularly the parahippocampal gyrus, but also in the frontal and parietal regions. The occipital lobe and the motor cortex are generally spared.

Histologically, there are several main abnormalities seen in Alzheimer's disease. **Amyloid**, composed of Aβ-peptide, is deposited in the cerebral cortex as spherical deposits termed **senile plaques** (*Fig. 21.34a*). Intraneuronal inclusions comprising bundles of abnormal filaments termed **neurofibrillary tangles** develop in cortical neurons (*Fig. 21.34b*). Tangles are frequently flame-shaped and occupy much of the space within the neuronal cytoplasm, being largely composed of a microtubule-binding protein called Tau protein. Cortical nerve-cell processes become twisted and dilated (**neuropil threads**) owing to the accumulation of the same filaments that form the tangles. The

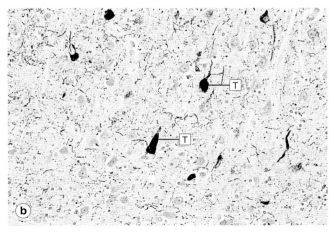

Fig. 21.34 Alzheimer's disease. (a) Plaques (immunochemistry – Aβ protein). (b) Tangles and neuropil threads (immunochemistry – Tau protein). Immunohistochemical staining shows accumulations of abnormal proteins in Alzheimer's disease. Amyloid plaques composed of Aβ peptide are seen scattered in the cortex (a). In (b) tangles (**T**) composed of Tau protein can be seen as flame-shaped structures in neurons. The fine brown linear staining is nerve-cell processes filled with Tau protein, termed neuropil threads.

Fig. 21.33 Alzheimer's disease. This shows slices from two brains. On the left is a normal brain from a 70-year-old; on the right is the same region from a 70-year-old with Alzheimer's disease. The diseased brain is atrophic with loss of cortex and white matter, most marked in the hippocampal region (**H**).

pathological diagnosis of Alzheimer's disease is based on the presence of lesions in high density in a patient with clinical dementia.

Neurochemical analysis of brains from patients with Alzheimer's disease has shown widespread neurotransmitter defects, particularly loss of acetylcholine from the cortex. Treatment protocols that supplement cholinergic transmission have shown promising results in trials.

Dementia may be associated with Parkinsonism or frontal lobe degeneration

Dementia with Lewy bodies is the second most common cause of dementia and has clinical features that overlap with those of Alzheimer's disease and Parkinson's disease. Patients have a cortical dementia resembling Alzheimer's disease, but also have mild features of rigidity and bradykinesia (slowness). Lewy bodies, the neuronal inclusions characteristic of Parkinson's disease, are seen in both the substantia nigra and the cerebral cortex.

Frontotemporal dementias account for about 10% of all cases of dementia and are characterized by the develop-

ment of impaired frontal lobe function, with memory impairment combined with a syndrome of disinhibition and mutism. Macroscopically, there is atrophy of the frontal and temporal lobes of the brain, and histological examination reveals neuronal loss, with some subtypes having neuronal inclusions. The importance of frontal patterns of dementia is that many cases are late-onset autosomal dominant conditions. In some families mutation in the Tau protein gene or the progranulin gene is responsible.

Neuronal system atrophies are neurodegenerative diseases affecting several neuronal groups

A number of uncommon neurodegenerative diseases show loss of neurons from several nuclei in the brain, brain stem, cerebellum and spinal cord, and are named according to the pattern of involvement. There are large numbers of such syndromes, each having different genetic and pathological causes. Clinically, patients have symptoms and signs that relate to the neuronal groups involved, including rigidity, chorea, cognitive decline and weakness.

Molecular pathogenesis of Alzheimer's disease

It is possible to divide cases of Alzheimer's disease into four main clinical groups, some of which are beginning to be associated with molecular genetic abnormalities that have been linked to genes on chromosomes 21, 19, 1 and 14:

- Sporadic late onset (most common).
- Familial late onset (uncommon).
- Familial early onset (rare).
- Associated with Down's syndrome.

Molecular analysis of the amyloid of Alzheimer's disease shows that it is derived from a normal cell-membrane protein of unknown function, coded on chromosome 21 and termed **Alzheimer precursor protein** or **APP**. Mutations in the gene coding for this protein explain some very rare cases of early-onset familial disease, as well as three copies of the gene explaining the association of Alzheimer's disease with Down's syndrome (trisomy 21). The protein found in the plaque amyloid is a fragment of APP, referred to as Aβ protein. The reason why there is abnormal accumulation of Aβ protein to form amyloid in plaques in sporadic Alzheimer's disease remains unknown.

The presence of apolipoprotein apoE4, a normal form of apolipoprotein, is believed to account for the linkage

of Alzheimer's disease to chromosome 19. Individuals homozygous for the gene coding for the ApoE4 variant are predisposed to the development of sporadic late-onset disease. However, this is believed to be a susceptibility gene, leading to increased susceptibility for the development of disease rather than a direct pathological mechanism. It is not inevitable that all those homozygous for the gene coding for the ApoE4 variant will develop AD.

The gene responsible for linkage to chromosome 14 is termed presenilin-1, and mutations in it account for the majority of cases of early-onset familial Alzheimer's disease. A homologous protein termed presenilin-2 is coded for by a gene on chromosome 1, mutations in this gene also causing some cases of familial early-onset Alzheimer's disease. The presenilin proteins are involved in the metabolism of APP as well as intracellular calcium handling.

Molecular investigation of the microtubule-binding protein Tau found in tangles has not yet revealed why they form, nor the link with Aβ protein deposition in plaques.

There is active search for a biomarker for use in diagnosis. So far a simple 'test' for AD is not available.

Fig. 21.35 Cerebellar atrophy. There is marked atrophy in the vermis of the cerebellum.

Fig. 21.36 Wernicke's encephalopathy. In this coronal section of brain the mammillary bodies (arrows) show petechial hemorrhages characteristic of acute Wernicke's encephalopathy caused by thiamine deficiency.

Among the main types of multisystem atrophy are **spinocerebellar degenerations**, a group of familial diseases with several inheritance patterns, which are characterized by loss of cerebellar cortical neurons and degeneration of spinal cord tracts. The best known of these is **Friedreich's ataxia**, a spastic cerebellar ataxia with degeneration of posterior columns and corticospinal and spinocerebellar tracts which is an example of a triplet-repeat expansion genetic disorder caused by GAA triplet repeat expansions of between 200 and 900 copies in the first intron of the frataxin gene.

Cerebellar cortical atrophies are diseases in which the main abnormality is loss of Purkinje cells from the cerebellar cortex, with lesser involvement of other neuronal groups. Patients present with cerebellar ataxia, usually in the third decade. Many cases are familial, with defined gene mutations (*Fig. 21.35*).

In **multiple system atrophy** patients have prominent cerebellar ataxia, extrapyramidal rigidity and bulbar paresis, caused by loss of neurons from the cerebellar cortex, substantia nigra and pons, respectively. Characteristic inclusions containing α-synuclein are seen in glial cells.

METABOLIC AND TOXIC DISEASE

Metabolic and toxic disorders of the nervous system are common

Several major diseases of the CNS have a metabolic or toxic causation, a reflection of the vulnerability of the nervous system to injury.

Several **vitamin deficiency states** are associated with damage to the nervous system. Vitamin B_1 (thiamine) deficiency causes **Wernicke's encephalopathy** (*Fig. 21.36*). Vitamin B_{12} deficiency is commonly associated with **pernicious anemia** (see pages 106 and 252). In the nervous system this causes degeneration of the lateral and posterior columns of the spinal cord, termed subacute combined degeneration of the cord, leading to paresthesias, ataxia, and sensory abnormalities.

Hepatic encephalopathy is a clinical state that arises in patients with severe liver failure. Patients develop impaired consciousness, which may progress to coma. Disease is thought to be due to the presence of excitatory transmitter substances in the blood, which have not been detoxified by the liver, e.g. GABA.

Carbon monoxide poisoning is commonly seen, either as an accident (usually involving faulty heating equipment) or as a result of attempted suicide. In patients who survive the acute poisoning and are resuscitated, delayed damage to the brain may occur, signs usually becoming apparent 24–36 hours after exposure. There is necrosis of the globus pallidus, demyelination of the hemispheric white matter and, frequently, diffuse cortical laminar necrosis (see page 459).

The brain and peripheral nerves are frequently damaged in alcoholism

Acute alcohol intoxication causes neuronal depression and may lead to death through respiratory depression.

Chronic alcoholism is associated with several diseases of both the central and the peripheral nervous system. It has been difficult to determine whether this is due to direct toxicity or whether it is caused by the nutritional and vitamin deficiencies commonly seen in patients dependent on alcohol.

The brains of alcoholic patients show generalized **cerebral cortical atrophy**, which sometimes causes cognitive decline. Cerebellar ataxia in patients with alcoholism is usually caused by **cerebellar degeneration** associated with severe atrophy of the cerebellar cortex.

Wernicke's encephalopathy is caused by thiamine deficiency, commonly seen in patients dependent on alcohol. It presents clinically as a triad of confusion, ataxia, and abnormal eye movements with ophthalmoplegia. Pathologically, there are petechial hemorrhages from small vessels in the mammillary bodies (see *Fig. 21.36*), which are associated with necrosis and loss of neurons, leading to eventual shrinkage and gliosis. Acute Wernicke's encephalopathy may prove fatal unless B-complex vitamins (including thiamine) are administered. Damage to the limbic system from repeated episodes of Wernicke's encephalopathy causes a permanent impairment of recent memory, termed **Korsakoff's psychosis**.

Exposure of the fetus to alcohol, when the mother is dependent, leads to growth retardation and cerebral malformations (fetal alcohol syndrome).

DEVELOPMENTAL ABNORMALITIES

Developmental abnormalities of the CNS are common, affecting 1% of newborns. They can be divided into two main groups: primary developmental abnormalities, which are the direct result of a genetic abnormality, and secondary developmental abnormalities, which are due to disruption of development by an intrauterine disease process such as infection or ischemia, or toxic factors.

Most malformations of the nervous system have no ascertainable cause

Establishing the cause of a developmental abnormality of the nervous system is important from the perspective of reproductive counseling for parents. Unfortunately, 60% of developmental abnormalities of the nervous system have no identifiable causative factor. Of the remainder, 20% are mixed environmental and genetic, 5% are due to single gene defects, 5% are due to chromosomal abnormalities, and 10% are due to exogenous factors such as infection, toxins, or poor nutrition. *Fig. 21.37* lists the main causative factors and associated malformations.

Neural-tube defects are the commonest form of CNS developmental abnormality

Defects in the closure of the neural tube are the most common cause of congenital malformation of the nervous system. Such defects may affect either the cranial or the spinal closure of the neural tube, and may be an open defect or one closed by meninges and skin.

The most severe and common form of cranial neural-tube defect is **anencephaly**. The cranial vault is generally not formed, although the face and eyes are usually well developed. The brain is replaced by a disc of abnormally developed neural tissue. A less severe cranial neural-

Fig. 21.37 Causes of developmental abnormalities of the brain

Chromosomal abnormalities	
Down's syndrome (trisomy 21)	Abnormal gyral formation and defective arborization of neuronal processes
Trisomy 13–15 (Patau's syndrome)	Forebrain abnormalities with midline facial clefts
Trisomy 17–18 (Edwards' syndrome)	Gyral maldevelopment
Single gene abnormalities	
Autosomal recessive gene	Meckel syndrome (encephalocele)
	Roberts' syndrome (encephalocele)
Multifactorial	
Genetic and environmental	Anencephaly, meningocele, encephalocele
Infections	
Rubella	Microcephaly, focal necrosis of brain areas
Cytomegalovirus	Necrosis and developmental failure
Toxoplasmosis	Necrosis and developmental failure
Teratogens	
Thalidomide	Anencephaly and meningomyelocele
Aminopterin	Anencephaly and encephalocele

tube defect is the development of an **encephalocele**, in which a defect in the bone of the skull is associated with cystic outpouching of meninges, which may contain brain.

Neural-tube defects of the spinal cord are most common in the lumbar region. The severity of the defect is variable (*Fig. 21.38*). The main defects include:

- **Spina bifida occulta.** Abnormal development of the bony arch of the spinal column. Meninges and cord normal. There may be an associated sinus track to the skin surface, or subcutaneous lipoma.
- **Meningocele.** Abnormal development of the bony arch of the spinal cord, with cystic outpouching of meninges covered by skin. Spinal cord may be normally or abnormally formed.
- **Meningomyelocele.** Abnormal development of the bony arch of the spinal cord, with cystic outpouching of meninges, including nerve roots and incorporating abnormally developed spinal cord.
- **Myelocele.** Abnormal development of the bony arch of the spinal cord, with exposure of abnormally developed spinal cord.

The neurological deficit associated with spinal neural-tube defects is related to the degree of severity of abnormality of the spinal cord and nerve roots. Other developmental abnormalities may be present, particularly hydrocephalus caused by Arnold–Chiari malformation (see pages 464 and 478).

A major complication is recurrent urinary tract infection leading to chronic pyelonephritis and renal failure. Diagnosis can be made in utero by ultrasound scanning or by detecting raised levels of α-fetoprotein (AFP) in serum or amniotic fluid.

Less common abnormalities of the CNS are summarized in *Fig. 21.39*.

Fig. 21.38 Spinal neural tube defects. (a) Normal. (b) Spina bifida occulta. (c) Meningocele. (d) Meningomyelocele. (e) Meningocele in a newborn child.

Fig. 21.39 Developmental abnormalities of the CNS

Agyria and pachygyria	Brain is smooth or has few gyri due to failure of migration of neuroblasts into developing brain
Heterotopia	Ectopic foci of gray matter due to premature arrest of migrating neuroblasts in developing brain
Holoprosencephaly	Single large ventricle with non-division of forebrain
Porencephaly and schizencephaly	Cystic cavities in the brain with gliosis following infarction caused by intrauterine vascular occlusion
Ulegyria	Gliotic shrunken gyri caused by hypoxic necrosis
Microcephaly	Small brain with many causative factors

Arnold–Chiari malformation type II is the second commonest form of CNS developmental abnormality

In Arnold–Chiari type II malformations there is herniation of the brain stem and the lower part of the cerebellum into the foramen magnum, blocking drainage of CSF and causing hydrocephalus. This abnormality is nearly always associated with development of a lumbar meningomyelocele.

Hypoxia is a major cause of perinatal brain damage

The neonatal brain is vulnerable to a wide variety of injurious agents, the most important being hypoxia associated with the trauma of birth. The two main abnormalities found are hemorrhage and necrosis.

Perinatal hypoxia is a major cause of neurological damage in the newborn, with an incidence of about 3 per 1000 live term births. Although many die, around one-third develop cerebral palsy, epilepsy or mental retardation.

Hypoxic ischemic encephalopathy is the term applied to brain damage caused by neonatal asphyxia. The main lesions encountered are hemorrhages into the brain and ventricles from the germinal matrix adjacent to the lateral ventricles; necrosis of brain leading to cystic gliosis (ulegyria, porencephaly, hydranencephaly); and necrosis of white matter in cerebral hemispheres (periventricular leukomalacia).

Birth trauma may cause tearing of dural veins, leading to subdural hematoma.

INBORN ERRORS OF METABOLISM

The nervous system is involved in several inborn errors of metabolism, either primarily or as a consequence of systematized disease. The main disorders in this group are those of myelin formation, termed **leukodystrophies**, and **storage disorders** (see Chapter 25) due to lack of normal enzyme activity causing accumulation of a metabolic product in nerve cells.

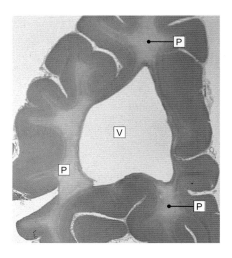

Fig. 21.40 Leukodystrophy. In this section from the frontal lobe of a child with leukodystrophy there is massive loss of myelin from the white matter, leaving it palely stained (**P**). The lateral ventricle (**V**) is dilated as a compensation for loss of tissue.

Leukodystrophies are genetically determined defects in myelin metabolism

Leukodystrophies generally present in childhood as cognitive or motor decline, but can also be seen, albeit less commonly, in adult life. They are caused by genetically determined metabolic abnormalities in the formation or metabolism of myelin. Macroscopically, brains are small and there is loss of myelin with gliosis (*Fig. 21.40*). The main types of leukodystrophy are:

- **Adrenoleukodystrophy.** X-linked recessive disease caused by deficiency of peroxisomal enzymes involved in oxidation of long-chain fatty acids.
- **Metachromatic leukodystrophy.** Autosomal recessive disease caused by lack of activity of aryl sulfatase A.
- **Krabbe's disease (globoid-cell leukodystrophy).** Autosomal recessive disease caused by galactocerebroside β-galactosidase deficiency.

The diagnosis of these metabolic defects in myelin formation is made by assay of enzymes detectable in blood leukocytes or cultured fibroblasts.

Neurometabolic storage disorders are genetic diseases causing accumulation of abnormal material in the brain

Several of the inborn errors of metabolism (see Chapter 25) are characterized by storage of abnormal material in the nervous system. The majority of diseases are associated with mutations in defined genes and most commonly arise in childhood. Among the main types are:

- **Gangliosidoses** are autosomal recessive disorders causing neuronal storage of gangliosides, e.g. Tay–Sachs disease.
- **Mucopolysaccharidoses** cause abnormal storage of mucopolysaccharides in brain and other tissues, the main types being Hurler's syndrome (gargoylism) and Hunter's syndrome.
- **Gaucher's disease** is caused by deficiency of β-glucocerebrosidase, resulting in the accumulation of glucocerebroside in brain and macrophages in other organs (see page 576 and *Fig. 25.23*).
- **Ceroid lipofuscinoses** are disorders in which there is neuronal storage of lipofuscin-like lipids. The main type is Batten's disease.
- **Niemann–Pick disease** is caused by deficient sphingomyelinase activity, only some varieties having neurological involvement.

Diagnosis of neurometabolic storage diseases is made by showing the abnormal enzyme activity in tissues or, increasingly, by identification of a mutation in a defined gene. Type OMIM into a search engine on the internet and you can look up specific gene defects in the Online Mendelian Inheritance in Man database.

Wilson's disease is an autosomal recessive disorder of copper metabolism

Wilson's disease is an autosomal recessive disorder in which there is excessive accumulation of copper in the brain, liver and kidneys. Neurological disease usually presents in adolescence with psychiatric disease (onset of psychosis), movement disorder (spasticity, rigidity, dysarthria, painful muscle spasms) or odd eye movements.

Advanced cases of neurological disease are now uncommon because of effective treatment. In severe cases there is shrinkage of the basal ganglia, with loss of nerve cells and gliosis. The gene, which is located on chromosome 13, codes for a copper transport ATPase.

PHAKOMATOSES

The phakomatoses are familial disorders in which there are developmental abnormalities associated with hamartomatous or neoplastic growths. The main types of disease are neurofibromatosis 1 (NF1), neurofibromatosis 2 (NF2), tuberous sclerosis, and von Hippel–Lindau syndrome.

NF1 is an autosomal dominant disease that causes tumors of peripheral nerves

NF1, formerly called 'von Recklinghausen's syndrome,' is an autosomal dominant disorder that affects 1 in 3000 individuals. The main clinical features are the development of benign tumors of peripheral nerves, termed **neurofibromas** (see page 487), and the presence of pigmented skin lesions called **café au lait spots**. Less prominent are hamartomas of the iris, optic-nerve gliomas, and bone abnormalities. Patients characteristically develop multiple polypoid skin nodules, which can vary from 1 mm to 5 cm in diameter. There is a risk of developing malignant nerve tumors (**neurofibrosarcomas**). The gene defect in NF1 is located on chromosome 17 and codes for neurofibromin, which acts as a tumor suppressor and is present at high concentrations in nervous tissues

NF2 is an autosomal dominant disease that causes tumors on acoustic nerves

NF2 is an autosomal dominant disorder affecting 1 in 25 000 individuals. The clinical features are the development of bilateral benign tumors (also termed **schwannomas**) of the eighth cranial nerve, which are also known as **acoustic neuromas**, hence the alternative name of bilateral acoustic neurofibromatosis (BANF). There is also a tendency to develop other brain tumors, meningiomas and gliomas. Patients present with tinnitus, deafness, or signs of a mass lesion compressing the brain stem. The gene defect for NF2 is located on chromosome 22 and codes for the protein merlin (also called schwannomin).

Tuberous sclerosis is an autosomal dominant disease causing epilepsy and mental retardation associated with hamartomas of the brain

Tuberous sclerosis is an autosomal dominant condition affecting 1 in 100 000 individuals. This is a multisystem disorder that can feature a wide range of manifestations, including epilepsy, mental retardation, skin lesions called angiofibromas, and retinal hamartomas. A minority of patients develop cardiac tumors termed **benign rhabdomyomas**, as well as renal tumors (**angiomyolipomas**). *Formes frustes* of tuberous sclerosis are common in which a full clinical phenotype does not develop.

The brain shows characteristic lesions termed tubers (after which the syndrome is named), which appear as firm, white nodules, 1–3 cm in size, at the crest of gyri. The tubers are hamartomatous overgrowths of neurons and astrocytes. A characteristic feature is thickening of the tissues beneath the ventricular linings of the brain, which has been likened to 'drips of candle wax.' Some patients can develop an unusual brain tumor termed subependymal giant cell astrocytoma (SEGA). There is more than one genetic cause for this phenotype. One gene on chromosome 9 (TSC1) codes for a protein termed hamartin. Another gene for tuberous sclerosis (TSC2) is located on chromosome 16 and codes for a protein termed tuberin. The gene products hamartin and tuberin form a dimer which normally inhibits signaling in a kinase pathway.

von Hippel–Lindau disease causes multiple benign hemangioblastomas and predisposes to renal carcinoma

von Hippel–Lindau disease (VHL) is a familial disorder in which affected individuals are genetically predisposed to develop multiple benign tumors of the brain and spinal cord, termed hemangioblastomas. Hemangioblastomas are well-circumscribed tumors that most commonly develop in the cerebellum, but also in the brain stem and spinal cord. These lesions may secrete erythropoietin and cause polycythemia. Angiomas of the retina may also be present, and there is a predisposition to the development of carcinoma of the kidney and pheochromocytoma of the adrenal.

The VHL tumor-suppressor gene is located on chromosome 3. Mutations and deletions in the gene have been detected in patients with von Hippel–Lindau disease, as well as in some sporadic renal-cell carcinomas. Patients with this diagnosis require intense follow-up for multiple and recurrent tumors.

The VHL gene product, pVHL, is involved in the control of angiogenesis, and has a role in degrading the transcription factor HIF (hypoxia-inducible factor) in the presence of oxygen. Failure to degrade HIF appears to contribute to tumor development.

TUMORS OF THE NERVOUS SYSTEM

Primary neoplasms of the CNS are important as they commonly affect young patients; in incidence they are second only to the leukemias, accounting for about 10% of cancer deaths in those aged between 15 and 35 years. Overall, they account for only about 2% of all deaths from cancer and, in general, are uncommon. Tumors are derived from the various tissues that make up the CNS:

- **Metastases.** Overall, the most common cause of a neoplasm affecting the brain.
- **Meningeal.** Tumors derived from epithelial cells of the meninges, termed 'meningiomas.'
- **Neuroepithelial.** Tumors loosely termed 'gliomas', which are derived from astrocytes, oligodendrocytes, ependyma, neurons or primitive embryonal cells.
- **Non-neuroepithelial.** Tumors including cerebral lymphomas, germ-cell tumors, cysts and tumors extending from local growth in the skull and pituitary.

METASTASES TO CNS

Metastatic tumors are commonly seen in the brain and vertebral column

Metastases to the CNS are very common: outside specialist clinical neuroscience units they are encountered more often than primary brain tumors.

As well as focal neurological signs, metastases to brain cause signs of raised intracranial pressure. The main primary sites of metastatic tumor to brain are lung, breast and skin (melanoma). Macroscopically, metastases are often multiple and commonly begin as lesions at the junction of the cortex and white matter. Cerebral edema is often extensive around metastases, accounting for the main problem of raised intracranial pressure.

Metastatic tumor commonly affects the spinal cord as extradural deposits, causing compression. The most common are metastases from carcinomas of the prostate, kidney, breast and lung, together with lymphoma and myeloma.

TUMORS OF MENINGEAL ORIGIN

Meningiomas are benign tumors derived from epithelial cells of the meninges

Meningiomas are tumors derived from meningothelial cells, the epithelial cells of the meninges. They are common intracranial tumors, and have a female preponderance.

Meningiomas are typically rounded lesions that arise from the dura and grow slowly to compress the underlying brain (*Fig. 21.41*). Most are fleshy and rubbery in consistency, but a minority are tough and fibrous. Tumors can vary in diameter from 1 or 2 cm up to 7 cm. Although most lesions are solitary, they may be multiple. Infiltration of the skull by tumor may occur, causing local bony thickening. Meningiomas typically present with either focal neurological signs or with features of raised intracranial pressure.

Tumors arise anywhere in the meninges, the most frequent sites being next to the falx, over the cerebral convexities, or over the sphenoid wings. Less commonly, meningiomas arise from the spinal dura and compress the spinal cord.

Histologically, tumors are composed of meningothelial cells, which may have a wide variety of histological patterns. A characteristic feature is the presence of small foci of calcification (**psammoma bodies**). The natural history of these tumors depends on the histological pattern.

- The vast majority are classed as benign meningiomas. These are slow-growing expansile lesions with a low risk of recurrence after surgical removal.
- A small proportion are classed as atypical meningiomas, have many mitoses, cell pleomorphism and necrosis, and an increased risk of local recurrence after surgery.
- A rare group are classed as malignant meningiomas. These are rapidly growing tumors that behave as locally invasive malignant tumors resembling sarcomas.

TUMORS OF NEUROEPITHELIAL ORIGIN

Tumors of neuroepithelial origin are common primary brain tumors, broadly grouped under the term **gliomas**. The main types are derived from astrocytes, oligodendrocytes, ependyma, choroid plexus, neurons, and embryonal cells. Tumors range from benign, slow-growing lesions to malignant, rapidly growing tumors known as **anaplastic gliomas**. Gliomas have a tendency for diffuse infiltration of adjacent brain, which makes surgical removal difficult and leads to frequent local recurrence.

Fig. 21.41 Meningioma. These two sections from different levels in the same brain show a meningioma (**M**) compressing the frontal lobe and distorting underlying brain.

Astrocytomas are diffuse lesions that range from benign to highly malignant

Astrocytomas may arise in the cerebral hemispheres, brain stem, spinal cord or cerebellum, and are derived from astrocytic cells. They vary from tumors with no histological features of atypia and a slow pace of growth (**astrocytoma**) to lesions with high cellularity, mitoses, pleomorphism and a rapid pace of growth (**anaplastic astrocytoma**).

Macroscopically, astrocytomas appear as ill-defined, pale areas of softening in the tissue of the nervous system, which blend into adjacent normal brain (*Fig. 21.42*).

These tumors may arise in children or adults, most presenting with focal neurological signs or raised intracranial pressure. Because of the diffuse nature of most astrocytomas, complete surgical removal is rarely possible and treatment by surgical debulking and radiotherapy is usual. Tumors do not metastasize, but can spread locally by diffuse infiltration of adjacent brain. Low-grade tumors are associated with many years' survival, anaplastic astrocytomas having a survival of 4–5 years. Low-grade tumors usually evolve into high-grade tumors with time.

Pilocytic astrocytomas are a special type of astrocytoma, usually seen in the cerebellum in childhood. They have an excellent prognosis following surgical removal. Typically they are seen as a cystic lesion with a solid nodule of tumor in the cyst wall.

Glioblastomas are highly malignant tumors derived from astrocytes

The most common form of glioma, glioblastomas are highly malignant astrocytic glial tumors with a rapid pace of growth. The incidence is greatest around the age of 65 years, but lesions also occur less commonly in childhood and adolescence.

Macroscopically, tumors are necrotic hemorrhagic masses, arising principally in the cerebral hemispheres (*Fig. 21.43a*), less frequently in the brain stem, and only rarely in the cerebellum or spinal cord. Tumors are composed of a mixture of astroglial cell types with many mitoses and nuclear pleomorphism. Necrosis is present, and this is a feature that delineates this type of lesion from the anaplastic astrocytoma (*Fig. 21.43b*).

Fig. 21.43 Glioblastoma. A large glioblastoma (**G**) arises from one cerebral hemisphere and has grown to fill the ventricular system. Such malignant tumors are associated with necrosis and hemorrhage. Histology (b) shows necrosis (**N**) and microvascular proliferation (**V**)

Fig. 21.42 Low-grade astrocytoma. A low-grade astrocytoma (**A**) has arisen in the frontal lobe, distorting surrounding brain. It is extremely difficult to tell where tumor starts and ends because of the diffuse infiltrative nature of such lesions, precluding surgical removal in most cases.

Tumors may present as glioblastomas or may have evolved into glioblastoma from a previously diagnosed lower-grade astroglial tumor. They usually cause death by rapid local growth, but may also spread within the neur-axis. They have a median survival of around 10 months from diagnosis.

Oligodendrogliomas usually occur in the cerebral hemispheres of adults

Oligodendrogliomas and anaplastic oligodendrogliomas are glial tumors composed of cells morphologically resem-bling oligodendrocytes. They arise in the cerebral hemi-spheres and have only rarely been described in the brain stem, cerebellum or cord. Macroscopically, tumors are very similar to astrocytomas, arising as ill-defined grayish white lesions that merge with adjacent brain. Histologically, tumors are composed of cells with rounded nuclei and pale vacuolated or pink-staining cytoplasm resembling oligo-dendrocytes (*Fig. 21.44*). These lesions may be divided into low-grade and anaplastic oligodendrogliomas on the basis of cellularity, mitoses, pleomorphism, and vascular proliferation. It is not uncommon to find mixed glial lesions with both astrocytic and oligodendroglial features (**oligoastrocytomas**).

There are distinct cytogenetic changes in this type of glioma which distinguish them from astrocytic tumors. Deletion of chromosomal regions from 1p and 19q are associated with a response to chemotherapy. Low-grade tumors in the temporal lobe have a favorable prognosis, whereas high-grade tumors recur locally and can also invade the meninges and spread in the CSF pathways.

Fig. 21.44 Oligodendroglioma. Oligodendrogliomas are composed of cells with rounded nuclei and vacuolated cytoplasm. Despite the name and the morphological resemblance to oligodendroglia, cell biological studies show no markers for oligodendrocytes in such tumors. The name is retained for historical reasons.

Ependymomas, most commonly seen in childhood, often occur in the spinal cord and ventricles

Ependymomas and anaplastic ependymomas are tumors derived from ependymal cells. They are most common in the first two decades of life, accounting for around 10% of all intracranial tumors in childhood. The most common sites are the spinal cord and the region of the fourth ventricle.

Histologically, ependymomas form tubules resembling the central canal of the spinal cord (*Fig. 21.46*). Although most ependymomas demonstrate no cellular atypia, ana-plastic ependymomas show cells with mitoses, pleomor-phism, and vascular endothelial proliferation, and are associated with a worse prognosis.

Myxopapillary ependymomas are a variant of ependy-moma seen in the filum terminale of the spinal cord. They behave as locally infiltrative lesions.

Cell biology of gliomas

Progression of tumors with time from low-grade astrocytomas to anaplastic astrocytoma through to glioblastoma is well established. This progression has been related to the development of serial molecular genetic defects, each contributing to further derangement of growth control (*Fig. 21.45*).

In the histological diagnosis of brain tumors it is often difficult to give an accurate assessment of the grade of an astroglial tumor. It is hoped that characterization of gliomas by their molecular genetic abnormalities may lead to better assessment of likely behavior.

Fig. 21.45 Oncogene defects seen in astroglial tumors	
Low-grade astrocytoma	p53 mutation. Loss of alleles from chromosome 17.
Anaplastic astrocytoma	p53 mutation. Loss of alleles from chromosomes 17 and 19.
Glioblastoma	p53 mutation. Loss of alleles from chromosomes 17, 19 and 10. EGF-R amplification.

Fig. 21.46 Ependymoma. These tumors form tubular structures (**T**) resembling the central canal of the spinal cord.

Fig. 21.47 Medulloblastoma. Medulloblastomas arise in the cerebellum and appear as masses of soft, white tissue (**T**), often in the vermis (as here).

Choroid plexus tumors are mainly benign papillomas

The most common tumor of the choroid plexus is the choroid plexus papilloma, derived from epithelial cells. Arising most frequently in childhood, these papillary, frond-like tumors most often develop in the lateral ventricle. Choroid plexus papillomas are benign and closely resemble normal choroid plexus, whereas the less common choroid plexus carcinomas are invasive malignant epithelial tumors with both solid and papillary areas.

Tumors containing neuronal elements are mainly benign

Several tumors of the nervous system contain neuronal cells; lesions may be composed solely of neuronal elements or may be mixed tumors with both neuronal and glial elements.

Gangliocytoma and **ganglioglioma** are neoplasms mainly seen in childhood. These well-circumscribed lesions are usually seen in the temporal lobe, where they can present as temporal-lobe epilepsy. Histologically, tumors contain differentiated neuronal ganglion cells and have a good prognosis after removal.

Central neurocytoma is a tumor that occurs in the lateral ventricles of young adults. It is composed of small neuronal cells and has an excellent prognosis after removal.

Embryonal tumors of the CNS are rapidly growing malignant lesions

The embryonal tumors of the CNS are common in childhood, forming a large proportion of primary tumors. They are composed of primitive small cells, which resemble the multipotential cells of the developing fetal brain, and are

Fig. 21.48 PNET. Primitive neuroectodermal tumors are composed of small cells with a high mitotic rate. In some, neuroblastic rosettes (**R**) form, indicating primitive neuronal maturation.

also called **primitive neuroectodermal tumors (PNETs)**. As a group, they are rapidly growing lesions composed of small cells with many mitoses. As well as being prone to local spread, they have a tendency to spread via CSF pathways.

The main tumor in this group is the **medulloblastoma**, which arises in the cerebellum and is composed of primitive small cells with multiple lines of differentiation (*Fig. 21.47*). As a result of modern treatment with surgery, radiotherapy and chemotherapy, the 10-year survival rate is over 50%.

Histologically, tumors are composed of sheets of small anaplastic cells with rod-shaped and rounded nuclei (*Fig. 21.48*). Evidence of neuronal and glial differentiation may be seen. Less common PNETs are cerebral neuroblastomas (composed of primitive neurons) and ependymoblastomas (composed of primitive ependyma).

NON-NEUROEPITHELIAL TUMORS OF THE CNS

Lymphomas of the nervous system are increasing in incidence as a complication of immunosuppression

Primary lymphomas of the nervous system are usually non-Hodgkin's lymphomas of B-cell type. These tumors generally arise sporadically, are increasing in incidence, and can also be associated with immunosuppression, particularly in patients with AIDS.

Lesions are ill defined and multifocal, usually being seen deep in the hemispheric white matter. Histology shows brain infiltrated by atypical lymphoid cells. These tumors have a very poor prognosis, with most patients dead 5 years after diagnosis.

Solitary plasmacytomas may also arise in the brain. These lesions are composed of sheets of plasma cells and may be associated with monoclonal light chains in CSF or serum.

The nervous system is a site for the origin of germ-cell tumors, mainly from the pineal gland

Germ-cell tumors identical to those seen in the ovary and testis may arise in the brain, most occurring in the pineal gland. The full range of germ-cell tumors is seen, i.e. germinoma, embryonal carcinoma, yolk-sac tumor, choriocarcinoma, teratoma and mixed germ-cell tumors. Most are malignant and are prone to spread via the CSF pathways, requiring treatment by radiotherapy and chemotherapy. Treatment may be monitored by detection of tumor markers in the CSF.

Developmental cysts of the nervous system may present as space-occupying lesions

Many different types of cysts and tumor-like lesions involve the CNS. For example, **dermoid** and **epidermoid cysts** are lined by squamous epithelium and filled with keratin. They are slowly expanding cysts, common in the temporal lobe region.

Colloid cysts of the third ventricle are solitary cysts lined by columnar epithelium. Filled with mucoid material, they arise in the third ventricle, commonly producing hydrocephalus by blocking the foramen of Monro.

Arachnoid cysts arise from the leptomeninges and are filled with CSF. They cause compression of the underlying brain.

Craniopharyngiomas are infiltrative epithelial tumors arising from the region of the pituitary fossa

Composed of squamous-cell-like epithelium, craniopharyngiomas are derived from remnants of Rathke's pouch, the

Fig. 21.49 Craniopharyngioma. A craniopharyngioma has both solid (**S**) and cystic (**C**) areas. The cyst is filled with thick fluid containing lipid derived from breakdown of the lining epithelium.

embryological source of the anterior pituitary gland. Accounting for 3% of intracranial tumors, they are most common in childhood. Tumors compress the pituitary gland and damage the overlying hypothalamus and optic chiasm, presenting with either hypopituitarism or visual problems. Macroscopically, lesions have cystic and solid areas, frequently growing into adjacent brain and around major blood vessels (*Fig. 21.49*), often with calcification.

Although craniopharyngiomas are benign, local recurrence is often a problem because of inability to completely excise infiltrative tumors.

DISEASES OF PERIPHERAL NERVES

Peripheral nerves are composed of several fascicles, each surrounded by the perineurium, which is composed of epithelial-like perineurial cells. Within the endoneurium, individual axons are supported by Schwann cells, which may form myelin.

There are three main pathological types of damage to peripheral nerves: primary axonal degeneration, primary demyelination, and destruction of both axon and myelin.

Provided the cell body of the nerve remains intact, damage to the peripheral axon or myelin may be repaired by regeneration.

Peripheral nerve damage can be divided into axonal damage or demyelination

In **axonal degeneration** nerve-cell bodies are unable to maintain long axonal processes. The result is degeneration of axons, starting at the periphery and progressing up towards the neuronal cell body. This process is often termed a **dying-back neuropathy** and is commonly due to toxic and metabolic damage to nerve-cell bodies. Loss of axons can be inferred by reduced amplitude of nerve impulses when measured electrically from affected nerves.

Clinical features of peripheral nerve diseases

Diseases of peripheral nerves are termed **neuropathies** and are clinically manifest by sensory or motor abnormalities, which may be predominantly motor, predominantly sensory, or mixed, depending on which diameter of nerve fibers is affected by a disease process.

Clinically, several terms are used to describe peripheral nerve disease. The term 'neuritis' is often used, but does not usually imply an inflammatory pathology.

- **Polyneuropathy** is generalized symmetrical involvement of peripheral nerves.
- **Focal peripheral neuropathy** is disease affecting peripheral nerves in a haphazard manner, the term 'mononeuropathy' being applied when one nerve is affected, and 'multiple mononeuropathy' being used to describe asymmetrical disease of several nerves.
- **Radiculopathy** is disease affecting a nerve root.

Disease of peripheral nerves is clinically investigated by electrophysiology. When diagnosis is uncertain, nerve biopsy may be performed; the most common site is from the sural nerve in the foot, as it leaves no significant neurological deficit.

Regeneration in the peripheral nervous system

The sequence of events that follows sectioning of axons in a nerve is termed **Wallerian degeneration** and, under favorable circumstances, this is followed by axonal regeneration.

1. When an axon is severed or damaged, the axon and myelin distal to the injury degenerate. The degenerate myelin and axon are removed by macrophages and Schwann cells. The target tissue, e.g. muscle, is denervated and atrophies.
2. Schwann cells in the distal nerve proliferate and enlarge within the still-intact basement membrane tube enclosing them.
3. The nerve-cell body becomes swollen, the nucleus enlarges, and there is an increase in the quantity of cytoplasmic intermediate filaments, termed **central chromatolysis** (a structural change reflecting regeneration). The stump of the proximal axon swells and several small axon sprouts grow out down the column of proliferated Schwann cells, which acts as a guide for the regenerating axon. The axons grows 2–3 mm per day, eventually reinnervating the denervated tissue.
4. The axon is remyelinated, but new myelin segments between nodes of Ranvier are shorter than in the original nerve.

The capacity of axons for regeneration allows surgical repair of peripheral nerves by nerve anastomosis after severance. Grafting of a portion of nerve is required when there has been scarring, as axons can only grow down the intact basement membrane tubes of Schwann cells, not through a collagenous scar.

In **segmental demyelination** the disease process spares axons but damages Schwann cells and myelin. Loss of myelin can be inferred by slowing of conduction velocity when measured electrically. Loss of myelin is mainly seen in immune-mediated disease, as well as with several toxins.

Provided that the cell body is intact, and that there is no scarring in the nerve, axons and myelin may regenerate, allowing recovery from damage to peripheral nerves (see pink box).

The main infections of nerves are herpes zoster and leprosy

In herpes zoster infection, virus lies dormant in the neuronal cell bodies of dorsal root ganglia, but becomes reactivated and tracks down nerves to cause infection of the skin in the sensory dermatome (**shingles**).

Mycobacterium leprae mainly affects peripheral nerves in the tuberculoid form. Destruction of both axons and myelin occurs, particularly in cutaneous nerves, causing skin ulceration and loss of digits with senory loss.

Laceration, compression and entrapment are common mechanical causes of nerve dysfunction

One of the most common causes of peripheral nerve dysfunction is mechanical trauma. Laceration of nerves is seen after penetrating trauma and is associated with some bone fractures. The nerve distal to the laceration undergoes Wallerian degeneration. If surgical anastomosis is performed, axons may regrow to reinnervate the denervated tissues.

Entrapment and compression of nerves is commonly seen in several sites:

- Nerve roots are compressed in intervertebral foramina by prolapsed intervertebral discs or osteophytes due to osteoarthritis of the spine (see pages 548 and 556).
- The median nerve is compressed by swellings in the carpal tunnel at the wrist (see page 555).
- The ulnar nerve can become compressed in the flexor carpal tunnel at the medial epicondyle of the humerus.
- The common peroneal nerve can be compressed at the neck of the fibula.

Compressed nerves develop segmental demyelination and abnormal conduction, but with prolonged damage there is additional axonal degeneration.

Acute immune-mediated demyelination is the most common cause of an acute peripheral neuropathy

Guillain–Barré syndrome, also known as **acute post-infectious polyradiculoneuropathy,** is the most common form of acute neuropathy. It is an immune-mediated demyelination of peripheral nerves, usually seen 2–4 weeks after a viral illness, but also triggered after a variety of infective processes. Histologically, nerves show infiltration by lymphoid cells, with phagocytosis of myelin by macrophages.

Widespread demyelination in peripheral nerves causes motor weakness, often leading to respiratory failure, with less prominent sensory changes. Remyelination usually occurs over a period of 3–4 months, and in most cases is associated with recovery.

Chronic demyelinating polyradiculoneuropathy is a chronic form of immune-mediated demyelination in which repeated episodes of demyelination and remyelination cause proliferation of Schwann cells, often leading to physical swelling of peripheral nerves (hypertrophic neuropathy).

Peripheral neuropathy may occur as a paraneoplastic syndrome, several cases being due to the formation of autoantibodies to the tumor, which cross-react with myelin.

Neuropathies may be caused by toxins, causing either demyelination or axonal degeneration

Many toxins cause damage to peripheral nerves, either by damaging myelin or by causing damage to neurons, leading to axonal degeneration:

- **Chronic alcohol abuse** is a common cause of peripheral neuropathy, which may be due to the direct toxic effects of alcohol as well as the effects of vitamin deficiency.
- **Drugs**, e.g. isoniazid, sulfonamides, vinca alkaloids, dapsone and chloroquine, are important causes of neuropathy.

- **Occupational exposure to chemicals** such as lead, arsenic, mercury and acrylamide.

Most toxins produce a dying-back axonal neuropathy that results in symmetrical sensory/motor neuropathy with a 'glove and stocking' distribution, reflecting loss of the ends of the longer axons.

Diabetes is the most common metabolic disorder causing neuropathy

Several metabolic disorders are associated with the development of a peripheral neuropathy, the most common being diabetes.

Diabetes mellitus is associated with four main patterns of neuropathy: symmetrical predominantly sensory peripheral polyneuropathy, autonomic neuropathy, proximal painful motor neuropathy, and cranial mononeuropathy (mainly third, fourth and sixth nerves).

The sensory and autonomic neuropathy is due mainly to a combination of axonal degeneration and segmental demyelination, whereas the motor neuropathy and cranial mononeuropathy are caused by vascular disease in blood vessels supplying nerves.

Vitamin deficiency is an important cause of peripheral neuropathy, particularly B_1 (thiamine) and B_{12} deficiency.

Amyloid (see Chapter 25) may infiltrate peripheral nerves and cause a neuropathy. In addition to secondary amyloid associated with systemic inflammatory diseases or myeloma, several types of familial amyloid cause a specific neuropathy due to a defect in the gene coding for transthyretin (prealbumin).

Vascular disease is a common cause of peripheral nerve damage

Vascular disease is an important cause of peripheral nerve disease, resulting in focal necrosis of major nerve trunks and loss of myelinated axons.

The most common causes of vascular damage to nerves are **atherosclerosis** and **arteriosclerosis**, particularly affecting arteries supplying nerves in the lower limbs of patients who have critical ischemia. This is most common in patients with diabetes.

Vasculitis may cause nerve infarction, presenting as a multiple mononeuropathy in, for example, polyarteritis nodosa, SLE, Wegener's granulomatosis and rheumatoid disease.

Hereditary diseases are important causes of peripheral neuropathy

Several peripheral neuropathies have a hereditary basis, many of which are of known cause. The mechanism for the development of neuropathy varies in each case. Porphyria, Fabry's disease, leukodystrophies, abetalipopteinemia and familial amyloidosis syndromes are all hereditary diseases that can be associated with peripheral neuropathies.

Mutations in genes expressed in Schwann cells and the axons cause **Charcot–Marie–Tooth (CMT) disease**, a group of hereditary motor and sensory neuropathies. Patients can be classified into two main groups depending on neurophysiology, as follows:

- CMT1 – demyelinating pattern with slow nerve conduction velocities.
- CMT2 – axonal pattern with normal nerve conduction velocities but reduced motor or sensory amplitudes.

Within each group, defined mutations and different patterns of inheritance have been described that further characterize disease. In some diseases inherited neuropathy also involves autonomic nerves.

The main tumors of peripheral nerve are benign nerve-sheath tumors

The main tumors of peripheral nerve arise from the nerve sheath and are termed schwannomas and neurofibromas. Uncommonly, malignant peripheral nerve-sheath tumors can develop (neurofibrosarcomas and malignant schwannomas).

Schwannomas, which are usually solitary tumors, can occur on any peripheral nerve. They are rounded lesions, typically 1–2 cm in diameter when removed, composed of spindle-shaped cells with features of Schwann cells. Schwannomas affecting the eighth cranial nerve are termed acoustic neuromas and may be part of the neurofibromatosis 2 syndrome (see page 479).

Neurofibromas, which may be solitary or multiple, are nodular or plexiform in type. Nodular neurofibromas are discrete tumors that form a defined mass, whereas plexiform neurofibromas diffusely affect nerves over a wide area, making surgical removal very difficult. Nodular neurofibromas are fusiform or rounded tumors composed of spindle cells that resemble perineurial cells. Plexiform neurofibromas often appear as boggy areas of ill-defined swelling and are composed of nerves expanded by a proliferation of perineurial cells and extracellular matrix material. Multiple neurofibromas are seen as part of the neurofibromatosis 1 syndrome (see page 479).

Malignant nerve-sheath tumors may arise de novo or may occur as malignant change in an existing benign tumor, usually in cases of neurofibromatosis. They behave as soft-tissue sarcomas (discussed in Chapter 24).

Post-traumatic neuroma is a regenerative phenomenon of attempted axonal sprouting

When a nerve is severed, by either trauma or surgery, the cut end develops a collagenous scar associated with attempted regeneration of axons. In most cases this is asymptomatic, but in some instances the attempt at regeneration forms a nodule that is painful to pressure. Histologically the nodule consists of collagen, proliferated Schwann cells and sprouting axon terminals. This common clinical problem, termed an amputation neuroma, sometimes arises in the stumps of leg amputations as a cause of pain when using a limb prosthesis.

The same collagenous scarring prevents successful regrowth of axons down a nerve after trauma; such lesions have to be surgically removed and the cut ends of nerve anastomosed, often with a nerve graft, to allow reinnervation.

MUSCLE DISEASES

Diseases of muscle fall into three main groups

In clinical practice, most non-neoplastic diseases of muscle present because of weakness, wasting, or pain in muscle. There are three main groups.

Muscular dystrophies are inherited diseases of muscle that generally result in progressive degeneration. They are classified according to inheritance pattern, the clinical pattern of muscle groups involved and, as the genes responsible become characterized, increasingly by molecular genetic techniques.

Myopathies are a group of conditions of diverse etiology, grouped together because of a predominant impact of disease on the muscle. There are four main subgroups:

- Inflammatory myopathies, in which there is a primary inflammation of muscle, often amenable to therapy (very common).
- Secondary myopathies, in which a systemic disease process causes pathology in muscle, often amenable to therapy (common).
- Metabolic myopathies, in which a primary metabolic problem has a major impact on muscle function (uncommon).
- Congenital myopathies, which are distinguished from the dystrophies in that they are generally non-progressive (rare).

Neurogenic disease, particularly disease of peripheral nerves or motor neurons, causes secondary atrophy of skeletal muscle.

Skeletal muscle has only a limited repertoire of pathological responses

Atrophy of muscle fibers occurs mainly with disuse, ischemia, denervation, steroid therapy, and malnutrition. It may affect one subtype of fiber preferentially, usually type 2.

Muscle biopsy

Muscle biopsy is an important investigation in certain neuromuscular diseases in which there are clinical features of weakness, muscle wasting, or muscle pain (myalgia). The two main techniques are **open excision biopsy**, which provides a large sample but is relatively invasive, and **percutaneous needle biopsy**, which provides a small sample but can be repeated if needed.

The main biopsy sites are the vastus lateralis, deltoid or gastrocnemius muscles. As it requires specialized techniques, histological examination of a muscle biopsy is not performed in most clinical laboratories. The sample needs rapid preservation by snap-freezing in liquid nitrogen, which then allows histological sections to be cut for enzyme histochemical staining, enabling the delineation of fiber types. Immunohistochemistry or immunoblotting using antibodies to functional proteins in muscle may identify deficiencies related to specific inherited dystrophies. Electron microscopy is useful to look for mitochondrial abnormalities, as well as the structural changes that can take place in some of the congenital muscle diseases, so small samples need immediate glutaraldehyde fixation. Frozen tissue can also be used for biochemical studies, for example looking at the mitochondrial respiratory chain or glycogen storage.

Key Facts
Skeletal muscle

- Skeletal muscle is composed of individual striated muscle fibers, which can be divided into two main subtypes. Type 1 contain abundant mitochondria and are specialized for aerobic metabolism. Type 2 contain abundant glycogen and are specialized for anaerobic metabolism. Fiber types are identified by enzyme histochemistry.
- A normal muscle is composed of a mixture of the two types of fiber, which are arranged randomly.
- Innervation of muscle is at specialized motor end-plates that have acetylcholine receptors on the muscle surface.

Hypertrophy of muscle fibers occurs to compensate for loss or atrophy of other muscle fibers due to a disease process.

Change in fiber type distribution is detected by histochemical staining. It is usually seen in association with change in muscle innervation, when muscle fibers come to be arranged in groups rather than a random checkerboard pattern.

Necrosis of muscle is usually seen in single fibers and is a feature of many of the primary muscle diseases. Less commonly, large areas undergo necrosis, usually due to vascular pathology in main vessels.

Phagocytosis of dead muscle fibers by macrophages occurs following necrosis.

Regeneration of skeletal muscle fibers can take place from the population of muscle stem cells (satellite cells).

Fibrosis, often accompanied by infiltration with adipose tissue, is seen as a tissue reaction in many types of muscular dystrophy.

Primary inflammation occurs in the inflammatory myopathies.

Given that skeletal muscle has a limited set of responses, the histological diagnosis of muscle disease is based on evaluation of the combination of different types of pathological responses.

Muscle disease can be divided into two main groups according to the pathology. In **dystrophic and myopathic disease**, there is hypertrophy and atrophy of fibers, with single fibers undergoing degeneration, necrosis, and phagocytosis. There is variable fibrosis.

In **neurogenic disease**, atrophy of fibers is seen in groups, with fibers elsewhere showing compensatory hypertrophy. Fiber-type grouping is often seen on histochemical staining.

Congenital myopathies are a cause of childhood hypotonia

The congenital myopathies usually present in childhood as hypotonia (floppy baby syndrome) or muscle weakness. The majority of congenital myopathies are named after the structural abnormalities seen on muscle biopsy, e.g. central core disease, nemaline body myopathy, myotubular myopathy, congenital fiber-type disproportion. They are generally non-progressive, which distinguishes them from muscular dystrophies. Inheritance is variable. Although many types are compatible with a long life expectancy, others may cause disability because of secondary skeletal deformities or respiratory muscle involvement.

Muscular dystrophies are progressive, genetically determined, degenerative diseases of muscle

The muscular dystrophies are a group of genetically determined degenerative diseases of muscle. Pathologically, they are characterized by the destruction of single muscle cells over a prolonged period of time, with fiber regeneration and the development of fibrosis. The muscular dystrophies are classified according to the pattern of inheritance and, increasingly, defined molecular genetic abnormalities. It has become clear that mutations in genes coding for proteins involved in the contractile apparatus as well as those involved in anchoring muscle cells to the extracellular matrix are the main causes of dystrophy (*Fig. 21.50*).

Based on the protein involved, classes of disease can be grouped, for example abnormalities in dystrophin are dystrophinopathies; abnormalities in sarcoglycans are grouped as sarcoglycanopathies.

Duchenne dystrophy is the most common form of muscular dystrophy in childhood

Duchenne dystrophy is an X-linked recessive disorder, hence it is almost exclusively seen in males. It is caused by mutation in the gene coding for **dystrophin**, a protein that normally helps anchor the internal cytoskeleton of muscle fibers through the cell membrane and to the extracellular matrix. Lack of this protein renders fibers liable to tearing with repeated contraction. The onset of clinical features is in early childhood, affected children showing muscle weakness with a high serum creatine kinase level (caused by necrosis) and clinical calf hypertrophy (due to fatty replacement of muscle). The disease has a very poor prognosis, most affected individuals dying in their late teens. Heart muscle is also affected, leading to cardiomyopathy. Becker dystrophy is related to partial lack of dystrophin.

Histologically, there is muscle fiber necrosis, phagocytosis of dead fibers, and replacement of muscle by fibrous and fatty tissue. Immunostaining for dystrophin reveals that it is absent from fibers (*Fig. 21.51*). Diagnosis can be assisted by performing molecular genetic analysis of the dystrophin gene.

Myotonic dystrophy is an autosomal dominant disorder

Myotonic dystrophy is the most common inherited muscle disease of adults, affecting 1 in 8000 of the population. It is characterized by muscle weakness, myotonia (inability to relax muscles), and several non-muscle features including cataracts and frontal baldness in males, cardiomyopathy, and low intelligence. It is inherited as an autosomal dominant disorder and usually becomes apparent in adolescence, with facial weakness and distal weakness in the limbs. Death is commonly due to involvement of the respiratory muscles.

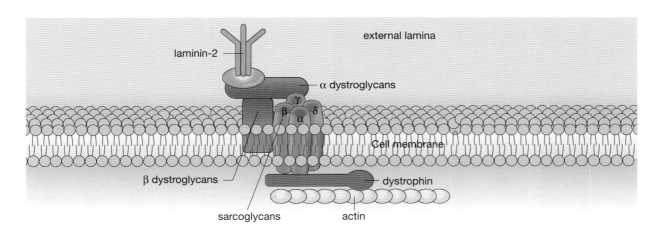

Fig. 21.50 Structural proteins involved in dystrophy. This diagram shows the main proteins involved in muscular dystrophy, many are part of a complex that anchors the internal cytoskeleton to the extracellular matrix. Mutations may cause either absence or reduction in a protein, leading to defective function and muscle fibre damage that causes fibre necrosis.

Fig. 21.51 Dystrophin abnormalities. This shows staining of muscle for dystrophin (brown). In Duchenne dystrophy this staining would be absent as no protein is produced. In Becker's dystrophy, staining is reduced or patchy.

Molecular pathology of myotonic dystrophy

Myotonic dystrophy is an autosomal dominant neuromuscular disease. The gene for the disorder is on chromosome 19; the mutation has been identified as an unstable trinucleotide CTG repeat in a sequence related to a gene coding for a cAMP-dependent protein kinase, widely expressed in many tissues. The mechanism through which this mutation causes myotonia is unknown.

The CTG repeat varies in length between affected siblings, generally increasing through generations in parallel with increasing severity of the disease. This is the basis of **anticipation**, whereby clinical disease is more severe in later generations of an affected family as a result of progressive increase in size of the gene expansion. Congenital myotonic dystrophy, a severe disease of the newborn, is exclusively maternally inherited.

The gene for myotonic dystrophy is located on chromosome 19, coding for a protein kinase (see pink box). Histologically, affected muscles show abnormalities of fiber size, with fiber necrosis, abundant internal nuclei, and replacement by fibrofatty tissue.

Inflammatory myopathies are diseases with an underlying abnormal immune response

The inflammatory myopathies are characterized by primary inflammation of muscle, with resulting fiber necrosis. The inflammatory infiltrate is mainly composed of T cells and monocytes as part of an abnormal autoimmune response. There are three main types of inflammatory myopathy.

Polymyositis presents clinically with weakness of proximal limb muscles and facial muscles, ptosis, and dysphagia. Although the precise stimulus causing disease is unknown, there are well-recognized clinical associations, the most common being the presence of connective tissue diseases such as SLE, rheumatoid disease or scleroderma (see Chapter 25). Polymyositis may also be a non-metastatic manifestation of malignancy, in which case it may be part of the clinical syndrome of **dermatomyositis**, in which muscle disease is accompanied by a characteristic skin rash.

Muscle biopsy shows lymphocytic infiltration of muscle with fiber necrosis. Muscle fibres abnormally express MHC class I protein. Disease may respond to immunosuppressive treatment with steroids or azathioprine.

Inclusion body myositis is clinically similar to polymyositis but occurs mainly in elderly patients. Muscle biopsy shows inflammation of muscle, fiber necrosis and the presence of vacuoles and filamentous inclusions in fibers (seen by electron microscopy). Diagnosis of this disorder is important because it is slowly progressive and has a poor response to immunosuppressive treatment.

Secondary and metabolic myopathies are common in clinical practice

Diseases of muscle secondary to either systemic disease or metabolic abnormality are frequently seen in clinical practice. There are many types and only the clinically most common are presented here.

Type 2 fiber atrophy myopathy is the most common pathological finding in biopsies from patients with muscle weakness. The type 2 fibers undergo selective atrophy, which can be detected on histochemical staining. This pattern of muscle abnormality is non-specific and may be secondary to several problems, the main ones being disuse, malignancy, steroid administration, Cushing's disease, thyroid disease and connective tissue diseases.

Endocrine myopathy describes the association of muscle weakness and wasting with endocrine disease. The main cause is corticosteroid excess (therapeutic or in Cushing's disease), which results in atrophy of type 2 fibers. Similar changes can occur with thyroid disease.

Carcinomatous myopathy describes the association of muscle weakness and wasting with systemic neoplasia. The tumor may cause non-metastatic manifestations in muscle through type 2 fiber atrophy myopathy, the development of polymyositis or dermatomyositis, or denervation due to a paraneoplastic neuropathy.

Fig. 21.52 Mitochondrial myopathy. (a) Trichrome stain. (b) Electron microscopy. In affected muscle (a), aggregates of mitochondria can be seen by light microscopy, staining red with special stains, hence the term 'ragged red fibers' (**R**). Ultrastructure (b) often shows crystalline inclusions in mitochondria, termed 'parking-lot inclusions', because of their orderly pattern.

Mitochondrial myopathy is due to heritable genetic abnormalities affecting mitochondrial function. Diseases are due to either mitochondrial (maternal inheritance) or nuclear genetic abnormalities (mendelian inheritance). Disease syndromes are characterized by muscle weakness, particularly extraocular muscles, with or without other neurological and metabolic disturbances. Muscle biopsy reveals abnormal pleomorphic mitochondria, often with crystalline inclusions on electron microscopy (*Fig. 21.52*). Molecular genetic analysis may show specific abnormalities in the mitochondrial genome, but the nuclear genetic causes are mostly uncharacterized.

Glycogenoses may affect muscle. The two main types of glycogenosis affecting muscle are acid maltase deficiency (type 2) and McArdle's disease (myophosphorylase deficiency, type 5). Both are diagnosable on muscle biopsy.

NEUROGENIC DISORDERS OF MUSCLE

Neurogenic disorders may present as muscle disease

Clinically, weakness of muscle may be caused by denervation due to disease of either peripheral nerves or anterior horn cells. Denervation is easily recognized on muscle biopsy as it causes atrophy of large groups of fibers. If reinnervation occurs, the normal random distribution of type 1 and type 2 fibers is replaced by large groups of a single fiber type, termed **fiber-type grouping**.

Spinal muscular atrophy is a heritable degeneration of spinal motor neurons

The childhood spinal muscular atrophies (SMA) constitute the second most common autosomal recessive disorder after cystic fibrosis. There is muscle wasting due to degeneration of the anterior horn cells in the spinal cord. Muscle biopsy shows large groups of abnormally small muscle fibers that have never been innervated (*Fig. 21.53*).

Fig. 21.53 Spinal muscular atrophy. In biopsy, large areas of muscle are composed of minute non-innervated fibers, contrasting with larger pink fibers that have been innervated.

Inheritance is autosomal recessive due to a defective gene located on chromosome 5. **Werdnig–Hoffman disease** presents as a floppy baby at birth. In the severe acute form, affected children usually die in the first year of life; an intermediate form is associated with longer survival. Less common late-onset variants of spinal muscular atrophy are also described.

DISORDERS OF MUSCLE FUNCTION

Myasthenia gravis is an autoimmune disease caused by antibodies to the acetylcholine receptor

Myasthenia gravis is a disease characterized by muscle weakness, ptosis and dysphagia. A main differential diagnosis is with an inflammatory myopathy, which can have identical clinical features. It is an autoimmune disease caused by generation of autoantibodies to the acetylcholine receptor located in the postsynaptic membrane of muscle motor end-plates. These antibodies prevent synaptic transmission by blocking the receptor sites.

Diagnosis can be made by giving a therapeutic trial of a short-acting anticholinesterase drug, which increases acetylcholine concentrations in the synaptic cleft and allows transmission.

An important association with this condition is pathology of the thymus gland. About 25% of cases have a thymoma (see page 317), others having thymic gland hyperplasia. Thymectomy may improve the myasthenia in a proportion of cases. There is no diagnostic pathology seen by routine light microscopy in muscle biopsy.

Diseases caused by defective ion transport in muscle

Several diseases of muscle have been shown to be due to abnormal ion transport across muscle membranes. The main syndromes are manifest by sudden reversible attacks of paralysis and flaccidity (**periodic paralysis**), abnormal relaxation of muscles (**myotonia**), or **fatiguability**.

Hypokalemic periodic paralysis is most common in women. Attacks of paralysis typically occur on waking in the morning and can last for many hours. There is a fall in the serum potassium level to 2–2.5 mmol/L. Mutations in the muscle dihydropyridine (DHP)-sensitive calcium channel α_1 subunit have been found.

Hyperkalemic periodic paralysis is most common in childhood and adolescence. Attacks are precipitated when the individual is at rest following a period of exercise, but are short-lived (1–2 hours). There is elevation of the serum potassium to 5–7 mmol/L during an attack. Fixed muscle weakness develops in most patients with time. This syndrome is caused by mutations in the gene for the α subunit of the skeletal muscle Na^+ channel located on chromosome 17.

Paramyotonia congenita (PC) is an autosomal dominant non-progressive muscle disorder characterized by cold-induced stiffness followed by muscle weakness. The weakness is also caused by a dysfunction of the sodium channel in muscle fibers, caused by mutation in the sodium channel gene located on chromosome 17.

Autosomal recessive generalized myotonia (Becker's disease) and **autosomal dominant myotonia congenita (Thomsen's disease)** are characterized by skeletal muscle stiffness manifest by difficulty in relaxing grip. These diseases are the result of muscle membrane hyperexcitability due to mutation in the gene for a skeletal muscle chloride channel protein on chromosome 7. Defective ion transport causes failure of muscle relaxation.

Lambert–Eaton myasthenic syndrome (LEMS) is characterized by abnormal fatiguability. It is an autoimmune disorder of neuromuscular transmission, often found in patients with lung cancer. Autoantibodies bind to presynaptic voltage-dependent calcium channels at motor nerve terminals to cause functional loss. This in turn causes reduced release of acetylcholine in response to nerve stimulation. Small-cell lung carcinoma cells express calcium channels, suggesting that autoantibody production is triggered by these tumor antigens.

Malignant hyperthermia is an inherited disorder in which exposure to certain drugs, especially those used in anesthesia, leads to sustained muscle contraction, hypermetabolism and pyrexia; this may be fatal. Disease is due to defects in the gene coding for a sarcoplasmic reticulum release channel called the ryanodine receptor; ryanodine is an artificial ligand which bonds to the channel. Mutation in this gene can also cause central core disease, one of the congenital myopathies. Some patients with muscle weakness and thymoma have autoantibodies to the ryanodine receptor, simulating myasthenia gravis.

Case-based questions

Case 1 – A man off his bike

A 22-year-old man is taken to the emergency room from an ambulance accompanied by his friends, members of a motorcycle gang called 'The Spores.' He has come off his bike on a bend and hit a tree. On examination he is unconscious, making no response to painful stimuli. He was wearing a helmet, which came off in the accident. He has a fractured right femur and poor movement of the right side of his chest, with a clinical hemothorax. There is a bruise with a superficial laceration over the right temporal area of his scalp. Blood is coming out of his right ear. His right pupil is dilated and does not respond to light. His left pupil is of normal size and contracts in response to light.

He is intubated and ventilated, the hemothorax is drained, and he is made hemodynamically stable. A CT scan shows a right-sided extradural hematoma associated with a fracture of the temporal bone of the skull vault. An emergency operation is performed and the extradural hematoma evacuated. He is given intravenous mannitol and dexamethasone after the operation. However, his condition does not improve and, following appropriate criteria, 5 days later he is pronounced brainstem dead.

1. What is the reason for a dilated and unreactive right pupil?
2. What is the origin of the extradural hematoma?
3. Why does he not make a recovery despite prompt treatment of the hematoma?
4. What is the clinical significance of the bleeding from the ear?

Case 2 – Collapse and hemiplegia

A man is brought to hospital as an emergency, having collapsed at the bank where he is a financial advisor. He is unconscious, and it is evident that he has a dense, left-sided hemiplegia. His wife attends and reveals that her husband, who is aged 63, has been on medication for high blood pressure for the past 10 years, although he does not always take his tablets. His blood pressure is 150/100. ECG shows left ventricular hypertrophy. His full blood count is normal, as are measurements of serum urea and electrolytes. A CT scan shows a large hematoma, 3 cm in diameter, in the region of the right internal capsule/basal ganglia region.

1. What is the most likely cause of this intracerebral hematoma?

2. What are the other common sites for primary intracerebral hemorrhages?
3. What are other, less common, causes of intracerebral bleeding?

Case 3 A miserable boy with a stiff neck

A 4-year old boy is brought by his parents to the hospital emergency room. Early in the afternoon he had complained of being unwell, and so was put to bed by his mother. Two hours later, when she had gone to check on how he was, his mother had found him virtually unrousable. On examination he is febrile and barely rousable, although he is making responses to painful stimuli. He has marked neck stiffness. There are no focal neurological signs. Blood cultures are taken and high-dose dexamethasone is given just before high-dose intravenous antibiotics. A CT scan shows no mass lesion in the brain.

A lumbar puncture is performed. CSF is turbid and is sent for analysis. There are very large numbers of neutrophils. CSF sugar is low. Gram stain shows many Gram-negative coccobacilli with filamentous forms. A diagnosis of acute purulent meningitis is made and treatment started with appropriate antibiotics.

1. What organisms commonly cause meningitis at this age?
2. What are the possible outcomes and complications following acute meningitis?

Case 4 A woman with lots of neurology

A farmer's 36-year-old wife is sent by her family doctor for a neurological opinion and investigation. She has developed weakness and incoordination of her right leg associated with some numbness. One year earlier she had an episode of blurred vision associated with pain behind her right eye. Her doctor suspects that she might have multiple sclerosis.

On examination she has loss of proprioception in her right leg associated with brisk reflexes and ankle clonus. She has reduced appreciation of light touch and pain in both legs. No other focal signs are seen.

Full blood count and ESR are normal. Serum B_{12} is normal. CSF shows a mild increase in lymphoid cells and a moderately elevated protein level. Electrophoresis of CSF shows oligoclonal immunoglobulin bands. Visual evoked potentials show delay of the positive wave in the right eye by 25 ms, compared to the left which is normal. MRI scanning shows abnormal areas of signal in white

▶

▶ matter at the angles of the lateral ventricles, in the cerebellar peduncles, and in the lower thoracic spinal cord.

A diagnosis of multiple sclerosis is made.

1. **What is the pathogenesis of multiple sclerosis, and what sort of clinical progression might be expected in this patient?**
2. **What is the name of the lesions seen in the brain and what do they look like?**
3. **What was the reason for the blurred vision and pain behind the eye?**

Case 5 A man with early morning headaches

A 62-year-old coal miner is seen because he has developed weakness of his left hand. He has been getting severe headaches over the past 5 weeks, often present when he wakes in the morning and made worse when he bends over. On examination, he has moderate weakness of his left arm and hand but no sensory changes. He has bilateral papilledema. A CT scan shows a lesion about 3 cm in diameter in the right parietal lobe of the brain which enhances after contrast.

He is treated with dexamethasone and admitted to hospital a week later, when he says that his headache has improved dramatically. A stereotactic biopsy of the lesion is performed and biopsy samples are sent for histology.

The pathology report reveals that the lesion is a glioblastoma multiforme. The tumor is composed of very pleomorphic astroglial cells with numerous mitoses. There is proliferation of vascular endothelium and extensive tumor necrosis.

1. **How will this tumor behave clinically?**
2. **What is the prognosis?**

3. **Why was dexamethasone given prior to operation, leading to improvement in headache?**

Case 6 A man with progressive weakness

A retired naval commander, now aged 73, is admitted to hospital. He has increasing weakness in his hands and shoulders such that he finds it hard to lift his arms above his head. He has also developed weakness of his thighs and cannot pull himself up to stand unaided. On examination he has moderate weakness in the shoulder and pelvic girdle muscles. Investigations show a normal full blood count and ESR. His serum creatine kinase shows a slight elevation above normal. Administration of a short-acting anticholinesterase drug has no benefit on his muscle strength.

A needle muscle biopsy is performed from the vastus lateralis and sent to the laboratory for enzyme histochemistry and histology. The pathology report reads as follows:

Needle biopsy of muscle: There is abnormal fibre size variation with many scattered atrophic fibres. A small number of fibres are necrotic and undergoing phagocytosis. There is a focal infiltrate of lymphoid cells. Several muscle fibres show rimmed vacuoles and eosinophilic inclusions. Electron microscopy shows that these inclusions are filamentous. The appearances are those of inclusion-body myositis.

1. **What is the natural history of this disease?**
2. **What other inflammatory myopathies are there?**
3. **What are the reasons for administering anticholinesterase?**

Brief answers to these case-based questions are given on pages 594–5. More detailed answers and other study resources are available online at www.studentconsult.com.

Ophthalmic pathology 22

INTRODUCTION

The eye, the anatomy of which is shown in *Fig. 22.1*, is designed to focus light onto the specialized photoreceptors of the retina. Diseases of the eye are common and frequently present to family practitioners, arising from the whole range of pathological causes, including several systemic diseases.

This chapter will consider diseases affecting the eyelids, conjunctiva and cornea, and disorders affecting the pigmented uveal tissues, the lens, the retina and vitreous. The pathology of glaucoma, eye trauma, and space-occupying lesions of the orbit will be discussed.

DISEASES OF THE EYELIDS, CONJUNCTIVA AND CORNEA

Inflammatory and neoplastic diseases of the eyelids are common

The structure of the eyelid is shown in *Fig. 22.2*. The tarsal plate is a tough collagenous sheet in which the sebaceous-like meibomian glands are located. Minor skin-appendage glands are associated with the eyelashes. The conjunctiva, which is a two-layered columnar epithelium containing mucin-secreting goblet cells, lines the eyelids (palpebral

Fig. 22.1 Normal anatomy of the eye. The anterior and posterior chambers are filled with aqueous and are anterior to the lens. The vitreous is a specialized support tissue, not merely a gelatinous fluid.

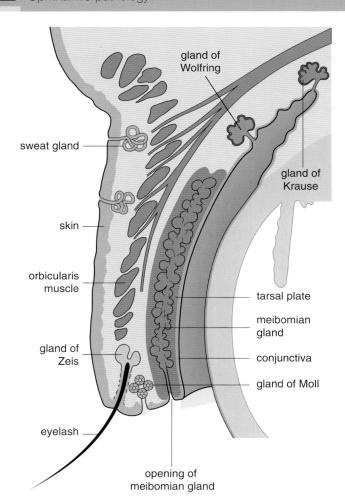

Fig. 22.2 Normal anatomy of the eyelid. The eyelid contains meibomian glands, which may become inflamed to form a chalazion. Cysts may develop from any of the skin appendages or mucous glands.

Fig. 22.3 Chalazion. A chalazion (meibomian cyst) develops as a result of blockage and inflammation of a meibomian gland. At first, lesions are red and tender, but later form firm nodules in the lid. Most resolve with local antibiotic ointment, but some require curettage. Lesions that do not resolve should be regarded with suspicion, as uncommon malignant tumors of the lid may present in this manner.

Fig. 22.4 Chalazion. A chalazion represents a histiocytic inflammatory response (**H**) to lipid material (**L**) released from damaged meibomian glands.

conjunctiva) and covers the anterior part of the globe (bulbar conjunctiva) up to the corneal epithelium (the limbus).

Diseases of the eyelids and conjunctiva are extremely common, ranging from self-limiting infections to malignant tumors.

Blockage and infection of a meibomian gland causes swelling and acute inflammation of the affected gland. A **chalazion** is a firm swelling in the eyelid, which bulges under the palpebral conjunctiva (see *Fig. 22.3*). Caused by rupture of a meibomian gland, histologically it consists of a foreign-body histiocytic chronic inflammatory response to lipid-rich material derived from the destroyed gland (*Fig. 22.4*).

The conjunctiva is frequently the site of infections causing **conjunctivitis**. Adenovirus types 3 and 7 cause follicular conjunctivitis, whereas types 8 and 19 cause epidemic kera-

toconjunctivitis. Allergic conjunctivitis is common in association with allergy to pollens. Bacterial conjunctivitis may also occur due to *Haemophilus* or, uncommonly, there may be neonatal infection with gonococcus. Granulomatous inflammation of the conjunctiva may be caused by several diseases, particularly sarcoidosis (see pages 567–9) and TB, and may arise with allergies such as hayfever. Involvement of the skin of the eyelid with molluscum contagiosum gives rise to typical umbilicated lesions (see page 511).

Proliferation of subepithelial support tissues gives rise to **pingueculas**, which are small areas of yellow thickening of the bulbar conjunctiva. Caused by cumulative exposure to damaging environmental stimuli such as sun, wind and dust, they increase in incidence with age. Similar areas that encroach over the limbus onto the cornea are termed **pterygia**.

The eyelids are the site of several tumors and cysts. The main tumors of the eyelid are derived from skin and skin appendages, and are histologically similar to those arising elsewhere in the skin (*Fig. 22.5*). Cysts may develop as a result of blockage and dilatation of skin appendages and minor glands in the eyelid.

- **Xanthelasmas**, plaque-like, yellow lesions seen in the skin around the eyelids, are collections of lipid-filled histiocytes in the dermis. They may be associated with hyperlipidemic states.
- **Conjunctival melanocytic nevi** are the most common tumor of the conjunctiva. They are classified in a similar way to those seen in the skin (see page 523).
- **Primary acquired melanosis** is the term used to describe flat, stippled pigmentation of the conjunctiva which develops in the elderly. Histologically such lesions may be entirely benign or may show cytological atypia when they may be a precursor lesion of conjunctival malignant melanoma.
- **Conjunctival papillomas** are benign, red polypoid lesions that arise from the palpebral or bulbar conjunctiva; some have a viral etiology.
- **Basal-cell carcinomas** are common tumors that involve the skin of the eyelid up to the lid margin (see *Fig. 22.5*). They are locally invasive and identical to those arising in other sites.
- **Squamous-cell carcinomas** arise from the skin of the eyelid or, less commonly, from the conjunctiva, where they may be preceded by intraepithelial carcinoma.
- **Malignant melanomas** can arise in the conjunctiva or from the skin of the eyelid. Both intraepithelial and invasive lesions are seen, which are like those described in the skin (see page 524).
- **Lymphomas** may develop in the conjunctiva, and these have the characteristics of a lymphoma of mucosal-associated lymphoid tissue (MALT).
- **Sebaceous gland carcinomas** are uncommon but highly malignant tumors arising from the meibomian glands.

Corneal diseases commonly cause scarring and loss of visual acuity

The cornea is covered by a non-keratinized squamous epithelium and is composed of a stroma with a lining endothelium. The endothelium is vital to normal corneal function because it actively pumps fluid out of the corneal stroma. The stroma is composed of highly organized parallel layers

Fig. 22.5 Eyelid tumor. In this case, this ulcerated lesion on the lid margin was a basal-cell carcinoma.

of collagen. Deposition of abnormal collagen leads to an opaque scar termed a **leukoma**.

Arcus senilis, seen as a yellow-white line at the corneal margin, is due to the accumulation of lipid in between the corneal stromal lamella. It is normal with aging, but when it arises in young patients is associated with hyperlipidemia.

Squamous metaplasia of the surface corneal epithelium may occur, causing corneal opacification. This is usually secondary to lack of normal lubrication by tears, e.g. in dry-eye syndromes, or when diseases prevent the eyelids covering the cornea. It can also be caused by vitamin A deficiency.

The important diseases of the cornea result in structural changes leading to opacification and impairment of visual acuity.

Minor trauma to the cornea can cause painful loss of surface epithelium, termed corneal abrasion. This may be complicated by secondary infection, but in most cases heals with regeneration.

Infective or inflammatory disorders of the cornea, which are collectively termed **keratitis**, can result in scarring leading to opacification. Infection is most commonly due to viruses (herpes simplex), *Chlamydia trachomatis* (causing trachoma) and bacteria.

Corneal edema is caused by loss of, or damage to, corneal endothelium. As the cornea becomes opaque due to the accumulation of interstitial fluid from failure of endothelial function, blurring of vision occurs. In severe cases, extremely painful bullae form beneath corneal surface epithelium, with secondary superficial scarring.

Keratoconus is characterized by abnormal thinning of central corneal stroma, leading to conical protrusion of the cornea associated with central scarring. This condition is associated with atopy and allergic conjunctivitis.

Corneal dystrophies are uncommon diseases (often inherited) that result in the deposition of abnormal material within the cornea, causing opacification. There are many different subtypes, which are categorized according to the site and nature of the abnormal material deposited, e.g. **lattice dystrophy** shows amyloid and **macular dystrophy** shows mucopolysaccharide accumulation.

Corneal transplantation is possible, replacing a damaged cornea by a healthy graft. Failure of grafts is mainly related to loss of endothelial cells in the donor graft causing development of corneal edema.

DISEASES OF THE UVEA

The uvea is an intermediate layer between the sclera and the retina. It contains blood vessels, nerves, support cells and melanocytes. Functionally the uvea is divided into three special areas: the choroid (beneath the retina), the ciliary body, and the iris.

Uveal inflammation is associated with several systemic diseases

The uvea is the site of several inflammatory processes, collectively known as **uveitis**. Depending on the preferential site of inflammation, these may be manifest as **choroiditis**, **iritis**, **cyclitis** (inflammation of ciliary body), **iridocyclitis** or, when all sites are involved, **generalized uveitis**.

Uveitis is one of the causes of an acutely painful, red, inflamed eye. Histologically, there is lymphocytic and sometimes granulomatous inflammation of the uvea. In **iritis** this causes exudates in the aqueous, which are visible as keratic precipitates. In **choroiditis**, inflammatory exudation can cause detachment of the retina, whereas inflammatory destruction of the pigment epithelial layer causes degeneration of overlying photoreceptors, which normally depend on this layer for support.

Uveitis can be caused by several disease processes, the most common being **immune mediated** and associated with other systemic diseases, such as sarcoidosis, rheumatoid disease, ankylosing spondylitis, Reiter's syndrome, and inflammatory bowel disease. Infection with **cytomegalovirus** or *Toxoplasma*, often as a complication of immunosuppression, can cause severe choroiditis leading to blindness. The larvae of *Toxocara canis* can reach the eye to cause severe inflammation in the choroid, spreading to the retina (**chorioretinitis**) and vitreous, at which stage blindness results.

Melanocytic tumors commonly arise in the uvea and may be benign or malignant

The melanocytes of the uvea are the cells of origin for benign melanocytic nevi as well as ocular malignant melanomas.

Most **benign melanocytic nevi** arise in the iris and are seen as abnormal areas of pigmentation. They often change in appearance with time, which brings them to medical attention. Most lesions are proliferations of spindle-shaped melanocytes.

Ocular malignant melanomas can arise anywhere in the uvea (5% arise in the iris, 10% in the ciliary body, and 85% in the choroid). Depending on the site of origin, tumors cause different types of symptom leading to impaired vision. Macroscopically, tumors are darkly pigmented lesions, typically 1–2 cm in diameter, which cause detachment of the overlying retina (*Fig. 22.6*). There are two main histological patterns of ocular melanoma:

- **Spindle-cell melanomas** tend to have little pleomorphism and few mitoses, and are usually localized to the globe. If they are excised completely, 10-year survival is around 90%.
- **Epithelioid melanomas** show large cells with pleomorphism and many mitoses. This type is associated with a 10-year survival of 35%, orbital invasion frequently being encountered at time of diagnosis.

Spread of ocular melanomas occurs directly into the orbit, or hematogenously to cause systemic metastasis. Late manifestation of metastatic disease from excised orbital melanomas is a well-recognized phenomenon.

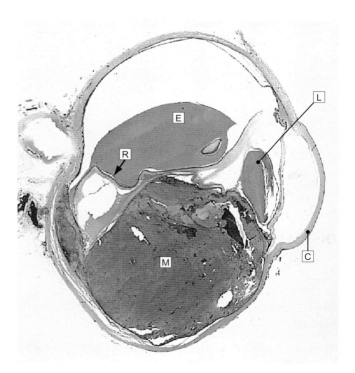

Fig. 22.6 Uveal malignant melanoma. Histological section of globe (lens (**L**), cornea (**C**)) showing mass of melanoma (**M**). The retina (**R**) has become detached with a subretinal exudate (**E**).

LENS ABNORMALITIES

Dislocation of the lens may be spontaneous or traumatic in origin

The lens is normally suspended by fibers of the ciliary zonule, which are composed of the protein fibrillin, and attached to the ciliary body. When dislocation of the lens occurs, which may be spontaneous or traumatic, the lens becomes detached from its normal position. In anterior dislocation the lens falls forward, obstructs the pupil, and causes acute glaucoma (see page 501). In posterior dislocation the lens falls back towards the vitreous, with loss of visual acuity.

Spontaneous dislocation is predisposed to by Marfan's syndrome, caused by mutation in one of the genes for fibrillin. Traumatic dislocation is seen with both penetrating and non-penetrating injuries (see page 502).

Cataracts, which are areas of opacification in the lens, have a wide range of causes

The normal lens is composed of a capsule, lens epithelial cells, and a central mass of tightly packed cells that have lost their nuclei and contain highly stable transparent proteins termed 'crystallins.' In cataract formation there is degeneration of lens crystallins, which become opaque. Structural changes in the lens occur, with hyaline globules, liquefaction, and focal calcification. Degenerate lens material may gain access to the aqueous, where it is phagocytosed by macrophages and may cause blockage of the trabecular meshwork, leading to secondary open-angle glaucoma (see page 502).

The main cause of cataracts is thought to be metabolic derangement in lens nutrition, which is derived from diffusion from the aqueous. There are several predisposing factors. The most common cataracts are those that develop with age (**senile cataracts**). Predisposing conditions include trauma, diabetes mellitus, corticosteroid therapy, inflammation in the globe (e.g. uveitis), glaucoma, and irradiation of the eye. Congenital cataracts may develop after rubella infection in utero.

DISEASES OF THE RETINA AND VITREOUS

Retinal diseases are mainly inflammatory, vascular or degenerative in etiology

The retina is the specialized neural layer of the eye. It contains the photoreceptors (rods and cones), which detect light, and the interneurons, which integrate input into the retinal ganglion cells (which give rise to the axons in the optic nerve). The ends of the retinal photoreceptors are embedded in the pigment epithelium of the uvea, which provides essential metabolic support. At its surface the retina is separated from the vitreous by a basement membrane, underlining the fact that the vitreous is not merely a ball of fluid, but a complex transparent support tissue that contains cells as well as specialized matrix proteins.

The retina can be secondarily damaged by several disease processes, such as disorders of vasculature (discussed below) and inflammatory diseases of the choroid, or there may be secondary damage from the high pressure in the globe caused by glaucoma (see page 501). Primary retinal diseases are degenerative or, uncommonly, infective.

Age-related macular degeneration (ARMD) is one of the most common causes of severe loss of vision in the elderly. AMD is characterized by progressive loss of central vision caused by degenerative and neovascular changes in the macula region.

- Early AMD shows protein/lipid masses termed drusen in the choroid beneath the retinal pigment epithelium. This stage is not associated with significant loss of acuity.
- Late AMD shows atrophy of the retinal pigment epithelium (geographic atrophy) and growth of new blood vessels into the retina from the choroid, which may bleed. This stage is associated with significant loss of acuity.

Several gene loci are now linked to increased risk for the development of AMD.

Pigmentary retinopathy is a term applied to a group of diseases in which there is retinal degeneration associated with melanin pigment migrating from the choroid to be sequestered in macrophages located around retinal vessels. The main type encountered is the hereditary disease **retinitis pigmentosa**. Other causes are secondary to primary neurometabolic storage diseases (see pages 92 and 478).

Infection by *Toxoplasma*, **cytomegalovirus** and **herpes** is seen in immunosuppressed patients, particularly those with AIDS, and is growing in importance as a cause of blindness.

Loss of retinal ganglion cells due to retinal disease causes optic nerve atrophy, seen as a small pale optic disc on fundoscopy. This indicates severe irreversible retinal damage, as retinal neurons cannot be replaced once lost.

Vascular diseases of the retina are a common cause of blindness

Vascular disorders are a major cause of eye disease, having their main impact on the retina. The main predisposing factors for vascular disease are hypertension and diabetes mellitus. Retinal complications of diabetes mellitus are now one of the most common causes of blindness in western countries.

Among the main vascular diseases is **benign hypertension**, which is associated with the development of hyaline thickening in retinal vessels. In accelerated-phase hypertension, flame hemorrhages, exudates, and areas of retinal ischemia develop, causing microinfarcts termed **cotton-wool spots**.

Diabetic retinal disease causes thickening of the basement membrane of capillaries and hyaline arteriolosclerosis. **Microaneurysms** occur as dilatations of arterioles and capillaries with abnormally fragile and permeable walls. Exudates develop, with 'blot hemorrhages' from leaking capillary vessels. Areas of ischemia cause **cotton-wool spots**. Retinal ischemia causes secretion of angiogenesis factors, inducing formation of new vessels (**proliferative retinopathy**).

Neovascularization is the term used to describe the formation of new vessels on the inner surface of the retina (leading to hemorrhages) and on the anterior surface of the iris (leading to secondary closed-angle glaucoma).

Retinal artery occlusion occurs with blockage of the central retinal artery as a result of embolism or, less commonly, from vasculitis such as giant-cell arteritis (see page 169). The retina undergoes necrosis and there is loss of retinal ganglion cells, leading to optic atrophy and proliferation of retinal glial cells (**retinal gliosis**).

Retinal vein occlusion is predisposed to by polycythemia and chronic glaucoma. Thrombosis leads to suffusion of the retina with blood, resulting in widespread hemorrhage.

In retinal detachment the retina is separated from the pigment epithelium, thereby losing metabolic support

Retinal detachment occurs when the neural retinal layer becomes separated from the retinal pigment epithelium. Provided that the photoreceptor layer is brought back into contact, the retina may regain function; however, prolonged detachment leads to loss of metabolic support from the retinal pigment epithelium, with degeneration of photoreceptor cells and permanent loss of function.

There are three main reasons for retinal detachment:

- **Traction on the retina** from abnormalities in the vitreous. This occurs with organization of previous trauma or with development of neovascularization. In diabetic proliferative retinopathy this is termed **vasoproliferative retinopathy** (VPR).
- **Shearing of the retina** may cause the formation of small retinal tears and the development of detachment. These tears are predisposed by degenerative conditions of the retina or vitreous and develop when the vitreous focally loses contact with the retina at the vitreoretinal junction. This loss of contact is predisposed to in patients with severe myopia.
- **Pressure on the retina** from accumulation of fluid in the subretinal space, commonly from inflammatory exudate, hemorrhage, or neoplasm.

Retinoblastoma is an uncommon tumor of childhood

Retinoblastoma is a very rare malignant tumor of the retina, occurring in children under the age of 5 years. Its importance lies in the fact that it is inherited in about a third of cases, and molecular genetics have shown it to be predisposed to by loss of a specific tumor-suppressor gene termed RB. Patients with the heritable form have a high incidence of bilateral disease, whereas patients with sporadic disease tend to have unilateral tumor.

Composed of primitive neuroblast-like cells, lesions macroscopically appear as a mass of white tissue that arises in the retina and replaces the vitreous. Tumors behave aggressively, with spread to the orbit and along the optic nerve to the CNS. Children present with enlargement of the globe, or with a white pupil due to tumor in the vitreous.

Pathology of common fundoscopic abnormalities

Papilledema is swelling of the optic disc, a clinical sign seen on fundoscopy. However, this is not simply edema as seen in other tissues. The swelling is due to pressure on the optic nerve as it enters the CSF-filled optic nerve sheath, usually the result of a focal lesion causing raised intracranial pressure. The increased pressure on the optic nerve leads to impairment of the normal flow of cytoplasm along the axon, causing the axons to become dilated and swollen. More severe pressure on the optic nerve impairs venous return and leads to development of secondary hemorrhages in the retina.

Hard exudates are lipid-rich accumulations of plasma proteins, which leak out of vessels and accumulate in the outer plexiform layer.

Cotton-wool spots are areas of microinfarction in the retina. The spots are the ballooned ends of damaged retinal axons.

Flame hemorrhages are caused by disease affecting arterioles. The flame shape is caused by blood tracking in the superficial nerve-fiber layer.

Blot hemorrhages are caused by capillary rupture deep in the outer plexiform layer of the retina.

Silver wiring of vessels is caused by arteriolosclerosis of retinal vessels, which demonstrate replacement of their walls by hyaline material.

GLAUCOMA

In glaucoma there is raised intraocular pressure, which damages the retina

A very common syndrome in which there is increased intraocular pressure, glaucoma affects 2% of the population over the age of 40 years. It is important in that if it remains untreated, blindness develops.

The maintenance of normal intraocular pressure is achieved through the continuous secretion of aqueous by the ciliary body being balanced by its removal from the anterior chamber by filtration from the trabecular meshwork at the periphery of the iris into the canal of Schlemm. In glaucoma the balance is disturbed, nearly always by an abnormality in the filtration and removal of aqueous.

There are two main clinical syndromes. **Chronic glaucoma** occurs with gradual increase in intraocular pressure, leading to slow, gradual deterioration in visual acuity if untreated. **Acute glaucoma** is associated with a rapid increase in intraocular pressure, which causes severe pain and redness in the eye, and rapid deterioration in visual function (this can be permanent if not urgently treated).

The effects of raised intraocular pressure are **cupping and atrophy of the optic disc**, detected on fundoscopy, and **degeneration of retinal ganglion cells**. Clinically, there is progressive peripheral visual-field loss, leading to blindness in untreated cases. In acute glaucoma there is breakdown of the endothelium, leading to edema of the cornea and formation of painful corneal bullae. In chronic glaucoma the sclera may stretch to form bulges termed **staphylomas**.

In glaucoma there is interference with filtration of aqueous at the trabecular meshwork

There are several common causes of glaucoma, divisible into primary and secondary.

Primary glaucoma is caused by two main abnormalities in the drainage of aqueous:

- Closing-up of the trabecular meshwork, which normally leads to the canal of Schlemm, can occur as a degenerative process, the incidence of which increases with age; it is mainly encountered in those over the age of 40, often being familial. Because the drainage angle is normal, this is termed **primary open-angle glaucoma** (*Fig. 22.7a*).
- With age, some patients develop narrowing of the angle between the iris and the cornea, causing functional blockage to aqueous drainage. This may be predisposed by the normal reduction of the size of the eye with aging, and the normal increase in the size of the lens with age. An acute attack occurs particularly when the pupil is dilated, as the iris thickens with contraction. Acute attacks may therefore be precipitated by being in the dark. Because the drainage angle is abnormal, this is termed **primary closed-angle glaucoma** (*Fig. 22.7b*).

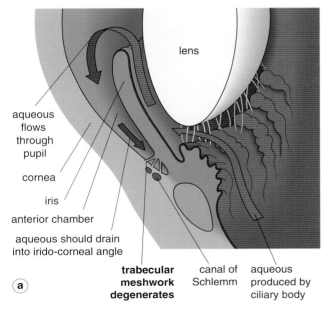

lens

aqueous flows through pupil

cornea

iris

anterior chamber

aqueous should drain into irido-corneal angle

trabecular meshwork degenerates   canal of Schlemm   aqueous produced by ciliary body

(a)

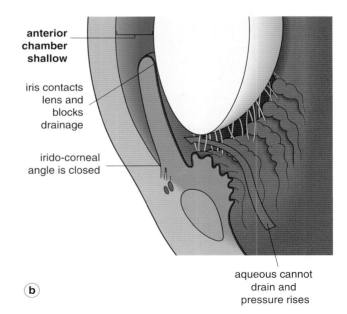

anterior chamber shallow

iris contacts lens and blocks drainage

irido-corneal angle is closed

aqueous cannot drain and pressure rises

(b)

Fig. 22.7 Glaucoma. (a) Primary open-angle glaucoma. With age, the channels in the trabecular meshwork degenerate. However, aqueous continues to be produced, so the pressure in the eye increases. As the angle between the cornea and iris root is normal (open), this is termed open-angle glaucoma. (b) Primary closed-angle glaucoma. If the anterior chamber becomes shallow, the drainage angle is functionally closed. If the pupil dilates, this further compromises the drainage of aqueous and may precipitate an acute attack of glaucoma.

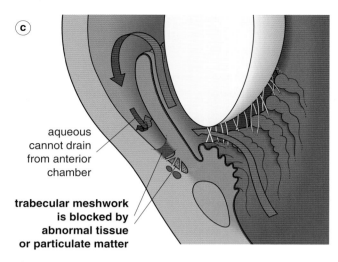

(c)

aqueous
cannot drain
from anterior
chamber

**trabecular meshwork
is blocked by
abnormal tissue
or particulate matter**

Fig. 22.7 (c) Secondary glaucoma. If abnormal tissue (e.g. new blood vessels) blocks the trabecular meshwork, then aqueous cannot drain and glaucoma may develop; this is termed secondary closed-angle glaucoma. If particulate matter (such as inflammatory cells) occludes the trabecular meshwork, it is termed secondary open-angle glaucoma, as the iridocorneal angle remains open.

Secondary glaucoma is caused by diseases that obstruct the drainage of aqueous. For example, there may be adhesions between the iris and cornea that are caused by uveitis or are secondary to vascular proliferation due to retinal ischemia (**secondary closed-angle glaucoma**). Alternatively, there may be blockage of the trabecular meshwork by particulate material in the aqueous, especially degenerate lens material, pigment from melanocytic lesions, or macrophages accumulating in response to hemorrhage or inflammation (**secondary open-angle glaucoma**) (*Fig. 22.7c*).

Congenital glaucoma seen in childhood with enlargement of the globe, is very rare. It is mainly due to developmental defects in the drainage of aqueous.

TRAUMA TO THE EYE

Trauma to the eye is a common cause of visual impairment

Mostly preventable by the use of suitable eye protection, trauma is a common cause of eye disease. Damage may be immediately apparent, or may develop after the injury as a secondary complication.

- **Contusion of the globe** can cause intraocular hemorrhage or tearing of the retina and uvea.
- **Dislocation of the lens** may occur with severe trauma
- **Penetrating injuries** (those that pass into the cornea) cause permanent scarring if there is damage to Bowman's membrane, whereas **perforating injuries** (those that pass through cornea) can be complicated

by hemorrhage or infection. Healing of a corneal perforation may be complicated by adhesion of the iris to the back of the cornea at the site of injury.
- **Secondary glaucoma** is an important complication of bleeding into the anterior chamber.
- **Siderosis bulbi** is caused by retention of an iron-containing foreign body in the globe. Iron pigment is deposited within the tissues of the eye, causing retinal degeneration.
- **Sympathetic ophthalmitis** is an uncommon T-cell-mediated immune response causing granulomatous inflammation in a normal eye that has been stimulated by damage to the other eye. The trigger for this immune reaction is exposure of retinal antigens (normally sequestered by a blood–retinal barrier) to the immune system after trauma to the globe. Histologically, there is severe granulomatous inflammation of the eye. The development of this condition can be prevented if the damaged eye is removed.

DISEASES OF THE ORBIT

Diseases of the orbit present with displacement of the eye (**proptosis**) or orbital pain. The main causes for swelling in the orbit are thyroid eye disease, vascular lesions, inflammatory diseases, and tumors. Clinical evaluation includes imaging of the orbit to establish the site and nature of the swelling, followed in many cases by biopsy. Thyroid disease (Graves' disease) may cause orbital swelling and proptosis owing to the accumulation of extracellular matrix material in the orbital tissues.

Orbital inflammatory diseases are of diverse etiology

Orbital inflammatory diseases present as swelling of the orbit, proptosis, and orbital pain. There are many causes for inflammation in the orbit, and biopsy is sometimes performed to establish a cause and to distinguish lesions from infiltration by tumor. These conditions were once called orbital pseudotumors, a name that should be avoided as a mass (tumor) is not always evident on investigation. Arteritis, connective tissue diseases, fungal infection, and specific inflammatory conditions related to the sclera can all present in this manner.

Vascular lesions are the most common cause of orbital swellings in adults

Vascular lesions and tumors are a common cause of orbital mass lesions. Rapid increase in size may be caused by thrombosis within a lesion.

Cavernous hemangiomas are well-circumscribed lesions 1–2 cm in diameter. The most common orbital tumors seen in adults, they are usually easy to remove surgically.

Capillary hemangiomas are poorly circumscribed lesions, most commonly seen in childhood. Their extensive involvement of orbital tissues makes surgical treatment very difficult.

Lymphangiomas may involve the orbit and, based on the extent of orbital involvement, can be divided into superficial, deep, and combined types.

Hemangiopericytomas are tumors derived from the vascular-related pericytes. They vary in malignant potential, 30% being locally recurrent, even if histologically benign.

In addition to these lesions, less well-defined AVMs and varicose veins are also encountered within the orbit.

Lymphoma is the most common type of primary malignant orbital tumor

The most common primary tumor of the orbit is non-Hodgkin's lymphoma. The majority are low-grade B-cell tumors. Burkitt's lymphoma, a high-grade lymphoblastic B-cell tumor, is the most common orbital tumor in some parts of Africa.

Macroscopically, tumors form masses within the orbit, often involving the extraocular muscles. Many arise from the lacrimal gland. Benign reactive lymphoid infiltrates of the orbit are also seen and must be distinguished from lymphomas by immunohistochemistry.

Orbital tumors of mesodermal and neural origin may be benign or malignant

Orbital tumors may arise from neural or mesodermal tissues. Different tumors, both benign and malignant, are encountered in different age groups.

Extension of an ocular tumor into the orbit is a frequent development, the main ocular tumors being retinoblastoma in childhood (see page 500), and uveal melanoma in adults (see page 498).

Rhabdomyosarcoma of the orbit is a tumor of childhood, being of the embryonal subtype. Although highly malignant, treatment with radiotherapy and chemotherapy shows a 3-year survival rate of 93%.

Fibrous histiocytoma is the most common mesenchymal tumor of the orbit in adults. It is a spindle-cell tumor composed of fibroblast-like cells and histiocyte-like cells with a collagenous matrix, classified into benign, locally aggressive, and malignant types. As they are poorly circumscribed, these tumors often recur, with a recurrence rate of 30% for benign lesions, 57% for locally aggressive lesions, and 64% for malignant lesions.

Fibro-osseous lesions from the skull often encroach on the orbit, particularly fibromatoses, primary bone tumors, fibrous dysplasia of bone, and Langerhans' cell histiocytosis (histiocytosis X) (see page 327).

Benign nerve-sheath tumors account for about 2% of all orbital tumors. They are either well-circumscribed schwannomas (neurilemmomas) or less easily excised plexiform neurofibromas.

Meningiomas of the orbit arise from the arachnoidal meningothelial cells of the optic nerve sheath and are similar to those that occur in the CNS.

Optic-nerve gliomas are astrocytomas of low-grade malignancy, classed as juvenile pilocytic astrocytomas. Histologically they are spindle-cell tumors with a fine fibrillarity.

Metastatic tumors in the orbit are most commonly from breast, lung, kidney and prostate

Metastatic tumor commonly involves the orbit, tumors of the breast, lung, kidney and prostate being the most commonly reported. The diagnosis of the primary site of a metastatic deposit can be aided by immunocytochemistry to determine the presence of marker substances within tumor cells. This is particularly useful with small samples removed from the orbit in cases in which the pathologist is not aided by architectural features of the tumor.

Clinically, diffuse invasion of the orbital tissues produces proptosis, pain from involvement of nerves, and paralysis of eye movements. In severe cases the eye is immobile (a frozen orbit).

Developmental lesions of the orbit are common in childhood

In childhood, developmental lesions account for many orbital swellings. Among the most common types are dermoid cysts lined by squamous epithelium, with skin appendages such as sebaceous glands, hair follicles, and sweat glands in the wall. These account for 46% of all orbital tumors in childhood, and for 24% of all tumors in all age groups.

Brain heterotopias may affect the orbit and are part of the spectrum of neural-tube defects (see pages 476–8). Anterior encephalocele may involve the orbit, with meninges, glial tissue or brain tissue present in the orbit.

Lacrimal gland swellings may be inflammatory or neoplastic

Enlargement of lacrimal gland may be due to specific or non-specific inflammation (including granulomatous diseases), or to primary (benign and malignant) and metastatic neoplasms.

Infection (commonly due to bacteria) of the lacrimal gland or ducts may cause swelling. Blockage of the duct may occur with local overgrowth of *Actinomyces*, forming the basis for a calculus composed of filamentous organisms.

Cysts of the lacrimal gland or associated ducts are common. Some are developmental dermoid cysts, whereas others are retention cysts caused by duct blockage.

Sjögren's disease is associated with autoimmune infiltration and enlargement of the gland by lymphoid cells, with gland loss causing dry eyes.

Sarcoidosis (see pages 567 et seq.) is associated with expansion of the gland by non-caseating granulomas.

Lymphoma of the lacrimal gland is the most common primary tumor (usually low-grade B-cell non-Hodgkin's lymphoma of MALT type).

Case-based questions

Case 1 – A man with deteriorating vision

A 58-year-old electrician has been referred by his optician to the eye clinic. He has noticed some deterioration in his vision and was noted by his optician to have early cupping of the optic disc. The pressure in his eye was measured by tonometry and found to be elevated, and a diagnosis of glaucoma is made. Examination of the iridocorneal angle shows that it is open, with a normal anterior chamber.

1. **What is the pathogenesis of primary open angle glaucoma?**
2. **What other types of glaucoma are there?**
3. **What is the natural history of untreated glaucoma?**

Case 2 – A painful lump in the eyelid

A 38-year-old man is referred to the eye clinic because of a red, painful swelling in his upper eyelid. This had developed over a 2-week period. On examination an area of thickening is noted in the upper eyelid. When the lid is everted an ill-defined area of yellow discoloration is seen beneath the conjunctiva. A clinical diagnosis of a chalazion is made.

1. **How do you explain the nature of a chalazion to the patient?**

Brief answers to these case-based questions are given on page 595. More detailed answers and other study resources are available online at www.studentconsult.com.

Skin disease 23

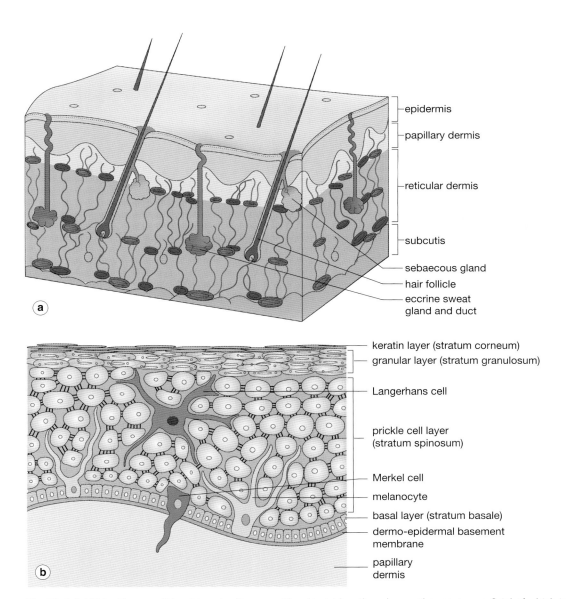

epidermis
papillary dermis
reticular dermis
subcutis
sebaecous gland
hair follicle
eccrine sweat gland and duct

a

keratin layer (stratum corneum)
granular layer (stratum granulosum)
Langerhans cell
prickle cell layer (stratum spinosum)
Merkel cell
melanocyte
basal layer (stratum basale)
dermo-epidermal basement membrane
papillary dermis

b

Fig. 23.1 (a) Skin-diagram (b) epidermis-diagram. The skin (a) has three layers, the most superficial of which is the **epidermis** (b), the dermis and the deep subcutis. The **dermis** is collagenous, with elastin fibres, loose and fine in the papillary dermis, but dense and compact in reticular dermis. The **subcutis** is mainly adipose tissue. The dermis contains the sweat glands which open onto the surface; hair follicles originate in dermis or subcutis, and the sebaceous glands discharge into them before they open onto the surface. The epidermis (b) comprises a stratified squamous epithelium generated by a dividing basal layer. The cells of the main prickle cell layer are linked by desmosomes; the cells flatten near the surface and acquire granules of keratohyaline which produce the surface keratin layer. Also present are basal melanocytes (which produce melanin), Merkel cells (which are receptors connected to nerves) and Langerhans' cells (which are antigen-recognition cells)

INTRODUCTION

Most epithelial surfaces, e.g. those lining the respiratory, alimentary and urinary tracts, show a very limited range of disease processes, rarely more than half a dozen common inflammatory disorders, and a similar number of neoplastic or growth disorders. In contrast, the skin exhibits many hundreds of different inflammatory patterns and probably 30 or 40 tumors or tumor-like lesions, the great majority of which are common. The breadth of dermatopathology is therefore immense; fortunately, much of the detail lies within the province of the specialist clinical dermatologist and dermatopathologist, and is not essential for medical students and non-specialist doctors.

The study of dermatopathology is further complicated by the fact that the pathogenesis of many of the skin conditions is unknown. In addition, the nomenclature of the various skin lesions, particularly for inflammatory skin diseases, is an arcane mixture of Latin and Greek that disguises the fact that the nomenclature is purely descriptive of the visual appearance of the rash. Thus, euphonious but uninformative names such as 'pityriasis lichenoides et varioliformis acuta' exist.

DERMATITIS

'Dermatitis' is the name given to inflammatory lesions in the skin, irrespective of whether they involve dermis or epidermis; in most cases both components of the skin are involved.

Some patterns of inflammatory skin disease have characteristic features, e.g. lichenoid dermatitis, psoriasiform dermatitis (see below), which enable them to be identified more accurately, both clinically and histologically. Other patterns are caused by microorganisms such as bacteria (e.g. impetigo, folliculitis), fungi (e.g. athlete's foot, ringworm), viruses (e.g. herpes, varicella) or other organisms (e.g. scabies), but many are **non-specific**. The most common pattern of non-specific dermatitis is traditionally called **eczema**, and may have many causes.

Non-specific (eczematous) dermatitis may be acute, subacute or chronic

In acute dermatitis the skin becomes red (erythema), itchy and tender, with tiny blisters called **vesicles** forming in the epidermis (*Fig. 23.2*). The vesicles burst, discharging clear, yellow fluid, and then crust over. The reddening of the skin is due to a chronic inflammatory cell infiltrate around blood vessels in the upper dermis; leakage of fluid from the vessels may produce swelling of the upper dermis, which may cause the lesion to be slightly raised above the level of normal skin.

Vesicles develop because fluid accumulates between the epidermal cells (**spongiosis**), eventually forming small fluid-filled collections. Some of the chronic inflammatory cells around the vessels in the upper dermis may migrate into the epidermis. The vesicles enlarge until they burst onto the surface.

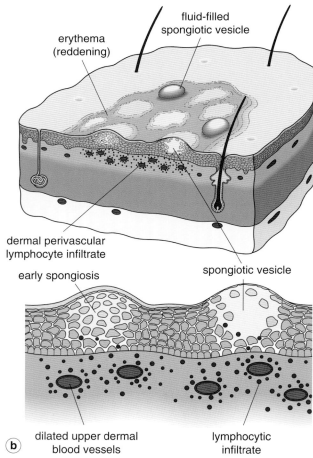

Fig. 23.2 Acute dermatitis. (a) Typical acute dermatitis with reddening (erythema) of the skin and numerous tiny vesicles, some of which have burst as a result of scratching because of severe itch. (b) The histological basis of erythema and of vesicle formation.

Because the lesion is itchy in the acute stage, it is almost invariably scratched by the patient. As a result, secondary changes occur due to repeated trauma rather than the background skin disease. Repeated trauma to lesions of acute eczema leads to **chronic dermatitis**.

Chronic non-specific dermatitis is usually the result of chronic trauma to the lesions of acute dermatitis. The skin is thickened, often cracked, and covered by thick, opaque scale (*Fig. 23.3*). This scale is a greatly thickened layer of

rete ridge   dermal
elongation   collagenization   hyperkeratosis   acanthosis

Fig. 23.3 Chronic dermatitis. (**a**) Close-up of chronic dermatitis with raised areas of skin thickening due to chronic scratching of a healing acute dermatitis. (**b**) The histological basis of chronic dermatitis.

surface keratin (**hyperkeratosis**), which overlies an epidermis markedly thickened by increase in the number of cells in the various layers (particularly stratum spinosum and the granular layer). Such thickening, termed **acanthosis**, is a common feature of many types of chronic inflammatory skin diseases of many types.

The epidermis also shows elongation and accentuation of the rete ridge system, an arrangement that, in normal skin, is designed to resist shearing forces. The dermis shows increased fibrosis, with prominent thick-walled vessels.

Constant scratching and picking at itchy inflammatory lesions in the skin leads to localized lesions with greatly thickened epidermis and thick horny keratin scale on top, together with localized fibrous thickening of the dermis. Called **prurigo nodularis**, the lesions often continue to be picked and traumatized so that there is surface ulceration, a lesion sometimes called 'picker's nodule.'

The term **subacute dermatitis** is sometimes used to describe skin inflammation in which there are features of chronic dermatitis (acanthosis, hyperkeratosis, dermal fibrosis, etc.), but with the addition of active spongiosis and vesicle formation.

The cause of non-specific dermatitis usually has to be inferred from the distribution and nature of the rash rather than from histological differences

Among the most common types of non-specific dermatitis seen in community practice is **atopic dermatitis**. Often starting in infancy and childhood but persisting into adult life, this pattern is associated with a strong family history, e.g. the patient and other family members may have asthma, hayfever or a predisposition to urticarial skin rashes. The atopic state, and its mechanisms, are discussed in Chapter 7.

Gravitational dermatitis (*Fig. 23.4a*) affects the ankle and lower leg of patients with varicose veins, and is sometimes called **varicose eczema**. The dermatitis features are superimposed on chronic changes in the skin due to inadequate venous drainage, e.g. thick-walled dermal vessels or extravasation of red blood cells (leading to brown pigmentation by hemosiderin).

Irritant contact dermatitis (*Fig. 23.4b*), which is due to contact of the skin with strong agents such as detergents and alkalis, most commonly affects the hands. The disease is particularly common in housewives who do not wear gloves when handling strong detergents, and in some people who have occupational exposure.

Allergic contact dermatitis is usually a reaction to metals such as nickel, materials in cosmetics, dye mixtures and rubber. It tends to occur in people who have a probable inherited predisposition, and the lesions are localized to the site of contact, e.g. around the wrist in response to nickel in the back or strap of a watch.

Fig. 23.4 Common clinical patterns of dermatitis. (a) Gravitational dermatitis. (b) Irritant contact dermatitis due to immersion of hands in strong detergent. (c) Seborrheic dermatitis in a young girl.

In **seborrheic dermatitis** (*Fig. 23.4c*) the reddened and inflamed skin is covered by thick waxy or white scale. In infants this is largely confined to the scalp (**cradle cap**), whereas in adults the face is also involved. Obese elderly people may develop this pattern in skin creases. This condition has recently been linked with *Pityrosporum* yeasts.

Other specific patterns of dermatitis include lichenoid, pityriasiform, and psoriasiform types

In addition to the eczematous pattern just described, there are other patterns of dermatitis which are grouped together because they share clinical and histological features. The most common are:

- **Lichenoid dermatitis**, the most common example of which is **lichen planus**.
- **Pityriasiform dermatitis**, the most common example of which is **pityriasis rosea**.
- **Psoriasiform dermatitis**, the most common example of which is classic **psoriasis**.

Lichen planus is the most common type of lichenoid dermatitis

Lichen planus is a common inflammatory skin disease that often affects the flexor aspects of the forearm, wrist and ankle. It also occurs on the trunk, as well as affecting various mucosal surfaces, particularly in the mouth and vulva; it occasionally arises on the penis. On the skin the lesions are raised, itchy papules, often purplish red in color, which sometimes form flat and shiny raised plaques (*Fig. 23.5*). The cause is unknown and the lesions often persist for many months or even years. When each lesion resolves, it frequently leaves a pigmented patch of flat skin.

The main histological abnormality in lichen planus is damage to the basal layer of the epidermis, destroying both basal cells and any contained melanocytes. It is this destruction of basal melanocytes that allows melanin to drop down into the dermis, where it accumulates in dermal macrophages, giving a healed lesion a brown discoloration. Associated with the destruction of the basal layer is a characteristic pattern of lymphocytic infiltration, which is closely applied to the dermoepidermal junction in the upper dermis. This pattern of inflammation is called **lichenoid** and can occasionally be seen in other skin conditions.

Lichen planus affecting the buccal and genital mucosae has a tendency to lead to separation of the epidermis from the underlying submucosa, as a result of destruction of the basal layer of the epidermis. The ensuing erosion leaves naked areas of inflamed submucosa (see Figs 19.3 and 12.4); this change rarely occurs in skin. Another variant of lichen planus, **follicular lichen planus**, causes destruction of the basal layer of hair follicles, which may result in hair loss; follicular lichen planus is one of the causes of inflammatory **alopecia** (see pages 531–2 and 562).

Destruction of the basal layer of the epidermis associated with a lichenoid pattern of upper dermal inflammatory cell infiltrate can be seen in some cutaneous reactions to drugs – '**lichenoid drug reaction**,' which may show some, but not all of the typical clinical features of classic lichen planus.

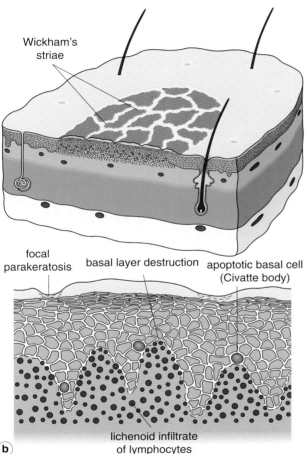

Wickham's striae

focal parakeratosis   basal layer destruction   apoptotic basal cell (Civatte body)

lichenoid infiltrate of lymphocytes

Fig. 23.5 Lichen planus. (a) Clinical appearance of raised, red plaques with thick, opaque, white lines (Wickham's striae). (b) The histopathological basis of lichen planus.

Other examples of lichenoid dermatitis include **lichen sclerosus,** which is particularly common on the skin of the vulva (see Chapter 19, page 414) and the glans penis (where it is still sometimes called **balanitis xerotica obliterans** (see Chapter 18, page 411).

Pityriasiform dermatitis is characterized by fine surface scale, due to parakeratosis

Despite its name (pityriasis is derived from the Greek word *pityron*, meaning 'bran' because of the supposed resemblance of the skin scale to fine flakes of bran), the surface scale formation in the pityriasiform skin diseases is much less marked than in psoriasis (see page 510). A number of skin diseases are called 'pityriasis,' although they share few clinical and histological features:

- **Pityriasis rosea** is the most common (see below).
- **Pityriasis versicolor** is a common pattern of fungal skin disease, presenting as patches of skin discoloration with fine surface scale.
- **Pityriasis lichenoides acuta** and **chronica** are both quite uncommon, only the chronic form having significant surface scale.
- **Pityriasis rubra pilaris**, of which there are many patterns, with variable degrees of scaling. Hair follicles plugged with keratin are a common feature.

Pityriasis rosea is the most common pityriasiform dermatitis seen in family practice

Pityriasis rosea is a common skin condition in young people, a typical pityriasis lesion being a red patch with a rim of scale. The first lesion is usually a large patch, up to 2 cm in diameter ('herald patch'), but subsequent lesions are usually smaller; all are characterized by an area of scale that begins in the center of the lesion, spreading peripherally as the lesion enlarges (*Fig. 23.6*). The generalized eruption usually follows 1–2 weeks after the onset of the enlarging herald patch, beginning on the chest and abdomen and later spreading to the limbs. The rash lasts for a couple of weeks before slowly resolving, but recurrences are not uncommon. The disease often follows a period of nonspecific malaise or a systemic viral infection.

Fig. 23.6 Pityriasis rosea. This close photograph of two pityriasis rosea lesions shows redness and irregularity of the skin surface, with a peripheral ring of white scaling.

The most common type of psoriasiform dermatitis is classic psoriasis

Psoriasis (*Fig. 23.7*) is a chronic intermittent disease in which red, raised plaques covered by thick, white scale

thick parakeratotic scale on red background

patches of parakeratosis containing neutrophil nuclear debris

dilated clubbed papillae containing dilated capillaries

neutrophil infiltrate

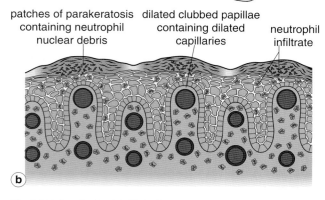

Fig. 23.7 Psoriasis. (a) Clinical appearance showing typical red patches covered with thick, white scale; note the nail involvement. (b) The histopathological basis of psoriasis.

appear on the knees, elbows, trunk and scalp. They may also occur in skin creases, where the silvery-white surface scale is often less obvious and may even be absent. A characteristic feature is that when the scale is lifted off, it reveals small areas of punctate bleeding.

Histologically, the scale is composed of flakes of thickened surface keratin, which contain remnants of the nuclei from the superficial squames from which they are derived (**parakeratosis**). The epidermis shows a characteristic pattern of abnormality, with long rete ridges separated by markedly edematous papillary dermis in which there are large numbers of dilated capillaries. It is these capillaries that bleed when the scale is lifted, for the epidermis overlying the swollen papillary dermis is often very thin. Another characteristic feature of psoriasis is that the major inflammatory cell involved is the neutrophil polymorph; these cells migrate through the epidermis and may be trapped beneath the thickened horny layer (Monro microabscesses). In some types of psoriasis very large numbers of neutrophil polymorphs migrate through the epidermis, accumulating beneath the parakeratotic scale to form neutrophil collections visible to the naked eye as yellowish purulent blobs (**pustules**). Known as **pustular psoriasis**, this pattern commonly affects the palms and the soles. Psoriasis may also affect the nail bed, leading to pitting, thickening and eventual destruction of the nail.

Inflammatory skin disease with some of the clinical and histological features of psoriasis can also be seen in some other conditions ('**psoriasiform dermatitis**'), e.g. the skin lesions in Reiter's syndrome.

INFECTIONS OF THE SKIN

Infections of the skin may be due to viruses, fungi or bacteria, viruses being the most common causative organisms.

Viruses can have both direct and indirect effects in skin infections

The **indirect effects** of generalized viremia are much more common than the direct effects, and are very variable in pattern, distribution and severity. Many viremias are associated with the development of a transient red (**erythematous**) rash with no specific features, although in the case of parvovirus infection the erythema is most marked and may be confined to the cheeks and buttocks (**slapped cheek syndrome**). Other common viral skin lesions include those of measles and rubella, in which the clinical appearance of the rash, its distribution, and associated systemic symptoms are diagnostic.

Three main groups of viruses affect the skin **directly**, producing lesions in which the virus particles are present (often in large numbers), sometimes in the form of intracellular inclusions.

- **Herpes virus** produces blistering lesions of the epidermis, with viral inclusions in the epidermal cells (*Fig. 23.8*). Examples include herpes simplex type 1 (**non-genital herpes**), herpes simplex type 2 (**genital herpes**), and herpes zoster-varicella (**chicken pox** and **shingles**).
- **Pox virus** produces multiple, pale, domed lesions on the trunk and face of children, adolescents and young adults (**molluscum contagiosum**) (*Fig. 23.9*). These are due to localized nodular thickening of the epidermis, the epidermal cells being packed with large viral inclusions.

- **Human papillomavirus** produces proliferative epidermal lesions (**viral warts**), the nature of which differs from site to site, varying from exophytic filiform fronded lesions (*Fig. 23.10a*) or small flat plaques (e.g. planar warts on the face) to deeply inverted hyperkeratotic lesions (e.g. plantar warts on the sole of the foot) (*Fig. 23.10c*). In the skin of the perineum, human papillomavirus produces florid papillomatous exophytic growths called **condyloma acuminata** (*Fig. 23.10b*); the virus may also infect the genital and anal mucosa in both males and females, and is regarded as an etiological factor in the development of carcinoma at these sites.

Fig. 23.8 Herpes virus. (a) Typical herpes virus vesicle in chicken pox. (b) Histology of chicken pox, showing destruction of epidermal cells, many of which contain viral inclusions (arrow).

Fig. 23.9 Molluscum contagiosum. (a) Clinical appearance showing raised nodules with a central keratotic core. (b) Histology showing part of a lesion, the keratotic core being composed of infected epidermal cells containing large red or purple viral inclusions.

Fig. 23.10 Human papillomavirus. (a) Typical filiform skin wart. (b) Perineal condylomata acuminata. (c) Plantar wart (verruca).

511

Fungi are common commensals on the skin surface and may give rise to skin disease

Superficial fungal infections of the skin are the most common type of pathogenic fungal infection. In the vast majority of cases the fungal hyphae or yeast forms reside in the keratin layer on the skin surface, and are associated with a minimal inflammatory response in the epidermis and upper dermis (*Fig. 23.11*).

These infections are commonly seen in community practice, the nature of the lesion being dependent on the type of causative organism and the particular area of skin involved. Common diseases such as athlete's foot (caused by *Trichophyton* and *Epidermophyton*) and ringworm (caused by *Microsporum* or *Trichophyton rubrum*) are conditions most familiar to the general public (*Fig. 23.12*).

Occasionally the fungi populate the hair follicles, in which case the inflammatory reaction may be more vigorous, resulting in a destructive folliculitis. This is becoming more common, particularly in immunosuppressed patients (e.g. those with AIDS).

Fig. 23.11 Dermatophytic fungi in horny layer of epidermis. The fungal hyphae, which are stained magenta, are confined to the keratinous horny layer (DPAS stain).

Fig. 23.12 Common fungal infections of skin		
Disease	**Site**	**Features**
Athlete's foot	Toes and feet	Redness, erosion and scaling
Ringworm	Face and trunk	Ring lesion with red scaly edge
Tinea capitis	Scalp	Hair loss and scaling
Tinea cruris	Groin	Red, scaly rash with brown patches
Tinea unguium	Finger/toe nails	Thick, crumbling nails
Pityriasis versicolor	Trunk, mainly upper	Flat patches of increased or decreased pigmentation

Subcutaneous fungal infections usually result from introduction of pathogenic fungi into the subcutaneous tissues following a penetrating injury

Subcutaneous fungal infections are relatively uncommon in the western world. The foot is the most common site, and people who spend much of their day barefoot are particularly prone.

Infection usually presents with extensive soft-tissue swelling, and the soft tissues become very hard. In the foot, there may be evidence of underlying bone destruction. In response to the presence of the fungi deep abscess cavities form, frequently discharging as sinuses onto the surface (*Fig. 23.13*). In such cases there is usually a very florid acute inflammatory reaction with suppuration, and the material that discharges from the sinuses is pus from the abscess cavities; fungi are often discharged with the pus. The most common type of infection is called 'Madura foot,' the causative organism of which is *Madurella*.

Fig. 23.13 Subcutaneous fungal infection. This chronic discharging abscess from the foot contains islands of pus **P** surrounded by a thick fibrous wall **F**. Fungal colonies (**arrows**) lie within some pus islands.

Bacterial infections of the skin are usually due to staphylococci or streptococci

Both staphylococci and streptococci can produce a condition called **impetigo**, which is highly contagious and spreads rapidly through populations, e.g. in schools. Large epidermal blisters (**bullae**) develop (*Fig. 23.14*), which may be filled either with clear fluid or with neutrophil polymorphs to form a pus-containing blister (**pustule**). In infants, some staphylococci produce a potent toxin that can lead to extensive disruption of the epidermis, with widespread confluent blistering and separation of the upper layers of the epidermis (**staphylococcal scalded skin syndrome**).

Infection of hair follicles by bacteria, usually *Staphylococcus aureus*, produces tiny pustules located in the necks of the follicles (**superficial folliculitis**) (*Fig. 23.15a*). Deep, severe follicle infection leads to an expanding collection of pus, which destroys the follicle and extends into surrounding dermis to form a **boil**.

Fig. 23.14 Impetigo. Clinical appearance showing typical yellow, crusting blisters.

Fig. 23.16 Erysipelas and cellulites. (a) Erysipelas of the face caused by streptococcus. Infection of the dermis has produced spreading inflammatory reddening of the skin. (b) A more severe bacterial cellulitis involving both dermis and subcutis. This is so severe that it is incipient necrotizing fasciitis; again, streptococcus is the causative organism.

Erysipelas is a spreading acute inflammation of the deep dermis and upper subcutis by streptococci, most commonly seen on the face (*Fig. 23.16b*).

Cellulitis is a similar infection but involves the dermis and subcutis. Sometimes the bacteria extend into deep subcutis, fascia and underlying muscle, where they proliferate rapidly and secrete toxins which lead to extensive spreading necrosis of the involved tissues. This is called **necrotizing fasciitis** and is difficult to control even with massive doses of antibiotics. It occurs particularly in the limbs (sometimes following a penetrating injury) and may necessitate amputation to prevent overwhelming septicemia. The most common causative organisms of both cellulitis and necrotizing fasciitis are streptococci and staphylococci, but anaerobic organisms may also be responsible for necrotizing fasciitis. A specific form of deep infection of muscle is **gas gangrene**, caused by *Clostridium perfringens* and some other clostridium.

Tuberculous infection of the skin is now rare, but other mycobacteria can cause skin disease

Infection of the skin by *M. tuberculosis* produces the slowly progressive chronic skin lesion called **lupus vulgaris**, in which there is giant-cell granulomatous inflammation in the dermis, leading to destruction of dermal collagen and skin appendages. The lesions are now mainly seen in elderly people, who often claim that they have been present for many years. In such lesions there may be extensive fibrous scarring, skin appendage destruction, and epidermal atrophy, although the epidermis may occasionally be irregularly thickened and raised, mimicking squamous carcinoma (pseudocarcinomatous hyperplasia).

Other mycobacteria may gain access to the dermis through small cuts, setting up chronic inflammatory granulomatous inflammation, often with ulceration. Examples include mycobacteria contracted through bathing (*M. balnei*) or through contact with infected tropical fish and their aquaria (see also pages 117 and 119).

Fig. 23.15 Bacterial folliculitis in skin. Bacterial infection of a hair follicle has produced a tiny pus-filled abscess (**arrow**) with surrounding inflammatory hyperemia.

Worldwide, the most important and common mycobacterial infection of skin is **leprosy**. The dermis of patients may be extensively infiltrated by swollen macrophages, the cytoplasm of which is packed with the causative *Mycobacterium leprae* (**lepromatous leprosy**), producing numerous raised nodules (papules) and plaques. In another form of cutaneous leprosy known as **tuberculoid leprosy**, small granulomas can be found in all layers of the dermis, but are particularly common around nerves, and may produce nerve damage. The causative organism can rarely be found in this form, the clinical lesions of which are very variable; they may be raised, reddish purple patches or flat areas (macules) in which there is loss of sensation and often loss of skin pigment.

The most important protozoal infection of the skin is caused by *Leishmania*

Infection of the skin by *Leishmania* is usually acquired following a sandfly bite. The organism is introduced into the dermis, where it excites an initially macrophagic reaction; the macrophages phagocytose the organisms, producing a small, raised, red nodule. At a later stage, a very heavy lymphocytic and plasma-cell infiltrate produces a much larger skin nodule (known as an 'oriental sore'), which fre-

Fig. 23.18 Cutaneous leishmaniasis. This girl had been bitten on the forehead while sunbathing on holiday in Cyprus; the lesion had slowly enlarged over 2 months. For histology, see *Fig. 8.38*.

quently ulcerates. The causative organism is *L. tropica*. Other forms of leishmania infection occur in the tropics and may involve mucous surfaces such as the mouth and nose. There may be skin nodules in systemic leishmaniasis due to *L. donovani* (see also page 132).

The most common parasitic infection of the skin in the UK, Europe and USA is scabies

Caused by the mite *Sarcoptes scabiei*, scabies presents with a very itchy raised lesion, which is often red and scaling. Lesions sometimes show a linear pattern caused by the mites burrowing a track in the epidermis, with inflammatory changes in the dermis beneath. Occasionally the mite can be found at the head of the track. The presence of the mite excites an inflammatory reaction in which eosinophils are numerous in both the epidermis and the underlying dermis. It is the eosinophils that are responsible for the severe itching of the scabies lesion.

Fig. 23.17 Lepromatous leprosy. (a) Shows the dermis to be infiltrated by large numbers of pale foamy macrophages (lepra cells) which contain the organism *Mycobacterium leprae*. (b) is stained by a special stain which demonstrates the bacteria (red).

Fig. 23.19 Skin – scabies. The mite **M** is burrowing in the superficial layers of the epidermis. There is an inflammatory reaction to its presence, both in the epidermis (**arrow**) and in the upper dermis.

BLISTERING DISEASES OF THE SKIN

Many skin diseases mainly affect the epidermis, causing the formation of a blister either in or immediately beneath the epidermis. If the blisters are small (<5 mm in diameter), they are known as **vesicles**; if they are larger (>5 mm in diameter), they are termed **bullae**.

Blister formation requires the separation of the keratinocytes in the epidermis from each other, or from the underlying basement membrane, or the separation of part or all of the basement membrane from the underlying dermis. This separation is accompanied by the accumulation of fluid at the site of separation.

Depending on where the separation occurs, blisters can be divided into:

- **Intraepidermal blisters**, where separation occurs in the keratinocytes above the basal layer.
- **Basal (or subepidermal) blisters**, where separation occurs in or below the basal layer.

Intraepidermal blisters can be further classified according to the process which has produced the separation of the keratinocytes (see below), whereas basal blisters can be usefully subdivided according to the type of inflammatory cell floating in the blister fluid, mainly neutrophils or eosinophils.

Intraepidermal blisters may form through one of three different mechanisms

Intraepidermal blisters may form as a result of:

- Excess fluid accumulating in the spaces between the keratinocytes (**spongiosis**).
- Breakdown of the normal structural attachments between adjacent keratinocytes, followed by shrinkage and rounding of the keratinocytes (**acantholysis**).
- Rupture of swollen degenerate or necrotic keratinocytes (**reticular degeneration**).

Spongiosis (*Fig. 23.20a*) is by far the most common cause of intraepidermal blister formation, but it tends to produce much smaller blisters (**vesicles**) than the other mechanisms; it is the cause of blistering in many forms of acute dermatitis, including atopic dermatitis, seborrheic dermatitis and contact dermatitis (see page 103).

Acantholysis (*Fig. 23.20b*) is the cause of blister formation in **pemphigus vulgaris**, in which large, flaccid bullae form on reddened skin, generally affecting the middle-aged and elderly. Blisters arise spontaneously in buccal mucosa and skin, but can be induced by rubbing apparently normal skin (Nikolsky's sign). The disease is thought to be immunologically mediated (see pink box on page 576).

Reticular degeneration blisters (*Fig. 23.20c*) are associated with necrosis of epidermal keratinocytes, often following a phase of marked keratinocyte swelling (ballooning degeneration). It is the pattern responsible for viral blisters such as herpes and varicella, and viral inclusions are present in the degenerating and dying keratinocytes. It may also be seen in some forms of blistering drug reaction, e.g. erythema multiforme (see page 520).

Fig. 23.20 Patterns of epidermal blistering. (a) **Spongiosis**, due to fluid accumulation. (b) **Acantholysis**, due to separation of abnormal epidermal cells. (c) **Reticular degeneration**, due to rupture of bloated epidermal cells.

Mechanisms in pemphigus vulgaris

Direct immunofluorescence can demonstrate both IgG and C3 in the intercellular spaces between keratinocytes in all levels of the epidermis (particularly in the stratum spinosum). Pemphigus vulgaris patients have a serum antibody (pemphigus antibody), which can be demonstrated by indirect immunofluorescence on normal squamous epithelium. It is postulated that the pemphigus antibody binds to the intercellular region of the epidermis, and the binding stimulates complement activation and proteolytic enzyme release, damaging the cell attachments and leading to separation and acantholysis.

The severity of the skin lesion appears to be directly proportional to the titer of antibody in the serum.

The likely cause of a basal blister can often be determined by the nature of the associated inflammatory cells

Blisters forming around the basement membrane often do so in an area that shows infiltration by inflammatory cells, and the nature of the inflammatory cell gives a clue to the likely diagnosis. Basal blisters can be divided into those in which the predominant inflammatory cell is:

- The **eosinophil** – in both blister fluid and adjacent upper papillary dermis. The most common causes are **pemphigoid,** a blistering disease of the elderly (see *Fig. 23.22*) and **herpes gestationis** (a rare but important blistering disease occurring in mid or late pregnancy.
- The **neutrophil**, in both blister fluid and the tips of the dermal papillae. The most common cause is **dermatitis herpetiformis**, an itchy blistering disease in young and middle-aged adults, which is associated with celiac disease (see *Fig. 23.21*).
- The **lymphocyte**, mainly in the dermis underlying the blister. This is much rarer than the above, and is largely limited to some cases of erythema multiforme (see page 227) and in the rare blistering variant of lichen planus (see page 508).

Fig. 23.22 Pemphigoid. (a) Clinical features showing incipient blister formation in an area of reddening. The epidermis has already begun to separate in the pale central area. (b) Histology showing complete separation of the epidermis from the dermis, and a heavy infiltrate of eosinophils.

Fig. 23.21 Dermatitis herpetiformis. This skin, from the extensor surface of the forearm of a young man, shows many tiny papules and two small vesicles. He also had celiac disease.

Some basal blisters form in areas in which there is no inflammatory cell infiltrate; the most common example is the friction blister formed by shearing forces in non-specialized skin, e.g. ankle blisters caused by badly fitting shoes. **Epidermolysis bullosa** is a rare but important disease characterized by basal blisters in which there is no inflammatory cell infiltrate around the basement membrane or in blister fluid.

Epidermolysis bullosa is not a single disease but is the name given to a group of basal blistering diseases

The disorders are linked in that they all involve separation of epidermis from dermis in the region of the epidermodermal basement membrane, usually with the formation of blisters. The separation is characteristically in response to minimal trauma, and is greatly disproportionate to the often trivial shearing forces to which the area of skin has been exposed. For this reason, epidermolysis bullosa is sometimes called 'mechanobullous dermatosis.'

There are over 20 types, which differ in clinical presentation, age at onset, body site involved etc., but only a few are common. Even the most common types are rare, however, but are important because some are potentially fatal and also have led to an increase in our knowledge of the molecular biology of the epidermo-dermal basement membrane. With the exception of one type (called epidermolysis bullosa acquisita) all the diseases are inherited as either autosomal dominant or autosomal recessive disorders (see pink box on page 518).

There are three main groups within the epidermolysis bullosa complex, but there are several clinical variants within each group. An important distinction between these groups is the site of separation (see *Fig. 23.23*) in the basement membrane region (see Fig. 23.23), and in the molecular biology (see pink box on page 518).

Epidermolysis bullosa simplex is inherited in an autosomal dominant pattern. Separation occurs above the basement membrane, within the basal cytoplasm of the basal cell layer of the epidermis. The basement membrane and adjacent dermis are not damaged, so the blisters heal without scarring or deformity, and the disease has a good prognosis. There are many variants, but the most common type mainly involves the hands and feet.

Junctional epidermolysis bullosa is also known as the lethal variant. It is present at birth and also affects other squamous epithelia, e.g. in the esophagus, leading to blistering in sites other than the skin. Again there are several variants, of varying degrees of severity, but the most severe generalized type leads to death in infancy. Inheritance is autosomal recessive, and separation occurs within the lamina lucida of the basement membrane, separating and damaging the hemidesmosomal attachments of the basal cells to the basement membrane.

Dystrophic epidermolysis bullosa is inherited in either an autosomal dominant or autosomal recessive pattern. Separation occurs in the dermis just below the basement membrane, by separation of the anchoring fibrils. These types lead to considerable scarring and disfigurement.

Epidermolysis bullosa

Fig. 23.23 This diagram shows the sites of separation in the various types of epidermolysis bullosa.

Molecular biology of epidermolysis bullosa

Epidermolysis bullosa simplex shows autosomal dominant inheritance. The separation occurs in the lower part of the basal cell layer, above the basement membrane. The mechanism is believed to be:

Junctional epidermolysis bullosa shows autosomal recessive inheritance. The separation occurs within the membrane. The mechanism is believed to be:

Dystrophic epidermolysis bullosa may be either autosomal dominant or recessive, different mechanisms operating in each.

Dominant

Recessive

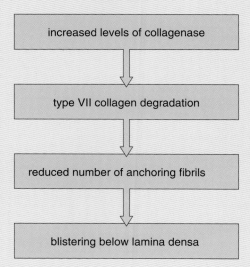

Increased activity or numbers of mast cells in the skin produces dermal edema and itching known as urticaria

Urticaria has many causes, the most familiar of which is 'hives' or 'nettle rash.' In addition, many patients with an atopic tendency or family history (see page 520) have a predisposition to develop urticaria, although the stimulus that provokes it may be difficult to identify; sometimes certain foods, heat, cold or sunlight are implicated. Degranulation of mast cells releases substances that increase vascular permeability, transudation of fluid into the dermis (leading to edema) and activation of platelets and eosinophils (leading to itch). In atopy the mast-cell degranulation is probably immunologically mediated by interaction of an antigen with IgE, which is bound to the mast-cell membrane (type I hypersensitivity reaction, see page 101), but many cases are probably non-immunologically mediated.

Localized accumulations of mast cells in the skin can produce multiple brownish raised patches, which urticate on pressure (**urticaria pigmentosa**); less commonly, there may be a solitary tumor-like nodule (**solitary mastocytoma**), usually in young children.

Small vessel vasculitis may be confined to the skin, or the skin can be one of many tissues affected

The most frequently involved vessels are the small capillaries, arterioles and venules in the upper dermis. Vasculitic damage to the walls leads to extravasation of red cells into the upper dermis, producing the lesions known as **petechiae** (when minute) or **purpura** (when larger). Some lesions may be slightly raised and nodular (palpable purpura); the lesions may be widespread, but the lower limb (particularly the area below the knee) is by far the most common site.

The most common causes of a vasculitic rash of this type are drug reaction (*Fig. 23.24*), systemic connective tissue disease (e.g. SLE), and bacteremia or septicemia (particularly acute meningococcal type, see *Fig. 8.10*).

Although the skin lesion is the most obvious manifestation, there may be evidence of other system involvement, e.g. joint and abdominal symptoms in Henoch–Schönlein purpura. When larger blood vessels are involved, the vasculitis occurs in the mid and deep dermis or subcutis. Larger, deeper, ill-defined nodules develop, again commonly on the lower limb. The most common cause is **polyarteritis nodosa**.

Some vasculitic lesions in the lower limb lead to necrosis of epidermis and dermis, producing an ulcer that is characterized by a raised, purplish edge.

Most acute purpuric vasculitic lesions of the skin show destruction of the vessel wall, with an associated neutrophil polymorph infiltrate (**neutrophilic or 'leukocytoclastic' vasculitis**), occasionally with fibrinoid necrosis of the vessel wall. Sometimes the infiltrate in the vessel wall is largely composed of lymphocytes (**lymphocytic vasculitis**) without fibrinoid necrosis. This pattern shows less red-cell extravasation, and purpura is not such an important clinical feature; often the lesion appears to be a localized area of erythema. Lymphocytic vasculitis is particularly seen in association with systemic connective tissue disease (e.g. SLE, rheumatoid arthritis), and as a drug reaction, with viremia (see also Chapter 10, page 107).

Fig. 23.24 Vasculitic skin rash producing purpura. In this case the purpura was due to a neutrophilic vasculitis, which occurred as part of an adverse drug reaction.

Many skin lesions are iatrogenic, due to ingested drugs

Skin lesions of this nature are becoming increasingly common and show a wide variation in appearance, pattern and duration. The most common pattern is a **toxic erythema**, clinically and histologically identical to that seen as an indirect effect of virus infection (see pages 510–1).

Skin reactions to drugs can mimic almost any other type of inflammatory skin disease. Common patterns are:

- **Lichenoid drug eruptions**, resembling lichen planus both clinically and histologically.
- **Vasculitic eruptions**, usually a small-vessel neutrophilic vasculitis in the upper dermis, producing purpura.

- **Urticarial eruptions**, producing blotchy, raised, itchy rashes.
- **Blistering and exfoliating eruptions**, particularly erythema multiforme (*Fig. 23.26*) and toxic epidermal necrolysis. The latter is the most severe – and often fatal – drug reaction in the skin, leading to extensive shedding of epidermis, together with severe metabolic disorder.
- **Erythema nodosum**, a characteristic deep dermal and subcutaneous reaction that produces firm, reddish purple nodules, usually on the legs (*Fig. 23.25*).

In general, skin rashes due to drugs develop at least a week after first exposure, improving within 3–4 days of stopping the drug; the rash recurs within 20 days of re-exposure. However, certain drug rashes persist for a very long time after the drug is stopped, e.g. the extensive erythematous rash that follows the ingestion of captopril and enalapril.

It is not sufficiently appreciated that drug reactions in skin are frequently due to non-prescription drugs bought over the counter (e.g. aspirin) or to agents included in foods (e.g. some coloring agents). A very detailed clinical history must be taken.

Many systemic diseases have cutaneous manifestations

Many systemic diseases have skin lesions as part of their general picture, and the first manifestation of disease may be the skin lesions. The most important group are the systemic autoimmune diseases such as SLE and systemic sclerosis. These diseases are dealt with in more detail in Chapter 25, and the skin lesions are discussed there (see pages 561 and 564).

Other systemic diseases in which there are important cutaneous manifestations are **diabetes mellitus** and **sarcoidosis**.

In diabetes mellitus some patients develop shiny red or yellowish depressed plaques on the leg, owing to degeneration of dermal collagen, known as **necrobiosis lipoidica** (*Fig. 23.27*).

In **sarcoidosis**, cutaneous sarcoid granulomas are very common and can have many different clinical patterns, although the presence of non-caseating giant-cell granulomas is common to them all. Patients with sarcoidosis may also present with, or develop, erythema nodosum (see page 568).

Internal malignant disease may be associated with the development of a range of skin lesions (such as dermatomyositis), many of which are bizarre both clinically and histologically.

Fig. 23.25 Erythema nodosum. Typical erythema nodosum on the shins (in this case the result of an adverse reaction to sulfonamide therapy).

Fig. 23.26 Erythema multiforme. In this case the erythema multiforme was due to an adverse reaction to antibiotics.

Fig. 23.27 Necrobiosis lipoidica. These advanced lesions had been present for many months on the shins of this diabetic.

TUMORS OF THE SKIN

Tumors of the skin can be divided into those derived from the cells of the epidermis, those from the skin appendages, and those from the connective tissues in the dermis.

The epidermis contains a number of different cell types, namely, keratinocytes, melanocytes, Langerhans' cells, and Merkel's cells. Tumors in the epidermis most commonly originate from keratinocytes or melanocytes.

Keratinocyte-derived tumors of the epidermis are of two main types: basal-cell carcinoma and squamous-cell carcinoma

Both basal-cell carcinoma and squamous-cell carcinoma are predisposed to by exposure to light and ionizing radiation, and are therefore most commonly seen in exposed areas such as the head and neck, and the dorsum of the hands. Both types arise most frequently in the elderly, and multiple lesions are not uncommon.

Basal-cell carcinoma, which occurs in three main patterns, is a locally invasive tumor that does not metastasize

The three main patterns are nodular basal-cell carcinoma, superficial basal-cell carcinoma and morpheic basal-cell carcinoma.

Nodular basal-cell carcinoma is the most common pattern, occurring most frequently in those over the age of 50 years. Arising on areas exposed to light, such as the face and forehead, it is relatively rare on the trunk and limbs. It presents as a firm, raised nodule, often showing central ulceration, with a raised, pearly edge, which may show numerous telangiectatic vessels (*Fig. 23.28*a,b). It is composed of clusters of small, dark cells resembling those of the basal layer of the epidermis. The edge of each cluster often shows a regular palisaded pattern. In the larger more protuberant lesions, cystic change is frequently seen.

Superficial basal-cell carcinoma usually appears as a flat, red plaque, often with an irregular edge (*Fig. 23.28*c,d). It is most common on the face, but this variant can occur on the trunk. Sometimes there are raised areas within the tumor, representing the development of a nodular basal-cell carcinoma within the existing superficial lesion. Histologically, there are usually many small buds or nodular downgrowths of basal cells from the overlying epidermis.

Fig. 23.28 Basal cell carcinoma. (a) and (b) show the clinical and histological appearances of **nodular pattern** basal cell carcinoma. Note the raised, well-circumscribed nodule with central ulceration (**arrows**). (c) and (d) show the clinical and histological appearances of **superficial pattern** basal cell carcinoma (see text).

Fig. 23.29 Basal-cell carcinoma: morpheic pattern. Histology showing narrow, compressed cords of basal cells in a dense fibrous stroma.

This superficial pattern may be multifocal, e.g. occurring in the irradiation field over the vertebrae in patients previously given radiotherapy for ankylosing spondylitis.

Morpheic basal-cell carcinoma appears as a flat, thickened, whitish or yellowish plaque, which may be sunken and firm, with focal areas of ulceration. In contrast to nodular basal-cell carcinoma, it has indistinct edges and the tumor may extend in the dermis for some way beyond the visible or palpable borders. Histologically, small clumps and cords of basal cells are separated by a dense fibrous stroma (*Fig. 23.29*).

All basal-cell carcinomas can be cured if completely excised. However, local recurrence is a problem, particularly in the morpheic and superficial types, which are less clearly defined to the naked eye. Neglected basal-cell carcinomas cause considerable local destruction of the soft tissues and, occasionally, the bones of the face (hence their old name of 'rodent ulcer'). Although most seem to originate from the basal cells of the epidermis, some appear to arise from the necks of hair follicles, and can be confused with a tumor of hair follicles known as 'trichoepithelioma'.

Invasive squamous carcinoma of the skin may arise in pre-existing epidermal dysplastic lesions

Two patterns of intraepidermal dysplasia are recognized. One is **actinic keratosis** (also known as **solar keratosis**), which occurs most commonly on the face, scalp and backs of the hands (i.e. light-exposed skin). It arises as irregular plaques or patches (frequently multiple), up to 1 cm in diameter, with a rough, hard hyperkeratotic surface. Histologically, the cells in the lower half of the epidermis show marked dysplasia and atypia.

The other pattern shows epidermal atypia, with pleomorphism and mitoses, throughout all layers of the epidermis to the surface (*Fig. 23.30a*). This is regarded as squamous carcinoma in situ (**intraepidermal carcinoma**) and, like actinic keratoses, occurs on light-exposed skin, but may also occur on skin that is normally covered, e.g. on the trunk.

Clinically, lesions appear as flat or raised reddish-brown plaques, sometimes with surface keratinous scale, and occasionally with focal ulceration.

The incidence of malignant invasive change supervening in intraepidermal carcinoma is very much greater than that in actinic keratoses.

Most squamous carcinomas of the skin are locally invasive and well differentiated, with the formation of keratin nests; occasionally, poorly differentiated non-keratinizing squamous carcinoma can develop in an area of pre-existing intraepidermal carcinoma. Unlike basal-cell carcinoma, invasive squamous carcinoma (*Fig. 23.30b*) has the potential for metastasis, usually metastasizing to regional lymph nodes initially.

Fig. 23.30 Intraepidermal carcinoma and invasive squamous carcinoma. (a) Histology of intraepidermal carcinoma showing thickening of the epidermis by pleomorphic dysplastic epidermal cells, without invasion into the dermis. (b) Invasive squamous-cell carcinoma of the skin showing the characteristic raised keratotic edges.

Melanocytes in the basal layer of the epidermis are an important source of tumor-like hamartomas (nevi) and invasive malignant tumors (malignant melanoma)

Melanocytic nevi (commonly known as 'moles') are extremely common and most individuals have a few somewhere on the skin, some people having very large numbers. They are regarded as hamartomatous malformations, and five main patterns are recognized.

In **junctional nevus** (*Fig. 23.31a* and *d*) the abnormal clumps of melanocytes are confined to the epidermis and are located in the basal layer. Clinically the lesions are flat (macular) and uniformly and deeply pigmented. They usually develop in childhood and adolescence.

Compound nevi (*Fig. 23.31b* and *e*) are raised, pale brown, slightly nodular lesions with an irregular surface, but the pigmentation is uniform. They are most common in adolescents and young adults. Histologically, there are clumps of melanocytes in both the epidermis (similar to those seen in junctional nevi) and the upper dermis. Those intradermal nevus cells that are closest to the junctional nests are histologically similar to the intraepidermal nevus cells. However, in the deeper levels they are smaller and more compact, a feature that is said to indicate maturation of the nevus cells. It is believed that the natural history of intraepidermal junctional nevus cells is for them to drop into the dermis and to become smaller and more compact the longer they have been in the dermis. It is not uncommon for coarse hairs to emerge from compound nevi (hairy mole).

Intradermal nevi (*Fig. 23.31c* and *f*) are also raised, but are normally smoothly domed, and may be flesh-coloured or slightly brown. They are usually seen in adults and are rare in adolescents and children. They appear to be entirely composed of nevus cells within the dermis, and there is no nested junctional component, although there may be a slight increase in melanocytes in the basal layer.

(a) junctional   (b) compound   (c) intradermal

(d)   (e)   (f)

Fig. 23.31 Types of benign melanocytic nevi. The distribution of melanocytes in junctional, compound and intradermal nevi. (a) In junctional nevus there are rounded nests of melanocytes, some of which contain melanin granules in the cytoplasm, in the lower epidermis at the dermoepidermal junction. (b) In compound nevus there is a junctional nevus component, combined with an intradermal mass of benign melanocytic nevus cells. (c) An intradermal nevus is entirely composed of melanocytic nevus cells in clusters within the upper dermis; there is no junctional component, and the intradermal melanocytes are usually small and entirely benign. (d) This flat pigmented lesion is regular in outline; it is a junctional nevus in a 17-year-old girl. In someone younger it would probably be more deeply pigmented. (e) This benign nevus is less intensely pigmented than the junctional nevus. It is becoming slightly raised as more of the melanocytes drop down from the epidermis into the upper dermis. The presence of coarse hairs is a frequent finding. (f) The clinical photograph shows a typical raised, slightly brown and wrinkled polypoid benign intradermal nevus. The color is uniform, as is the physical outline.

Blue nevi are entirely intradermal lesions, in which usually very heavily pigmented melanocytes are scattered in an ill-defined nodule separated by coarse bands of collagen. On cut surface these are brown due to the pigment, but they appear blue-black when viewed through the epidermis. They are usually first noted in childhood and can grow slowly, but are rarely more than 1 cm in diameter. Occasional very large blue nevi may be present on the buttocks, whereas the smaller blue nevi are most common on the head and arms. Malignant change is extremely rare.

Spitz nevus or **juvenile nevus**, as its name implies, is seen mainly in children, presenting as a raised, reddish brown, smooth-surfaced nodule. Although clinically they appear innocuous, histologically these melanocytic lesions show frightening degrees of pleomorphism and atypia and can be histologically confused with malignant melanoma.

The vast majority of nevi are entirely benign, but malignant change can occasionally supervene

It is the junctional component of junctional/compound nevi that is most at risk of conversion to malignancy. In benign nevi the junctional melanocytes are arranged either in nests or in a linear (lentiginous) pattern. The individual melanocytes show no evidence of pleomorphism or mitotic activity, and have the cytological characteristics of benign cells. Occasionally, both cytological and architectural atypia develop, the individual cells showing marked nuclear pleomorphism with increased numbers of mitoses; architectural atypia frequently takes the form of loss of roundness of the junctional cell nests, which often become flat and follow the general contour of the epidermal rete ridges.

Clinically, such nevi appear larger than usual (>1 cm in diameter) and have irregularity of edge, surface and pigmentation. This irregularity of surface texture and outline, and the development of variable degrees of brown pigmentation, may develop in a nevus which has formerly been smooth and uniform in surface, outline and colour. These changes in a pre-existing mole should be regarded as an indication of possible early malignant change, and excision biopsy should be performed as a matter of urgency. There is no place for shave, punch or incision biopsies (see pages 533 and 579). Such atypical nevi may be single, but some people have many, and there is often a family history (**dysplastic nevus syndrome**).

Lentigo maligna is a pattern of junctional melanocyte proliferation affecting the faces of the elderly

Clinically the lesions appear as flat, variegated, brown-black areas of pigmentation on the faces of elderly men and women. They gradually increase in size and have an irregular outline. Histologically, the basal layer of the epidermis is largely replaced by an almost continuous line of large atypical melanocytes, which sometimes partially extend down skin appendages such as hair follicles. Occasionally a solid, raised nodule arises within such an area, often indicating the development of a supervening early nodular malignant melanoma (**lentigo maligna melanoma**).

Malignant melanoma is increasing in incidence in white-skinned races

Malignant melanoma is predominantly a tumor of adults, but it does occasionally occur in children. It may arise within the junctional component of a pre-existing melanocytic nevus (see 'dysplastic nevus' and 'lentigo maligna'), or may apparently develop of its own accord within otherwise normal skin. The most important predisposing factor is excessive exposure to ultraviolet (UV) light, and the increasing incidence of malignant melanoma has been ascribed to both the reduced filtering power of the thinning ozone layer, and increased social exposure to sunshine. The tumor is uncommon in dark-skinned races, possibly because of the protective effect of increased epidermal melanin against UV irradiation. Women are slightly more likely to develop a tumor than men, the legs being a common site in women, and the trunk (particularly the back) being a common site in men. Malignant melanoma may occur in other mucosal surfaces, e.g. the mouth and nose.

Malignant melanomas of the skin present as irregular pigmented lesions

Compared to benign pigmented melanocytic lesions, malignant melanomas are often larger (with a history of recent increase in size), with an irregular border leading to asymmetry, and variable pigmentation. Ulceration may be present. Some forms are flat, others manifesting as raised nodular lesions. Malignant melanomas can be classified into three main groups:

- **Lentigo malignant melanoma.** A nodular lesion arising in a pre-existing facial lentigo maligna.
- **Superficial spreading malignant melanoma.** Usually a flat lesion with variable pigmentation and irregular edges. This is the most common type, accounting for about 75% of all malignant melanomas; it is in this group that the recent increase in incidence has been most marked.
- **Nodular malignant melanoma.** Presents as a raised brown-black nodule, usually without preceding benign melanocytic lesion. These account for about 5% of all malignant melanomas (see *Fig. 23.32f*).

A further group that is worth recognizing is the so-called **acral lentiginous malignant melanoma.** This is confined to the hands and feet, and some occur beneath the finger nails and toe nails (**subungual melanoma**). Although it is most common in elderly Caucasians, it is particularly common in Orientals. Histologically, it resembles superficial spreading malignant melanoma.

Superficial spreading malignant melanoma may be either in situ or invasive

In superficial spreading malignant melanoma in situ the atypical melanocytes are confined to the epidermis (*Fig. 23.33*). In contrast, with invasive superficial spreading malignant melanoma, in addition to the in situ change, clusters of malignant melanocytes invade the dermis. In the invasive type, the prognosis largely depends on the depth of dermal invasion (see blue box on page 526). In most cases, at the time of excision biopsy to establish the diagnosis the invasion is very superficial; the prognosis for these tumors is good if they are adequately excised.

Fig. 23.32 **Patterns of malignant melanoma.** (a) Melanocytes in normal skin. (b) Lentigo maligna. (c) Malignant melanoma in situ (melanocytic intraepidermal neoplasia). (d) Thin malignant melanoma with microinvasion of dermis. (e) Nodular malignant melanoma with vertical growth pattern. (f) Malignant melanoma (note the spreading pigmentation and the raised central nodule).

Fig. 23.33 **Superficial spreading malignant melanoma.** (a) This pigmented lesion of the skin shows marked irregularity in outline and in degree of pigmentation. This was originally a dysplastic compound nevus, which has transformed into a superficial spreading malignant melanoma. A biopsy has been taken from the most obviously malignant area. (b) There are malignant melanocytes invading upwards into the epidermis (pagetoid change – see arrows). At bottom left of the picture, melanocytes can also be seen beginning to invade downwards into the dermis (arrow).

Malignant melanoma in the skin can metastasize via lymphatics and blood vessels

Malignant melanoma can metastasize **by lymphatics** to the lymph nodes draining the area in which the primary lesion occurs, e.g. inguinal nodes in leg lesions. Sometimes clusters of melanoma cells become trapped in lymphatic vessels in the skin on the way to the lymph nodes, setting up metastases within the skin (**satellite deposits**).

Bloodstream spread can also occur, common sites for bloodstream metastasis being the liver, lung and brain. However, melanoma is notorious for producing bloodborne metastases in bizarre sites, such as the myocardium.

For malignant melanoma to metastasize, it has to gain access to the lymphatics and blood vessels in the dermis. The more extensive the growth and the deeper it extends into dermis, the more lymphatics and blood vessels it can invade. The risk of metastasis, and hence the prognosis, is thus largely dependent on the depth of invasion. The two ways of expressing this are Clarke's levels and the Breslow thickness (see blue box).

Proliferation of Langerhans' cells in the skin is rare and largely confined to young children

Langerhans' cells are slightly increased in number in a large range of inflammatory skin diseases, and may be found in

Prognostic factors in invasive malignant melanoma

Patients can be divided into three groups according to the risk of metastasis.

- **Low risk**. The best prognostic criterion is a Breslow thickness of less than 0.76 mm. The Breslow thickness is the measured thickness (on a histological section) from the deepest level of the malignant melanoma to the granular layer of the overlying epidermis.
- **Moderate risk**. Tumors with a Breslow thickness of between 0.76 and 1.5 mm.
- **High risk**. Tumors with a Breslow thickness of greater than 1.5 mm.

Clarke's levels express the depth of invasion of the tumor according to structural levels in the skin. For example, level 1 is confined within the epidermis, level 2 shows invasion of papillary dermis only, and later levels express varying degrees of invasion of the reticular dermis and subcutis. However, Clarke's levels are not as consistently reproducible as the Breslow thickness, which is the measurement of choice.

their normal location in the epidermis as well as around upper dermal blood vessels. There is a group of conditions called **Langerhans' cell histiocytosis** (also known as **histiocytosis X**), in which there is extensive proliferation of Langerhans' cells, either alone or in conjunction with other cells such as eosinophils, fibroblasts and lymphocytes.

There are three components to the Langerhans' cell histiocytosis group: **Letterer–Siwe disease** (a disease of infants, usually presenting with a skin rash), **Hand–Schüller–Christian disease** (in which there are localized accumulations in bone, producing osteolytic lesions, together with pulmonary infiltration and occasional lymph node involvement), and **eosinophil granuloma** (in which there is usually a solitary osteolytic lesion in bone, composed largely of Langerhans' cells with eosinophils). There is considerable overlap between these three syndromes, but Letterer–Siwe disease is the most clear-cut. It is largely confined to infants, presenting with a variable skin rash that often resembles seborrheic dermatitis. It behaves in a malignant fashion, with extensive infiltration of the upper dermis and many other systemic tissues by large abnormal Langerhans' cells.

Tumors of Merkel cells are rare, highly malignant, and usually found in the elderly

Merkel cells are neuroendocrine cells in the basal layer of the epidermis, associated with peripheral nerve endings by synaptic connection. Tumors of Merkel cells usually occur in the elderly, mainly around the head and neck, with the arm being the next most common site. Lesions principally occur in sun-damaged skin as raised painless nodules that grow rapidly. They have a poor prognosis and metastasize widely and early.

TUMORS OF SKIN APPENDAGES

The skin appendages that most frequently give rise to tumors are the pilosebaceous apparatus and the eccrine ducts and glands. Tumors of apocrine glands are rare.

Two common tumors are derived from hair follicles: trichoepithelioma and pilomatrixoma

Trichoepithelioma commonly presents as a skin-covered nodule, less than 1 cm in diameter, on the faces of teenagers and young and middle-aged adults. Both clinically and histologically, these lesions resemble small nodular basal-cell carcinomas. The difference in age incidence is the main distinction between the two.

Pilomatrixomas occur mainly in children, arising on the face, neck and shoulders. They are raised, knobbly, dermal tumors up to 2 cm in diameter, which are often very pale or white with thin epidermis stretched over them.

Tumors or tumor-like nodules derived from the sebaceous component of the hair follicle most frequently occur on the face. The most common is **sebaceous hyperplasia**, in which there is a number of yellow papules, usually on the forehead, cheeks and the area around the nose. They mainly affect elderly men and, less commonly, women; clinically they may be mistaken for small basal-cell carcinomas.

Tumors derived from eccrine sweat glands and their ducts are not common, but there are many different types

The main types are:

- **Syringoma.** Multiple, small, pale white nodules or papules on the lower eyelids and cheek, usually in women.
- **Eccrine poroma.** A raised, solitary, fleshy tumor, usually situated on the sole but occasionally seen in the palm.
- **Hidroacanthoma simplex.** Usually located on the lower leg in elderly people, often confused clinically with basal-cell carcinoma or seborrheic keratosis.
- **Clear-cell acanthoma.** A flat or slightly raised reddish lesion on the legs.
- **Clear-cell or eccrine hidradenoma.** Usually located on the head or neck of young adults. Arises as a solitary nodular tumor which may appear cystic. Solid lesions are usually flesh-colored or slightly red; cystic lesions may have a bluish tinge.
- **Cylindroma.** One of the most common tumors, the majority occurring on the head, scalp and neck as slow-growing, pink, raised nodules. They are particularly common in women, and multiple cylindromas may occur with an autosomal dominant mode of inheritance. Multiple tumors on the scalp are sometimes called 'turban tumor'.

Most skin cysts are derived from skin appendages

The most common skin cyst derived from a skin appendage is the so-called **pilar cyst**, which occurs on the scalp of the elderly as a well-circumscribed, round tumor. Histologically, lesions are lined by squamous epithelium similar to that of hair follicles and contain thick, white, compacted keratin. They may be multiple.

Epidermal cysts are also believed to be derived from hair follicles and are very similar to pilar cysts. They are mainly seen on the face, neck and upper trunk in young and middle-aged adults, and may occur in an area previously damaged by severe acne. Similar epidermal cysts may be seen at the angle of the eye in children (**external angular dermoid**) and are regarded as congenital malformations. Epidermal cysts may also be seen anywhere on the body following penetrating injury and are believed to be derived from squamous epithelium from the epidermis, implanted during trauma (**inclusion dermoid**). The skin and subcu-

taneous tissue around some epidermal cysts may show reddening and swelling, and the lesion becomes tender. This is commonly called 'infected epidermoid cyst,' but the inflammation is caused by leakage of keratin into surrounding tissues following trauma and is not associated with infection.

TUMORS AND TUMOR-LIKE ENLARGEMENTS OF THE DERMIS

Although many of the lesions originating from the cells in the dermis appear to be tumor-like, they are in fact hamartomatous malformations rather than true neoplastic proliferations. The most common are: **angioma** and angioma-like proliferations (e.g. pyogenic granuloma), **fibrohistiocytic lesions** (e.g. dermatofibroma), **neurofibroma** and **neurilemmoma** (Schwannoma), and **leiomyoma**.

Dermal lesions due to abnormal blood vessels are common, most being developmental malformations rather than true neoplasms

The most frequently seen vascular lesions in the dermis are hamartomatous, and the most common examples include capillary hemangioma, cavernous hemangioma and port-wine stain.

Capillary hemangiomas are common in babies (strawberry nevus) and are usually located on the trunk, buttocks or face. They are not present at birth, but manifest in the first few months of life; they spontaneously enlarge and then regress over the first couple of years of life. These firm, dark-pink tumors protrude from the surface of the skin and are usually 2–3 cm in diameter.

Cavernous hemangiomas are clinically similar to capillary hemangiomas, occurring in the same location and in

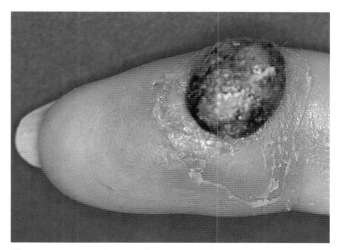

Fig. 23.34 Pyogenic granuloma. Typical site and appearance of pyogenic granuloma, a raised angioma-like lesion, in this case due to trauma from a rose thorn.

the same group. However, they tend to be larger, less clearly defined, and show no tendency to involute.

Port-wine stain usually presents at birth as a flat, purplish red or pink area on the face and neck. It occasionally arises on the limbs. These lesions show no tendency to regress and may continue to grow; they are sometimes associated with intracerebral vascular malformations (Sturge–Weber syndrome).

Pyogenic granuloma is a common, raised, red, vascular-looking lesion (*Fig. 23.34*). Histologically, it appears to be composed of highly vascular granulation tissue with inflammatory cells in the stroma. Often showing surface ulceration, it grows rapidly up to 1–2 cm in a matter of weeks until they are pedunculated red nodules. It is most common on the head and neck, and also involves the buccal and gingival mucosa (see Chapter 12), particularly in young pregnant women. It also occurs on the limbs, particularly around the lower arms and hands, and there is sometimes a history of penetrating trauma.

The most important true tumors of vascular origin in the skin are glomus tumor, angiosarcoma and Kaposi's sarcoma

Glomus tumors most commonly occur in the fingers, particularly underneath the nails. They are small, reddish nodules (sometimes slightly blue), which are exquisitely tender, particularly when pressed, but may also be spontaneously painful. They are derived from special arteriovenous anastomoses called 'glomus bodies,' which are most frequently found in the hands.

Angiosarcoma is a highly malignant tumor in the skin. It is usually seen in elderly people, arising mainly in the head and neck region, particularly the scalp and forehead. Lesions appear as slightly raised purplish red patches or plaques, which spread and then undergo ulceration.

Kaposi's sarcoma was formerly uncommon in the western world, being mainly confined to Central Africa. However, occasional cases were seen in elderly Caucasians, usually men, and principally in the hands and feet.

Kaposi's sarcoma has become a much more important tumor because of its high incidence in young adults (mainly men) who have AIDS; in this group the lesions are often multiple and grow rapidly, sometimes involving the oral mucosa, with a tendency to metastasize widely. They usually begin as a small, reddish patch, which enlarges and becomes a raised plaque or nodule (see page 170).

Fibrous histiocytic tumors are the most common true tumors of the dermis

The cell of origin is considered to be the myofibroblast, a connective tissue cell that shows features of smooth muscle and fibroblast, together with some histiocytic characteristics.

Fibrous histiocytic tumors arise most commonly on the limbs in middle-aged adults, and are slightly more common

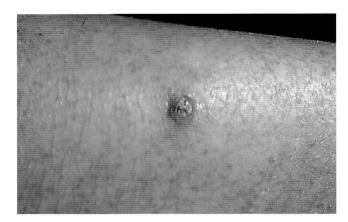

Fig. 23.35 Dermatofibroma. This close photograph shows a raised reddish-brown lesion with a central depression. It is one of the variants of dermatofibroma.

in women. The lesions are solitary raised nodules, usually brownish in color, and the overlying epidermis may show some thickening and hyperkeratosis.

The most common histological pattern is that of **dermatofibroma,** in which the dermal nodule is ill defined (*Fig. 23.35*) and composed of spindle-shaped myofibroblasts, lying between dermal collagen bands and expanding the dermis. Of the two less common variants, one (histiocytoma cutis) contains a much higher proportion of lipid-filled histiocytic cells, giving the lesion a yellow color on cut surface; this is particularly common around the ankle. The other variant, the so-called 'sclerosing hemangioma,' is more densely sclerotic, with increased numbers of vessels. Often hemosiderin from leaked blood gives the lesion a brownish cut-surface appearance.

Dermal fibrous histiocytic tumors of this type are entirely benign, but there are two with histological similarities that behave as malignant tumors. **Dermatofibrosarcoma protuberans** is a much larger, slowly growing dermal tumor which is irregular in outline and has multiple nodules within it. **Malignant fibrous histiocytoma** is one of the most common malignant soft tissue tumors that affect the deep tissues (particularly of the thigh and buttock), but some malignant fibrous histiocytomas appear to arise in subcutaneous fat and may initially present as a deep skin tumor.

Non-neoplastic fibrous lesions of the dermis are common

The most common non-neoplastic fibrous lesions of the dermis are **keloids**. These occur as raised, firm, collagenous lesions, often covered by smooth, rather thin epidermis. They grow slowly and become harder with time. They are usually found around the head, neck, upper chest and upper arms of young people (there is a female preponderance), and young women of Afro-Caribbean origin are particularly prone. Lesions follow a history of trauma, e.g. keloids on the earlobe are commonly the result of ear piercing, and

Fig. 23.36 Keloid. (a) Keloid in earlobe following ear piercing. (b) Keloid in scar, common in the upper trunk in young women.

Fig. 23.37 Multiple neurofibromas in von Recklinghausen's disease. Very large numbers of soft, fleshy dermal tumors are present, together with some less protuberant subcutaneous tumors.

keloidal change in surgical scars is an important cosmetic problem in the areas of the body where keloid change tends to occur (*Fig. 23.36*). They probably represent excessive reactive collagen formation by fibroblasts after trauma, with the proliferation of fibroblasts and collagen deposition extending beyond the original site of trauma. In this way they are distinguished from hypertrophic scarring, in which a slowly resolving scar remains localized to the area of trauma.

The **fibromatoses** are diffuse proliferations of fibrous and fibrohistiocytic tissues in the subcutis and adipose tissue. There are many types, most of which are rare. The most frequently seen is **palmar fibromatosis (Dupuytren's contracture)**, in which there is fibrous thickening of the tissues in the palm of the hand, usually in the form of a single long cord (see Fig. 24.27). This leads to fixed flexion deformities of the fingers, most commonly the fourth or ring finger, giving rise to puckering of the palmar skin, a palpable rigid bar of firm tissue running to the finger, and a claw-like deformity of one or more fingers. It occurs most commonly in adult Caucasian males and has a particularly high incidence in alcoholics. There may also be plantar fibromatosis, in which a similar thickening occurs on the soles of the feet but rarely, if ever, produces flexion deformity of the toe.

Neurofibromas may be solitary or multiple; neurilemmoma is a solitary tumor

Neurofibromas are characteristically soft, raised, fleshy dermal tumors which are often pedunculated.

In **von Recklinghausen's disease** (NF1) there are large numbers of such tumors in many areas of the skin (*Fig. 23.37*), and similar lesions are present in the internal organs. They are complex benign tumors containing Schwann cells, but elements of endoneurium and perineurium are also present (see also page 487). Malignant change may occasionally supervene in one of the larger skin tumors in von Recklinghausen's disease, but the solitary tumors are benign.

Schwannomas (neurilemmomas) are solitary tumors of the Schwann cells of peripheral nerves, and usually lie in the line of a peripheral nerve (see page 487). They are usually located in the subcutis rather than the dermis. They occur in middle-aged adults, with an equal gender incidence, and are seen mainly on the limbs and head and neck. They are benign, but may undergo degenerative change if long-standing (ancient Schwannoma).

Leiomyomas in the skin are derived either from the walls of dermal vessels or from arrector pili muscles. They present as raised, red lesions up to 1 cm across, and are both painful and tender. Those derived from arrector pili may be multiple and usually arise on the trunk and limbs in young adults; those derived from blood vessel smooth muscle are usually solitary, and may be larger than 1 cm in diameter.

The most common lymphoma to present in the skin is cutaneous T-cell lymphoma (CTCL)

B-cell lymphoma in the skin usually occurs as part of a systemic lymphoma. It manifests either as a solitary, raised, reddish purple nodule or as a series of coalescing nodules, particularly in the head and neck.

T-cell lymphoma may present in the skin, sometimes remaining in the skin for many years before becoming systematized. The florid lesions of T-cell lymphoma in the skin are known as **mycosis fungoides**, appearing as multiple, raised, red nodules or indurated plaques. However, many patients have a long history of red skin patches with a wrinkled, scaly surface (often for many years), which occasionally become slowly more raised to form reddish confluent plaques (*Fig. 23.38a*).

Histologically, these are manifestations of infiltration of upper dermis and epidermis by increasing numbers of malignant T lymphocytes (*Fig. 23.38b*), and are known respectively as the 'patch' and 'plaque' stages of CTCL. By the time the patient has developed a nodular lesion of mycosis fungoides, the dermis contains nodular infiltrates of malignant T lymphocytes.

Some patients with CTCL present with general widespread reddening of the skin (erythroderma), and a few have lymphadenopathy and malignant T lymphocytes in the peripheral blood (**Sézary's syndrome**).

There are many conditions that mimic CTCL both clinically and histologically, and the diagnosis of the disease may be difficult until the late stages, when plaques and nodular tumors are prominent.

IMPORTANT MISCELLANEOUS SKIN CONDITIONS

There are many common and important lesions of the skin that are very difficult to fit into the categories used above, mainly because their etiology and pathogenesis are not known. They can be divided into non-neoplastic squamous keratoses, disorders of hair and hair follicles, and chronic skin ulcers.

Seborrheic warts, keratoacanthomas and cutaneous horns are benign epidermal proliferations characterized by excess keratin production

Seborrheic keratoses are extremely common, increasing in number with age. They are almost invariably multiple and present as slightly raised, greyish brown keratotic lesions, the larger examples of which may have an obviously warty surface (*Fig. 23.39*). They are due to proliferation of epidermal cells resembling those that occupy the basal layer, and there is excessive production of keratin. They are invariably benign.

Fig. 23.38 Cutaneous T-cell lymphoma (mycosis fungoides). (a) The skin shows a mixture of red patches and raised plaques due to skin infiltration by malignant T lymphocytes. (b) Histology shows large numbers of pleomorphic T lymphocytes in the dermis and invading the epidermis.

Fig. 23.39 Raised benign seborrheic keratosis (seborrheic wart). These are often covered by a thick layer of warty, grey keratin.

Fig. 23.40 Keratoacanthoma. Typical lesion with a raised, red edge. It is filled with creamy grey masses of keratin. These can be clinically mistaken for squamous-cell carcinoma of the skin.

Fig. 23.41 Acne vulgaris. Severe acne, some lesions showing pustule formation and crusting.

Keratoacanthoma most commonly occurs in the elderly, particularly on the face. A characteristic and frightening feature is that clinically they resemble squamous-cell carcinomas and grow extremely rapidly, changing in a matter of weeks from a slightly raised, red papule to a large domed nodule with raised, firm edges and a central mass of keratin (*Fig. 23.40*). At certain stages in their growth keratoacanthomas also share histological features with squamous-cell carcinoma, and the differential diagnosis can be very difficult. Most keratoacanthomas regress spontaneously within months, but those that persist should be excised because of the difficulty of distinguishing them from squamous-cell carcinomas.

Cutaneous horns are hard, protruding lumps of keratin that arise from an area of abnormal epidermis. The underlying epidermal abnormality is usually benign, e.g. a viral wart or seborrheic keratosis, but occasionally cutaneous horns can arise on an area of intraepidermal carcinoma.

Disorders of the hair and hair follicles are very commonly encountered in community practice

Hair follicles are the site of both keratin retention and bacterial and fungal infection (**superficial folliculitis**). Acute superficial folliculitis is usually due to *Staphylococcus aureus*. It is most common in the beard area in adolescent and young adult males, but may also occur elsewhere, e.g. the thighs and buttocks. Clinically it presents as minute, yellowish, rounded pustules, often with a central hair. **Deep folliculitis** occurs when the infection (also usually staphylococcal) occurs deep in the hair follicle. This causes an expanding mass that destroys the follicle, producing a 'boil'.

Acne vulgaris, which most commonly affects adolescents, is a form of chronic folliculitis associated with excess keratin accumulation in the pilosebaceous duct. The infective lesion probably arises in obstructed hair follicles, which produce small, raised, white nodules (whiteheads or blackheads). Rupture of these nodules releases a mixture of keratin, sebaceous-gland secretion and bacteria into the surrounding dermis, where there is a mixed inflammatory reaction, both acute inflammatory and chronic granulomatous (*Fig. 23.41*). Sometimes acne forms large tender keratin-filled cysts (**cystic acne**). The cause is not known, but high circulating androgens are thought to be significant.

Rosacea is a follicle-related disease in which there is marked reddening of the skin of the face, associated with telangiectatic dilatation of upper dermal vessels and a perivascular chronic inflammatory infiltrate which, when heavy, leads to persistent indurated reddening of the skin. Papules or pustules frequently develop, and are based on markedly dilated hair follicles in which fragments, live or dead, of the mite *Demodex folliculorum* are commonly found. The most floridly lumpy forms of rosacea are those that occur when the follicles rupture, their contents exciting a giant-cell granulomatous reaction (granulomatous rosacea), or when the lesion occurs in an area of marked sebaceous gland hyperplasia, commonly the noses of elderly men (**rhinophyma**).

Abnormal hair loss is called alopecia and there are many types

Hair loss from the scalp is a normal aging change, with exaggerated or early loss in those in whom there is a family predisposition (particularly men). There are many causes of hair loss outside the normal range, the most common being **alopecia areata**. Other types of alopecia include **alopecia totalis and universalis** (loss of all head hair and all body hair, respectively), **trichotillomania** (traumatic hair loss due to avulsion, usually self-inflicted, of the hair from the follicle for esthetic or psychological reasons), and **scarring alopecia** (usually the result of inflammatory destruction of hair follicles due to some other disease, e.g. lupus erythematosus or lichen planus, affecting the hair follicles).

Alopecia areata is the most common type of pathological hair loss

In alopecia areata there is sudden onset of round or oval patches of baldness in the scalp, leaving unusually smooth, almost shiny skin. The patches persist for many months, but in most cases the hair grows back within 12–18 months, although further patches may develop. A few progress to alopecia totalis.

The disease is multifactorial, and there is often a family history; more than half of the patients have a history of atopic eczema, asthma, or an autoimmune disease (particularly of the thyroid). It is common in association with Down's syndrome. There appears to be a sudden loss of anagen (growing) hairs, and the follicles enter the resting catagen/telogen phase, during which time there is a perifollicular infiltrate by lymphocytes.

The most common ulcers of the skin occur on the lower legs and are associated with chronic venous insufficiency

Most common in middle-aged and elderly women with varicose veins, chronic venous insufficiency in the lower legs and gravitational dermatitis, 'varicose' or 'venous' ulcers are a common and persistent problem in community practice.

They are shallow but often spreading ulcers, forming on a background of chronic gravitational dermatitis and pigmentation in the fragile atrophic skin around the ankles and lower shin (*Fig. 23.42*). They show little tendency to heal spontaneously, and secondary infection is common; some

Fig. 23.42 Chronic leg ulcers. The characteristic location and appearance of chronic leg ulcers, on the medial side of the leg, just above the ankle. In this case the ulcers are due to chronic venous insufficiency (note the brown pigmentation in surrounding skin). This is an important cause of morbidity in the elderly, but may also occur in middle-aged women with varicose veins, and in the obese. Healing is slow, and the skin remains fragile and predisposed to further ulceration even after complete healing.

of the topical applications used to treat or prevent bacterial infection produce a contact dermatitis, leading to deterioration of the ulcer.

Occasionally, chronic skin ulcers have a slightly raised purplish edge; these ulcers may be the result of vasculitic lesions in dermal vessels.

Arterial ulcers commonly involve the distal leg

Leg ulcers may also be due to arterial insufficiency, and are particularly common in diabetics (see *Fig. 25.16*, page 572) They occur in elderly people with severe atherosclerosis of the leg arteries and poor foot pulses; there may also be a history of intermittent claudication (see page 162). In diabetics the ulceration is often a result of combined arterial disease and peripheral neuropathy, when loss of peripheral sensation (particularly over the bony protuberances of the foot) leads to persistent unrecognized shearing trauma, followed by ulceration which cannot heal normally because of the poor blood supply. Arterial ulcers on the lower leg can be difficult to distinguish clinically from venous ulcers, but they tend to be more painful and may have a bluish-purple rim.

Dermatitis artefacta is associated with severe psychological disturbance

Self-inflicted skin lesions are commonly seen in dermatological practice. In its simplest (and commonest) form, this involves nothing more than the patient persistently scratching and picking at itchy skin lesions such as eczema or urticaria, often giving raised thickened skin nodules which persist ('picker's nodule'). In these cases the patients happily confess to their role in the causation and perpetuation of the lesion. In true dermatitis artefacta the patient denies all knowledge of their role. The range of lesions, and the methods of producing them, are legion, from the dropping of strong acid or alkali onto the skin to produce blisters or shallow necrotic ulcers, to self-injection with a variety of liquids including milk, suspensions of feces, etc. The diagnosis and management of these cases can be difficult, and the motivation of the patient is not always apparent without detailed psychiatric assessment. Broken love affairs, unhappiness in their occupation, and avoidance of work or domestic responsibility are some of the background problems.

Skin biopsy

Most dermatological disorders are easily diagnosed by a competent dermatologist on their clinical features alone, but some have an atypical appearance or an unusual distribution, leading to doubt about the diagnosis. In these cases, histological examination of a skin biopsy may be useful. The various biopsy techniques are:

- **Curette biopsy**: in which the skin lesion (usually raised) is scraped off piecemeal with a curette and the fragments are sent for histological examination. This is not recommended if an accurate histological diagnosis is required.
- **Shave biopsy**: in which a raised skin lesion is 'shaved off' with a sharp blade. This is sometimes carried out as a part-diagnostic/part-therapeutic maneuver for raised melanocytic lesions such as compound nevi, but is unsafe if there is any clinical doubt about the malignant potential of the lesion, as excision is rarely complete.
- **Punch biopsy**: a 3, 4 or 6 mm punch-biopsy sample is obtained. This method is useful to sample a uniform

skin lesion, particularly in an inflammatory disease such as psoriasis or discoid lupus erythematosus.
- **Incision biopsy**: in which a biopsy of a large skin lesion is taken by scalpel in the form of a sliver which includes both normal and abnormal skin.
- **Excision biopsy**: in which a small skin lesion is completely excised, usually as an ellipse with normal skin all around, for diagnostic purposes. However, where the lesion is solitary, and particularly when a skin tumor is suspected, an excision biopsy is also curative. This is the method of choice for all solitary skin tumors, particularly melanocytic lesions, basal-cell carcinomas, squamous-cell carcinomas and skin appendage tumors. If there is a clinical doubt about the extent of local spread, the lesion can be excised with a large area of normal skin.

Although histological examination of the biopsy forms the basis of laboratory diagnosis, immunofluorescent examination (e.g. pemphigoid, dermatitis herpetiformis) and electron microscopy (e.g. T-cell lymphoma) may be useful.

Case-based questions

Case 1 A miserable child with an itchy rash

A miserable and distressed 5-year-old child is brought to the family practitioner by a distraught and weary mother, who complains that the child has itchy rashes on the arms and forehead. Neither mother nor child has had a good night's sleep for many days because of the child's misery from the constant itching, which had not responded to creams and lotions purchased over the counter at the local pharmacy. On examination there were red, weeping and crusting lesions on the forehead and flexural aspects of the arms, particularly extensive and severe in the flexural crease of the elbows. On the upper arm there was an area of non-weeping thickened skin. The child also suffered from asthma

1. **What is the most likely diagnosis?**
2. **What other symptoms, besides asthma, is the child likely to have?**

3. **What is the likely long-term outcome in this case?**
4. **What is the explanation for the thickened patch of non-inflamed skin on the upper arm?**

Case 2 An old woman with large blisters

An 83-year-old woman is referred by her family practitioner to a Dermatology clinic because of a severe blistering rash. The blisters are worst on her lower abdomen, but there are also some on the medial aspect of both thighs. The blisters are domed and tense, up to 5 cm in diameter, mostly filled with clear fluid but a few contain bloodstained fluid. The patient said that the lesions started as very itchy red patches in which the blistering occurred after a few days. The dermatologist performed a punch biopsy from a very early lesion, an itchy red patch in which an early blister was forming. The dermatopathologist's report on the biopsy said 'The punch biopsy shows a basal blister containing clear fluid

▶

in which there are scattered eosinophils. There is also a heavy infiltrate of eosinophils in the upper dermis at the base of the blister and in surrounding skin. The appearances in this biopsy are those of ***** *****'.

1. **Supply the missing words from the pathology report.**
2. **Does the biopsy diagnosis fit with the clinical features?**
3. **Is biopsy necessary to establish the diagnosis?**

Cases 3, 4 and 5 Three men with skin tumors

A dermatology teacher illustrates to a group of medical students three men who are attending for skin surgery. One man (case 3) has a raised nodule on the side of his nose, about 5 mm in diameter, with a central depressed ulcerated area, present for 2 months. Another (case 4) has a flat pink and white plaque on his forehead, about 10 mm in diameter, with an irregular pink edge and a depressed central white area. It had been present for 7 months, slowly enlarging. The third man (case 5) had a lesion on his chest wall, present for over 2 years, slowly enlarging to its present size of 20 mm in maximum diameter. It took the form of a scaling red patch, with tiny foci of ulceration and scab formation.

The dermatologist tells the students that all three men, despite the great variation in clinical appearance, have basal cell carcinoma.

1. **Can the dermatologist be correct?**
2. **In which of the men will the surgery be easiest and most curative?**
3. **In which case will the surgery be most difficult, and why?**
4. **Should the tumors excised be submitted for histological examination?**

Case 6 A man with a lesion on his back

This lesion was removed from the back of a 23-year-old single man. It had recently bled.

Q 6.1 What is the diagnosis?

Q 6.2 What is the prognosis, and why?

Brief answers to these case-based questions are given on pages 595–6. More detailed answers and other study resources are available online at www.studentconsult.com.

Orthopedic and rheumatological pathology

REVISION OF BONE ARCHITECTURE AND RHEUMATOLOGICAL PATHOLOGY

Fig. 24.1 Bone architecture. (a) Diagram of long bone. (b) Compact cortical bone, H&E. (c) Trabecular medullary bone, H&E. The diagram (a) shows the structure of a typical long bone, with a central shaft region (diaphysis) and two variably bulbous ends (epiphyses) which are modified for articulation with adjacent bones by a surface coating of smooth articular cartilage. Elsewhere, the outer surface of the bone is covered by a thin fibrous periosteum. The strong and rigid outer component of the bone is composed of compact cortical bone which encloses a medullary cavity which is criss-crossed by a complex network of interconnected trabecular bone, with bone marrow between the trabeculae. The cortical bone (b) is composed of haversian systems **H** (or osteones), each with a central vascularized haversian canal (arrows) surrounded by concentric rings of compact lamellar bone. There is a layer of outer circumferential lamellae **OCL** on the exterior just beneath the fibrous periosteum **P**. The trabecular bone (c) is a network of interconnecting struts composed of lamellar bone (see below), arranged to produce maximum strength in the direction of greatest weight-bearing.

Bone is composed of specialized collagen (osteoid), which is mineralized by the deposition of hydroxyapatite

Bone is composed of a collagen-containing extracellular matrix (**osteoid**) synthesized by **osteoblasts**, which is mineralized by calcium-containing salts. There are two main patterns of bone deposition (*Fig. 24.2*).

In normal **lamellar bone** the osteoid collagen is deposited in a mechanically strong, parallel stratified pattern. The collagen is deposited in a direction dependent upon the maximal stresses to which the bones will be exposed, giving the maximum strength for the minimum bone bulk.

In abnormal **woven bone** the osteoblasts deposit osteoid collagen in a haphazard pattern. With its random arrangement of osteoid collagen fibers, this woven pattern is far less efficient and much weaker than lamellar bone, with a greater tendency to fracture under stress.

Bone is constantly being refashioned by osteoblastic new bone formation and osteoclastic removal of old bone

Osteoclasts are highly specialized cells capable of removing bone; they are multinucleate giant cells derived from the monocyte–macrophage series. Combined activity of osteoblasts and osteoclasts can produce reshaping of bone in order to meet new directional stresses. Unbalanced pathological increase in osteoclastic activity leads to destruction of bone, a feature of some metabolic bone diseases (discussed later in this chapter). The control of osteoblast and osteoclast activity, and hence the balance between bone formation and destruction in normal remodeling, is not completely understood, but many factors play a role (see Pink box).

Several factors are involved in bone formation and destruction

Parathyroid hormone (PTH) is secreted by the parathyroids in response to a fall in blood calcium, and restores the plasma calcium level by directly or indirectly stimulating osteoclastic bone resorption. PTH also increases both resorption of calcium ions and phosphate ion excretion by the kidney.

Vitamin D acts as a hormone, promoting the mineralization of bone (see page 538). Vitamin D deficiency leads to **osteomalacia**, a disease in which there is failure of mineralization of osteoid collagen (see page 538).

Calcitonin, a hormone produced by the parafollicular cells of the thyroid, is secreted in response to a rise in plasma calcium and has the opposite effects to PTH. It depresses osteoclast activity, thereby reducing bone resorption, and is used as a therapeutic agent to suppress abnormally increased osteoclast activity in diseases such as Paget's disease (see page 539).

Many other factors exert some influence on bone formation, e.g. growth hormone, corticosteroids, androgens and estrogens, insulin and some vitamins, local growth factors, cytokines and prostaglandins.

METABOLIC BONE DISEASE

Metabolic bone disease comprises four fairly common conditions in which there is an imbalance between osteoblastic (bone forming) and osteoclastic (bone destroying) activity.

In **osteoporosis** there is a slowly progressive increase in bone erosion, which is not adequately counteracted by new bone formation. Thus, the cortical bone is thinned, and the bone trabeculae are thinned and reduced in number, leading to general reduction in bone mass, but without distortion of architecture.

In **osteomalacia**, osteoblastic production of bone collagen is normal but mineralization is inadequate. This leads to trabecular bone that is only partially mineralized and therefore soft and weak.

In **Paget's disease of bone** there is excessive uncontrolled destruction of bone by abnormally large and active osteoclasts, with concurrent inadequate attempts at haphazard new bone formation by osteoblasts, producing physically weak woven bone.

In **hyperparathyroidism**, excessive secretion of PTH produces increased osteoclastic activity. There is excessive destruction of cortical and trabecular bone, with inadequate compensatory osteoblastic activity.

Fig. 24.2 Woven and lamellar bone. Polarizing light micrograph showing recently formed woven bone (**W**). The haphazard collagen arrangement contrasts with the regular lamellae of lamellar bone (**L**).

Patients with chronic renal failure develop the bone disease known as **renal osteodystrophy** as a result of mixed metabolic disturbance (mainly the combined effects of osteomalacia and hyperparathyroidism). The mechanisms are discussed below.

Osteoporosis is characterized by reduced bone mass and is the most common metabolic bone disease

Osteoporosis is characterized by a generalized reduction in the mass of bone, the bone being composed of abnormally thin trabeculae. It is widespread in the elderly and is an important cause of morbidity and even mortality, the weakened bone being particularly predisposed to fracture with minimal trauma. In established osteoporosis, thinning of the cortical bone is combined with thinning and reduction in number of bone trabeculae (*Fig. 24.3*). The consequences of osteoporosis are related to the general weakening of both cortical and trabecular bone.

Bone pain, particularly in the back, is a common symptom, and imaging often shows a so-called 'compression fracture'

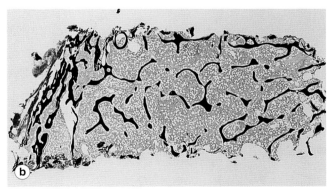

Fig. 24.3 Osteoporosis. (a) Micrograph of a resin section of a bone biopsy from the iliac crest, showing normal cortical and trabecular bone. It has been stained with a silver method, which stains calcified bone black. (b) Micrograph of bone from a patient with osteoporosis. When compared with (a), which shows the bone mass of a normal patient of the same age, it is obvious that the cortical zone is narrower, and that the trabeculae are thinner and less numerous.

of one or more vertebral bodies. Multiple compressions of vertebrae can lead to an overall loss of height, which may be compounded by uneven compression of vertebrae leading to bending of the spine anteroposteriorly (**kyphosis**).

Fractures of the neck of the femur and of the wrists are common complications of osteoporosis in the elderly; the cause is often relatively trivial (usually a fall). Elderly patients with a fractured neck of femur are an important component of the orthopedic workload, representing a substantial cost to the health services because of the often long and difficult postoperative return to mobility.

There are several different predisposing factors for the development of osteoporosis (see Key Facts box below).

It is most commonly encountered in postmenopausal women, when it is termed **senile osteoporosis**. It is believed that a major reduction in bone mass occurs in the 10 years after the onset of menopause, implying a hormonal influence for estrogen in maintaining bone mass.

Osteoporosis localized to one or both lower limbs is a common finding in people with paralysis due to neurological disease, in which case it is considered to be a form of **disuse atrophy**. Reduction in general mobility and activity may be a factor in osteoporosis in the elderly.

Osteoporosis is seen as a common complication of prolonged **corticosteroid therapy**. It is particularly important when the corticosteroids are being administered for diseases such as rheumatoid arthritis, in which there is also an element of disuse atrophy owing to a reduction in mobility. Osteoporosis can also be seen in some other endocrine disorders, such as thyrotoxicosis and panhypopituitarism, and associations have been reported with liver disease and diabetes.

Key Facts
Predisposing factors in osteoporosis

- Old age: particularly in postmenopausal women.
- Disuse: particularly in limb paralysis and, temporarily, in an immobilized limb following fracture.
- Perimenopausal state: osteoporosis in postmenopausal women may be minimized by hormone replacement therapy.
- Prolonged corticosteroid therapy: particularly when given for rheumatoid arthritis and immunosuppression.
- Assorted endocrine disorders: there is a strong association with Cushing's disease and Cushing's syndrome, and a less strong association with thyrotoxicosis, diabetes and hypopituitarism.
- Miscellaneous factors include liver disease, particularly alcoholic liver disease.

Osteomalacia is due to failure of mineralization of osteoid; 'rickets' is osteomalacia affecting children

In osteomalacia there is normal deposition of bone osteoid by osteoblasts, and bone architecture is normal. However, there is inadequate mineralization, so that, for example, only the center of bony trabeculae is adequately mineralized, the periphery being composed of soft unmineralized osteoid (*Fig. 24.4*). In adults this results in bone pain, sometimes due to microfractures of cortical plate and trabecular bone; the cortical microfractures can sometimes be seen radiologically (Looser's zones) and are most common in the bones of the lower limb, which are also the site of

Fig. 24.4 Osteomalacia. Micrograph of iliac crest bone embedded in acrylic resin without prior decalcification from a patient with osteomalacia. Note the broad zone of unmineralized osteoid (red) and the central zone of mineralized bone (black), in this section stained by the von Kossa silver technique.

major bone pain. In severe long-standing untreated osteomalacia in adults, softening of the long bones may lead to bowing of the legs.

In children, in whom the skeleton is not fully formed, osteomalacia leads to characteristic structural deformities of the long bones of the leg (severe bowing), distortion of the skull bone (leading to bossing), and enlargement of the costochondral junctions of the ribs (producing a characteristic 'rickety rosary').

Osteomalacia is usually the result of abnormalities of vitamin D metabolism

The metabolism of vitamin D and its association with bone mineralization is illustrated in *Fig. 24.5*. Owing to its effect on calcium metabolism, an inadequate supply of vitamin D, for whatever reason, is the most important cause of osteomalacia. Vitamin D deficiency may be due to:

- **Inadequate dietary intake**. Formerly the most common cause of osteomalacia in children, this is now rare in the western world, except in people who have extreme diets, e.g. pure vegans.
- **Inadequate body synthesis of vitamin D**. As vitamin D is synthesized in the skin under the influence of UV light, extensive covering of the skin for social and cultural reasons may be an important contributory factor in osteomalacia.

The above two factors are responsible for the high incidence of osteomalacia in natives of the Indian subcontinent living in the UK and other European countries. In Caucasians living in the west, the most important causes are:

- **Malabsorption due to intestinal disease**, for example after extensive small-bowel resection, treated and untreated Crohn's disease, and untreated celiac disease.

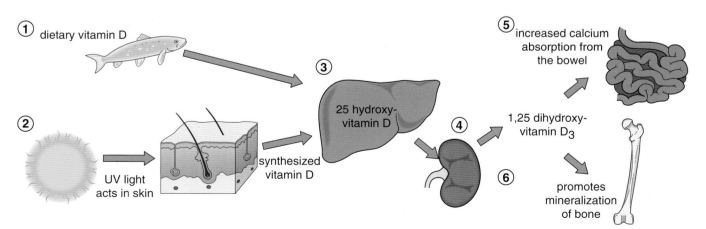

Fig. 24.5 Metabolism of vitamin D. Some vitamin D is dietary (1) e.g. from fish and fish oil, but most is synthesized in skin (2) by the action of UV light on the precursor 7-hydrocholesterol. Both dietary and synthesized vitamin D undergo hydroxylation in the liver (3) to form 25-hydroxyvitamin D, which is further hydroxylated in the kidney (4) to the major active substance 1,25-dihydroxyvitamin D_3, which increases absorption of calcium by the small bowel (5) and promotes mineralization of bone (6).

• **Renal disease**. In chronic renal failure, conversion of vitamin D to its active metabolite (1,25-dihydroxy-vitamin D_3) by renal tubular epithelial cells is impaired, and osteomalacia is one of the important metabolic bone diseases associated with renal failure.

Rarely, liver disease and some drug therapies may interfere with vitamin D metabolism and have a role in the development of osteomalacia.

Metabolism of vitamin D

Vitamin D_3, either from the diet or produced in the skin, is metabolized in liver and kidney to produce the active form, which has effects on bone and gut (*Fig. 24.5*).

Paget's disease of bone is a common disease of unknown cause affecting bones in the elderly

In Paget's disease there is excessive uncontrolled resorption of bone by large abnormal multinucleated osteoclasts. Excessive osteoclastic erosion occurs in waves, leading to localized destruction of trabecular and cortical bone; each wave of bone destruction is followed by a vigorous but uncoordinated osteoblastic response, producing new osteoid in an attempt to fill the defects left by the osteoclasts. Both the osteoclastic erosion and the osteoblastic response are random, haphazard, and unrelated to the functional stresses on the bone. As a result, the bone architecture is greatly distorted, and although there may be an increase in bone bulk, paradoxically it is weaker than normal. New bone formed as a repair attempt by the osteoblasts often has the characteristic woven, non-lamellar pattern indicative of rapid reparative deposition. Disruption of the bone architecture is followed by progressive fibrosis of the marrow spaces (*Fig. 24.6*).

Fig. 24.6 Paget's disease. Micrograph of a resin-embedded section of bone from a patient with Paget's disease. The bone trabeculae (green) are irregular and abnormally broad. They are composed of woven bone with haphazard deposition of osteoid (red). Osteoclasts (C) resorb bone, whereas osteoblasts (B) deposit new bone osteoid. There is associated fibrosis of marrow spaces (S).

Paget's disease may be widespread, affecting many bones, or confined to one area in a single bone (monostotic Paget's disease). Its cause is unknown, but a viral infection of osteoclasts has been postulated because of the observation that some abnormal osteoclasts in Paget's disease contain paracrystalline inclusions resembling paramyxovirus. However, no virus has been shown using sophisticated molecular techniques.

There are two common effects of Paget's disease. **Bone pain** is usually localized to the site of most active disease, Paget's disease characteristically waxing and waning. **Bone deformity** is usually seen only where there is extensive involvement of an entire bone or series of bones, e.g. there may be marked enlargement of the skull, or thickening, enlargement and bowing of the tibia. Most patients present with one or both of the above features, but some occasionally present with the complications of Paget's disease. For example, **nerve compression symptoms** are usually seen in association with Paget's disease of the skull, in which enlargement of the abnormal bone can lead to cranial nerve palsies.

In cases of **pathological fracture**, although the bone is increased in bulk, it is weaker than normal and more likely to fracture with trivial trauma. Imaging illustrates that the fracture has occurred at a site of bone abnormality, and there may be radiological evidence of Paget's disease elsewhere in the same or other bones.

Malignant tumor, usually osteosarcoma, may develop in areas of long-standing active Paget's disease. Osteosarcoma is normally a disease of children (see pages 544–6), and its development as a complication of Paget's disease is one of the very rare instances in which it is seen in the elderly.

Hyperparathyroidism produces bone erosion by stimulation of osteoclast activity

Parathyroid hormone (PTH) stimulates osteoclastic resorption of bone, with the release of calcium from the bone into the plasma. Its activity is normally finely controlled by a feedback mechanism whereby PTH secretion from the parathyroid gland is suppressed by a rise in plasma calcium concentration and stimulated by a fall. Failure of the feedback mechanism leads to excessive parathormone secretion, with continuing PTH output and excessive osteoclastic destruction of bone.

There are two main patterns of hyperparathyroidism. In **primary hyperparathyroidism** an autonomous parathyroid tumor, usually a parathyroid adenoma, secretes excess PTH continuously outside the control of the feedback mechanism. In **secondary hyperparathyroidism** a persistently low serum calcium level (due to excess calcium loss in the urine in chronic renal disease) leads to continuous stimulation of the parathyroids by the feedback mechanism. This results in hyperplasia of all the parathyroid glands and a constant excessive secretion of PTH.

The effects on bone of constant PTH stimulation are unremitting osteoclastic resorption of bone, followed by compensatory attempts by osteoblasts to deposit new bone. In addition to the diffuse bone resorption affecting all bones, single or multiple focal osteolytic lesions are occasionally present in bone. To the naked eye, these lesions appear to be filled with soft, semi-fluid brown material. These are the so-called **brown tumors**, which are composed of large masses of giant osteoclast-like cells and spindle cells associated with old and recent hemorrhage. Multiple brown tumors produce numerous osteolytic lesions in many bones, a condition sometimes called 'von Recklinghausen's disease of bone' or **osteitis fibrosa cystica**. Whether single or multiple, brown tumors are most common in primary hyperparathyroidism. In secondary hyperparathyroid bone disease due to renal failure there is usually associated osteomalacia due to vitamin D_3 abnormalities resulting from renal tubular disease.

In primary hyperparathyroidism the serum calcium level is often greatly increased (**hypercalcemia**) because of the continuous release of calcium from bone in the absence of an effective feedback mechanism. In secondary hyperparathyroidism it is the presence of a pathologically low serum calcium level that stimulates PTH activity and calcium release from bone; the serum calcium level is therefore low (**hypocalcemia**) or normal because any calcium mobilized from the bone is almost immediately lost through the abnormal kidneys.

Data Set
Renal bone disease

A 31-year-old man with polycystic kidney disease:

Plasma

Calcium	1.83 mmol/L	(2.2–2.6)
Phosphate	2.33 mmol/L	(0.7–1.4)
Albumin	32 g/L	(35–50)
Alkaline phosphatase	391 U/L	(80–280)
Urea	34 mmol/L	(1–6.5)
PTH	123 ng/L	(10–55)

Hypocalcemia is a common complication of chronic renal failure. Contributory causes include the lack of the active form of vitamin D, 1,25-dihydroxy-cholecalciferol, which is normally formed in the kidney by 1α hydroxylation of 25-hydroxy-cholecalciferol. Renal phosphate retention may also cause hypocalcemia, by precipitation of calcium phosphate. Hypocalcemia stimulates the release of parathyroid hormone (PTH). Secondary hyperparathyroidism and 1,25-dihydroxy-cholecalciferol deficiency result in metabolic bone disease, reflected in the raised alkaline phosphatase released from osteoblasts.

Renal osteodystrophy is a metabolic bone disorder associated with chronic renal failure

The term 'renal osteodystrophy' refers to metabolic and structural abnormalities of bone caused by the presence of chronic renal failure. There are two main components to renal osteodystrophy: **osteomalacia of renal origin** (due to failure of conversion of 25-hydroxyvitamin D_3 to the active principle, 1,25-dihydroxyvitamin D_3, in the kidney because of tubular damage) and **secondary hyperparathyroid effects** (secondary to low serum calcium because of a combination of vitamin D deficiency, excess calcium loss in urine, and phosphate retention).

The bone in renal osteodystrophy therefore shows a combination of secondary hyperparathyroidism changes, excessive bone erosion by osteoclasts, and failure of mineralization of osteoid collagen.

A further factor occurs in patients receiving long-term hemodialysis for chronic renal failure. Such patients often retain increased quantities of aluminium, which become deposited in the bone in the site in which mineralization by calcium should be taking place, blocking calcification of the osteoid, and thus playing a role in the osteomalacia.

BONE FRACTURE

Bone fractures heal by granulation tissue formation and fibrous repair, followed by new bone formation in the fibrous granulation tissue

Caused by physical trauma, bone fracture is one of the most common abnormalities of bone. The degree of fracture can vary widely, from a simple crack in the cortical bone to a complex multiple fracture with fragmentation and displacement of the bone pieces, associated with severe damage to the surrounding soft tissues and, sometimes, exposure of the bone fragments to the exterior through a large gaping wound (open 'compound' fracture).

The sequence of events in healing of a simple undisplaced fracture is illustrated in *Fig. 24.7*. For a fracture to heal efficiently it is important that all conditions are optimal; there are many factors that interfere with the satisfactory healing of fractures.

Delayed or abnormal healing of fractures can lead to non-union, in which the fractured bone ends do not join by bone

For proper fracture healing to take place it is essential that the fractured bone ends be in close apposition, that the fracture is immobilized, and that the patient's healing capacity is adequate.

Among the factors that detrimentally affect healing of bone is **poor blood supply** to the affected area. This is particularly important in certain areas, such as the scaphoid bone in the wrist and the neck of the femur, both of which

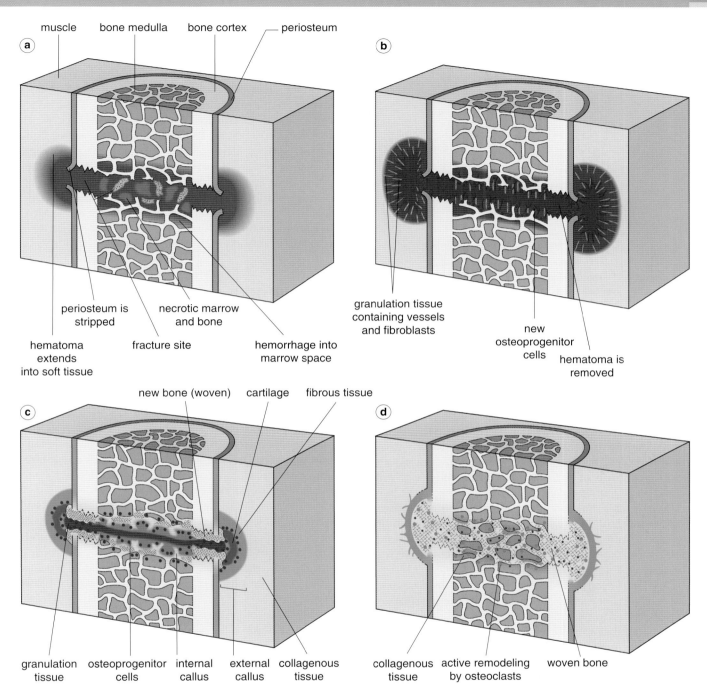

muscle   bone medulla   bone cortex   periosteum

a

b

periosteum is stripped   necrotic marrow and bone

hematoma extends into soft tissue   fracture site   hemorrhage into marrow space

granulation tissue containing vessels and fibroblasts   new osteoprogenitor cells   hematoma is removed

new bone (woven)   cartilage   fibrous tissue

c

d

granulation tissue   osteoprogenitor cells   internal callus   external callus   collagenous tissue

collagenous tissue   active remodeling by osteoclasts   woven bone

Fig. 24.7 Bone fracture. (a) Due to tearing of blood vessels in the medullary cavity, cortex and periosteum, a hematoma forms at the site of fracture. The periosteum is stripped from the bone surface. (b) Organization of the hematoma is associated with the migration of neutrophils and macrophages into the fracture hematoma; these cells phagocytose the hematoma and necrotic debris. This is followed by ingrowth of capillaries and fibroblasts from surrounding tissue, producing fibrovascular granulation tissue. New osteoprogenitor cells develop from mesenchymal precursor cells. (c) Osteoblasts derived from osteoprogenitor cells migrate into the granulation tissue and differentiate into osteoid-synthesizing units, which proceed to deposit large quantities of osteoid collagen in a haphazard way, producing a woven bone pattern. **External callus** bridges the fracture site outside the bone and, if there is a significant gap between the bone ends, it may include cartilage. **Internal callus** bridges the fracture in the medullary cavity and rarely contains cartilage. When bone ends are closely apposed, direct ossification between fractured ends occurs. (d) Callus is usually well established by the third week after fracture, but initial bony union is by woven bone, which is mechanically weak. Remodeling of callus occurs once the defect between the two bone ends is bridged by bony callus, taking many months. A combination of osteoclastic erosion and organized osteoblastic osteoid synthesis removes surplus calcified callus, replacing the inefficient bulky woven bone with compact organized lamellar bone.

residual scar
in muscle

remodeling of
medulla with some
residual fibrosis

cortex replaced by
lamellar bone

Fig. 24.8 Healed bone fracture. With time, remodeling creates new lamellar trabecular bone, which is orientated in a direction determined by the stresses to which the bone is exposed with mobilization. Even with remodeling, cortical irregularity and minor marrow space fibrosis persist at the site of fracture.

can be associated with avascular necrosis of fracture fragments. **Poor general nutritional status** (particularly where there is protein malnutrition or vitamin deficiencies) and **poor apposition of the fractured bone ends** (e.g. wide displacement, entrapped viable soft tissue between the bone ends, or excessive mobility) can also contribute to delayed or abnormal healing, as can **the presence of foreign bodies** or large quantities of necrotic bone, **the presence of infection** (particularly in open fractures) and **corticosteroid therapy**.

The aim of treatment in fractures is to ensure close apposition of the bone ends, followed by firm immobilization so that the fractured ends cannot move during the formation of granulation tissue and callus.

When fractured bone ends are not closely apposed, or if any of the above local complicating factors are present, ossification of the callus does not occur and the two bone ends are joined by fibrous tissue (**fibrous ankylosis**), which is unstable.

Fracture may occur with minimal trauma if the underlying bone is abnormal

For normal bone to fracture, the causative trauma usually has to be severe. In contrast, trivial trauma may cause fracture when the underlying bone is abnormal (**pathological fracture**).

Among the common abnormalities predisposing to pathological fracture are **osteoporosis** (particularly in the femur and vertebral column in the elderly), **osteomalacia** (the

fractures are often small microfractures without displacement), **Paget's disease of bone** (the pagetic bone being structurally weak despite the increase in bulk), and **primary** or **metastatic tumor**. Metastatic carcinoma in bone is an important cause of pathological fracture. Bone metastases from carcinoma of the breast, bronchus, thyroid and kidney produce bone destruction (osteolytic metastases), which predisposes to fracture. Primary tumors of bone or bone marrow, such as giant-cell tumor of bone and myeloma, also play a role, as do some non-neoplastic bone lesions such as bone cysts.

Congenital bone disorders can also predispose to pathological fracture. The most important disorder is osteogenesis imperfecta, in which multiple fractures occur, often in utero and in infancy, with minimal trauma.

ISCHEMIC BONE NECROSIS

Osteonecrosis is the generic term for ischemic bone necrosis of all types

When bone becomes ischemic, the hemopoietic cells of the bone marrow die first (within 12 hours), followed by the bone cells (osteoblasts, osteoclasts and osteocytes) in 12–24 hours, whereas the adipocytes of fatty marrow can survive for 4–5 days.

In general, osteonecrosis occurring in the shaft of a long bone, and in flat and irregular bones, is called **bone infarction,** whereas in the epiphyses of long bones it has traditionally been called **avascular necrosis**.

Bone infarction usually only involves trabecular bone and marrow in the medulla, as the cortical bone has an alternative blood supply via the periosteum, but avascular necrosis in the epiphysis of long bones may also involve the cortical bone, because the epiphyses are largely covered by articular cartilage and do not have the alternative periosteal blood supply.

Many diseases predispose to osteonecrosis, including hemophilia, sickle cell disease, thalassemia, chronic pancreatitis, Cushing's disease and exogenous corticosteroid therapy, as well as the autoimmune connective tissue disorders. However, the most common and important patterns of osteonecrosis are:

• Those seen secondary to bone fracture.
• The specific idiopathic osteonecrosis syndromes.

Subcapital fracture of the neck of the femur almost always tears a substantial component of the main arterial supply to the femoral head, leading to osteonecrosis in the head. Osteonecrosis (with failure to heal) is a well-recognized complication of fractures of some other bones, particularly the scaphoid bone of the wrist.

An important cause of idiopathic osteonecrosis (avascular necrosis) of the head of femur is **Legg–Calvé–Perthes disease** (see page 543).

Legg–Calve–Perthes disease is avascular necrosis of the femoral head (epiphysis) in children

The disease is of unknown cause, mainly affects boys, and first presents between the ages of 4 and 10 years with hip or groin pain, sometimes thigh or knee pain, associated with a limping gait. It is bilateral in 10–15% of cases although one hip usually gives trouble first, followed by the other hip some time later.

The main lesion is ischemic necrosis of a wedge-shaped area of bone in the subarticular zone of the head of the femur (*Fig. 24.9*). This is not detectable by X-ray in the early stages but is easily seen on MRI. Despite attempts to repair the necrotic bone, the process is too slow to prevent microfracture and collapse of the necrotic area of bone under the pressure of weightbearing. This produces deformity of the normally rounded femoral head, with irregular flattening of the epiphysis. Management and outcome depend on the amount of femoral head that is necrotic, and on the age of onset; in general, children who present before the age of 6 years and have only a small area of involvement do well with conservative treatment such as traction and bed rest, and have few long-term complications, mainly osteoarthritis in adult life. Older children, or those with more extensive femoral head damage, may

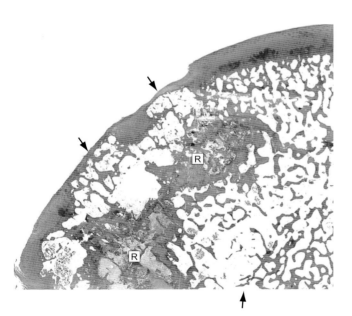

Fig. 24.9 Avascular necrosis of femoral head. This section shows part of a femoral head with early avascular necrosis, before significant flattening has occurred. The cortical bone and cartilage in the affected area is thinned and irregular (arrows), and much of the subcortical trabecular bone has been destroyed. Some attempt at repair (R) is occurring.

require prolonged immobilization with a plaster cast, or even surgery (e.g., osteotomy, bone graft or hip replacement).

INFECTION OF BONE

Infection of bone is called 'osteomyelitis' and usually involves the cortex, medulla and periosteum

The main causative organisms include *Staphylococcus aureus, Escherichia coli* (particularly in infants and the very elderly), *Salmonella* (particularly in patients with sickle-cell disease), and *Mycobacterium tuberculosis.*

In osteomyelitis the infective organisms gain access to the medullary cavity of the bone by two main routes:

- **Direct access through an open wound**. This is an important cause after trauma, particularly when trauma has been followed by an open fracture, and can lead to failed or delayed fracture repair. It is also an important cause in postoperative patients who have had surgery on bones.
- **Bloodborne spread** following bacteremia from a focus of sepsis elsewhere, e.g. acute pyelonephritis. Tuberculous osteomyelitis is the result of bloodborne spread from a primary tuberculous infective lesion in the lung.

Occasionally, bone infection can be a complication of sepsis in adjacent soft tissues or organs, e.g. mastoiditis complicating bacterial middle-ear infection.

In all forms of acute osteomyelitis (except for TB) the marrow cavity becomes filled with a purulent acute inflammatory exudate, leading to necrosis of medullary bone trabeculae. Destruction of the cortical bone may lead to the discharge of pus into extraosseous connective tissue, and the infection may track through to the skin surface, producing a chronic discharging sinus.

Because the infection is localized to the confined space of the marrow cavity, the pus has little chance to drain without surgical intervention; inflammation tends to become chronic, and organisms remain viable within the marrow cavity for many years. **Chronic osteomyelitis** results, with extensive bone destruction, marrow fibrosis and recurrent focal suppuration. With chronicity, there is reactive new-bone formation, particularly around the inflamed periosteum, leading to a thickened and abnormally shaped bone.

In **tuberculous osteomyelitis** the marrow cavity contains rapidly enlarging caseating granulomas that destroy trabecular and cortical bone.

BONE TUMORS

It is important to distinguish between tumors **of** bone and tumors **in** bone, as the most commonly seen tumors in bone are not derived from bone cells such as osteoblasts and osteoclasts, but are either:

- **Bloodborne metastases** of malignant tumors spread from other primary sites; or
- **Tumors of hemopoietic cells** located within the marrow spaces of bones, particularly myeloma.

Malignant tumors derived from the cells involved in bone formation and modeling are comparatively rare, the most common being **osteosarcoma** and **chondrosarcoma**. Less common primary tumors of bone are summarized in *Fig. 24.10*.

Some intraosseous lesions with the clinical and radiological manifestations of bone tumors are not true neoplasms but represent hamartomatous malformations, non-neoplastic proliferative disorders, or non-neoplastic cysts.

The most common malignant tumor in bone is metastatic bloodborne malignancy, usually metastatic carcinoma

Five common carcinomas have a particular predilection for metastasizing to bone: adenocarcinoma from the breast, carcinoma of the bronchus (particularly small-cell undifferentiated carcinoma), adenocarcinoma of the kidney, adenocarcinoma of the thyroid, and adenocarcinoma of the prostate (which often produces sclerotic reaction in bone).

Most metastatic tumor cells in bone marrow spaces lead to erosion of trabecular bone, either directly or through osteoclast stimulation, and to erosion of bone cortex (osteolytic metastases). This leads to bone weakness, predisposing to **pathological fracture**, which may be the first presenting feature. Carcinoma of the prostate often produces metastatic deposits in which there is stimulation of new bone formation (osteosclerotic metastases), particularly in the lumbosacral vertebrae.

Metastatic carcinoma in bone commonly produces bone pain, usually localized to the site of metastatic deposits. In addition to bone pain and fracture, it may produce symptoms due to three effects: **extensive replacement of**

Fig. 24.10 Important primary tumors of bone

Name	Presumed cell of origin	Age and sex incidence	Common sites	Behavior
Osteoid osteoma	Osteoblast	Adolescents M > F	Lower limb	Benign, osteosclerotic; painful
Non-ossifying fibroma	Uncertain	Child/adol M > F	Long bones of lower limb	Benign, osteolytic; occasionally multiple
Chondromyxoid fibroma	Uncertain	Adol/young adult M > F	Long bones esp. tibia	Benign osteolytic
Enchondroma	Chondrocyte	Young adults M > F	Bones of hands	Usually benign and expansile
Giant-cell tumor	Osteoclast	20–40 yrs M > F	Around knee	Mostly benign, may recur; rarely malignant
Chordoma	Notochord tissue	40+ yrs M > F	Sacrum	Local bone destruction and invasion
Osteosarcoma	Primitive osteoblast	(i) 10–25 yrs (ii) over 65 yrs M > F	(i) Around knee (ii) At site of Paget's disease	Highly malignant; early metastasis to lungs
Chondrosarcoma	Chondrocyte	30–60 yrs M > F	Spine and pelvis	Malignant; local spread and distant metastasis
Ewing's sarcoma	Primitive neuroendocrine	Child/adol M > F	Midshaft of long bones	Malignant; early and extensive metastasis

bone marrow, leading to leukoerythroblastic anemia; **symptoms due to hypercalcemia**, caused by release of calcium from bone by the destructive osteolytic process; and **nerve and spinal compression**, particularly in vertebral metastases.

Myeloma is a tumor of plasma cells that commonly presents as single or multiple bone tumors

The vast majority of plasma-cell tumors occur in bone (see page 314), arising in one of three patterns: **diffuse plasma-cell infiltration of marrow**, in which there is no discrete tumor formation; **solitary osteolytic bone lesion (solitary plasmacytoma)**, which is an unusual pattern; and **multiple osteolytic lesions in many bones (multiple myelomatosis)**.

Bone pain (and occasional pathological fracture) is an important clinical feature of myeloma. However, symptoms are not confined to bone because the neoplastic plasma cells produce abnormal amounts of immunoglobulin (usually IgG); this is of a single clonal type (monoclonal gammopathy), as it is produced by a single clone of neoplastic plasma cells. Many of the clinical features of myeloma are the result of the replacement of normal marrow cells by malignant plasma cells, together with the impact of the abnormal IgG (and its component heavy and light chains) on blood viscosity and renal function. Myeloma is discussed in greater detail in Chapter 15.

Fig. 24.11 Myeloma in bone. This bisected sternum shows multiple soft brown tumor masses (arrowed) of myeloma. There were multiple similar lesions in long bones, vertebrae, skull and ribs (multiple myeloma). The brown colour is characteristic of myeloma.

The most common malignant primary tumors of bone are osteosarcomas and chondrosarcomas

Osteosarcoma is a malignant tumor of osteoblasts which occurs in adolescent children, most commonly boys. The majority arise around the knee, either in the lower end of the femur or in the upper end of the tibia, although a small percentage occur in other long bones such as the humerus, or in the upper end of the femur.

The tumor causes gradually increasing pain around the knee, and is often well advanced at the time of clinical and radiological diagnosis. It originates in the medullary cavity close to the metaphyseal plate and spreads extensively within the medullary cavity, eventually eroding through cortical plate and extending into soft tissue (*Fig. 24.12*). The malignant osteoblasts produce varying amounts of osteoid collagen, some of which becomes mineralized (*Fig. 24.12*); this mineralization can be demonstrated radiologically and by other imaging methods, and is particularly apparent when the tumor is invading soft tissues.

Fig. 24.12 Osteosarcoma. An osteosarcoma is seen at the lower end of the femur. Tumor expands and destroys the bone (a). Histologically (b), neoplastic osteoblasts secrete pink-stained osteoid (arrows) between cells.

The tumor grows rapidly and metastasizes early via the bloodstream, usually producing pulmonary metastases. The prognosis has generally been poor (5–10% 5-year survival), but is improving with the adoption of earlier surgical treatment combined with radiotherapy and chemotherapy. Osteosarcoma in adults is largely confined to elderly patients with a long history of active Paget's disease of bone, the tumor occasionally developing in an area of Paget's disease.

Chondrosarcoma mainly occurs in adults, usually the middle-aged or elderly, and is particularly common in the bones of the pelvis

Chondrosarcomas are slow-growing tumors that often reach a large size, expanding the bone and eventually breaking through the periosteum into surrounding soft tissue, but usually maintaining a clearly defined border. Although malignant, they metastasize very late in most cases, the majority being low-grade well-differentiated tumors, histologically very similar to benign cartilaginous tumors; a few are high-grade poorly differentiated tumors with marked pleomorphism and high mitotic activity; they grow rapidly, with early bloodborne metastases.

Macroscopically, tumors have a glistening white appearance (*Fig. 24.13*). Radical local surgery may be curative in the low-grade group.

Fig. 24.13 Chondrosarcoma. A chondrosarcoma replaces much of the bone of the pelvis. The acetabulum (A) is still visible. Cartilage tumors have a glistening white appearance, similar to that of normal cartilage.

The most common benign bone-forming tumor is osteoid osteoma

Osteoid osteomas are found mainly in the long bones of the lower leg in adolescents and young adults. They present with bone pain localized to the area of the lesion. Usually <2 cm in diameter, they are radiologically characteristic, with a central dense area surrounded by a halo of bone lucency. Histologically they are composed of active osteoblasts, which deposit large irregular masses of osteoid collagen in a haphazard manner.

So-called **giant osteoid osteoma** or **benign osteoblastoma** is a larger tumor with similar histological features, mainly affecting the bones of the hands and feet and vertebrae; these are often more cellular than small osteoid osteomas, more locally aggressive, and can recur after incomplete excision.

Ivory osteoma is composed of densely compact bone of cortical type with haversian systems. It arises as small round nodules, usually in the skull bones.

Fig. 24.14 Osteoid osteoma. (a) Low-power picture showing a typical osteoid osteoma in the medullary bone of the tibia. At higher magnification (b), the tumor consists of irregular masses of recently formed osteoid **Ost** produced by numerous active but benign osteoblasts **Ob**.

The most common benign tumor of cartilage-forming tissue is the chondroma

Chondromas, most commonly found in the small bones of the hands and feet, may be single (solitary enchondroma) or multiple (enchondromatosis). The tumors arise in the metaphysis and may originate from residual nests of cartilage cells left behind as bone growth proceeds. They are composed of cartilaginous matrix containing scattered benign chondrocytes. A solitary chondroma at the periphery rarely undergoes malignant change, but this occasionally happens in multiple enchondromatosis. The term 'enchondroma' is used to indicate that these tumors arise within the bone, to distinguish them from the benign osteochondroma, which grows as a nodular exophytic lesion.

Benign osteochondroma grows as an exophytic nodule from the metaphysis of a long bone

Benign osteochondromas, also known as **cartilage-capped exostoses**, may be solitary (as a sporadic abnormality in childhood and adolescence) or multiple (as in the autosomal dominant condition **hereditary multiple exostoses**). They are composed of a nodule of protuberant bone covered by a cap of cartilage and an outer layer of perichondrium (*Fig. 24.15*). In children the cartilage layer may be thick, but this thins as the patient ages. Lesions are found most commonly in the humerus, femur and upper end of the tibia. Chondrosarcomatous change is rare in single sporadic lesions, but is more common in hereditary multiple lesions.

Giant-cell tumor of bone, sometimes called 'osteoclastoma', arises in the epiphysis of a long bone

Giant-cell tumors of bone are osteolytic lesions that occur in young and middle-aged adults, being generally more common in women. The bone is replaced by a mass of large multinucleated giant cells resembling large osteoclasts, which are embedded in a supporting spindle-celled stroma. The lesions expand into the metaphysis and, with enlargement, may erode the cortical bone. However, they rarely penetrate the periosteum or articular cartilage. These locally aggressive tumors are difficult to treat because of frequent recurrence at the site of inadequate local excision, particularly if an attempt has been made to eradicate the tumor by curettage. Because of their apparent osteoclast component, and the presence of hemorrhage and cystic change associated with bone destruction, giant-cell tumors of bone can be difficult to distinguish from the **brown tumor of hyperparathyroidism** and also from an unusual lesion called **aneurysmal bone cyst**. The latter can usually be distinguished by the different site, most commonly in the vertebrae or in the shaft of a long bone. Unlike giant-cell tumors, aneurysmal bone cysts can usually be cured by curettage.

Ewing's sarcoma is a highly malignant tumor in children and teenagers

Ewing's sarcoma belongs to the family of undifferentiated tumors called **peripheral primitive neuroectodermal tumors (pPNET)**. It is most common between the ages of 10 and 20 years, but can occur in younger children and in adults up to the age of 35. The tumor can occur in any bone, but the majority occur in the pelvic bones, the shafts of the long bones of the lower limb, and the ribs.

The tumor arises in the medullary cavity and can spread extensively within it, destroying trabecular bone as it goes, as well as eroding cortical bones from within. When the cortical bone is eroded by tumor there is marked reactive thickening in the adjacent periosteum. Destruction of bone by tumor causes pain at the site, and pathological fracture is a common feature.

The tumor is composed of small undifferentiated round cells, sometimes with some spindle-celled areas; the cells are mainly nucleus, and the small amount of cytoplasm is often pale or vacuolated owing to the presence of abundant glycogen.

There are gene abnormalities in the tumor cells in almost all cases, the most common being a translocation between chromosomes 11 and 22 in 85–90% of cases.

An almost identical tumor, called the **Aspin tumor**, affects the chest wall and ribs in children (particularly boys) in the same age group. The histology and gene abnormalities seen in Ewing's tumor are also present in Aspin tumor.

Before chemotherapy the prognosis was very poor, with death following metastatic spread, but the introduction of chemotherapy, often combined with surgical excision or debulking, has led to 5-year survival rates of 75–80%, and long-term cures in more than half of patients.

Fig. 24.15 Cartilage-capped exostosis. Histology of an exostosis shows a cartilage cap (C) overlying bone (B).

DISEASES OF JOINTS, TENDONS AND SOFT TISSUES

Bones are joined together by **joints**, which allow varying degrees of movement between the adjacent bone ends; some joints permit considerable movement, others only limited movement. The most important type of joint that permits considerable movement is the **synovial joint**, illustrated in *Fig. 24.16*. Excessive joint movement is limited by a strong joint capsule and an enclosing ligament, assisted by attached muscles and tendons. In joints in which there is only limited movement the bones are joined by fibrous or cartilaginous tissue, e.g. the fibrocollagenous and cartilaginous intervertebral discs between adjacent vertebral bodies.

Patients with diseases in the joints and associated tendons and soft tissues may present to the orthopedic surgeon, rheumatologist or, in the case of acute post-traumatic lesions, in Accident and Emergency departments. Furthermore, such patients are numerous in general community practice, comprising a significant percentage of the persistent uncured attenders at clinics of all types. Thus, these diseases are an important cause of morbidity in patients of all ages (with the exception of very young children), although the nature of the disorder is different at different ages. For example, osteoarthritis of the hip is the most common disease in the elderly, whereas in adolescents and young adults the consequences of trauma to tendons, ligaments and joints are most common. Constant repetitive actions involving the same series of joints over a long period of time (often in the course of the patient's occupation) can lead to repetitive strain symptoms, with mixed features of joint, tendon and ligament disease (see page 556).

Inflammatory disease of joints (arthritis and synovitis) has four main causes

Inflammatory disease of joints, which is grouped under the terms **arthritis** and **synovitis**, has four main causes:

- **Degeneration**, e.g. osteoarthritis.
- **Autoimmity**, e.g. rheumatoid arthritis, SLE, autoimmunity (see page 561) rheumatic fever (see page 187).
- **Crystal deposition**, e.g. gout and other crystalline arthropathies.
- **Infection**, e.g. septic arthritis, tuberculous arthritis.

Osteoarthritis is a common and important degenerative disease, with both destructive and reparative components

Osteoarthritis may arise as a primary disorder, as well as secondary to other joint malfunctions (particularly abnormal loading or structural deformities). The pathological changes involve cartilage, bone, synovium and joint capsule, with secondary effects on muscle (*Fig. 24.17*). The main factors in the development of osteoarthritis are aging, abnormal load on joints, crystal deposition, and inflammation of joints.

In general, osteoarthritis affects joints that are constantly exposed to wear and tear. It is an important component of occupational joint disease, e.g. osteoarthritis of the fingers in typists, and of the knee in professional footballers.

Previous abnormality of the joint predisposes to the early development of severe osteoarthritis (sometimes called 'secondary osteoarthritis'); causes include:

- Congenital abnormality of joints.
- Trauma to joints (including trauma resulting from lack of sensory innervation).
- Inflammatory joint disease.
- Avascular necrosis of bone.

Clinically, osteoarthritis can be classified according to the main presenting features, namely:

- **Primary generalized osteoarthritis** is usually associated with the development of Heberden's nodes on the fingers and is commonest in postmenopausal women.
- **Erosive inflammatory osteoarthritis** describes forms of osteoarthritis in which there is severe inflammation and erosion of cartilage, with rapid progression.

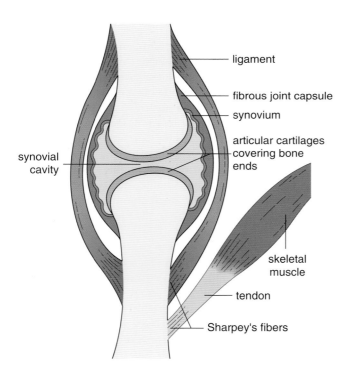

Fig. 24.16 Synovial joint. Diagram of a simple synovial joint showing the two articulating bone ends separated from each other by synovial fluid and enclosed within a fibrocollagenous capsule. Surrounding ligaments and tendinous muscle attachments prevent excess movement.

labels: ligament; fibrous joint capsule; synovium; articular cartilages covering bone ends; skeletal muscle; tendon; Sharpey's fibers; synovial cavity

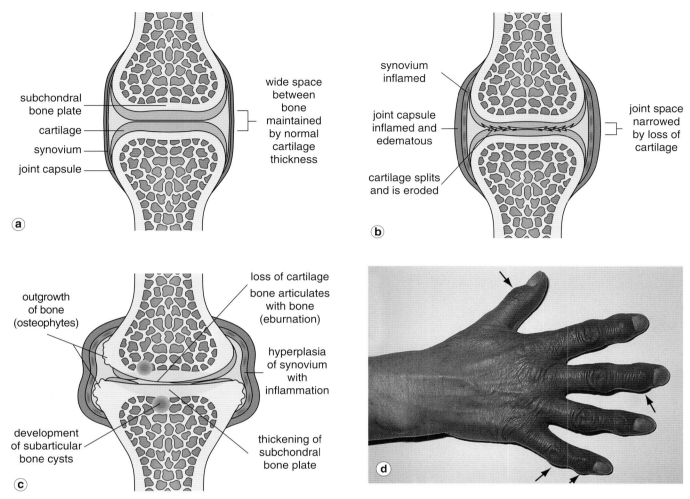

Fig. 24.17 Pathological changes in osteoarthritis. (a) In a normal synovial joint the distance between the bone ends seen on radiography is maintained by the thickness of articular cartilage. (b) The early change in osteoarthritis is **destruction of articular cartilage**, which splits (fibrillation), becomes eroded, and leads to narrowing of the joint space on radiography. There is inflammation and thickening of the joint capsule and synovium. (c) With time, there is **thickening of subarticular bone** caused by constant friction of the two naked bone surfaces, leading to a highly polished bony articular surface (eburnation). **Small cysts** develop in the bone beneath the abnormal articular surface. **Osteophytes** form around the periphery of the joint by irregular outgrowths of bone. There may be **reactive thickening of the synovium** due to inflammation caused by bone and cartilage debris. Inflammatory changes are also often seen. **Atrophy of muscle** is caused by disuse following immobility of the diseased joint. (d) In osteoarthritis of the hands, osteophytes on the interphalangeal joints of the fingers are termed 'Heberden's nodes' and appear as small nodules (arrows).

- **Hypertrophic osteoarthritis** describes forms with florid osteophyte formation and bone sclerosis, with a slow progression and relatively good prognosis.

Irrespective of the site, osteoarthritis causes pain and limitation of movement at the affected joint, sometimes associated with visible swelling; this is due partly to the presence of bony osteophytes and partly to fluid accumulation in the joint cavity and synovial fibrosis. In osteoarthritis affecting the cervical vertebrae (**cervical spondylosis**), osteophytes compressing emerging spinal nerves are responsible for much of the symptomatology.

Rheumatoid disease is a systemic autoimmune disease that particularly affects the joints, leading to arthritis

Rheumatoid arthritis is a common and important cause of inflammatory joint disease, although it is but one manifestation of a generalized systemic disorder (see Chapter 25). It is characterized by the presence of a circulating autoantibody, 'rheumatoid factor' (**seropositive arthritis**), which distinguishes this form of disease from several other inflammatory joint diseases (**seronegative arthritis**).

Rheumatoid arthritis mainly affects peripheral synovial joints such as the fingers and wrists, but can also affect the knees and more proximal joints. Women are affected two to three times more commonly than men, and the usual

Fig. 24.18 Rheumatoid arthritis. (a) The early pathological change in rheumatoid arthritis is **rheumatoid synovitis**. The synovium is swollen and shows a villous pattern. There is a great increase in chronic inflammatory cells (mainly lymphocytes and plasma cells) in the synovial stroma, often with an exudate comprising **fluid**, which produces an effusion in the joint space, and **fibrin** which is deposited on the synovial surface. Soft tissue swelling from synovial inflammation can be marked. (b) With time, there is **articular cartilage destruction**; vascular granulation tissue grows across the surface of the cartilage (**pannus**) from the edges of the joint, and the articular surface shows loss of cartilage beneath the extending pannus, most marked at the joint margins. (c) The inflammatory pannus causes **focal destruction of bone**. At the edges of the joint there is osteolytic destruction of bone, responsible for 'erosions' seen on radiographs. This phase is associated with joint deformity. (d) The characteristic deformity and soft tissue swelling associated with long-standing rheumatoid disease of the hands.

age of onset is between 35 and 45 years. The affected joints become swollen, painful and warm, often with redness of the overlying skin. There are three main pathological changes, as illustrated in *Fig. 24.18.*

In long-standing chronic disease the articular cartilage may be largely destroyed and replaced by fibrous pannus; the underlying bone shows osteolytic erosions, and the synovium lining the joint capsule is greatly thickened and chronically inflamed. The loss of articular surface can lead to the development of secondary osteoarthritic changes, particularly in weightbearing joints such as the knee. Unlike most other autoimmune arthropathies, rheumatoid arthritis is chronic and progressive. It usually leads to eventual joint deformity, with secondary features (e.g. muscle wasting) owing to disuse of the disorganized joint.

The joint changes are often associated with the development of subcutaneous **rheumatoid nodules**; these, and other features seen in systemic rheumatoid disease, are discussed in Chapter 25.

Autoimmune arthritis also occurs in patients with SLE, rheumatic fever and systemic sclerosis

Several types of arthritis are associated with systemic autoimmune disease processes.

SLE is a systemic disease in which joint involvement is a frequent but minor feature. The arthropathy is often transient, affecting the same types of joint as rheumatoid disease (i.e. fingers, wrists and knees), but is rarely progressive and does not lead to joint deformity.

Rheumatic fever is described in Chapter 10 because of its severe impact on the heart. A transient flitting arthritis is a characteristic feature of the acute stage, and the larger joints (e.g. elbow, knee and ankle) are most frequently involved. Like the arthritis of SLE, it is transient and does not lead to chronicity and joint deformity. There may occasionally be subcutaneous nodules similar to those seen in rheumatoid arthritis, but they are localized to the region of the affected joint; these nodules are transient and do not persist as in rheumatoid arthritis.

Systemic sclerosis is a systemic connective tissue disease that mainly affects the skin, bowel, lung and kidneys; occasionally there is an associated arthritis, with features similar to those of mild rheumatoid arthritis.

The crystal arthropathies are caused by deposition of crystals in joints, causing arthritis

The crystal arthropathies are diseases characterized by the deposition of crystals in joints and soft tissues. Affected patients usually present with an episode of acute monoarthritis or oligoarthritis, inflammation being caused by the deposition of the crystals, sometimes called a 'chemical' arthritis. With time, inflammatory changes lead to development of a chronic arthritis with features of osteoarthritis (secondary osteoarthritis).

The nomenclature of this group of disorders is in a state of change: the term 'gout' is used as a clinical description for joints affected by crystal deposition, which must then be refined by demonstrating the type of crystal involved. There are two main types of crystal arthropathy: **urate gout** (gout) and **calcium pyrophosphate gout** (pseudogout).

Less common forms of crystal arthritis are caused by deposition of hydroxyapatite, which also causes periarthritis and tendinitis. Oxalate arthritis may be seen in patients with hyperoxaluria, and in some patients on hemodialysis.

The most important crystal arthropathy is caused by deposition of uric acid, causing true gout

Urate gout is characterized by deposition of urate crystals in joints and soft tissues, which is caused by the presence of hyperuricemia. Uric acid is normally derived from the breakdown of purines and is excreted in the urine. Urate gout is largely confined to men, although some women develop it after the menopause. It can present at any time between the ages of 20 and 60 years, most cases presenting with an acute attack of arthritis, often affecting the big toe.

There are two main reasons for hyperuricemia:

- **Underexcretion of uric acid**. Seen in the majority of patients with urate gout, but of uncertain origin. It is clinically associated with hyperlipidemia, renal failure, alcohol consumption, and some drugs (diuretics).
- **Overproduction of uric acid**. High cell turnover (leukemia and chemotherapy for tumors).
- Rare congenital enzyme defects of purine metabolism.

In the majority of patients with urate gout, disease is probably the result of polygenic factors leading to underexcretion of uric acid (primary gout). Only a small proportion of patients develop urate gout as a result of overproduction of uric acid.

Urate crystals are deposited in certain joints, particularly the metatarsophalangeal joint of the big toe, stimulating an acute inflammatory reaction leading to a painful acute arthritis (*Fig. 24.19*). Uric acid crystals are also deposited in the soft tissues around joints, where their presence excites a foreign-body giant-cell reaction. These soft tissue masses may enlarge to produce a palpable mass composed of white chalky material (**tophi**).

In the joint, the urate crystals are deposited on the surface of the articular cartilage to form a white powdery deposit, beneath which the cartilage shows degenerative changes. Attacks of acute gouty arthritis are intermittent and may be precipitated by dietary indiscretion. The pain of an acute attack is excruciating, and various inflammatory mediators (particularly interleukin (IL)-1) have been implicated in the

Fig. 24.19 Gouty arthritis. This is an opened joint showing a white deposit of urate crystals on the articular surface in gout (a). The most commonly affected site is the big toe (b); the metatarsophalangeal joint becomes inflamed, often developing secondary osteoarthritis with deformity.

pain, edema and redness seen in the acutely inflamed joint. The stimulus to inflammatory mediator release is probably the deposition of crystals in the joint cavity, synovium and periarticular soft tissues, and neutrophil polymorphs can be seen to phagocytose urate crystals in the joint fluid. The diagnosis is best made by examining aspirated synovial fluid from the joint for the presence of crystals.

Recurrent attacks of acute gout affecting the same joint eventually lead to articular cartilage destruction, chronic synovial thickening and a secondary osteoarthritis; this is called **chronic gouty arthritis**.

Urate crystals deposited in the kidney may lead to an interstitial nephritis and to renal calculi composed of uric acid. Precipitation of urates in renal tubules may produce acute tubular necrosis and acute renal failure in leukemic patients with massive purine release after chemotherapy.

Hyperuricemic gout has a familial tendency and is believed to be polygenically inherited (see page 70). It is associated with an increased predisposition to hypertension and coronary artery disease.

Fig. 24.20 Uric acid crystals forming tophi. (a) This photomicrograph shows characteristic fine feathery crystals of urate from a gouty tophus. (b) The crystals are particularly obvious and beautiful when viewed under polarized light.

Calcium pyrophosphate crystal arthritis is also known as 'pseudogout'

Crystals of calcium pyrophosphate dihydrate may be deposited in the articular cartilage of joints (**chondrocalcinosis**). The deposition may be entirely asymptomatic, but if the crystals are shed into the joint space, patients develop an acute arthritis similar to that seen in urate gout. The shedding of crystals may be precipitated by trauma or intercurrent illness, or may be spontaneous. The joint most commonly affected is the knee, followed by the wrist, shoulder and ankle. The diagnosis is made by demonstrating pyrophosphate crystals in aspirated joint fluid; as the disease may closely mimic true urate gout, it is often also called 'pseudogout'.

This type of crystal arthritis is most common in the elderly as a primary degenerative disorder, some cases being due to an autosomal dominant trait. Patients under the age of 60 with this form of arthritis may have a secondary form associated with hyperparathyroidism, hemochromatosis, or less common metabolic or endocrine disorders.

With time, damage to cartilage by pyrophosphate may lead to the development of secondary osteoarthritis.

Infective arthritis is mainly due to pyogenic bacteria and mycobacteria

Pyogenic bacteria may gain access to a joint either by bloodstream spread or, more commonly, by local trauma or spread from adjacent infective foci. Infective arthritis is a well-recognized complication of prosthetic surgery at the knee and hip (the most common sites for infective arthritis of all types and causes).

A wide range of bacteria may be responsible, but *Staphylococcus aureus*, streptococci and *Haemophilus* are the most important. Bloodborne infection by the gonococcus is an important cause in teenagers and young adults. Children and young adults are the most likely groups to develop septic arthritis, most cases in older adults being associated with penetrating injury such as open fractures, insertion of a surgical prosthesis, and non-sterile intra-articular injections of steroids for established autoimmune arthritis. Intravenous drug users are particularly likely to develop septic arthritis associated with Gram-negative bacteremia.

Almost all cases of infective arthritis affect a single joint only, but some cases of gonococcal arthritis and arthritis in intravenous drug abusers may affect more joints. The diagnosis can be established with certainty only by aspiration of fluid from the joint space, which is examined cytologically for evidence of pus and microorganisms, and then cultured.

Tuberculous arthritis is now rare, and is the result of bloodstream spread from pulmonary TB. In adults the vertebral column is most often affected; tuberculous osteomyelitis leads to the collapse of affected vertebrae, particularly in the lumbar and lower thoracic spine (Pott's disease), and paravertebral collections of tuberculous caseous material occasionally track down the psoas muscle (**psoas abscess**) to point in the groin. In children, tuberculous arthritis mainly affects the hip and knee. Synovial biopsy shows caseating tuberculous granulomas.

Infective arthritis in syphilis and brucellosis is now rare. Arthritis due to the spirochete *Borrelia burgdorferi* (Lyme disease) and to some fungal infections such as blastomycosis occurs in outbreaks in the USA and Europe.

The seronegative spondylarthritides are characterized by peripheral joint inflammation without circulating rheumatoid factor

The seronegative spondylarthritides are a set of inflammatory arthritides that involve peripheral joints as well as the sacroiliac joint and spine; they are distinguished from rheumatoid disease by the absence of circulating rheumatoid factor. The cause and pathogenesis of these diseases are not known, but an autoimmune reaction is suggested by a high incidence of the antigen HLA B27. The most important conditions are **ankylosing spondylitis, psoriatic arthropathy, enteropathic arthropathy** and **reactive arthritis**.

Ankylosing spondylitis is almost as common as rheumatoid disease, but is often not clinically diagnosed. It typically presents in late adolescent and young adult Caucasian males, as an ankylosing arthropathy that begins in the lumbar vertebral spine and sacroiliac joints, extending upwards to involve the thoracic and cervical vertebrae. In addition, there is often involvement of peripheral joints, mainly the hips and knees. The disease progresses slowly and unremittingly. In the early stages there is inflammation (with a heavy lymphocytic infiltrate) of the ligaments around the vertebrae, which subsequently heals by dense fibrosis and ossification of the ligaments to form a rigid shell linking the periphery of the vertebral bodies. Eventually the vertebral column becomes fused, inflexible and rigid (bamboo spine). Systemic manifestations include recurrent iritis and aortic valve incompetence. Over 90% of men with ankylosing spondylitis have the HLA B27 antigen (less than 10% of the normal population have this antigen).

Reactive arthritis follows genital infection with *Chlamydia trachomatis* in some susceptible individuals, or arises after bacterial gastroenteritis due to *Salmonella*, *Yersinia* or *Campylobacter*. The HLA B27 antigen is present in 80% of affected patients.

Reiter's syndrome comprises arthritis, urethritis, and conjunctivitis. The arthritis usually affects the knee or the ankle, and the clinical and histological features of the arthropathy resemble those seen in rheumatoid arthritis, with chronic inflammatory synovitis. There is spontaneous resolution in some affected patients, but symptoms are still present in 80% of patients after 5 years. In a minority of cases severe spondylitis and features very similar to ankylosing spondylitis develop.

Fig. 24.21 Psoriatic arthropathy. The arthropathy associated with some cases of psoriasis can be severely destructive, leading to marked deformity, pain and loss of function, particularly in the hands. Note that the patient has severe active psoriasis of the skin of the hands and arms.

Psoriatic arthropathy occurs in 5–10% of patients with psoriasis. It tends to involve the distal interphalangeal joints (a characteristic feature), but there may be a more widespread symmetrical multi-joint involvement, with sacroiliitis and spondylitis. The joint changes are similar to those seen in rheumatoid arthritis, and osteolytic destruction of bone is particularly common in association with the arthritis involving the distal interphalangeal joints (*Fig. 24.21*). Patients who have associated spondylitis usually have the HLA B27 antigen.

Acute trauma to joints and associated tendons, ligaments and soft tissues is responsible for considerable morbidity

Direct trauma to joints may lead to **dislocation**, a condition predisposed to by lax ligaments. Although the trauma required to produce dislocation is usually severe, some patients have a predisposition to dislocation of certain joints, particularly the shoulder; in severe cases dislocation may occur without trauma when the joint is held in a certain position. Most dislocations that occur without associated fracture are the result of sports injuries, and are therefore seen in the young and otherwise healthy. Shoulders and finger joints are particularly commonly affected by sports injuries. When the dislocated bones have been relocated in their proper configuration in the joint, there may be residual inflammation because of direct trauma from the dislocated bone on the joint capsule and surrounding ligaments; this trauma sometimes leads to permanent weakness of the soft tissues surrounding the joint, predisposing to further episodes of dislocation.

Lacerations of the menisci in the knee joint may occur in either normal or degenerate menisci

The **menisci** of the knee joint are principally composed of dense compact collagen in which the fibers are arranged

Fig. 24.22 Torn knee meniscus. The specimen is a severely damaged knee meniscus showing the so-called 'bucket-handle' appearance. The inner part of the meniscus has completely separated away.

mainly in a circumferential pattern, probably to withstand the circumferential stress to which they are exposed. In addition, there are some radial fibers which probably hold the circumferential fibers together and resist splitting (which might result from excessive compression).

Lacerations of a structurally normal meniscus in young people are almost invariably the result of sporting injury, usually severe rotational stress in a partly bent knee. They mainly involve the medial meniscus, the laceration commonly initially appearing as a split separating the circumferential fibers. The split tends to extend throughout the meniscus to produce the so-called 'bucket-handle tear' (*Fig. 24.22*). Occasionally there is a partial radial tear which may lead to irregular fragmentation on the medial aspect of the meniscus.

In the elderly, laceration of the meniscus usually occurs with minimal trauma in menisci that are abnormal as a result of myxoid degeneration of the collagen, leading to separation, fraying, and occasional cyst formation. Focal calcification of the menisci is a characteristic feature of pseudogout due to pyrophosphate crystal deposition (see pages 551–2).

Torn ligaments are a common consequence of overstretching at a joint

Ligament tears are usually the result of excessive physical exercise, and are therefore a common sporting injury, although the ligaments on the lateral aspect of the ankle are frequently damaged by acute overstretching during trivial stumbles (sprained ankle).

The intra-articular cruciate ligaments within the knee joint are frequently torn in sporting injuries (*Fig. 24.23*). Rupture of the cruciate ligaments leads to chronic instability of the knee; because these ligaments are long structures stretched between two bone surfaces, tearing leads to their pulling apart, and spontaneous natural healing is usually unsuccessful because of the distance between the separated ends. Current treatment options include replacement by various types of prosthetic ligament.

Fig. 24.23 Torn cruciate ligament. This photograph was taken during arthroscopic exploration of the knee. It shows the completely separated remains of a cruciate ligament, now shrunken and white following its detachment after rupture. It is from the knee of an English soccer player.

Acute tendon damage is usually due to either penetrating injuries or spontaneous rupture

Industrial or domestic injuries, particularly to the hand, are an important cause of laceration of one or more **flexor or extensor tendons of the hand**, with consequent loss of the ability to flex or extend the affected fingers. Spontaneous rupture of the Achilles tendon usually occurs as a sporting injury following acute overstretching. Healing is slow even when the torn ends of the long cylindrical tendons are closely apposed surgically. Tendon is very slow to heal because it is a densely collagenous fibrous tissue with a comparatively poor blood supply and very scanty fibroblasts. For good healing, accurate apposition of the torn ends is essential. The gap is filled by vascular granulation tissue, with eventual fibroblast proliferation and deposition of new densely hyaline collagen. A further problem is that these long tendons frequently run in a surrounding synovial-lined tendon sheath, and healing by fibrosis of the damaged tendon sheath leads to fibrous adhesions between sheath and tendon, limiting the sliding movement of the tendon within the sheath. Repeat surgery to separate these adhesions and to mobilize the healed tendon is frequently necessary, as is strenuous physiotherapy.

'Tennis elbow' is due to repeated damage to the tendinous insertion of the extensor muscles of the forearm on the lateral aspect of the elbow

'Tennis elbow' (also called lateral epicondylitis) is pain and tenderness at the lateral epicondyle of the elbow joint where the common tendon of the extensor muscles of the forearm is inserted into bone. Minor tears in this tendon occur with certain strenuous movements (particularly vigorous single-handed backhand strokes in tennis), and repetition of these movements perpetuates the damage. Because tendon tissue is relatively acellular, healing is slow and incomplete. The repeatedly damaged tendon shows areas of myxoid degeneration of collagen, increased vascularity and replacement of dense tendon with looser collagenous scar, and there may be foci of calcification. In some cases there may be reactive thickening of the periosteum of the lateral epicondyle around the site of insertion.

Although tennis elbow is frequently the result of a sporting injury, it also occurs in manual workers whose job involves repeated rotation and gripping movements of the wrist and lower arm with the elbow partially flexed. Because of the different strains involved, 'golfer's elbow' involves the medial epicondyle of the elbow, with tendon damage similar to that seen in tennis elbow.

Carpal tunnel syndrome is a common condition affecting the hand, particularly in women

The flexor tendons of the fingers enter the hand at the wrist through a space called the **carpal tunnel**. This is floored by the carpal bones of the wrist and the roof is formed by a strong dense fibrocollagenous band called the flexor retinaculum. With the flexor tendons in the tunnel is the median nerve (*Fig. 24.24*), and compression of this nerve is responsible for the symptoms of the syndrome, mainly pain and paresthesia in the distribution of the median nerve (thumb, all of the index and middle fingers, and the radial half of the ring finger). In severe or late cases there may be loss of sensation in this distribution, wasting of the muscles of the thenar eminence, and occasionally pain up to the elbow. The syndrome is due to a reduction in the size of the space in the carpal tunnel and may result from degeneration and thickening of the flexor retinaculum, thickening of the synovium on the inner surface of the flexor retinaculum and the outer surfaces of the flexor tendons, a reduction of the fluid in the space, or a combination of all three.

It is about four times more common in women than in men, and can be a transient symptom in the later stages of pregnancy, the symptoms frequently occurring early in the morning and improving during the day. Persistent carpal tunnel syndrome is thought to be related to excessive use of the wrist in sport or the workplace, but some cases follow Colles' fracture of the wrist, rheumatoid arthritis, and in patients with renal failure on hemodialysis with long-standing arteriovenous shunts at the wrist.

de Quervain's tenosynovitis is due to thickening of the tendon sheath of the thumb abductors at the radiostyloid process

The tendons of the thumb abductors (extensor pollicis brevis and abductor pollicis longus) pass through a small

normal carpal tunnel

carpal tunnel syndrome

Fig. 24.24 Diagram showing carpal tunnel syndrome. (a) The contents of the normal carpal tunnel containing the long flexor tendons of the fingers and thumb, together with the median nerve, enclosed by the bones of the hand and the flexor retinaculum. The outer surface of the long flexor tendons is coated by a synovial sheath (blue) which is normally thin. (b) The features of carpal tunnel syndrome in which the median nerve is compressed and damaged, usually by thickening of the synovium over the long flexor tendons.

compartment roofed by a tight fibrous bridge just before the styloid process of the radius. This compartment is very variable in size and shape, and is sometimes divided into two compartments by a vertical septum.

Certain repetitive twisting movements at the wrist with the fingers and thumb flexed may produce localized thickening of the tendon sheaths of the two tendons, reducing the space within the compartment. The tendon sheaths show increased vascularity and marked edema, often followed by varying degrees of fibrous thickening. This produces pain and tenderness on the radial side of the wrist at the site of the compartment.

'Trigger finger' is due to thickening of the tendon sheaths of the long flexors of the fingers

The most commonly affected fingers are the middle and ring fingers, but in infants the thumb may be involved. In most cases the mechanism is thought to be repeated external trauma or chronic friction to the tendon and tendon sheath, leading to local thickening of the tendon sheath by fibrosis, edema and hypervascularity, and probably also to the annular ligament that overlies it at the base of the finger. As a result of the thickening the tendon finds it increasingly difficult to slide under the annular ligament, often making a popping noise as it passes through with difficulty. Repeated attempts to pass through lead to a worsening of the thickening of the two components, until eventually the tendon will not pass through unless manually assisted by forced extension of the finger. Eventually the tendon and finger become stuck in the flexed position.

Repetitive strain injury (RSI) particularly involves the upper limb

Repeated overuse of muscle, tendons and joints in the upper limb, particularly on a regular basis over a long period in an occupational activity, may lead to a combination of degenerative changes of the joints (osteoarthritis; see page 548) and degenerative changes in tendons and ligaments, often leading to laxity of ligaments and fibrous thickening of the tendon sheath (stenosing tenosynovitis). Although the individual components may be quite minor, together they can lead to significant morbidity, with joint pain and tenderness, limitation of movement, and swelling if there is a significant degree of osteoarthritis.

The details of all the pathological changes involved are not fully documented, but the symptom complex is known as **repetitive strain injury**. It is not yet clear whether the overuse is causative or merely exacerbates abnormalities already present. The etiological role of repetitive strain injury in such common wrist and hand conditions as carpal tunnel syndrome and de Quervain's tenosynovitis is still in dispute, but the recognition of the entity has led to better ergonomic design of seating, work desk heights and equipment, particularly in occupations involving keyboard work.

Intervertebral disc disease is a common and important cause of back pain and neurological symptoms

The intervertebral discs not only permit a limited degree of movement between adjacent vertebrae, they also act as shock absorbers and are constantly exposed to vertical compressive forces. Each disc is composed of cartilaginous end-plates, with densely collagenous annulus fibrosus surrounding a central slightly gelatinous nucleus pulposus

Fig. 24.25 Intervertebral disc. In disc prolapse the soft nucleus pulposus (NP) herniates through the tough annulus fibrosus (AF) to compress nerve roots.

(*Fig. 24.25*). The narrow cartilaginous end-plate is most prominent in the young.

Although abnormalities of the disc structure occur with increasing age (general shrinkage and reduction in the gelatinous nucleus pulposus), most clinically significant episodes of intervertebral disc disease occur in young people who have a normal bulky, non-shrunken disc and abundant nucleus pulposus. The symptoms usually follow some physical activity that raises the pressure of the nucleus pulposus inside the disc, such as lifting a heavy weight and forward flexion of the spine, and the nucleus pulposus material is forced under pressure against the annulus fibrosus, particularly posteriorly where it is comparatively thin and weak. The effect depends on the impact on the annulus fibrosus:

- In **disc fissure** some of the inner fibres of the annulus fibrosus are torn but the structure remains intact. However, sensory nerve twigs in the annulus are irritated by the nucleus pulposus, and there is localized back or neck pain.
- In **disc protrusion** the pressure is great enough to cause the annulus to thin and bulge, and the bulging may be extensive enough to bring the disc material into contact with an adjacent nerve root, leading to referred pain down the leg or arm.
- In **disc herniation** the area of annulus fibrosus is destroyed and nucleus pulposus material ruptures through to lie free, almost always compressing nerves and nerve roots.

The changes occur most commonly in the lumbar region and in the neck. When there is nerve root involvement in the lumbar region, referred pain and sensory impairment give the symptom complex called **sciatica**, and when the cervical discs are involved the pain and sensory symptoms radiate down the arm – **'cervical spondylosis'**.

BONE AND JOINT DISEASE IN CHILDREN

The tumors that particularly affect children (osteosarcoma, page 545 and Ewing's sarcoma, page 547) have already been dealt with.

Children have a general predisposition to fracture, largely because of their levels of physical activity in play and sport, and their limited ability to sense risk and danger. Also, they are more likely to be physically abused than any other group, and multiple or repeated fractures in a child should ring alarm bells.

Pediatric bone disorders resulting from abnormal skeletal development are important, particularly **achondroplasia** and **osteogenesis imperfects**. Some joint disorders are largely confined to children.

Achondroplasia is an inherited disorder of growth cartilage that results in dwarfism due to short limbs

Achondroplasia is an autosomal dominant condition caused by mutations in the fibroblast growth factor-3 (FGF-3) receptor located on chromosome 4. Mutations cause permanent activation of the receptor, leading to the arrest of bone growth. There is a high incidence of spontaneous mutation, accounting for its sudden appearance in a child with normal parents. The condition is recognizable at birth and is compatible with normal survival and lifespan. The trunk develops normally, but the head may be enlarged, with a depressed bridge of the nose and prominent forehead.

Osteogenesis imperfecta may lead to spontaneous fractures with minimal trauma in infancy and childhood and, occasionally, in utero

Osteogenesis imperfecta is due to mutations in the gene coding for type I collagen, resulting in abnormal collagen formation in osteoid. This leads to widespread weakness of bone, with multiple fractures frequently leading to severe deformity. Formation of the teeth is also affected, and the collagen of the sclera of the eye is poorly formed, giving rise to the characteristic physical sign of pale-blue sclerae. The pattern of inheritance can be either dominant or recessive, and there is marked variation in severity; the most severe cases are usually stillborn because of extensive intra-uterine fractures.

In community practice, Osgood–Schlatter's disease is a common cause of bone pain in children

Osgood–Schlatter's disease mainly affects children between 10 and 12 years of age. Patients present with pain just below the knee, and have a tender spot at the site of the

---

Molecular genetics of osteogenesis imperfecta

Osteogenesis imperfecta ranges in severity from a minor increase in the rate of fractures to the most severe form, which leads to intrauterine or perinatal death. It results from mutations in the genes that encode the chains of type I collagen, the major structural protein in bone osteoid.

There are over 20 genes coding for collagen, distributed over 10 chromosomes; more than 50 mutations in the COL1A1 and COL1A2 genes (responsible for coding for type I pro-collagen) are known to produce various types of osteogenesis imperfecta. Some are point mutations in which, for example, glycine is replaced by cystine or arginine. When such point mutations occur near the carboxy terminus, they seem to produce lethal disease; those near the amino terminus produce mild disease.

All collagen-gene mutations resulting in osteogenesis imperfecta are associated with reduced production of normal type I pro-collagen. When abnormal type I pro-collagen is produced, the phenotype can range from very mild to lethal, depending on the nature of the mutation. However, when minimally abnormal type I pro-collagen is produced, the phenotype is generally very mild, i.e. with normal stature and little or no bone deformity.

---

tibial tubercle at the upper end of the tibia. This is due to the tendon insertion separating from the front of the tibia, pulling away with it a small fragment of bone from the tibial tubercle; the bone fragment may undergo avascular necrosis as a result of this avulsion fracture.

Talipes is a fairly common congenital abnormality

The most common of this group of foot abnormalities is **talipes equinovarus** (club foot), in which plantar flexion and adduction of the foot is combined with inversion of the heel. In **talipes calcaneovalgus** the foot is dorsiflexed and the sole faces outwards. Both may be bilateral or unilateral, and are twice as common in boys. Most cases appear to be due to abnormal pressure molding of the fetus in utero, and oligohydramnios may be a predisposing factor. Some cases have a genetic basis, and there may be associated congenital abnormalities, e.g. developmental dysplasia of the hip and abdominal wall hernia.

Slipped capital epiphysis is an important hip disorder in children

Legg–Calvé–Perthes' disease has already been discussed and is illustrated on page 543. Another important cause of hip disease in children is slipped capital epiphysis, which presents with very similar symptoms of hip, thigh or knee pain, with limping.

This disorder occurs during the period of major long bone growth in adolescence, mainly between the ages of 10 and 16 years in boys and 12–14 years in girls. It is two to three times more common in boys, and obese adolescents are particularly vulnerable. The disease is usually bilateral, although only a small proportion of patients present with symptoms in both hips at the same time.

X-rays show that the femoral head has slipped in relation to the femoral neck, usually being displaced posteriorly and inferiorly.

In adolescents with this disorder the epiphyseal growth plate is thicker than normal, almost entirely due to expansion of the zone of hypertrophy. A shearing force linear fracture occurs through this zone, leading to disorganization of the normal vertical palisading architecture; this is followed by abnormal and irregular maturation of cartilage and abnormal endochondral ossification.

Congenital dislocation of the hip is now called developmental dysplasia of the hip (DDH)

In this condition the hip joint is structurally abnormal at birth, and the ball of the femoral head may slip out of the acetabular socket either completely (dislocation) or partly (subluxation) some time after birth. The underlying structural abnormalities may include unusual shallowness of the acetabular cup, or laxity and stretching of the retaining ligaments that surround and strengthen the joint capsule and normally assist in retaining the femoral ball in the acetabular socket.

There is a strong female preponderance (nearly 10:1) and the disorder is particularly likely to occur in breech presentations; often there is a family history. Treatment is aimed at maintaining the hip joint in a flexed and abducted position, with the ball in the socket, by using a splint or harness for some months. Without treatment, the hip is painful when the child begins to walk, and the gait is abnormal. Long-term complications include premature osteoarthritis in the affected hip.

DISORDERS OF SOFT TISSUE

The most commonly seen soft-tissue disorders in community practice are those due to trauma. They include **skeletal muscle injury** due to tearing of fibers, which is the result of overstretching after vigorous or extraordinary exercise. This is most frequently seen in young healthy adults participating in vigorous sports. There may be associated ligament and tendon damage (see pages 139–40, 555–7). **Blunt trauma** produces hematomas in muscle, subcutaneous fat and fascia; **open trauma** produces laceration of skeletal muscle and fascia with bleeding (usually the result of a road traffic accident or a severe fall). There is often an associated fracture of underlying bone.

Skeletal muscle can heal by fibrosis, although some functional fiber loss is experienced, together with disuse atrophy (which follows immobilization during healing).

Sometimes blunt trauma to muscles, particularly the bulky muscles of the proximal parts of the limbs, may be followed by a localized tumor-like mass of active fibroblastic proliferation within which some fibroblast precursors convert to osteoblasts and produce osteoid, which eventually calcifies into irregular bone. This condition, **myositis ossificans**, is most common in active young people, often following a sporting injury. Other localized fibroblastic proliferations may mimic soft tissue tumors, e.g. **nodular fasciitis**.

Tumors of soft tissue are rare except for subcutaneous lipoma

Benign tumors composed of adipose tissue are very common in the subcutaneous fat, but may also occur deep within muscle masses (**intramuscular lipoma**). They are slow-growing, soft, lobulated, well-circumscribed tumors on the trunk or limbs of adults, and are usually solitary but may be multiple. Multiple lipomas are often tender, histologically showing an increased number of blood vessels (**angiolipoma**) or increased amounts of fibrous tissue (**fibrolipoma**). The subcutaneous tumors are entirely benign and usually well circumscribed, although the deep intramuscular lipomas have ill-defined margins, are difficult to remove surgically, and recur frequently, with occasional malignant change to a **liposarcoma** supervening.

Liposarcoma may also occur in the retroperitoneal fat, producing a large tumor mass. In general liposarcomas vary greatly in their malignancy, from borderline malignant with a close resemblance to benign lipoma, to poorly differentiated tumors with high metastatic potential.

The most important group of connective-tissue tumors with malignant potential are those that show fibrohistiocytic differentiation. Believed to be derived from primitive fibroblasts that retain the potential to show histiocytic differentiation, their histogenesis is still uncertain. Benign **fibrous histiocytomas** are very common tumors in the dermis (see page 528), but **malignant fibrous histiocytoma (MFH)** is rare (although it is still the most common malignant soft-tissue tumor). They occur in adults, principally the elderly, and usually present as an enlarging painless mass located deep in the thigh and, occasionally, the lower leg. Some are deeply located in the muscle compartments, but others are more superficial, often being subcutaneous. These tumors are slowly infiltrative, with a high recurrence rate; a proportion show bloodborne metastatic spread. A variant of this tumor can occur in the retroperitoneum, producing a large mass that compresses the ureters and distorts the kidneys.

True tumors of skeletal muscle are very rare, although **rhabdomyosarcoma** is probably the most common primary soft-tissue tumor in infants and children.

Rhabdomyosarcoma is a highly malignant tumor of children and adolescents

Rhabdomyosarcoma is a malignant tumor of primitive striated muscle cells (rhabdomyoblasts) in which primitive striations may sometimes be seen, but sarcomeres are usually seen by electron microscopy and the cells show myogenic markers immunohistochemically. They are most common in the pelvic region (e.g. bladder, vagina, paratesticular tissue) and head and neck (e.g. nasal cavities, orbit), but are rare in the muscles of the rest of the body.

There are two main histological patterns, **embryonal rhabdomyosarcoma**, which is the common pattern in pelvic and head and neck tumors in young children, and the less common **alveolar rhabdomyosarcoma,** which is the type most frequently seen in the muscles of the limbs in adolescents.

Tumors derived from nerve sheath are common in soft tissues and in the subcutis

One of the most common tumors of soft tissues is derived from support cells of peripheral nerves and is termed a **peripheral nerve sheath tumor**.

Benign schwannoma (**neurilemmoma**) occurs in adults as a well-circumscribed, slow-growing tumor, usually in the subcutaneous tissue in the head and neck or upper limb. These lesions are completely benign, but surgical removal entails damaging the nerve to which they are attached.

Neurofibroma is a benign tumor that is usually solitary, but multiple in von Recklinghausen's neurofibromatosis. The solitary lesions most commonly occur in the subcutaneous tissue of young adults, whereas the multiple lesions occur in other sites as well, particularly in the cauda equina. Malignant change may occur in the multiple lesions, but is virtually unknown in solitary tumors. These tumors are also discussed in Chapter 21.

Superficial fibromatoses affect the palms, soles and the penis

There are three conditions characterized by diffuse irregular proliferation of fibroblast-like cells, probably myofibroblasts:

- Palmar fibromatosis (Dupuytren's contracture).
- Plantar fibromatosis.
- Penile fibromatosis (Peyronie's disease).

Dupuytren's contracture is a thickening of the fibrous fascia of the palms of one or both hands, producing palpable linear or nodular thickenings which eventually infiltrate skin and flexor tendons, the latter involvement producing flexion contractures, particularly of the fourth and fifth fingers (*Fig. 24.27*).

Plantar fibromatosis is a similar sequence of changes occurring in the sole, but flexion contractures are mild and rare.

Peyronie's disease is a similar fibromatosis in the shaft of the penis, usually on the dorsal or lateral aspects. Contracture in the late stages leads to abnormal curvature distortion of the penile shaft; because the dorsal and lateral areas are involved, the curvature is commonly upwards or to one side.

Fig. 24.26 Rhabdomyosarcoma in soft tissue. The tumor is highly pleomorphic and largely undifferentiated, but in some areas typical round or strap-shaped eosinophilic malignant rhabdomyoblasts **Rm** are present.

Fig. 24.27 Dupuytren's contracture. Thickening and contraction of palmar fascia has produced flexion contracture of the fourth finger. The arrow points to the short thick cord of fibrous tissue which has produced the flexion.

Case-based questions

Case 1 An elderly woman with leg pain

An elderly Asian woman, an immigrant to the UK from the Indian subcontinent, attended hospital with her husband, who acted as translator. She complained of constant pain in her legs, worst in the thighs; she had found walking progressively more painful and difficult over the last year. On examination there was bone and muscle tenderness in the thighs and lower legs. Questioning revealed that she was a vegetarian, spent most of her time in the house, and invariably wore traditional dress.

1. On the basis of clinical suspicion, what is the most likely diagnosis?
2. In this particular case, what are the most likely causative factors?

To confirm the clinical diagnosis, the following investigations were undertaken:

- Serum calcium, phosphate, and alkaline phosphatase levels.
- X-rays of pelvis and lower limb bones.

3. If the clinical diagnosis is correct, what would these tests show?
4. If the diagnosis is still in doubt, a trephine or Jamshidi needle biopsy of iliac crest bone may be undertaken. What would it show?
5. The physician also requested renal function tests. Why?
6. What treatment will be given?

Case 2 A boy with a painful swelling above the knee

An active boy of 10 was referred to an orthopedic specialist because of a persistent and worsening pain and swelling above the knee. The pain had first been noted 2 weeks previously when playing soccer with his friends, although it did not appear to follow any particular injury or strain. Despite analgesics and local measures such as cold compresses, the pain worsened and the swelling increased, such that he now walked with a distinct limp and was unable to run. An astute family practitioner referred the boy to hospital as an emergency.

1. What diagnostic possibility so concerned the family practitioner that he arranged an urgent specialist opinion?

The hospital specialist requested urgent imaging of the affected limb, which confirmed the suspected diagnosis, and also requested imaging of the lung

2. What would the imaging of the knee show, and why was imaging of the lung requested?
3. If the lesion was biopsied or excised, what would the histological examination show?

Case 3 A man with a painful toe

A 42-year-old man presented to his family practitioner with a painful swollen toe. He stated that he had been feeling generally 'off-color' for a couple of days, and was awoken in the early hours of one morning with an excruciating pain in the big toe of his left foot. He could think of no injury that could have brought it on. He had a sleepless night in which even the weight of the bedclothes on his toe was almost more than he could bear. Standard analgesics had little or no effect, and in the morning light he noticed that the skin around the affected toe joint was swollen, red, shiny and smooth. The pain abated somewhat over the following few days, but it was 3 days after onset before he could hobble to his family practitioner.

1. On the history and examination findings, the family practitioner made a diagnosis. What was it?
2. For confirmation of his diagnosis, the doctor ordered a blood test; what was it?
3. Why is this blood test related to the etiology of this disease?
4. What other manifestations of this disease may occur?
5. The family practitioner questioned the patient about his diet, alcohol consumption, and prescription drugs taken. Why?

Brief answers to these case-based questions are given on page 596. More detailed answers and other study resources are available online at www.studentconsult.com.

Important multisystem diseases

25

Some important diseases cause damage in many tissues and organs

Many diseases are specific to one organ or system, but some important diseases can cause damage in a number of systems. These are called **multisystem diseases**, and can be divided into four main categories:

- **Disorders with an immune or autoimmune basis**. In this chapter we discuss, in some detail, systemic lupus erythematosus (SLE), progressive systemic sclerosis, rheumatoid disease and sarcoidosis, although some aspects of each are also discussed in the chapters relating to other systems that are particularly affected (e.g. see Chapter 24 for the joint manifestations of rheumatoid disease, Chapter 17 for the renal lesions in SLE). Systemic vasculitis is also briefly summarized here, but is dealt with mainly in Chapter 10.
- **Disorders involving storage or deposition of abnormal substances**. Amyloid is still an important disease in this group, although its incidence is falling. The metabolic storage disorders such as the glycogenoses and lipidoses, hemochromatosis and Wilson's disease are examples of this type of multisystem disorder.
- **Disorders involving systemic metabolic defects affecting many tissues**. Diabetes mellitus is the most important example. It is dealt with here in recognition of its impact on many organs and tissues, rather than in association with the islets of Langerhans' of the pancreas in Chapter 16.

SYSTEMIC LUPUS ERYTHEMATOSUS

This is a very common (though frequently undiagnosed) condition in the general population, particularly in young and middle-aged women. It is one of the so-called 'connective tissue disorders' in which patients produce antibodies to a very wide range of their own tissues ('autoantigens'). The cause is unknown, but it has been postulated that the stimulus to the production of the abnormal autoantibodies may be sensitizing drugs or chemicals, or unidentified viral infection. Drugs and chemicals have been implicated because of the known development of SLE following the use of many drugs, particularly hydralazine.

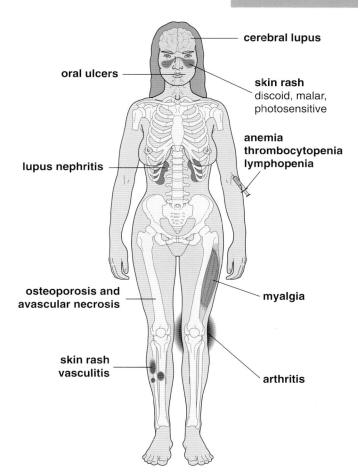

Fig. 25.1 Multisystem manifestations of systemic lupus erythematosus. SLE affects a wide range of tissues and organ systems.

Many tissues and organs are involved in SLE, but synovial joints, skin, kidneys and brain are the major target organs

The diagnosis of SLE is based on a combination of clinical features and the result of laboratory investigation, primarily the identification of the autoantibodies, and particularly those antibodies directed against nuclear DNA (see blue box on page 563). As so many different organs and tissues may be involved, the ways in which the disease can present are many and varied (*Fig. 25.1*). The range of features that can occur in SLE is shown well by the American Rheumatism Association List of Diagnostic Criteria for SLE (in order of specificity):

- Discoid skin rash.
- Neurological disorder.
- Malar skin rash.
- Skin photosensitivity.
- Oral ulceration.
- Renal abnormality (lupus nephritis).
- Evidence of immunological disorder.
- Hematological disorder.
- Serosal inflammation.
- Presence of antinuclear antibody.
- Arthritis.

Skin rashes of various types occur in about 80% of all patients with systemic lupus

One of the most common tissues affected in SLE is the skin. The most common patterns of skin rash are:

- **Chronic discoid LE:** round ('discoid'), red scaly telangiectatic plaques, usually on the face and scalp, and less commonly on the hands. Follicular plugging with keratin is common, particularly in the scalp and facial lesions. The lesions heal from the center, with the skin becoming atrophic, often with loss of pigment. Involvement of the scalp may lead to patchy hair loss (see pages 508 and 531–2); this is a cause of **scarring alopecia**.
- **Malar skin rash:** a symmetrical, slightly raised red erythematous rash on the cheeks and across the bridge of the nose. The characteristic distribution of broad patches on the upper cheeks joined by a narrower band across the nose has led to this being called the 'butterfly' rash.
- **Photosensitivity reactions:** rashes in light-exposed areas, worse when there has been increased sun exposure, may be of either of the above malar or discoid patterns, but may also be non-specific. Direct immunofluorescence of sun-exposed but non-lesional skin shows IgG, IgM and complement in the epidermal basement membrane in patients with SLE, irrespective of the clinical pattern of the skin disease. These represent immune complex deposits on the dermal side of the basement membrane, within the intercellular matrix and between collagen fibers.
- **Vasculitic skin lesions:** these occur as either an acute purpuric neutrophilic vasculitis in the upper dermis, or a lymphocytic vasculitis producing slightly raised erythematous patches, and are important features of skin rashes in lupus. Their significance is often missed because the rashes do not conform to the classic discoid or malar types described above.

The SLE variant that is known as **mixed connective tissue disease** (MCTD) has skin lesions less commonly

Fig. 25.2 SLE – malar skin rash. The rash from the cheek is red, raised and scaling; this is more severe than often seen because there is a superadded photodermatitis component.

than classic SLE, but many patients have a non-specific lymphocytic vasculitis at some stage in the illness, and eventually develop Raynaud's phenomenon.

Oral mucosal lesions in SLE produce superficial erosions and ulcers

Clinically and histologically, the oral lesions in SLE closely resemble oral lichen planus (see page 227–8) with red erosions, but they are found rather more commonly on the hard palate than is lichen planus. A characteristic histological feature of oral LE is the presence of extensive basal layer destruction, similar to that seen in lichen planus and in skin lesions. Oral mucosal lesions occur in about 20% of patients with SLE.

Neurological and psychiatric disorders are common in SLE, and may be the presenting symptom

The most common feature of neurological involvement in SLE is a non-organic psychiatric disorder of unknown cause; occasional cases that come to autopsy show either acute neutrophilic or lymphocytic vasculitis in the brain. Patients may also have a wide range of organic brain disorders, such as focal demyelination, microinfarction and neu-

Fig. 25.3 SLE – oral mucosal lesion. There is extensive superficial mucosal ulceration at the back of the buccal mucosa (arrow).

ronal loss, leading to a variety of symptoms. Grand mal epileptic seizures are an important clinical manifestation of cerebral lupus. Vascular occlusion is the result of antiphospholipid antibodies causing platelet aggregation.

It is important to remember that some of the neurological manifestations in SLE may be the result of the treatment rather than the disease, particularly corticosteroid therapy.

Kidney involvement in SLE is common, and is an important cause of morbidity and mortality

Renal involvement in lupus is common, and the severity can vary from minor abnormalities (such as asymptomatic albuminuria) to severe glomerular disease leading to renal failure. The main abnormalities in renal involvement in SLE are in the glomerulus, where there can be a wide range of structural abnormalities. There may also be extraglomerular vascular abnormalities and tubular damage, particularly interstitial nephritis.

Lupus nephritis may mimic other forms of glomerular disease by showing the following patterns: focal segmental mesangial glomerulonephritis, focal segmental proliferative glomerulonephritis with tuft necrosis, membranous nephropathy, and membranoproliferative pattern of lupus nephritis.

These patterns of glomerular structural abnormality are discussed and illustrated in greater detail on page 377. The basis of the glomerular damage in all patterns is the deposition of immune complexes in the glomerulus. The complexes may be deposited in the basement membrane (leading to basement membrane thickening), or in the mesangium (leading to mesangial expansion); immunofluorescence methods show that the immune complexes contain three types of immunoglobulin, IgG, IgA and IgM, and two types of complement, C3 and C1q.

The detection of this 'full house' of immunoglobulins and complement factors, together with the particular locations of the immune complexes in relation to the glomerular basement membrane, is important in distinguishing lupus glomerulonephritis from non-lupus patterns.

Fig. 25.4 SLE – glomerular lesion. Lupus nephritis is discussed in detail in Chapter 17. This lesion shows a mixed membranoproliferative (arrow) and tuft necrosis (**N**) pattern.

Hematological abnormalities are common in SLE

Patients with SLE frequently have hematological abnormalities, some having an unknown cause, and others having an autoimmune mechanism.

- **Normocytic hypochromic anemia**.
- **Autoimmune hemolytic anemia** (approximately 10% of cases), with red-cell antibodies and a positive Coombs' test.
- **Reduced peripheral white cell count**, usually due to disproportionate reduction of lymphocytes (lymphopenia).
- **Thrombocytopenia**, sometimes associated with the presence of antiplatelet antibodies.
- **Predisposition to thrombosis**, particularly if there are anticardiolipin/lupus anticoagulant antibodies.

Musculoskeletal symptoms may be the earliest presenting feature of SLE

SLE frequently presents clinically with musculoskeletal symptoms. Joint pain and other symptoms of arthritis occur in about 90% of all patients, and may precede the recognition of SLE by some years. The main rheumatological disorders of SLE are **arthritis**, **bone disease** and **myalgia**.

Arthritis, which is sometimes misdiagnosed as rheumatoid arthritis or asymmetrical polyarticular arthritis, usually begins in the fingers, wrists and knees. Avascular bone necrosis may contribute to the arthropathy. The synovial surfaces may show fibrin deposition, and the articular cartilage shows changes similar to those seen in mild rheumatoid arthritis.

Immunological investigation of suspected SLE

There is a cluster of antibodies that are aimed against the nuclei (antinuclear antibodies – ANAs) that can be used for diagnosis. These are not specific to SLE, as they can occur in some of the lupus-overlap syndromes with other connective tissue diseases.

- **Anti-dsDNA** (antibody against double-stranded DNA) is the most frequently detected and specific autoantibody.
- **Anti-ssDNA** (antibody against single-stranded DNA) may be found in SLE, but is also found in other diseases.
- **Anti-DNA histone** is found particularly commonly in drug-induced SLE.

Antibodies are useful in the detection of other types of systemic connective tissue disease.

Bone disease usually presents as disproportionately severe osteoporosis for the patient's age. It is difficult to separate the osteoporosis due to SLE from that due to the corticosteroids used in treatment. Avascular bone necrosis is common in SLE, appearing to be polyarticular, and usually being associated with the joints showing the most severe arthritis.

Myalgia in the form of pain in skeletal muscles is a very common feature of SLE, and is frequently neglected clinically as it is difficult to dissociate from the pain due to coexisting arthritis. Muscle biopsy in patients with significant myalgia frequently shows a lymphocytic vasculitis.

PROGRESSIVE SYSTEMIC SCLEROSIS (PSS)

Systemic sclerosis is one of the so-called connective tissue diseases and affects many systems and organs. It is three times more common in women than in men, and occurs mainly in middle-aged or elderly women. The main abnormality is an excess formation of fibrous tissue in tissues. The fibrous tissue is particularly collagenous, leading to rigidity of the affected tissue, often with the destruction of specialized cells. Vessel wall thickening and perivascular fibrosis are characteristic features of systemic sclerosis, and are responsible for slowly progressive ischemic damage in a wide range of tissues. The skin is the most commonly affected organ in systemic sclerosis, but the alimentary tract, lung, kidney and heart may also be involved (*Fig. 25.5*).

Skin involvement in systemic sclerosis is called 'scleroderma'

In systemic sclerosis the skin involvement consists of dermal thickening through the process of fibrous replacement of normal dermal structures. This thickening often extends into the subcutis, and leads to gradually increasing rigidity of the skin with tightening and atrophy of the overlying epidermis. The lesions affect particularly the fingers and the face: the fingers become hard, rigid and shiny (*Fig. 25.6*), and the face shows a characteristic tautness of the skin with overlying epidermal atrophy and indrawn margins of the mouth.

In the fingers there may be associated Raynaud's phenomenon, and, in old long-standing cases there may be calcification of the soft tissues, particularly around the finger joints (calcinosis cutis). The dermal fibrosis leads to destruction of skin appendages, so the skin becomes hairless and eccrine sweat ducts are damaged.

This pattern of skin involvement is usually associated with involvement of the internal organs, but there are a few cases where the scleroderma remains localized to the skin. **Morphea** is the name given to single (rarely multiple) skin lesions which have the histological and clinical features of localized scleroderma. Morpheic lesions are initially creamy-

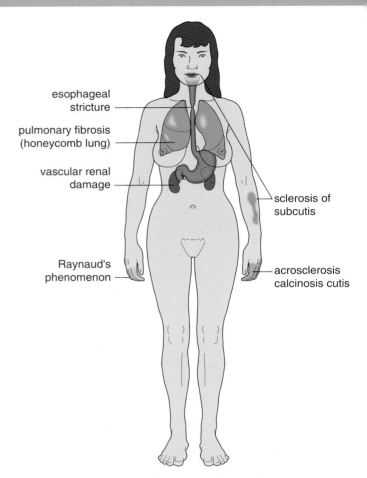

Fig. 25.5 Multisystem manifestations of systemic sclerosis. Systemic sclerosis affects a wide range of tissues and organ systems, often as a result of vascular obliteration.

Fig. 25.6 Systemic sclerosis. The fingers in some patterns of systemic sclerosis are narrowed, with tight shiny skin. Subcutaneous calcification (calcinosis cutis) can also be seen as white spots on the ends of the fingers.

coloured, thickened plaques on the trunk or limbs, sometimes with a purple edge in the actively growing phase. The lesions eventually become depressed with atrophic epidermis. Multiple areas may coalesce.

Involvement of the alimentary tract in systemic sclerosis particularly affects the esophagus

Proliferating fibrosis with collagenosis in the esophageal muscle wall leads to the destruction of the smooth muscle and its replacement by collagenous fibrous tissue; nerve fibers in the esophageal wall are also damaged by the fibrosis, and there is often thickening of the blood vessels. These changes result in a thickened, rigid esophageal wall, which is often incapable of coordinated contraction and therefore unable to produce efficient peristalsis. As a result, reflux esophagitis with inflammation and even ulceration are common, and these may lead to the presence of fibrous strictures.

Lung involvement in systemic sclerosis leads to extensive interstitial fibrosis and 'honeycomb lung'

Progressive fibrosis of the pulmonary interstitium leads to appearances similar to those seen in end-stage interstitial pneumonitis. Respiratory bronchioles, alveolar ducts and alveolar walls are progressively destroyed, until the lung is a fibrous network that contains large cystic spaces; this is termed 'honeycomb lung' (see page 208).

Kidney involvement in systemic sclerosis is largely the result of vessel abnormalities and their effects on the glomeruli

Kidney involvement in systemic sclerosis usually presents acutely with evidence of severe small vessel and glomerular damage. The appearances of the afferent arterioles are very similar to those seen in malignant hypertensive disease of the kidney, with an intimal proliferation of small arteries and arterioles leading to the almost complete occlusion of the lumen (see Fig. 17.28); this is also associated with fibrinoid necrosis of some of the afferent arterioles and of portions of the glomerular tuft. These renal changes in progressive systemic sclerosis are called **acute scleroderma kidney**.

SYSTEMIC VASCULITIS

Systemic vasculitis can affect blood vessels of all types

This topic is dealt with in greater detail in Chapter 10, pages 166–9. In the context of this chapter, vasculitis can be a stand-alone disease (for example polyarteritis nodosa) or a component of other autoimmune diseases such as systemic lupus erythematosus, progressive systemic sclerosis or rheumatoid disease.

Polyarteritis nodosa is characterized by necrosis of part or all of the walls of small and medium-sized arteries, associated with a neutrophil (and sometimes eosinophil) inflammatory reaction. These vascular lesions are scattered, and the clinical effects are the result of reduced arterial flow through the damaged artery, often due to associated thrombotic occlusion. This leads to infarction of the local area supplied by the artery; because many arteries are affected at the same time, there are multiple infarcts in many areas of the body. The most commonly involved sites are given in table form in *Fig. 10.27*. The kidney and gut are the most common sites (*Fig. 25.8*).

Fig. 25.8 Polyarteritis nodosa in ileum. (a) Multiple small infarcts in the wall of the ileum result from (b) segmental necrosis of the wall of medium-sized arteries.

Fig. 25.7 Systemic sclerosis – lung. Progressive lung damage in systemic sclerosis eventually leads to 'honeycomb' lung.

RHEUMATOID DISEASE

Rheumatoid disease is a multisystem connective tissue disease in which the dominant effects are on the joints, giving **rheumatoid arthritis**; the changes in the joints are described in Chapter 24.

The disease is more common in women than in men, and there is a genetic predisposition, although the cause or causes remain unknown. Rheumatoid disease also affects the skin, lungs, blood vessels, eyes, and the hemopoietic and lymphoreticular systems (see *Fig. 25.10* on page 567). The treatment for rheumatoid disease may itself cause pathology, e.g. steroid-induced osteoporosis, analgesic-related ulceration of the stomach, and drug-induced renal disease.

Rheumatoid arthritis is a symmetrical polyarthritis, characterized by the destruction of articular cartilage and its replacement by chronic inflammatory pannus

The histological changes in rheumatoid arthritis have been described on page 550. In most cases the disease first attacks the finger joints, followed, in order of frequency, by the metatarsophalangeal joints and the joints of the ankles, wrists, knees, shoulders, elbows and hips. However, the disease may also affect joints such as the temporomandibular joint, the synovial joints of the spine (particularly the upper cervical spine), and occasionally the joints of the larynx.

Skin is involved in rheumatoid disease by the formation of rheumatoid nodules or the presence of vasculitis

The most frequent skin lesion in rheumatoid disease is the **rheumatoid nodule** (*Fig. 25.9a*), a subcutaneous firm nodule located usually over the extensor aspect of the forearm but also found occasionally in the skin overlying other bony prominences. The nodules are composed of extensive areas of degenerate collagen surrounded by a giant-cell granulomatous reaction (*Fig. 25.9b*). They are seen in approximately 25% of cases of rheumatoid arthritis, particularly in patients with severe arthritic disease and other visceral involvement, such as pulmonary fibrosis. Occasionally, the nodules can antedate the development of arthritis.

The other important skin manifestation is the development of **vasculitis**. This is either an acute neutrophilic vasculitis presenting with purpura and occasional foci of ulceration, or a lymphocytic vasculitis producing a more low-key erythematous patchy rash. The cutaneous vasculitis may be part of a more generalized vasculitis affecting other organs, particularly **lymphocytic vasculitis**.

Fig. 25.9 Rheumatoid nodule. At the elbow there is a large raised subcutaneous nodule (a) on the extensor surface distal to the joint. Histologically (b) the nodule is composed of degenerate collagen (arrow) surrounded by a chronic inflammatory reaction with macrophages and giant cells, and walled off by fibrosis.

Rheumatoid disease can cause 'dry-eye syndrome' and degeneration of the sclera

In rheumatoid disease both the lacrimal and mucous glands may be affected by lymphocytic inflammation, leading to the destruction of the glands and to dry eyes (**keratoconjunctivitis sicca**). The lack of tears leads to secondary inflammation of the cornea. The degeneration of collagenous tissue may occur in the eye, analogous to that which is present in rheumatoid nodules, causing **scleritis**. In severe cases this progresses to cause perforation of the globe, termed **scleromalacia perforans**.

Pulmonary involvement in rheumatoid disease causes interstitial fibrosis

The most common form of pulmonary involvement in rheumatoid disease is **interstitial pneumonitis and fibrosing alveolitis**, which leads, eventually, to a pattern of interstitial pulmonary fibrosis very similar to that seen in progressive systemic sclerosis, 'honeycomb lung' (see page 208). In addition, patients may develop lesions that are very similar to the subcutaneous rheumatoid nodule, both within the lung and on the pleural surfaces.

Intrapulmonary rheumatoid granulomas are particularly common in patients who already have industrial lung disease due to the inhalation of various types of silica; the associa-

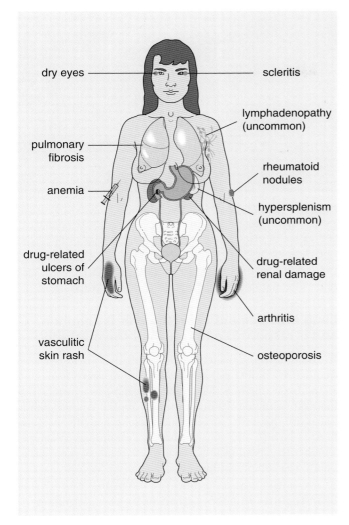

dry eyes

sceleritis

lymphadenopathy
(uncommon)

pulmonary
fibrosis

rheumatoid
nodules

anemia

hypersplenism
(uncommon)

drug-related
ulcers of
stomach

drug-related
renal damage

arthritis

vasculitic
skin rash

osteoporosis

Fig. 25.10 Multisystem manifestations of rheumatoid disease. Although the initial manifestation is usually an arthritis, rheumatoid disease is a systemic illness.

tion of coalminer's lung with rheumatoid granulomas in seropositive miners is called **Caplan's syndrome** (see page 210).

Anemia of chronic disorders is common in rheumatoid disease, and a minority of patients develop hypersplenism or lymphadenopathy

Anemia is very common in rheumatoid disease, usually being of the normocytic hypochromic type that is characteristic of chronic disease (see page 320). Despite the hypochromia there is no regular iron deficiency, but there is probably a defect of iron incorporation and utilization. The bone marrow may show follicular lymphocytic aggregates.

Lymph nodes may be enlarged in rheumatoid disease as a result of follicular hyperplasia. Enlargement of the spleen is usual, but it is rarely great enough to be palpable except

Laboratory diagnosis of rheumatoid disease

The laboratory diagnosis of rheumatoid disease is based on demonstrating the presence of antibodies known as **rheumatoid factors**. These factors react with antigenic sites on the C_H2 domain of the Fc portion of IgG. The most common type of rheumatoid factor is an immunoglobulin IgM molecule, which can form complexes with circulating IgG.

High rheumatoid factor titers are associated with severe progressive disease, particularly when there are systemic complications and rheumatoid nodules in the subcutis of the skin. There are two methods for demonstrating the presence of rheumatoid factors:

- **Rose–Waaler test**: based on the ability of IgM rheumatoid factor to agglutinate sheep red cells which have been coated with rabbit anti-sheep antibody.
- **Latex agglutination test**: in which the rheumatoid factor antibody agglutinates latex particles that have been coated with human IgG. This test is less specific than the Rose–Waaler test.

Radio-immunoassays and enzyme-linked immunosorbent assay (ELISA) can be used to measure rheumatoid factors of all types, including the most common IgM form.

in cases of **Felty's syndrome**, in which splenomegaly, lymphadenopathy, anemia and leukopenia are present in a patient with seropositive rheumatoid arthritis; there is an increased susceptibility to infection, and sepsis is an important and common cause of death in these patients.

SARCOIDOSIS

Sarcoidosis is a chronic granulomatous disease of unknown cause in which many tissues are infiltrated by non-caseating granulomas (see page 54). It is slightly more common in women than in men, and most patients present before the age of 40 years. The organs and systems most commonly involved clinically are the lymphoreticular system, the lungs, skin, eyes and the brain, although histological examination in sarcoidosis shows asymptomatic granulomas in many other organs and tissues, such as the heart, skeletal muscle, lacrimal glands and gastrointestinal tract (*Fig. 25.11*).

As so many systems and organs are involved, the clinical presentation patterns are wide and varied; there are also marked differences in the clinical expression of the disease on a geographical and racial basis.

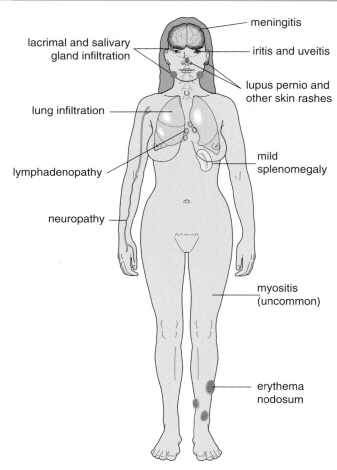

Fig. 25.11 Multisystem manifestations of sarcoidosis. The granulomatous infiltrate of sarcoidosis may be seen in most tissues.

Fig. 25.12 Sarcoidosis. This photomicrograph shows a lymph node containing numerous discrete sarcoid granulomas (**G**), composed of histiocytes. The granulomas may contain giant cells but do not show caseous necrosis (*cf.* tuberculous granulomas – *Fig. 4.20*).

The etiology and pathogenesis are completely unknown, although numerous immunological abnormalities can be detected in patients with sarcoidosis; however, these may be an effect of the disease rather than the cause. Nevertheless, particularly in lung involvement it is thought that one important factor is an enhanced cell-mediated immune response.

Lymphoreticular involvement in sarcoidosis is manifest as enlarged lymph nodes

The lymph nodes that are most commonly enlarged in sarcoidosis are the intrathoracic lymph nodes at the hilum of the lung. The enlargement of these nodes is invariably bilateral and almost symmetrical, and can be associated with diffuse pulmonary infiltration. Sarcoid enlargement of peripheral nodes, such as the axillary or cervical nodes, is less common.

The spleen is histologically involved in many patients, but enlargement of the spleen is clinically manifest only in about 5% of cases in Caucasians; it is more common in Afro-Caribbeans, probably being manifest in about 15% of

cases. Massive splenomegaly may be associated with secondary hematological features such as pancytopenia.

Lung involvement in sarcoidosis is common, and is responsible for much of the morbidity

In addition to the bilateral hilar lymphadenopathy, there is frequently a diffuse pulmonary infiltration which leads to a restrictive ventilatory defect and reduced gas transfer. The lung shows interstitial infiltration by typical sarcoid granulomas in the early stages, but these eventually heal by fibrosis. Much of the permanent pulmonary damage, whether structural or functional, is the result of progressive pulmonary interstitial fibrosis.

Skin lesions in association with sarcoidosis are very common

Skin manifestations occur in about one-quarter to one-third of all cases of sarcoidosis. There are two main patterns of involvement.

Erythema nodosum presents as characteristic, tender, red or purple subcutaneous lumps, usually on the shins and thighs, sometimes accompanied by fever and malaise, and frequently by associated arthralgia (see *Fig. 23.25*). It is an inflammatory lesion of the subcutaneous fat, usually associated with inflammation of a large vein. Although occasional giant cells are seen in relation to necrotic fat, true sarcoid granulomas are not seen. This pattern is particularly associated with the bilateral hilar lymphadenopathy pattern in the thorax, and is said to have a good prognosis.

Sarcoid granulomas in the skin may have several clinical manifestations, including brown papules (sometimes associated with hair follicles, leading to hair loss), reddish-brown fixed nodules and plaques, and a characteristic pattern called **lupus pernio**. In this pattern, which is associated with severe systemic involvement (including the nasal passages, lung and eye), there are persistent, rubbery, purple shiny plaques on the face, the tip of the nose and the ends of fingers and ears.

Eye involvement in sarcoidosis is a common presenting symptom, particularly in women

The most common type of ophthalmic involvement in sarcoidosis is an **acute uveitis**. This is often transient and mild, and is particularly associated with erythema nodosum and bilateral hilar lymph node enlargement. It is probable that uveitis occurs in over a quarter of all cases of sarcoidosis, but is subclinical in the majority.

More severe eye involvement occurs in **chronic uveitis**, which is persistent and more likely to lead to permanent impairment of vision. It is usually associated with more severe sarcoidosis, e.g. with extensive pulmonary infiltration and fibrosis, or with cutaneous lupus pernio.

Involvement of the central and peripheral nervous system in sarcoidosis is important and often underdiagnosed

Neurological involvement occurs in at least 10% of patients with sarcoidosis, and is particularly common in patients with diffuse pulmonary infiltration and eye lesions. Sarcoid granulomas that are developing and proliferating in the nervous system can produce a wide range of clinical effects, which are dependent on their location; some of the more common are:

- **Chronic meningitis** with cerebrospinal fluid abnormalities and non-caseating granulomas in the meninges.
- **Cranial nerve lesions**, often as a result of chronic sarcoid meningeal inflammation at the base of the brain.
- **Space-occupying lesions** in the cerebral hemispheres, pituitary or hypothalamus.
- '**Mononeuritis multiplex**', due to the involvement of many peripheral nerves.

DIABETES MELLITUS

Diabetes mellitus (DM) is a multisystem disease with both biochemical and structural consequences. It is a chronic disease of carbohydrate, fat and protein metabolism, resulting from inadequate action of the hormone insulin.

Two main types of **primary diabetes mellitus** are identified, mainly on clinical grounds (*Fig. 25.13*): **type I** (insulin-dependent diabetes mellitus – IDDM, or juvenile-onset diabetes), and **type II** (non-insulin dependent diabetes – NIDDM, or maturity-onset diabetes).

Type III diabetes refers to specific types of diabetes caused by rare genetic defects in islet insulin-secreting cell function and genetic defects in insulin action. **Type IV disease** refers to diabetes related to pregnancy.

Diabetes may also occur **secondarily** to generalized disease of the pancreas, e.g. chronic pancreatitis and hemochromatosis, or may be caused by the secretion of hormones that antagonize the effects of insulin, e.g. in Cushing's syndrome and acromegaly; such diabetes is called **secondary diabetes mellitus**.

Type I diabetes is an organ-specific autoimmune disease

As one of its synonyms implies, type I diabetes usually presents in childhood or adolescence, mainly as a result of the biochemical disorders leading to hyperglycemia and diabetic ketoacidosis. This type of diabetes is an autoimmune phenomenon; the majority of patients have circulating antibodies to the endocrine-cell population of the islet cells of the pancreas, including antibodies against the insulin-secreting cells. It is therefore an example of an **organ-specific autoimmune disease** (see page 104).

The pancreas in type I diabetes shows lymphocytic infiltration and destruction of the insulin-secreting cells of the islets of Langerhans. This destruction of insulin-secreting cells leads to an insulin deficiency, which in turn leads to hyperglycemia and other secondary metabolic complications.

Type II diabetes is the result of insulin resistance in peripheral tissues

Type II diabetes is four or five times more common than type I. Unlike type I, where there is an absolute absence of insulin, in type II diabetes the blood insulin levels are initially normal, or may even increase in the early stages, before eventually falling to below normal. The defect in the type II pattern is a combination of the effects of the relative deficiency of insulin compared to the need, and the phenomenon of **insulin resistance**, in which the tissues are unable to respond to insulin. Insulin resistance is thought to be due to an impairment of the function of receptors for insulin on the surfaces of target cells, meaning that glucose does not enter the cell.

Fig. 25.13 Comparison of type I and type II diabetes

Type I	Type II
Childhood and adolescence onset	Late middle-age/elderly onset
Thin	Obese
Ketoacidosis common	Ketoacidosis rare
Severe insulin deficiency	Relative deficiency and end-organ resistance
Islet-cell antibodies	No islet-cell antibodies
Autoimmune mechanism	No autoimmune mechanism
Genetic predisposition associated with HLA-DR genotype	Polygenic inheritance

A protein called **amylin** is produced in the insulin-secreting cells of the pancreatic islets, and is secreted with the insulin. In type II diabetes this protein accumulates in excess around the pancreatic islet cells, producing an amorphous deposit of material with the characteristics of amyloid (see page 572). Its role is not understood, but it may interfere with the subsequent secretion of insulin by the islet cells.

Pathogenesis of type II diabetes

The precise pathogenesis in type II diabetes is not known, although etiological factors such as age, obesity and a genetic predisposition are well recognized. Although type II diabetics do not have the HLA-DR4 genotype, there is a strong genetic factor: 90–100% of identical twins show concordance. Inheritance is considered to be polygenic (see page 70).

Pathogenesis of type I diabetes mellitus

Patients with type I diabetes are usually HLA-DR3 or HLA-DR4 positive, a feature demonstrated by other organ-specific autoimmune diseases. It is thought possible that a viral infection may be the trigger for the autoimmune destruction of insulin-secreting cells; viruses implicated include the common childhood viral infections, such as mumps, measles and Coxsackie B. One postulated mechanism is that the viruses induce mild structural damage to the islet cells of the pancreas, thereby altering their antigenicity, and that certain individuals with the genetic susceptibility to organ-specific autoimmune disease, e.g. the possession of HLA-DR4, then mount an autoimmune response against the damaged insulin-secreting cells. Another postulate is that an endogenous retrovirus is responsible for eliciting an immune response directed against islet cells.

Laboratory diagnostic criteria for diabetes mellitus

There are currently two widely used sets of diagnostic criteria for diabetes mellitus, based on assessment of plasma glucose levels. One is promoted by WHO (1985), and the other more recent criteria are promoted by the American Diabetes Association (2004) (see Fig. 25.14).

A condition of **impaired glucose tolerance** is defined as plasma glucose greater than 7.8 mmol/L fasting and 7.8–11.0 mmol/L 2 hours after a 75 g glucose load (WHO).

The American Diabetes Association recognizes the state of **impaired fasting glucose** defined as plasma glucose greater than 6.1–6.9 mmol/L (fasting).

These two states carry the implications of a higher than normal risk of developing diabetes mellitus and cardiovascular disease.

Fig. 25.14 Biochemical criteria in diabetes mellitus

WHO criteria	
Fasting plasma glucose	≥ 7.8 mmol/L
AND	
Plasma glucose	≥ 11.1 mmol/L 2 hours after a 75 g oral glucose load
American Diabetes Association	
Fasting plasma glucose	≥7.0 mmol/L
OR	
Random plasma glucose	≥ 11.1 mmol/L with appropriate clinical symptoms
OR	
Plasma glucose	≥ 11.1 mmol/L 2 hours after a 75 g oral glucose load

Morbidity and mortality in diabetes mellitus are now mainly the result of its structural complications

Whereas in the past the biochemical disturbances in diabetes mellitus usually led to an early death, the development of insulin treatment for type I diabetes and of various oral hypoglycemic agents (when combined with diet) for type II diabetes has greatly reduced mortality from hyperglycemia, hypoglycemia and the complications of ketoacidotic coma. Nevertheless, diabetes remains an important cause of morbidity and mortality owing to a series of common complications (*Fig. 25.15*). The major complications of diabetes are:

- Predisposition to infection.
- Increased severity of atherosclerosis and its complications.
- Extensive small vessel disease (arteriolosclerosis).
- Renal glomerular disease (see pages 366, 380).
- Retinal vascular disease (see page 500).
- Peripheral nerve damage (see page 486).

As a result of these complications, diabetics of both types have a predisposition to develop ischemic heart disease, cerebrovascular disease, peripheral gangrene of lower limbs, chronic renal disease, reduced visual acuity leading to blindness, and peripheral neuropathy.

Diabetics are particularly prone to infection

Patients with diabetes have an increased tendency to develop infections, usually bacterial or fungal in nature. The main target organs are the skin, the oral and genital mucosae, and the urinary tract.

In the skin, diabetics are particularly vulnerable to follicular infections by staphylococci, and the lesions tend to be more severe than in non-diabetics; boils are particularly frequent in elderly patients with type II diabetes. Other skin conditions that are more common in diabetics are superficial fungal infections, cellulitis and erysipelas (see Chapter 23).

Diabetics may have particularly severe oral or genital mucosal infections with *Candida*.

In the kidney, in addition to the other abnormalities due to small and large vessel disease, there is an increased predisposition to **acute pyelonephritis**, often associated with recurrent lower urinary tract infections, and sometimes complicated by **papillary necrosis** (see page 381).

Diabetics have very severe atherosclerosis

Although atherosclerosis is widespread and common, diabetics in general suffer much more severe and extensive atherosclerosis than non-diabetics of the same age and gender. Furthermore, in diabetics the atherosclerotic changes extend into much smaller artery branches than in non-diabetics. The main clinical sequelae of this are seen in:

- The heart, where coronary atherosclerosis is more severe and extensive than in non-diabetics, predisposing to ischemic heart disease.
- The brain, where atherosclerosis of the internal carotid and vertebrobasilar arteries and their branches predisposes to cerebral ischemia.
- The legs and feet, where severe atherosclerosis of the iliofemoral and smaller arteries in the lower leg predisposes to the development of gangrene. Ischemia of a single toe, or ischemic areas on the heel, are characteristic features of diabetic gangrene, which is due to the involvement of smaller, more peripheral arteries than is the case in non-diabetic generalized atherosclerosis.
- The kidney, where extension of atherosclerosis into the main renal arteries and their intrarenal branches makes a major contribution towards chronic nephron ischemia, an important component of the multiple renal lesions in diabetes (see below).

Microvascular disease is an important feature of diabetes, and is responsible for many of the pathological complications

In diabetes the small arterioles and capillaries show a characteristic pattern of wall thickening, which is due to a

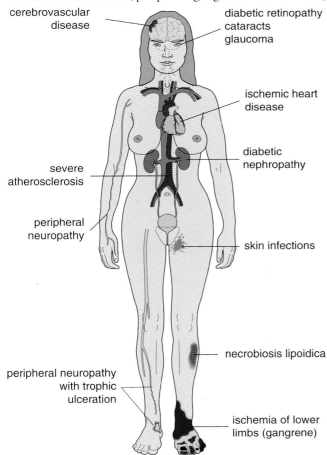

Fig. 25.15 Multisystem manifestations of diabetes mellitus. The most important complications are vascular disease, renal disease, and eye disease.

marked expansion of the basement membrane, termed **hyaline arteriolosclerosis** (see pages 164 and 461). This small vessel abnormality is widespread, and is responsible for ischemic changes which are symptomatic in the kidney, the retina, the brain and in peripheral nerves.

In the kidney, the capillaries of the glomerular tuft show marked basement membrane thickening associated with increased leakiness of the capillary wall. This permits the leakage of plasma proteins into the glomerular filtrate in amounts greater than can be reabsorbed in the tubular part of the nephron, leading to **proteinuria**, and eventually **glomerular hyalinization and the development of chronic renal failure**.

In the retina, the vessel wall changes lead to retinal hemorrhage and vascular proliferation. In the brain, the small vessel lesions lead to lacunar infarction and ischemic white matter degeneration. In peripheral nerves, the capillary wall changes are believed to be a major factor in the development of peripheral neuropathy.

Peripheral neuropathy is an important cause of intractable ulceration of the foot in diabetics

The various patterns of diabetic neuropathy are discussed briefly on page 486. The most common is symmetrical peripheral polyneuropathy, which particularly affects the hands and feet in a 'glove and stocking' distribution. This leads to impairment or loss of sensation, including the loss of pain sensation. The normal pain withdrawal from injury reflex is lost, and areas of the skin are repeatedly damaged by trivial trauma such as friction from tight-fitting footwear (see *Fig. 25.16*). This form of trophic ulceration becomes chronic, healing being impaired by a combination of repeated trauma and the ischemia almost invariably present in the feet of diabetics with severe coexisting vascular disease.

Fig. 25.16 Diabetic trophic ulcers. The combination of peripheral sensory neuropathy and ischemia caused by diabetic small vessel disease makes diabetics particularly prone to develop trophic ulcers at sites of pressure and friction. These are notoriously difficult to heal.

Diabetic nephropathy is an important cause of mortality in diabetics

The kidney is affected in many ways in diabetes. As well as the predisposition to urinary tract infection and the tendency to chronic ischemia associated with severe atherosclerosis, certain renal lesions are particularly associated with diabetes; these are glomerular basement membrane thickening, diabetic glomerulosclerosis (both diffuse and nodular), glomerular exudative lesions, and papillary necrosis. These are considered in more detail in Chapter 17. The end result is the development of chronic renal failure.

Diabetes is an important cause of acquired blindness in the western world

Diabetes can affect the eyes in five main ways:

1. **Background retinopathy** is due to small vessel abnormalities in the retina leading to hard exudates, hemorrhages and microaneurysms; this does not usually affect visual acuity.
2. **Proliferative retinopathy** is caused by the extensive proliferation of new small blood vessels in the retina. Sudden deterioration in vision can result from vitreous hemorrhage from the proliferating new vessels or the development of retinal detachment.
3. **Maculopathy** is caused by edema, hard exudates or retinal ischemia, and causes a marked reduction in acuity.
4. **Cataract formation** is greatly increased in diabetics.
5. **Glaucoma** shows an increased incidence in diabetics due to neovascularization of the iris, **rubeosis iridis** (see page 502).

AMYLOIDOSIS

Amyloidosis is a condition in which there is a deposition, in many tissues, of an abnormal extracellular fibrillar protein termed **amyloid**. Amyloid is derived from many different precursor peptides, with the precursors themselves often being fragments derived from larger proteins; it is deposited as a meshwork of rigid, straight fibrils 10–15 nm in diameter, being composed of the precursor peptides lined up in an antiparallel β-pleated sheet structure. It is therefore the physical arrangement of the constituent peptides that makes a protein an amyloid, rather than any specific peptide sequence.

Amyloid is detected histologically as a bright-pink hyaline material. It also takes up certain special stains, the most widely known being Congo red; electron microscopy shows it to have a fibrillar ultrastructure (*Fig. 25.17*).

Amyloid can be classified according to the nature of the precursor protein

Despite uncertainty about why amyloid is formed, there are well-characterized associations between particular diseases and the deposition of amyloid. In each case there is an accumulation of a precursor peptide which is processed into an amyloid protein. In some of these diseases there is an identifiable reason for the accumulation of the precursor peptide, and the amyloid is termed **secondary amyloid**. In other cases the cause of the accumulation is not known,

and the amyloid is termed **primary amyloid**. In addition, there are several inherited disorders, the **heredofamilial amyloidoses**.

Amyloid is deposited outside cells, and can be classified into localized or systemic patterns

Amyloid is deposited in the extracellular compartment of tissues, and in H&E preparations it is seen as a uniformly eosinophilic (pink-staining) material. It can be highlighted in histological sections by the use of special stains such as Sirius red and Congo red. Congo red staining is commonly used for diagnostic purposes, with amyloid staining orange and exhibiting a green coloration when viewed with polarized light (*Fig. 25.19*).

Amyloidosis may involve many tissues in the body as it is particularly deposited in the blood vessel walls and basement membranes. The progressive accumulation of amyloid leads to cellular dysfunction, either by preventing the normal processes of diffusion through extracellular tissues, or by the physical compression of functioning parenchymal cells. In some diseases amyloidosis is a systemic process affecting many organs simultaneously (**systemic amyloid**); there is also group of conditions in which amyloid only affects one organ or tissue (**localized amyloid**).

Fig. 25.17 Amyloid ultrastructure. Amyloid is composed of filaments of protein deposited extracellularly.

 Amyloidogenesis

Amyloid is derived in two main ways (*Fig. 25.18*):

- A precursor is produced in abnormally large amounts (examples are given).
- Polymorphisms of normal proteins give rise to peptides which are predisposed to form amyloid, termed amyloidogenic (the two most common examples are given). The nature of the peptide sequences required for this process is still uncertain.

It is thought that cells of the mononuclear–phagocyte system are responsible for processing the precursor peptide to form amyloid fibrils, often by producing fragments of the main precursor peptide.

In addition to the precursor peptide, amyloid contains another serum protein, called serum amyloid P, which may assist in nucleation.

Fig. 25.18 Amyloidogenesis.

Amino-acid sequencing of amyloid proteins in different disease states has enabled a classification of amyloid to be made on biochemical grounds (*Fig. 25.20*).

The commonest example of amyloid deposition is in the nervous system, in both Alzheimer's disease and normal aging. The amyloid is derived from a normal, neuronal membrane protein termed **Alzheimer precursor protein (APP)**, being formed from a peptide fragment termed **Aβ protein** or **A4 protein**.

Amyloid that is associated with an abnormal proliferation of plasma cells is made up of immunoglobulin light chains, with such amyloid deposition occurring in diseases such as myeloma and plasmacytoma (see page 314).

Reactive amyloid may be associated with long-standing chronic inflammatory processes. As in any inflammatory disorder, the associated systemic acute-phase response causes excessive production of serum amyloid A protein (a normal, acute-phase protein) by the liver. With time, and for uncertain reasons, some of this protein is deposited as amyloid. Diseases that lead to this type of secondary amyloid include tuberculosis, rheumatoid arthritis, bronchiectasis and chronic osteomyelitis.

Fig. 25.19 Histology of amyloid. (a) Amyloid appears as homogeneous bright pink-staining material. In this example, from the spleen, amyloid is deposited as rounded masses. (b) If amyloid is stained with Congo red and viewed under polarized light, it shows apple-green birefringence.

Fig. 25.20 Classification of amyloid

Localization	Clinical association	Precursor protein
Systemic amyloid		
	Plasma cell tumors	Immunoglobulin light chain (AL)
	Chronic inflammation	Serum amyloid A protein (AA)
	Familial Mediterranean fever	Serum amyloid A protein (AA)
	Familial neuropathy	Transthyretin (prealbumin) (ATTR)
	Dialysis associated	β_2-Microglobulin (Aβ_2M)
Localized amyloid		
	Senile cardiac amyloid	Transthyretin (prealbumin) (ATTR)
	Medullary carcinoma	Calcitonin (ACal)
	Islet-cell amyloid	Amylin (AIAPP)
	Alzheimer's disease	Aβ protein (A4 protein) (Aβ)
	Cerebral amyloid angiopathy	Aβ protein (A4 protein) (Aβ)

Diagnosis of amyloidosis

The diagnosis of systemic amyloidosis is usually confirmed by tissue biopsy. The most useful site for biopsy is the rectal mucosa, where amyloid can be detected in the submucosal vessels in 60–70% of cases of generalized amyloidosis. Amyloid may also be detected in renal biopsies or liver biopsies.

More recently, radiolabeled serum amyloid P can be injected into patients and imaged; it localizes to any amyloid deposits.

Tumors of peptide-secreting endocrine cells may form amyloid from the hormone peptide, e.g. in the calcitonin-derived amyloid in medullary carcinoma of the thyroid. In type II diabetes the excessive secretion of amylin by the β cells of the pancreas is associated with its deposition as **islet amyloid**. Uncommon familial types of amyloid are believed to be caused by gene polymorphisms in normal proteins. The amino-acid substitutions are believed to make the proteins – or their peptide fragments – susceptible to amyloid formation.

Amyloid is deposited mainly in the kidney, heart, liver, spleen and nerves

The kidneys are the organs most commonly functionally impaired by systemic amyloidosis, usually presenting with proteinuria or the nephrotic syndrome (see page 378).

Deposition of amyloid in the spleen can occur in either a diffuse pattern or a nodular pattern.

In the liver, amyloid is deposited in the space between the sinusoidal lining cells and the hepatocytes. Clinically, hepatic amyloidosis may be a cause of hepatomegaly. However, there is rarely significant clinical evidence of impaired liver function.

Amyloid involvement of the heart may be a manifestation of senile cardiac amyloid, which is derived from transthyretin (prealbumin). The most severe form of cardiac amyloid is seen in systemic amyloidosis, causing cardiomyopathy (see page 178).

INHERITED METABOLIC DISORDERS

Several multisystem diseases are the result of inherited metabolic defects, the vast majority of which are inherited as recessive traits. In some diseases the metabolic defect results in the accumulation of a metabolic product in cells, giving rise to the term **metabolic storage diseases**. In most cases the inherited defect is lack of an enzyme, leading to the failure to break down a substrate, which then accumulates in cells, eventually interfering with cell function. In many cases the substrate accumulates preferentially in lysosomal-derived vesicles (**lysosomal storage disease**), but in others it accumulates in cell cytoplasm.

Storage disorders can be classified according to the type of substance that accumulates

The main groups are:

- **Glycogenoses:** diseases characterized by the accumulation of glycogen in cells.
- **Mucopolysaccharidoses:** diseases due to the accumulation of mucopolysaccharides (MPS) in cells.
- **Lipidoses:** diseases due to the accumulation of sphingolipids.
- **Metal storage diseases**: particularly iron (hemochromatosis) and copper (Wilson's disease). As a major impact in both diseases is on the liver, these are also discussed in Chapter 14, and Wilson's disease also in Chapter 21.

Other, rarer, disease groups include the **mucolipidoses** (defects in lysosomal enzyme transport systems) and the **glycoproteinoses** (defects in enzymes that degrade glycoproteins)

Disease variously affects:

- The lymphoreticular system (spleen, liver, bone marrow, lymph nodes) resulting in splenomegaly and hepatomegaly.
- The nervous system, resulting in mental retardation or progressive failure of intellectual development.
- Endothelium, smooth muscle, skeletal muscle.
- Hepatocytes, resulting in hepatomegaly.

Diagnosis is based on the clinical recognition of disease complemented by the detection of the abnormal product in cells or, in some cases, the urine. The enzyme defect may be demonstrated in lymphoid cells or in cultured fibroblasts.

The glycogenoses result in abnormal accumulation of glycogen in tissues

The glycogenoses are a group of diseases in which there is an abnormal accumulation of glycogen in tissues; this is caused by diverse abnormalities of enzymes involved in the glycogen metabolism. There are over 12 subtypes, the majority of which have defined enzyme deficiencies (*Fig. 25.21*). Diagnosis is often made initially by demonstrating the presence of glycogen in tissue biopsy samples (*Fig. 25.22*), followed by demonstrating a lack of the appropriate enzyme activity. Increasingly, genetic techniques are being used to refine diagnosis.

Fig. 25.21 Main subtypes of glycogenosis

Type	Enzyme deficiency	Features
IA (von Gierke's)	Glucose-6-phosphatase	Hypoglycemia in early life with hepatomegaly
IC	Glucose-6-phosphate translocase	Neutropenia and infections
II (Pompe's)	Lysosomal acid maltase	Cardiac failure in early infancy with cardiomegaly and hepatomegaly
II (Adult onset)	Lysosomal acid maltase	Proximal myopathy or cardiomyopathy
III	Debrancher enzyme	Hypoglycemia, hepatomegaly, cirrhosis
IV	Branching enzyme	Hepatomegaly and cirrhosis
V (McArdle's)	Myophosphorylase	Muscle cramps, rhabdomyolysis, myopathy
VI (Her's)	Hepatic phosphorylase	Hepatomegaly
VII	Phosphofructokinase	Muscle cramps, myopathy

Fig. 25.22 Liver – glycogenosis. The liver cells are bloated with stored glycogen in this biopsy from an infant with type II (Pompe's) glycogenosis. There is also hepatocyte necrosis with pyknotic nuclear debris.

Most mucopolysaccharidoses produce a decline in physical and mental function

There are numerous subtypes, each differing clinically and associated with a lack of different enzymes, and hence different mucopolysaccharides (glycosaminoglycans) stored. They are grouped as MPS types I–VII, of which types I, II and III are the most common and important.

MPS I includes Hurler's syndrome, in which developmental delay occurs within the first year of life, followed by progressive mental and physical decline, and usually death before the age of 10 years. The mucopolysaccharide is stored in cells throughout the body, in the brain causing the mental decline, in the bones causing bony deformity, particularly noticeable in the facial bones, and also producing hepatosplenomegaly and cardiomegaly.

MPS II includes Hunter's syndrome, clinically similar to Hurler's syndrome but becoming manifest later in childhood, being less severe, and with survival into the early 20s.

MPS III includes Sanfilippo syndrome, of which there are four subtypes. All are associated with mental deterioration.

Most lipidoses have a major effect on the brain

In the lipid storage diseases, lipids of various types accumulate in cells and eventually interfere with cell function, and in most types there is central nervous system involvement. Thus many of these disorders (the Niemann–Pick group, Krabbe's disease, metachromatic leukodystrophy, the gangliosidoses, Batten's disease) are dealt with in Chapter 21.

The commonest lipidosis is **Gaucher's disease**, caused by a deficiency of the enzyme glucocerebrosidase. There are three main types, the commonest of which does not significantly affect the central nervous system, but symptomatology is due to the accumulation of lipid in liver, spleen and bone marrow (*Fig. 25.23*), leading to hepatosplenomegaly, bone pain and hematological disorders (anemia and thrombocytopenia). Brain damage is a feature of the other, rarer, types of Gaucher's disease.

Familial defects in lipid metabolism cause hyperlipidemias and are an important cause of atheroma

Hyperlipidemias are conditions in which there is an abnormally high level of one or more lipoproteins in the plasma. Where this is the result of a systemic metabolic disturbance it is termed **secondary hyperlipidemia,** the main causes being obesity, excess alcohol intake, diabetes mellitus, nephrotic syndrome and hypothyroidism. When hyperlipidemia is caused by a genetic predisposition to an

Fig. 25.23 Gaucher's disease. Macrophages in this bone marrow sample shows swollen granular cytoplasm as a result of storage of glucocerebroside.

abnormal lipid metabolism, the term **primary hyperlipidemia** is used.

Such primary hyperlipidemias have been shown to be due to a wide range of abnormalities in the genes that code for enzymes, apolipoproteins, or receptors involved in the lipid metabolism.

There are several types of hyperlipidemia, which can be characterized by the determination of the lipoprotein profile in plasma. The WHO classification is based on that proposed by Fredrickson, and divides cases into types I–V. Unfortunately, this does not indicate the cause of a hyperlipidemia (i.e. whether primary or secondary). Recent developments in the biochemistry of these disorders are allowing precise diagnoses to be made, based on metabolic or genetic characterization.

Fig. 25.24 Hyperlipidemias

Type	Inheritance	Features	Mechanism
Familial hypercholesterolemia	Autosomal dominant 1:500 population	Increased plasma cholesterol Increased plasma LDL Arcus senilis and tendon xanthomas Increased atheroma risk	Caused by abnormalities in LDL synthesis, transport, receptor binding or internalization. Many different mutations and genes involved
Familial combined hyperlipidemia	Autosomal dominant 1:300 population	Increased plasma cholesterol Increased plasma VLDL Increased plasma LDL Increased atheroma risk	Abnormally high levels of apolipoprotein B produced by liver, thought to be caused by defect in a regulatory gene
Familial hypertriglyceridemia	Autosomal dominant 1:600 population	Increased VLDL in plasma Increased atheroma risk in some cases	Possible polymorphisms in some of the genes coding for apo A and C. Patients with associated low HDL develop premature atheroma
Familial dysbetalipoproteinemia	Autosomal polymorphism Uncommon	Increased chylomicrons Increased IDL Palmar xanthomas Eruptive xanthomas Increased atheroma risk	Apolipoprotein E phenotype E2/2
Familial alphalipoproteinemia	Uncommon	Increased serum cholesterol Increased HDL Reduced atheroma risk	HDL increased
Familial chylomicronemia	Autosomal recessive Rare	Increased chylomicrons Xanthomas in some cases Pancreatitis in some cases	1) Reduced endothelial lipoprotein lipase 2) Reduced apo C-II levels

This table shows the main types of hyperlipidemia and the most important features of each. About 6:1000 of the population have an autosomal dominant predisposition to develop an abnormality of lipid metabolism that increases the risk of developing atheroma. In addition, others have a polygenic increased risk. Some of these cases will come to medical attention because of the trend for the routine screening of blood for cholesterol levels. Other cases will come to light having presented with a complication of atheroma at a young age, e.g. ischemic heart disease or cerebrovascular disease.

One of the most important consequences of certain types of hyperlipidemia (mainly WHO type IIa) is a raised serum cholesterol concentration, mainly a reflection of serum LDL, which predisposes to atheroma.

The main types of hyperlipidemia and their most important features are listed in *Fig. 25.24*.

In addition to the effects of hyperlipidemia, high levels of one particular lipoprotein termed lipoprotein (a) confers a high risk of the development of both ischemic heart disease and cerebrovascular disease, independent of LDL/cholesterol levels.

Case-based questions

Case 1 A young woman with a rash

A 27-year-old woman is referred to a nephrology specialist from a Dermatology clinic. The dermatologist writes:

> I would be grateful if you would see this young woman who I have seen in my clinic on two occasions. On the first visit she had a severe photosensitive rash on her face shoulders and arms following sunbathing; on the second occasion she had a symmetrical erythematous rash on her upper cheeks with some scaling. This second rash is typical of ******************, and I refer her to you because on both occasions, routine urine testing showed significant proteinuria. She also suffers from joint pain and stiffness.

1. **What do you think are the missing words in the dermatologist's letter?**
2. **Why did the finding of persistent proteinuria necessitate referral to a nephrology clinic in this case?**
3. **What investigations might the nephrologists consider?**

Case 2 A woman with Raynaud's phenomenon

A 23-year-old woman complains of thickening and shininess of the skin of all her fingers, which were often painful. She was no stranger to painful fingers, as she had suffered from intermittent Raynaud's phenomenon for about 3 years. She also thought that her face had got thinner recently, and she was unable to open her mouth to its fullest extent without discomfort.

1. **What is the most likely diagnosis?**

The physician questioned her about her breathing capacity, whether she had a history of heartburn or difficulty swallowing, and ordered, among other investigations, X-rays of the hands and chest, and a barium swallow.

2. **Explain the purpose of the specific questions he asked and the investigations requested.**
3. **To expand your knowledge in this area of medicine, look up CREST syndrome and mixed connective tissue disease.**

Case 3 An old man with ulcers on his feet

A 73-year-old man presented with ulcers on both heels and a smaller ulcer on the lateral aspect of his left fifth toe. He was not sure how long he had had the heel ulcers, as he had only noticed them when he noticed that his socks were sticking to them. He said that they were not painful, but were slowly getting bigger despite topical treatment with over-the-counter creams, ointments and dressings.

On direct questioning he described some loss of sensation in both feet and, to a lesser extent, his fingers and hands. Clinical examination showed shallow weeping ulcers on both heels, with a purplish rim of discoloration; there was a similar smaller lesion on the left fifth toe. Foot pulses were poor in the right foot, and scarcely detectable in the left. Neurological examination showed sensation loss in a glove-and-stocking distribution.

1. **Summarize the most likely link between the ulcers and the neurological findings.**
2. **What is the most likely underlying disease?**
3. **What factors predispose to failure of the ulcers to heal?**

Brief answers to these case-based questions are given on page 596. More detailed answers and other study resources are available online at www.studentconsult.com.

Appendix
Laboratory methods and terminology

Acidophilic

Staining with acidic dyes, for example eosin (see **hematoxylin and eosin**).

Autopsy

see **postmortem examination**

Basophilic

Staining with basic dyes, for example hematoxylin (see 'hematoxylin and eosin').

Biopsy methods

There are many ways in which samples can be taken for histological examination to establish an accurate tissue diagnosis:

- **excision biopsy.** The entire abnormal area is excised and submitted for microscopic examination; this is usually both diagnostic and curative, for example the complete excision of a neoplastic polyp in the colon.
- **incision biopsy** is undertaken where it is impossible or inappropriate to excise the whole of the diseased area; a sample is removed by incising the lesion with a scalpel to provide a substantial amount of tissue for microscopic examination.
- **needle biopsy** is undertaken for both superficial and deep lesions. A hollow needle is introduced into the lesion, upon which a small core of tissue occupies the needle lumen, from where it is removed gently and sent for microscopic examination. This technique is widely used in the examination of liver disease and kidney disease. Where the lesion to be sampled is fairly superficial, for example an abnormal enlarged lymph node in the neck, accurate guiding of the needle is simple; for deeper lesions the needle may need to be introduced under imaging control.
- **trephine biopsies** are usually confined to the removal of samples of bone, such as to investigate either disease of the bone itself or, in hematological disorders, the bone marrow. The trephine is like a hollow drill which is inserted by hand, the biopsy sample occupies the hollow centre of the trephine from which it can be extracted after removal.

- **Endoscopic biopsy** is performed by using fine biopsy forceps that are passed down the channel of an endoscope. The lesion to be sampled is viewed directly, and samples 1–2 mm in diameter are removed for histologic examination. This is mainly used in the upper and lower gastrointestinal tracts, the upper and lower airways, and the lower urinary tract.
- **Stereotactic biopsy** is a special technique in which imaging is used to locate precisely a deep-seated lesion with reference to surface landmarks or an attached frame. A needle can then be guided to biopsy an area with accuracy to within 1 mm. This is particularly used in biopsy of brain lesions.

Bone marrow aspiration

A trephine or needle is inserted into a bone marrow cavity, usually the sternum, iliac crest or tibia (in infants), and hemopoietic marrow is aspirated; smears are prepared and stained, and are then examined microscopically to determine the cell types present. This process is undertaken in the diagnosis of severe intractable anemia of unknown cause, leukemias (both proven and suspected), myelodysplastic syndromes, and many other conditions. As well as being used for initial diagnosis, marrow aspiration is used to assess the effectiveness of treatment in leukemia and lymphoma, and to diagnose early relapse.

Cervical cytology

This branch of cytology concentrates on the analysis of exfoliative cytology of the cervix as a means of detecting cervical neoplasia. Infective and inflammatory conditions of the female genital tract may also be detected by this technique. A special spatula is used to scrape cells from the endocervical junction and these are smeared on a slide, fixed, and sent to the laboratory. The Papanicolaou technique is used to stain smears, resulting in blue nuclei, pink superficial cells, and blue-green parabasal cells.

Clinical chemistry

Investigations are now carried out largely in automated systems, and many can be carried out on small samples of blood or other body fluids. In the majority of cases estimations can be made on 5 mL of clotted blood; these include frequent investigations such as urea and electrolytes, serum calcium, proteins, enzymes, hormone assays, and most drug level estimations. Occasionally it is necessary to place the blood in a container with an anticoagulant so that it does not clot; lithium–heparin and fluoride–oxalate are the most frequently used anticoagulants. For most estimations on body fluids, such as urine, all that is required is an untreated sample of the fresh fluid, but occasionally 24-hour samples of urine are required. Each laboratory has its own set of normal standards, according to the technique used in the estimations; similarly, some laboratories vary in the way in which they prefer their samples presented. Every student and practicing doctor should pay great attention to the instructions of their particular laboratory if samples, time and money are not to be wasted.

Cytogenetics

Culture of cells is performed and chromosome spreads made for analysis. Alterations in chromosome number or fine structure can be detected, and may be useful in analysis of congenital abnormalities, mental retardation, and certain tumors. Tissue must be rapidly transported in specialized tissue culture medium to the laboratory.

Cytological examination

In this technique a diagnosis is based on the appearances of isolated cells taken, or shed, from an abnormal area. The technique is used mainly in the diagnosis of malignant disease, using the cytological criteria indicating that a cell is both neoplastic and malignant (e.g. nuclear atypia, high mitotic rate, high nucleus to cytoplasm ratio). Cells can be obtained from an abnormal area by:

- **exfoliation methods**, in which cells are scraped from the surface of an abnormal area. This method is limited to disorders in which the abnormality is in an accessible epithelial surface, for example the cervix of the uterus, or the mucosal lining of the esophagus, stomach or proximal tracheobronchial tree. The specimen may be obtained either by using a specially designed spatula which scrapes the cells from the surface, or by a brush which is passed over the abnormal surface, superficial cells becoming adherent to the brush bristles. Cells are transferred to a microscope slide, fixed, and then stained with various stains to show the nuclear and cytoplasmic characteristics.
- **fluid aspiration** is a method in which fluid is aspirated from hollow viscera such as the pleural and peritoneal cavities, and the cell content of the fluid is examined microscopically. The cell population is frequently small, and various methods are used to provide a concentrated sample. Similar methods can be used to examine cerebrospinal fluid in the diagnosis of malignancy involving the brain and meninges, and sometimes clues about the nature of inflammatory diseases in the CNS can be obtained by noting the type of inflammatory cells present, for example neutrophils in bacterial meningitis, lymphocytes in tuberculous meningitis and viral meningoencephalitis. Naturally voided fluids, such as urine and sputum, can also be examined for cell content to detect atypical or reactive cells.

- **aspiration of cells from solid lesions** – 'fine needle aspiration' – is an important and clinically convenient method of diagnosing suspected malignancy without the necessity for a surgical maneuver involving excision or incision biopsy. A needle is inserted into a solid lump (usually in an organ or tissue close to the surface such as breast, thyroid, or superficial lymph node) and suction applied so that some of the cells in the lump pass into the needle. These are then expressed onto a microscope slide, fixed and stained for microscopic examination. As with most diagnostic cytological techniques, it is mainly used in the diagnosis of malignant tumors, looking for the cytological criteria of malignancy.

Fixation and staining of cytological preparations is discussed under 'fixation and fixatives' and 'special stains'.

Electron microscopy (EM)

This is used to supplement analysis performed by light microscopy. It is particularly valuable in the assessment of renal biopsies for glomerulonephritis when the location of immune complexes can be determined. It is used in the diagnosis of tumors by looking for fine detail of cell differentiation. Muscle biopsy relies on electron microscopy for the diagnosis of several important myopathies. Viral disorders can also be diagnosed by the analysis of characteristic viral particles. Tissue samples for EM should be fixed in a specially prepared, buffered glutaraldehyde fixative. Samples should be 1–2 mm in diameter to ensure adequate fixation.

Enzyme histochemistry

This is a technique for demonstrating the location of specific enzymes in tissue sections. It is particularly used for the analysis of skeletal muscle biopsies, allowing delineation of different fiber types. Fresh, unfixed tissue is essential (see also **frozen section**).

Erythrocyte sedimentation rate (ESR)

This is a test performed in hematology departments. Blood is allowed to stand in special tubes and the rate of sedimentation is measured and expressed in mm/h. If red blood cells are induced to form aggregates then the sedimentation time is rapid. Conditions in which there are acute-phase proteins in the blood, or when there are high concentrations of immunoglobulin, are particularly associated with a high ESR.

Fixation and fixatives

The histological diagnosis of disease processes is still largely based on the microscopic examination of a thin (3–5 μm) section of the tissue, which has been embedded in paraffin wax after the tissue has been fixed. The most common and widely used protein-linking substances that are used as fixatives are aldehydes, particularly formaldehyde and glutaraldehyde. Formaldehyde is used as a 10% aqueous solution (formalin), which is often buffered to prevent the fixative solution becoming acidic (as the formaldehyde spontaneously converts to formic acid).

Why does the tissue have to be fixed? Fixation achieves a number of objectives:

- first, it prevents the tissue undergoing autolysis (i.e. self-breakdown by the release of tissue enzymes when cells die). Autolyzed tissues lose all their architectural and cytological characteristics, rendering accurate microscopic diagnosis impossible. Fixation inactivates the enzymes responsible for autolysis, as well as killing microorganisms that may be present in the sample.
- second, fixation hardens the tissues by cross-linking the structural-protein component of the cells and stromal components, so that the architectural and cytological relationships are retained in a state which pretty-much resembles the true living state.
- third, fixation protects the tissues from the possible untoward effects of the various processes that it has to go through during the embedding of the tissue sample in paraffin or other supporting medium. When the tissues may need to be examined by special laboratory techniques (for example, electron microscopy or immunocytochemistry), special fixatives may be required.

Frozen section

A frozen section is performed by freezing a sample of fresh tissue rapidly in a special mounting medium, and then making histological sections in a machine called a cryostat (basically a freezer containing a microtome). The tissue is held at about −20°C, at which temperature it becomes hard enough to cut sections about 8 μm thick. These sections can be stained, and a rapid diagnosis can be made, for example while a patient is under anesthetic. Frozen sections are also used for some special examinations, particularly enzyme histochemistry and immunohistochemistry. A disadvantage of this technique is that sections lack the resolution obtainable with wax-embedded material.

Full blood count

This is the basis of initial hematological investigation, and is carried out mainly by machinery that provides figures for hemoglobin levels, red-cell numbers, size (diameter and volume), white-cell numbers and platelet numbers. Microscopic examination of the blood smear gives valuable information about the nature of red cells and white cells, particularly in the presence of abnormal forms of any of the cells. The cytological appearance of these cells may give a strong clue to the diagnosis, but not all films are examined microscopically because it is very time consuming, costly,

and labor intensive. In most cases, the staff of the hematology laboratory will make a decision on whether to examine a smear, which is based on the information given on the request form and on the figures obtained from the full blood count; they will always examine a film if requested to do so. To get the maximum information from a basic hematology request, it is vital that full clinical information be supplied on the request form.

Hematoxylin and eosin

This is the standard histological stain used in histology laboratories. Hematoxylin stains nuclei deep purple; eosin stains cytoplasm shades of pink. Structures that stain with eosin are termed eosinophilic or, because eosin is an acidic dye, acidophilic. Structures that stain with hematoxylin are termed basophilic as this is a basic dye.

Immunofluorescence

This is a technique for staining histological sections in order to detect the presence of a specific protein or antigen in the tissue. An antibody that is directed at the antigen is applied to the section, and detected by a fluorescent dye. Sections need to be viewed with a special fluorescence microscope. This is useful in the diagnosis of renal disease and skin diseases caused by autoimmune or immune-complex reactions.

Immunohistochemistry

This is a staining technique that allows the detection of specific proteins or antigens in tissue sections. Antibodies to specific proteins or antigens are applied to tissue sections and are detected by a colored reaction product. In most cases there is a brown reaction product generated by the detection of a marker enzyme, peroxidase – hence the term 'immunoperoxidase reaction.' This technique is routinely performed in most laboratories and allows very specific identification of cell types as well as tumor markers.

Necropsy
see **postmortem examination**

Neuropathology

Examination of the tissues of the nervous system is traditionally carried out in specialized laboratories. Postmortem examination of the brain takes many weeks, as fixation, tissue processing, and staining of large sections of brain is much more prolonged than for small tissue samples.

Postmortem examination

The investigation of disease should not end with the death of the patient. Postmortem examination should be carried out to confirm or establish the structural diseases present, to note the effect or failure of any treatment given during life and, most importantly, to establish a cause of death and a list of conditions present at the time of death for accurate registration. Considerable weight is placed on the officially registered cause of death when devising statistics on which to base the distribution of healthcare resources, and it is vital that the national figures are accurate. Unfortunately, many studies in western countries have shown that cause of death registration is frequently very inaccurate unless a postmortem examination has been performed. (Comparative studies in which practitioners were invited to list the cause of death before autopsy, and the pathologist asked to provide a cause of death afterwards, shows a very high level of inaccuracy without adequate postmortem examination.) A postmortem is therefore a vital component of clinical audit, but is sadly neglected in most countries, resulting in spurious and highly inaccurate figures for disease incidence and causes of death. There are important implications, as inappropriate allocation of healthcare resources is inevitable because of diagnostic inaccuracies. It should be the intention of clinical practitioners to request a postmortem examination on any death occurring in hospital, and it should be possible for practitioners in the community to request postmortem on any of their patients of whom they are not absolutely certain of the cause or mechanism of death.

Some deaths require a postmortem examination by law, for example those of medicolegal significance, where there is a possibility that death was not due to natural disease, or where death may be attributable to an accident or industrial disease. There are many such categories where postmortem examination is compulsory by law, and these cases come under the aegis of the Coroner in England and Wales, the Medical Examiner in the United States, and the Procurator Fiscal in Scotland.

Postmortem examination

A postmortem examination is carried out by dissection of the internal organs, which are usually removed through a single longitudinal incision extending from the neck to the suprapubic region in the anterior midline. The brain is examined after lifting the calvarium through an incision passing over the back of the head. In most cases a provisional diagnosis is established by naked-eye examination of the organs after dissection. Histological and microbiological examinations of tissue samples removed at postmortem are performed to establish an accurate diagnosis.

Unless the case has been referred by one of the medicolegal authorities, the written permission of the next of kin is required before a postmortem examination can be carried out. If it is the wish of the next of kin, it may be possible to carry out a 'limited postmortem' in which, for example, only the heart or brain is examined if the disease is believed to be localized to that area.

After the removal and dissection of the organs, they are replaced in the body cavities, which are cleaned, and then the skin incisions are sewn together. Reconstitution of the body is an important part of examination. When the deceased is dressed in a shroud, it is possible to view the body without visible signs of the examination having been performed.

Preservation of operative and biopsy specimens

Fixatives can provide their beneficial effects only if they penetrate the tissues. Most fixatives penetrate fairly slowly. Small tissue fragments, such as needle-biopsy samples, fix very quickly, and the architecture and cytology are usually very well preserved. However, large tissue samples fix more slowly as the immersed specimen can only be fixed by diffusion of fixative from the outer surface; furthermore, large specimens require large volumes of fixative. A compact organ such as the spleen, even if immersed in a large volume of fixative in a large container, will reach the laboratory a few hours after removal with only the outer 2–5 mm fixed; the remainder of the splenic tissue will have already undergone some degree of autolysis and subsequent architectural and cytological distortion. Therefore, the only part of the spleen that will show good preservation for microscopic analysis will be the splenic capsule and the underlying couple of millimeters of splenic parenchyma. The same applies to any solid organ; this is particularly important in the case of enlarged lymph nodes, where accurate diagnosis is dependent upon the high-quality preservation of cytology and architecture. There are four main rules for handling tissue samples and for presenting them to the histopathology laboratory (see following blue box).

Rules for handling tissues for the laboratory

Rule 1

If a pathological lesion is unusual, or is likely to require special techniques such as electron microscopy, ring the laboratory to check whether the specimen should be fixed or sent down fresh and, if fixed, which fixative should be used. This is becoming increasingly important with the wider use of immunocytochemical techniques and electron microscopy in the accurate diagnosis of lymphoma and certain tumor types. Some tissues, for example skeletal muscle, can be diagnosed only if unfixed and received promptly. Some tissue samples may need to undergo enzyme histochemistry or have frozen sections made to reach a diagnosis. If the laboratory requires the specimen fresh, arrange for immediate transfer of the specimen to a named person in the laboratory. Do not rely on a hospital portering system. Many biopsy specimens are ruined by the amount of autolysis and drying out that occurs when small specimens such as Tru-cut needle biopsies are delayed either in theatre, in the porter's pocket, or

▶

▶ because they are hanging around in the laboratory because no member of laboratory staff has been notified of its arrival. If a fresh specimen is to be sent, always warn the laboratory that it is on its way. All fresh tissue should be handled as if it were potentially infective. Samples should be placed in sealed containers and labeled with the nature of the specimen, the name and details of the patient, and the appropriate clinical details.

Rule 2

If a specimen is to be fixed, always ensure that the specimen is placed in sufficient fixative and in a large enough container to take the specimen and fixative solution (preferably four to five times the volume of the specimen) without distortion to the specimen. Remember that soft, unfixed tissues are pliable and can be squashed into quite a small container, but that the space left for fixative solution will be so small that insufficient fixative will be used and the specimen will remain largely unfixed. Also, if the specimen has been squashed, when it is hardened by the fixative it will retain the shape of the container into which it has been forced.

Rule 3

If the pathological lesion is at the centre of the excised specimen, it will not be fixed properly unless one surface of the lesion is exposed to the fixative; it is therefore advisable to transect the excised specimen through the lesion so that the fixative will hit the main pathology immediately upon immersion. For example, a carcinoma in the centre of a mastectomy specimen will show severe autolysis unless the specimen is transected through the pathological lesion. A word of caution here: although a simple transection through a lesion will facilitate fixation, repeated slicing or the use of a random hacking

technique, applied to the specimen by the surgeon before insertion into fixative, will render accurate reconstruction impossible after fixation. Although this will not interfere with the histological diagnosis, it may mean that the pathologist is unable to offer any valid comment on the extent of spread or completeness of excision of a neoplastic lesion. In many large laboratories, pathologists encourage receipt of fresh material within minutes of removal so that tissue can be fixed properly or, alternatively, preserved by other techniques.

A small tissue sample such as a needle biopsy will be completely fixed within a couple of hours, and embedding into paraffin wax can begin on the same day that the biopsy is taken, with a good chance that a histology report may be available by the following day (within 24 hours of the biopsy being taken). Larger specimens may take 12–24 hours to fix, even if every precaution to ensure good fixation has been taken. Because processing into paraffin cannot take place until the sample has been fully fixed, a histopathology report from a large specimen may take 3–4 days. This time can be shortened if the main pathological lesion in a large specimen is transected so that it is exposed to the formalin; the pathologist can then take a sample from the fixed part of the lesion, and a report on the nature of the lesion can be issued within 24 hours, even though the report on the remainder of the specimen may need to follow in 2–3 days' time.

Rule 4

All specimens must be fully labeled with patient details and the nature of the sample. A request card also labeled with patient details, the nature of the sample, and full clinical details of the case must accompany the samples.

Resin sections

Resin rather than paraffin wax (see **tissue processing**) can be used to embed tissue samples, as it allows much thinner sections and greater resolution of fine structure. This is particularly the case for the histology of bone, as it allows sectioning of the densely calcified matrix.

Special stains

Certain structures can be highlighted by use of special staining techniques. Common methods used in histopathology laboratories are:

- PAS stain (periodic–acid Schiff) detects mucin and mucopolysaccharides. It will also detect many fungi.

- reticulin stain detects reticulin and basement membranes.
- methenamine–silver stain detects basement membranes.
- trichrome stains distinguish collagen, cells, and elastic tissues.
- Masson–Fontana stain detects melanin.
- Perls' stain detects iron pigment
- Ziehl–Nielsen stain detects acid-fast bacilli such as *Mycobacterium tuberculosis*.
- gram stain detects bacteria.

Tissue processing

Once received by the laboratory, fixed tissues must be processed into paraffin wax. A pathologist examines specimens, and portions of tissue are taken for examination by histology. For small samples, such as needle biopsies, the whole specimen is processed. For large, resected specimens, small samples are dissected using a scalpel. In most laboratories, automated machines expose tissues to increasing concentrations of alcohol, xylene and finally paraffin wax at 60°C. Specimens are then embedded in wax in molds and allowed to harden. Sections are cut on a microtome at 3–5 µm thickness, mounted on glass slides, and stained for histological examination. The whole process from specimen to section (including adequate fixation) takes about 24 hours.

Viral diagnosis

Viral diseases can be diagnosed by microbiological, histological and immunological means. Histological examination of tissue samples is not used frequently, but can be useful in the diagnosis of viral disorders of the skin (e.g. herpes, and HPV infection producing warts). The diagnosis is based on the characteristic histological and cytological features of virus-infected cells, or the presence of characteristic viral inclusions. Electron microscopy can be used to visualize the viral particles. Immunocytochemical methods can also be used on tissue sections to identify certain types of virus, such as some strains of human papilloma virus.

Using microbiological and immunological methods, viral diagnosis can be established early in the course of the illness by fluorescence of viral antigen in smears of infected cells, by isolation in cell culture, and by the detection of virus-specific IgM in the serum.

The detection of antibodies during the period of convalescence enables the viral infection to be diagnosed retrospectively by the demonstration of changing titers of antibody during the illness and subsequent convalescence. For this reason, at least two serum samples need to be taken, one during the illness, and at least one during the convalescence period; the presence of detectable antibody on a single occasion indicates only that the patient has been exposed to the virus in the past. Changing antibody levels are necessary to establish current or recent infection.

Answers

Brief answers to the case-based questions are given in this chapter. More detailed answers and other study resources are available online at www.studentconsult.com.

Chapter 10 Blood Circulatory System

Case 1

The most likely causes of critical limb ischemia relate to arterial occlusion.

Atherosclerotic peripheral vascular disease Aortic, ileofemoral and popliteal complicated atheroma related to atheroma risk factors.

Thromboembolism Origin from heart (atrial fibrillation, mural thrombus following myocardial infarction, vegetations from endocarditis). Origin from abdominal aortic atheroma, especially if associated with aneurysm or origin from popliteal atheromatous disease.

Vasculitis Less likely in this patient, given that he has two atheroma-related cardiovascular risk factors.

Given the likely pathological causes of arterial occlusion, in planning the investigation of this patient the following are relevant:

Examine peripheral vascular system The peripheral vascular system is examined in detail to confirm arterial occlusive disease and look for evidence of an aneurysm.

ECG – to detect atrial fibrillation or signs of myocardial infarction (may be old and associated with left ventricular aneurysm).

AP chest X-ray may show an abnormal contour to the heart, or aneurismal, dilated thoracic aorta.

Imaging of the peripheral vessels will detect occlusion.

Ultrasound examination of the heart and abdomen can detect mural thrombus, vegetations on cardiac valves and aneurysmal dilatation of arteries.

Other risk factors for atherosclerotic vascular disease (in addition to the smoking and hypertension) should be assessed and managed accordingly.

Case 2

The complications of myocardial infarction can be divided into immediate, early and late. This patient falls into the category of an early complication of MI.

VF arrest The commonest cause for collapse at this stage would be a ventricular arrhythmia, usually ventricular fibrillation.

Further ischaemia Recurrent infarction (infarction in a different artery) within 48 hours may occur in up to 40% of patients.

Failing ventricle Cardiogenic shock due to poor myocardial function can lead to a progressive decline in cardiac output.

Mitral valve regurgitation Papillary muscle dysfunction, and a more severe extension of this, papillary muscle rupture.

PEA arrest There are three relevant causes of a pulseless with electrical activity arrest (PEA arrest, also sometimes called electromechanical dissociation (EMD) arrest):

- Massive pulmonary thromboembolism can occur in post MI patients.
- Cardiac rupture with hemopericardium is predisposed to by softening of the infarcted left ventricular myocardium.
- Tension pneumothorax: if the patient required a central line, then an iatrogenic pneumothorax may be a complication.

Stroke or bleed If there has been mural thrombus developing over the infarct, then left ventricular thrombus occurs in 20% of cases after infarction, leading to embolic phenomena.

Case 3

1. Abdominal aortic aneurysms are usually caused by atheroma.
2. Histological changes occuring in the wall of the aorta. The histological changes of atheroma are:
   - Deposition of lipid in the intima of the vessel.
   - Production of collagenous fibrosis in the intima.
   - Loss of elastic and replacement of the muscle of the vessel wall by collagen.
   - Thrombus formation in the aneurysm cavity.

3. Embolization of atheroma debris or thrombus from within the aneurysm sac

Rupture of the aneurysm, leading to massive retroperitoneal hemorrhage.

4. Other main types of aneurysm and their causes:
   - Syphilitic aneurysms of the ascending aorta and arch
   - Berry aneurysms affect the cerebral arteries due to congenital defect in the vessel wall.
   - Mycotic aneurysms are caused by inflammatory destruction of the vessel wall by bacteria within infected thromboemboli.

Chapter 11 Respiratory System

Case 1

1. The most likely diagnosis for initial symptoms is a hospital-acquired pneumonia.
2. Predisposing factors for the development of a chest infection are a reduced ability to clear bronchial secretions due to smoking, general anesthesia and immobility.
3. Pathological changes in the lungs are likely to be those of bronchopneumonia. Macroscopically, lungs contain firm airless areas and pus in peripheral bronchi. Microscopically, acute inflammation of bronchi and an acute inflammatory exudate in the alveoli.
4. Most hospital-acquired pneumonia is caused by Gram-negative organisms. The antibiotic chosen for initial therapy, albeit reasonable for first-line treatment of a community-acquired chest infection, would not be the first choice for a hospital-acquired infection. Common complications of bronchopneumonia include pleurisy, septicemia and lung abscess.

Case 2

1. The results of the spirometry (restrictive ventilatory defect) and the episodic nature suggest extrinsic allergic alveolitis. Specific questions should be asked about occupation, hobbies and pets.

   Although extrinsic allergic alveolitis is the most likely cause, other causes of pulmonary interstitial fibrosis need to be considered.

2. Serological studies may show an increase in IgA and IgG in typical extrinsic allergic alveolitis. Specific antibodies may be detected by precipitin tests.
3. Following acute exposure to the antigen there is a type III hypersensitivity response, with the formation of immune complexes, complement activation and inflammation.
4. With repeated antigen exposure a type IV hypersensitivity response occurs, with the formation of

small granulomata. This results in interstitial fibrosis with progressive cough and dyspnea, eventually leading to end-stage honeycomb lung and cor pulmonale.

Case 3

1. This person is most likely to have chronic obstructive pulmonary disease (COPD). The three main pathologies contributing to COPD are emphysema, chronic bronchitis and bronchiolitis. The clinical feature in this case is an infective exacerbation of chronic obstructive pulmonary disease. The clinical features of right-heart failure and right-ventricular hypertrophy on ECG suggest pulmonary hypertension and the development of cor pulmonale.
2. The airways in chronic bronchitis show mucous plugging and hyperplasia of mucin-secreting glands in their walls. There will be inflammatory changes due to the respiratory tract infection.
3. The main risk factors that have been suggested for COPD are lifetime smoking exposure, recurrent chest infections in childhood, atopy and asthma, and occupational exposure to dusts (especially mining).

Chapter 12 Oral and ENT Pathology

Case 1

1. Acute necrotizing ulcerative gingivitis.
2. Poor dental hygiene and smoking.
3. Commonly *Fusobacterium* and *Borrelia* spp.
4. Cancrum oris, a severe, necrotizing infection of the lips and face, can occur in children.

Case 2

1. Frictional keratosis or smoker's keratosis.
2. To exclude dysplasia (leukoplakia).

Case 3

1. Squamous cell carcinoma of the tongue.
2. Wide, local excision of the tumor, often a hemiglossectomy.
3. Regional lymph nodes in the neck.

Case 4

1. Benign pleomorphic salivary adenoma of the parotid gland.
2. A wide resection margin is required, as the tumor can recur, but care must be taken not to damage the facial nerve.
3. Yes, the history is that of a benign lesion.

Case 5

1. Otitis media with effusion (OME).
2. The major complication is permanent damage to the middle ear with deafness and impairment of language development.

3. Obstruction of the eustachian tube.
4. The most common organisms are haemolytic streptococci. Virus infection often causes bilateral disease.
5. Antibiotic therapy and/or grommet insertion.

Case 6

1. Singer's nodules.
2. Singer's nodules are smooth, round nodules on the true cord representing areas of submucosal fibrosis.

Case 7

1. This is most likely to be an invasive squamous cell carcinoma.
2. Smoker's keratosis, possibly associated with carcinoma in situ.
3. The initiating event is heavy smoking leading to smoker's keratosis that eventually progresses to invasive squamous cell carcinoma.
4. There is the potential for local spread and metastatic disease to local and regional lymph nodes.

Chapter 13 Alimentary Tract

Case 1

1. Inflammatory bowel disease with Crohn's disease is the most likely diagnosis; in view of the presence of anal disease, Crohn's disease is much more likely than ulcerative colitis. The symptoms of infective-type colitis may mimic inflammatory bowel disease, but in that situation the history is usually days or weeks rather than months.
2. Crohn's disease.
3. Tuberculosis, other rarer granulomatous infections and, rarely, foreign-body type reactions.
4. These include enteropathic arthritis, ankylosing spondylitis, iritis, aphthous stomatitis, sclerosis cholangitis, erythema nodosum and pyoderma gangrenosum.
5. The main complications are consequences or bowel inflammation, stricture/fistula formation and the complications of repeated bowel resections.

Case 2

1. Duodenal or gastric ulceration with or without reflux oesophagitis
2. An imbalance between the effects of acid and pepsin attack and the mucosal defenses of the bowel wall.
3. The major complication is perforation of a vessel with subsequent gastrointestinal hemorrhage.
4. Fiberoptic endoscopy is the investigation of choice.
5. An endoscopic biopsy may show acute and/or chronic inflammation associated with regenerative changes. The inflammation may be associated with gland atrophy,

small intestinal metaplasia and, in some cases, infection with *H. pylori*.
6. Medical therapy with proton pump inhibitors or H₂ receptor antagonists is the first-line treatment, often accompanied by *Helicobacter* eradication therapy.

Case 3

1. The symptoms of 'heartburn' are suggestive of gastroesophageal reflux disease (GORD).
2. The endoscopic and biopsy appearances confirm a Barrett's oesophagus.
3. It is important to exclude dysplasia and invasive malignancy.

Case 4

1. Celiac disease is the most likely diagnosis.
2. These results are very suggestive of celiac disease due to the low levels of vitamin B₁₂ and the hypersensitivity reaction to α-gliadin.
3. The final diagnosis is celiac disease, provided the patient's symptoms respond to a gluten-free diet and the histological changes relapse on re-challenge.
4. Treatment is by adhering to a strict gluten-free diet.

Case 5

1. The most likely diagnosis is colorectal adenocarcinoma.
2. This is a Dukes' C carcinoma (T3, N1, M0; stage IIIB). There is about 30% 5-year survival with this type of disease.
3. There is much evidence to suggest that most carcinomas of the colon arise in pre-existing adenomas (adenoma–carcinoma sequence).
4. Colorectal carcinomas metastasize mainly to regional lymph nodes and liver.

Chapter 14 Liver, Biliary Tract, and Pancreas

Case 1

1. There are three main patterns of alcohol-related liver damage:
   - **Fatty liver** – accumulation of fat in hepatocytes.
   - **Acute alcoholic hepatitis** – a true hepatitis, with focal necrosis of liver cells. Mallory's hyaline may form in hepatocytes.
   - **Alcoholic cirrhosis** – characterized by liver fibrosis and nodules of regenerating hepatocytes.
2. Alcoholic cirrhosis affects fewer than 10% of patients suffering from chronic alcoholism.
3. (i) Obtain informed consent.
   (ii) An important complication of liver biopsy is bleeding and biopsy is contraindicated if coagulation is poor. Check prothrombin time, hemoglobin concentration and platelet count. These can be abnormal in liver disease because of failure of the

protein synthetic functions of the liver or reduced absorption of vitamin K.

Case 2

1. There are three common features in cirrhosis, irrespective of causation:
   - Long-standing destruction of liver cells, often associated with chronic inflammation.
   - Fibrosis characterized by defined bands of collagenous tissue separating nodules of hepatocytes.
   - Regeneration of hepatocytes to cause nodules.
2. Prominent fatty change and the presence of Mallory's hyaline are suggestive of alcoholic liver damage.
3. The main consequences of cirrhosis are:
   - Reduced hepatocyte function – decreased synthesis of proteins and failure of detoxification. This relates to clinical features of poor coagulation (bruises), ascites and oedema (low serum albumen), spider nevi and gynecomastia (failure to eliminate estrogen).
   - Disturbance of blood flow through the liver, causing portal hypertension. This relates to ascites and splenomegaly, predisposed by increased hydrostatic pressure in the portal circulation. Esophageal varices may also develop and predispose to a risk of gastrointestinal hemorrhage.
   - Reduced immune competence and increased susceptibility to infection.
   - Increased risk of development of hepatocellular carcinoma.
   - Increased risk of development of portal vein thrombosis.

Case 3

1. The most likely diagnosis is primary biliary cirrhosis (PBC). The investigations so far based on liver function tests suggest early symptomatic disease.
2. An understanding of the pathogenesis and natural history of the disease allows an explanation to be given to the patient.

This patient is symptomatic, and so it is appropriate to say that disease has probably been developing for the past 4–5 years. It is likely that this patient's disease will progress, leading to advanced disease over a period of 6–10 years.

It would be appropriate to obtain consent for a liver biopsy to evaluate the stage of the disease, as this will help with planning management.

Treatment using ursodeoxycholic acid may improve liver function, but liver transplantation is often necessary.

Case 4

1. Mechanical obstruction of pancreatic ducts:
   - Gallstones
   - Trauma
   - Postoperative (e.g. ERCP)
     Metabolic/toxic causes:

   - Alcohol
   - Drugs (e.g. thiazide diuretics, azathioprine, steroids)
   - Hypercalcemia
   - Hyperlipidemia
     Vascular/poor perfusion:
   - Atherosclerosis, vasculitis
   - Hypothermia
     Infections:
   - Mumps and other viruses (EBV, CMV).

   In this patient the most likely cause of acute pancreatitis relates to alcohol abuse.

2. Inflammation and necrosis of the pancreas are caused by the liberation of digestive enzymes; this results in extensive enzyme-mediated local tissue necrosis, particularly fat necrosis. Three patterns of pancreatic necrosis have been defined:
   - Periductal necrosis, particularly that associated with gallstones, and alcohol.
   - Periobular necrosis seen in shock and hypothermia.
   - Panlobular necrosis.
3. Most patients with acute pancreatitis recover. A complication is the development of a cyst filled with serosanguinous fluid, termed a pancreatic pseudocyst. Chemical peritonitis and shock may develop, predisposing to adult respiratory distress syndrome. A long-term complication may be the development of chronic pancreatitis.

Chapter 15 Lymphoid and Hemopoietic Tissues

Case 1

1. There are several potential causes of granulomatous inflammation within lymph nodes. An understanding of the causes allows planning of further clinical investigations.
   - Mycobacterial infection – mycobacterium tuberculosis as well as atypical mycobacteria
   - Sarcoidosis.
   - Cat-scratch disease.
   - Toxoplasmosis.
   - Fungal infection (e.g. *Histoplasma*).
   - Other bacteria (e.g. *Yersinia* or *Brucella*).
   - Crohn's disease.
   - Rarer causes (e.g. reaction to Hodgkin's disease).

   Some of these possible causes are unlikely in this patient, given the site of the enlarged nodes. For example, cat-scratch disease would be expected in nodes draining the site of a relevant cat-inflicted injury. Yersinial infection and Crohn's disease typically involved mesenteric nodes.

2. Part of the lymph node should have been sent for culture, including for TB. Mycobacterial organisms may take 4–6 weeks to grow. Other investigations (which may already have been done) should include a chest X-ray, sputum microscopy and culture and a

Mantoux test. Staining of the node for acid-fast bacilli as well as fungi should be performed.

3. A granuloma is a collection of histiocytes, epithelioid macrophages, and possibly giant cells with or without a mantle of lymphocytes. It is a manifestation of cell-mediated immunity and a type IV hypersensitivity response.

Case 2 – Lymphadenopathy detected on a chest X-ray

1. The diagnosis of HD requires the presence of neoplastic Reed–Sternberg (RS) cells (or variants thereof) within an appropriate cellular background.

Histologically, five types of Hodgkin's disease have been defined (**WHO classification**).

Nodular lymphocyte-predominant disease – the nodes are replaced by reactive lymphoid cells, among which are a small population of Reed–Sternberg cells. Most patients present with stage I or II disease.

Mixed-cellularity disease mainly affects adults in later life. Lymph nodes are replaced by an infiltrate of Reed–Sternberg cells, with a cellular response composed of lymphoid cells, eosinophils, plasma cells and histiocytes. Over 50% of patients present in stage III or IV.

Nodular sclerosis is the most common type of Hodgkin's disease, mainly affecting young adults. In most cases the mediastinal nodes are involved at presentation. The key feature is that the infiltrate is divided into nodules by broad bands of collagen.

Lymphocyte-rich Hodgkin's disease is characterized by Reed–Sternberg cells set in a diffuse background of lymphoid cells.

Lymphocyte-depleted disease is rare and mainly seen in the elderly. The infiltrate is composed of many pleomorphic Reed–Sternberg cells, and shows few reactive lymphoid cells.

2. Stage I – Disease confined to one group of lymph nodes or extranodal site (IE).

Stage II – Disease confined to several nodal groups on the same side of the diaphragm, with limited involvement of an adjacent extranodal site (TIE).

Stage III – Disease is present in lymph node groups on both sides of the diaphragm, or with limited involvement of an adjacent extranodal site (IIIE), or with involvement of the spleen (1115).

Stage IV – Disseminated involvement of one or more extranodal tissue, such as the liner or bone marrow, with or without nodal involvement.

These groups are further subdivided on the absence (A) or presence (B) of symptoms, which include: unexplained fever (>38°C), night sweats, and unexplained weight loss greater than 10% of body weight in the preceding 6 months.

3. The best prognosis is seen with lymphocyte-predominant and nodular sclerosis Hodgkin's disease, the worst with lymphocyte-depleted disease. Bad prognostic features within each subgroup include increasing age, increasing stage, and the presence of systemic symptoms.

Case 3

1. Although the clinical features and X-ray findings together with a raised ESR and raised Ca2 are highly suggestive of myeloma, the diagnosis must be confirmed by serum electrophoresis for the detection of a monoclonal immunoglobulin protein (paraprotein) and bone marrow biopsy to detect an increased number of monoclonal plasma cells.

2. There are many possible causes of renal failure in myeloma, and several are readily reversible. They include:
   - Dehydration
   - Hypercalcemia
   - Hyperuricemia
   - Urinary-tract infection
   - Damage to tubular epithelium by light-chain casts
   - Infiltration of kidney by plasma cells
   - Amyloid.

3. One of the major problems in myeloma is the paraprotein. In the presence of high levels of this protein the production of normal gammaglobulin is reduced, leading to recurrent bacterial infections. The abnormal protein can also give rise to a hyperviscosity syndrome.

Case 4

1. In acute leukemia replacement of bone marrow by blast cells causes reduced red cell production, leading to anemia and the related symptoms of fatigue and lethargy. Granulopoiesis is impaired, and this increases predisposition to bacterial infections (fever). Production of platelets by megakaryocytes becomes compromised, leading to a bleeding tendency (petechial hemorrhages and bleeding gums).

2. Examination of the peripheral blood will show an elevated white cell count in about half of cases of acute leukemia. The diagnosis is established by bone marrow aspirate or trephine biopsy, which will show the replacement of normal hemopoietic tissue by abnormal blast cells. A detailed immunochemical and molecular profiling is performed to precisely categorize the nature of the blast cells and type the leukemia.

3. Acute leukemias are broadly divided into:
   - Acute lymphoblastic leukemia (ALL) seen mostly in children.
   - Acute non-lymphoblastic leukemia (ANLL) seen most often in adults.

In ALL, the morphology (FAB type) of the leukemic cells and the presence or absence of specific cell-surface antigens allows a prognosis to be given.

The ANLLs are divided into eight FAB types with varying degrees of granulocytic, erythroid or megakaryocytic differentiation of the blast cells.

Chapter 16 Endocrine System

Case 1

1. CT/MRI investigations should examine the contents of the sella turcica, and a biochemical profile of the pituitary gland is required. A visual field assessment should be performed to confirm the pattern of visual loss.
2. The visual defect is caused by compression of the optic chiasm by expansion of the pituitary gland.
3.

Adenoma	Hormone affected	Symptoms
Somatotroph cell	GH	Early = Acromegaly Late = Metabolic disturbances
Mamotroph cell	PRL	Galactorrhoea, amenorrhoea, hypogonadism
Gonadotroph cell	LH & FSH	Hypopituitarism, menstrual irregularities etc
Thyrotroph cell	TSH	Hyperthyroidism
Adrenocorticotroph cell	ACTH	Cushing's disease
Null cell		Chiasmal pressure symptoms, Hypopituitarism

GH = Growth hormone, PRL = Prolactin, LH = Leuteinising hormone, FSH = Follicle stimulating hormone, TSH, Thyroid stimulating hormone, and ACTH = Adrenocorticotrophic hormone.

Case 2

1. The most likely diagnosis is hyperthyroidism, probably Graves' disease.
2. Thyroid function tests are the initial investigation of choice.
3. The most likely cause in a woman this age is Graves' disease, an autoimmune disorder where stimulating IgG antibody binds to thyroid acinar cells, mimicking the effects of TSH and resulting in excess thyroxine production.

Case 3

1. Solitary nodules in the thyroid may be a disproportionately large nodule of a multinodular goitre, a thyroid adenoma, or a malignant thyroid tumor.

2.

Investigation	Result
Thyroid function tests	Normal
Thyroglobulin	Raised
Radioactive iodine scan	An inactive or 'cold' nodule
Ultrasound scan	The nodule is solid in consistency
FNA cytology	Malignant cells typical of papillary cell carcinoma are present
Chest CT	No tracheal compression or retrosternal extension of the tumor is seen

3. A short clinical history and an asymmetrically enlarged, hard thyroid nodule with adjacent cervical lymphadenopathy are all suggestive of cancer.
4. Papillary cell carcinoma has a good prognosis in young people, with a 5-year survival rate of 80%.

Case 4

1. The clinical history is suggestive of a pheochromocytoma, which is a rare but treatable cause of hypertension.
2. It is necessary to perform a 24-hour urine collection to measure catecholamines and their metabolites (VMA, metadrenalins).

   An MRI/CT scan is required to localize the lesion.

3. A pheochromocytoma is a component of multiple endocrine neoplasia II (MEN II) which occurs in association with parathyroid tumors and medullary cell carcinoma of the thyroid.

Case 5

1.
   - Scaphoid fracture
   - Angina
   - Overweight
   - Diabetes mellitus
   - Cataracts
   - Diabetic retinopathy
2. Elderly diabetics often have multiple pathologies, including:
   - Peripheral vascular disease (peripheral gangrene)
   - Diabetic neuropathy (tingling and numbness in the feet)
   - Arterial disease (can lead to myocardial infarction)
   - Skin infections (e.g. *Staphylococci*)
3.
   - Vascular disease such as angina and myocardial infarction
   - Retinopathy that can lead to loss of vision
   - Ulceration of the feet (due to combination of diabetic neuropathy and peripheral vascular disease)

- Skin infections (*Staphylococcal*)
- Impotence.

4. Symptoms may be divided into acute, subacute, and delayed as follows:

   Acute
   - Thirst, polyuria, weight loss (also in young patients). Puritis vulvae or balanitis (due to *Candida* infection) and visual blurring are common in the elderly.

   Subacute
   - As above, but slow in onset with the addition of malaise and tiredness.

   Delayed
   - Present with the complications of NIDDM (see above).

Case 6

1. The features are those of increased circulating glucocorticoid (Cushing's syndrome), which has several common causes.
2. The three most useful tests are a dexamethasone suppression test, a 24-hour free urinary cortisol estimation and circadian rhythm tests.
3. The systemic effects of glucocorticoids include:
   - Pigmentation (ACTH-dependent only – due to the N-terminal residues of ACTH mimicking MSH).
   - Weight gain with central obesity
   - Amenorrhea
   - Poor libido
   - Thin skin with easy bruising
   - Hirsutism
   - Osteoporosis: pathological fractures or vertebrae and ribs
   - Polyuria/polydipsia
   - Hypertension
   - 'Buffalo hump'
   - Striae.
4. Failure of significant plasma cortisol suppression suggests an ectopic source of ACTH, such as a small cell carcinoma of the lung, or an adrenal tumor.

Chapter 17 Diseases of the Urinary System

Cases 1 and 2

1. The acute nephritic syndrome.
2. Crescentic glomerulonephritis (rapidly progressive glomerulonephritis (see *Fig. 17.22*)
3. Acute diffuse proliferative glomerulonephritis, **without** crescent formation (see *Figs 17.16 and 17.17*).
4. Rupture of glomerular capillary walls → stimulates crescent formation → rapid proliferation of crescent compresses and destroys glomerular tuft. Cycle occurs in more than 75% of glomeruli.
5. *Complete recovery* – disappearance of deposits, regression of endothelial and mesangial cell proliferation, and re-establishment of patency of capillary lumina with re-establishment of glomerular filtration.

Proteinuria persists – as above but incomplete regression of mesangial cells, which continue to produce slightly excessive amounts of mesangial matrix. Very slowly progressive destruction of glomeruli by this persistent excessive production of mesangial matrix → progressive glomerular hyalinization and destruction.

Cases 3 and 4

1. The nephrotic syndrome. Most likely cause at this age is minimal change nephropathy (*Fig. 17.25*).
2. *Glomerulus* – normal by light microscopy, but loss of podocyte foot processes by EM.
   Tubules – swelling and pallor of convoluted tubular epithelial cells (lipoid nephrosis).
3. In the absence of microscopic hematuria, focal glomerulosclerosis or membranous nephropathy are most likely.
4. Most likely are glomerular lesions of diabetic nephropathy (see *Fig. 17.29* and related text), some patterns of SLE nephropathy (see *Fig. 17.26* and related text), and membranous nephropathy (see *Fig. 17.18*).

If there is associated microscopic or macroscopic hematuria, other glomerular disorders enter the differential diagnosis (see full answer on website).

Case 5

1. Electron microscopy and immunochemistry.
2. *Electron microscopy* – immune complex deposits in mesangium and paramesangial regions.
   Immunochemistry – IgA deposited in mesangium and paramesangial regions (see *Figs 17.23 and 17.24*).
3. Focal and segmental proliferation of mesangial cells with production of excess mesangial matrix, leading to focal and segmental loss of glomerular function. In 25% of cases this destruction is continuous and affects increasing numbers of segments of more and more glomeruli until chronic renal failure develops.

Case 6

1.
   - Inadequate glomerular perfusion to allow ultrafiltration to take place, thus no ultrafiltrate/urine formed
   - Ischemic necrosis of epithelial cells lining proximal and distal tubules (**acute tubular necrosis** – see *Fig. 17.34* and related text).
2. Inadequate renal perfusion by oxygenated arterial blood because of prolonged hypotension and hypovolemia following severe acute blood loss.
3. Good. Once his hypotension and hypovolemia have been treated, glomerular perfusion and ultrafiltration will resume, and the damaged tubules will become

relined by metabolically active epithelial cells. Normal renal function will resume.

Chapter 18 Male genital system

Case 1

1. Acute torsion of the testis.
2. If over 6 hours, the testis will be completely infarcted, and external or surgical detorsion will fail to save it. Orchidectomy required.
3. Manual detorsion.
4. Surgical detorsion after opening the scrotum succeeded because the length of history was only 2 hours.

Case 2

1.
- Primary testicular tumor (at this age, either mature teratoma, or yolk sac tumor).
- Hydrocele (less likely because palpation showed swelling was testicular).
- Infective orchitis (unlikely because swelling is painless).

2. Yolk sac tumor because of history of rapid onset.
3. *Imaging* – to confirm presence and size of testicular mass, and to search for evidence of lymph node metastases in pelvic and para-aortic node groups, and for evidence of lung metastases.

   Tumor-cell markers – HCG, AFP and LDH.

4. Raised AFP makes the diagnosis of yolk sac tumor almost certain.

Cases 3 and 4

1. Patient 3 – seminoma, because over 35.
   Patient 4 – mixed germ cell tumor, because under 35.
2. Tumor cell markers HCG, AFP and LDH would be measured preoperatively.
   Patient 3 – no increase in markers in most cases, but LDH may be raised if there are already extensive metastases, and there may be a small rise in HCG if the seminoma is one that contains scattered trophoblastic cells.
   Patient 4 – may be raised HCG (if mixed tumor contains trophoblastic elements) or AFP (if it contains yolk sac elements).

Case 5

1. Adenocarcinoma of prostate.
2. Metastatic carcinoma in lumbar vertebrae.
3.
- *Full blood count* – to assess any marrow infiltration by metastatic tumor (e.g. leukoerythroblastic anemia).

- *PSA (prostate-specific antigen)* – greatly raised if there is metastatic tumor.
- *Imaging* – looking for evidence of metastatic spread to bones (particularly vertebrae and pelvic bones). Chest X-ray for lung metastases, and possibly a liver scan.

4. Adenocarcinoma arises in the periphery of the gland, away from the urethra, so transurethral biopsy may miss the tumor.

Chapter 19 Gynecologic and Obstetric Pathology

Case 1

1. The ovarian cysts of endometriosis are often called 'chocolate' cysts because of the color and the consistency of the semi-viscous brown contents.
2. The reason for the development of endometriosis is uncertain, but several theories have been proposed, including retrograde menstruation, metaplasia of the peritoneal lining and mesenteric spread of endometrium along lymphatics or blood vessels.
3. The primary treatment is the suppression of the endometrial tissue by endocrine agents including analogs of GnRH.
4. Complications include fibrosis and adhesions, caused by the presence of free blood, the latter possibly leading to infertility or the possibility of ectopic pregnancy.

Case 2

1. As many as 20% of postmenopausal women with ovarian thecomas develop endometrial carcinoma.
2. Carcinoma of the body of the uterus spreads locally into the myometrium and along the fallopian tubes. Lymphatic spread is to the internal iliac and para-aortic lymph nodes.
3. Stage I carcinomas are confined to the body of the uterus, stage II carcinomas have, in addition, infiltrated into the cervix, stage III carcinomas involve the side walls of the pelvis and stage IV carcinomas have spread outside the pelvis or involve the rectum or the bladder. The prognosis for this patient is good as stage I carcinomas have a 75% 5-year survival.

Case 3

1. Other common causes of lower, female, genital tract infections include *Candida albicans*, *Gardnerella vaginalis*, herpes simplex virus, *Gonococcus*, *Mycoplasma spp* and human papilloma virus.
2. *Trichomonas vaginalis* is usually sexually transmitted.
3. Metronidazole is the present treatment of choice for urogenital *Trichomonas* infections.

Case 4

1. Leiomyomas usually present with abnormal, often heavy, menstrual bleeding and consequent anemia.

Malignant change is thought to be very rare in leiomyomas, and most malignant smooth muscle tumors arise de novo.

2. A leiomyoma is recognized by a lack of cellular atypia and mitoses.

Case 5

1. These account for approximately 10% of ovarian neoplasms.
2. The ovarian mass has probably undergone ischemic infarction secondary to torsion. This can lead to cyst rupture and peritonitis.
3. The four main groups of germ cell tumours can be grouped as:
   - Solid teratomas (malignant immature teratoma, mature benign tumours and monodermal tumours)
   - Dysgerminoma
   - Yolk-sac tumours
   - Ovarian choriocarcinoma.

Case 6

1. Approximately 40% of conceptions fail to implant and convert into recognized pregnancies.
2. Causes of first trimester abortions include: abnormal chromosomal karyotypes, other genetic mutations, neural tube and other structural defects, transplacental infection, some autoimmune diseases.
3. Some animal zoonoses can cause spontaneous abortion, the most relevant to veterinarians are *Brucella, Toxoplasma* and *Listeria*.

Chapter 20 Breast Disease

Case 1

1. Breast cancer is the most common malignancy in women, with 1 in 10 women in the United States developing breast cancer at some time in their life (1 in 12 in the UK).
2. Fine-needle aspiration cytology is used as part of a 'triple approach' to diagnose breast lesions. It is relatively painless, complication-free, and has an extremely low false-positive rate. Cytological features of malignancy include pleomorphism and increased cell size and loss of cohesion of the cells.
3. Carcinoma of the breast spreads in a characteristic fashion, which explains several of the common clinical manifestations of disease. Breast carcinomas spread locally into the overlying skin, causing tethering, and into the underlying pectoralis muscles, causing fixation. In addition, lymphatic and blood vessels may he invaded. In this way, tumor-cell emboli reach the local lymph nodes in the axilla and also the internal mammary node. Bloodstream spread to bones may cause pathological fractures, spinal-cord compression and anemia; spread to other organs may be seen, including lung, pleura, ovary and brain.

4. Your discussion with the patient would need to reflect the reality that she has poor prognosis disease. This is a high-grade (grade 3) and advanced-stage tumor.
5. Your discussion with the patient would include possible endocrine therapy, if the tumor profile was appropriate. Prognosis is related to **hormone receptor status.**

Case 2

1. Histological grade is determined by assessing three components of a breast carcinoma:
   - The extent of the tumor which is forming tubules.
   - The degree of pleomorphism and the cell size of the tumor cells.
   - The mitotic count.

Some authorities use a method of assessing nuclear grade, instead of histological grade, which is also well-correlated with prognosis.

2. As well as histological grade, the staging of the tumor is of significance in predicting prognosis in patients with breast cancer. An accurate assessment of the size of the carcinoma is also predictive of outcome. Other variables of statistical significance in predicting survival are the presence or absence of vascular invasion and the histological type of carcinoma. Hormone receptor status is also related to prognosis, tumors expressing oestrogen receptors having a better prognosis than those that do not.
3. The patient has an excellent prognosis. She has a small, grade 1 carcinoma of tubular type with no evidence of metastases in her axillary lymph nodes. Her life expectancy is equivalent to that of an age-matched control, i.e. the same as if she had not had carcinoma.

Case 3

1. It has been reported that over 40% of grossly normal breasts examined histologically at autopsy show features of FCC. Clinical symptoms are said to be reported in 10% of women, often in their 30s or 40s.
2. There are two components to fibrocystic change, divided into non-proliferative and proliferative. Epithelial proliferation is the component which confers an increased risk of subsequent carcinoma developing. Epithelial hyperplasia of usual type confers a 2-fold increase in the risk of developing carcinoma. If this shows atypia (atypical ductal hyperplasia) the risk increases to 4–5 times that of the general population.
3. The axillary tenderness is most likely due to a reactive lymphadenopathy as a result of an inflammatory response to a ruptured breast cyst. This clinical situation causes obvious diagnostic difficulties and malignancy must always be positively excluded by further investigation in a patient with a breast mass and enlarged lymph nodes.

Chapter 21 Nervous System and Muscle

Case 1

1. Understanding this clinical sign depends on a knowledge of the pathology of an intracranial space-occupying lesion and the concept of cerebral herniation. The space-occupying hematoma on the right side has caused transtentorial herniation of the parahippocampal gyrus over the free edge of the tentorium cerebelli. This causes stretching of the third cranial nerve on the same side, resulting first in a sluggishly responding pupil, and then a paralysed dilated pupil.

2. The fracture of the skull has torn the middle meningeal artery, causing acute extradural hematoma.

3. Brain pathology from head injury can be divided into two groups: primary and secondary. Secondary damage occurs after the initial impact and is caused by hypoxia, hypotension, and brain swelling. This patient has multiple trauma, with unconsciousness, a hemothorax and a major leg fracture. It is therefore likely that he has sustained severe secondary brain damage.

4. After head injury, bleeding from the ear strongly suggests a fracture of the base of the skull, usually involving the middle cranial fossa.

Case 2

1. The commonest cause of cerebral hemorrhage is hypertensive vascular damage. Prolonged hypertension results in arteriosclerosis and the development of microaneurysms, termed Charcot–Bouchard aneurysms, which predispose to vessel rupture, resulting in a hematoma.

2. The common sites for hypertensive intracerebral hematoma are the sites supplied by fine perforating vessels: the basal ganglia, internal capsule, thalamus, cerebellum and pons.

3. In patients over the age of 70, 10% of cerebral hemorrhages are caused by the presence of cerebral artery amyloid composed of Aβ protein (amyloid angiopathy). This causes hematomas seen in the periphery of cerebral hemispheres (lobar hemorrhages).

Less common causes of a cerebral hematoma are bleeding into a tumor, rupture of vascular malformations, cerebral vasculitis, bleeding associated with disordered coagulation, and bleeding occurring in association with leukemias.

Case 3

1. The main causes of acute purulent meningitis differ in different age groups:
   - Neonates: *Escherichia coli*, streptococci, *Listeria monocytogenes*.
   - Children: *Haemophilus influenzae*, *Neisseria meningitidis*.
   - Adults: *Neisseria meningitiidis, Streptococcus pneumoniae* type 3.
   - Elderly: *Streptococcus pneumoniae* type 3, *Listeria monocytogenes*.

In this case, the age and Gram-negative coccobacilli suggest *Haemophilus influenzae* infection. The incidence of *Haemophilus* meningitis in children has fallen in areas with a high uptake of Hib vaccination.

2. Acute bacterial meningitis is a severe life-threatening illness. Thrombosis of small cerebral vessels leads to diffuse cerebral ischemic damage and death. If treated early, before vascular damage occurs, there may be resolution of disease, but complications caused by organization of the inflammatory exudate may lead to obstruction of the CSF drainage pathways and the development of hydrocephalus. Cerebral abscess may also develop.

Case 4

1. Multiple sclerosis (MS) is a disease in which there are relapsing episodes of immunologically mediated demyelination in the CNS. It is likely that the disease is the result of a genetic susceptibility predisposing to the mounting of an inappropriate immune response that causes damage to oligodendrocytes.

There is great variation in outcome. Some patients have a relatively benign form of disease, experiencing only minor disability and few episodes of demyelination. Others have frequent repeated episodes of myelin loss, progressing such that in the late stages of disease they are rendered blind, paraplegic, and incontinent, with cognitive dysfunction caused by loss of hemispheric white matter (progressive relapsing–remitting MS). The least common form is characterized by unremitting rapid progression from onset (primary progressive MS).

2. The lesions of multiple sclerosis are confined to the brain and spinal cord. Areas of demyelination are termed 'plaques.'

3. This is termed optic neuritis and is a very common manifestation of multiple sclerosis.

Case 5

1. Glioblastomas are highly malignant astrocytic glial tumors with a rapid pace of growth. Like most gliomas, they diffusely infiltrate the brain, and there is extensive local spread. With growth, the tumor comes to occupy a significant volume of the brain and death is usually due to the effects of raised intracranial pressure.

2. There is a very poor prognosis with this type of tumor. There is a median survival of around 10 months from diagnosis.

3. Much of the swelling associated with brain tumors is the result of abnormally leaky blood vessels, causing

cerebral edema. Dexamethasone prevents this and reduces cerebral swelling, thereby reducing intracranial pressure. In this case the headache was due to raised intracranial pressure and improved when the peritumoral edema was treated by dexamethasone.

Case 6

1. Inclusion-body myositis is clinically similar to polymyositis but occurs mainly in elderly patients. Muscle biopsy shows inflammation of muscle, fibre necrosis and the presence of vacuoles and filamentous inclusions in fibres seen by electron microscopy. This disorder is important to diagnose as it is slowly progressive and, unlike other types of inflammatory myopathy, has a poor response to immunosuppressive treatment. This is an underdiagnosed condition.
2. Polymyositis presents clinically with weakness of the proximal limbs, facial muscles, ptosis and dysphagia. Polymyositis may be associated with the presence of connective tissue diseases such as SLE, rheumatoid disease or scleroderma, and may also be a non-metastatic manifestation of malignancy. Dermatomyomyositis is clinically similar to polymyositis and includes the presence of a vasculitic skin rash.
3. This clinical presentation could have been due to myasthenia gravis, a treatable condition caused by autoantibodies directed to the acetylcholine receptors in motor endplates. Muscle strength transiently improves if anticholinesterase is administered. The usual drug given is edrophonium hydrochloride (Tensilon).

Chapter 22 Ophthalmic Pathology

Case 1

1. Closing up of the trabecular meshwork which normally leads to the canal of Schlemm, can occur as a degenerative process. It increases in incidence with age, being encountered mainly after the age of 40 and often being familial. Because the drainage angle is open this is termed primary open-angle glaucoma.
2. Glaucoma can be divided into primary and secondary:
   - Primary open-angle glaucoma (see above).
   - Primary closed-angle glaucoma develops in patients who have a congenitally shallow anterior chamber and who develop narrowing of the angle between the iris and the cornea, causing functional blockage to aqueous drainage. This particularly occurs when the pupil is dilated, as the iris thickens with contraction, hence acute attacks may be precipitated by being in the dark.
   - Secondary closed-angle glaucoma is caused by adhesions between the iris and cornea, for example caused by uveitis or secondary to vascular proliferation due to retinal ischemia.

- Secondary open-angle glaucoma is caused by blockage of the trabecular meshwork by particulate material in the aqueous, particularly degenerate lens material, pigment from melanocytic lesions, or macrophages accumulating in response to hemorrhage or inflammation.
- Congenital glaucoma is very rare, (seen in childhood with enlargement of the globe) and is mainly due to developmental defects in the drainage of aqueous.

3. The effects of raised intraocular pressure are cupping of the optic disc (detected on fundoscopy), and degeneration of retinal ganglion cells. Clinically, there is progressive peripheral visual field loss, leading to blindness in untreated cases. In acute glaucoma there is breakdown of the endothelium leading to edema of the cornea and the formation of painful corneal bullae. In chronic glaucoma the sclera may stretch to form bulges termed 'staphylomas.'

Case 2

1. Blockage and infection of a meibomian gland causes swelling and acute inflammation of the affected gland. A **chalazion** is a firm swelling in the eyelid, which bulges under the palpebral conjunctiva. Caused by rupture of a meibomian gland, it histologically consists of a foreign-body histiocytic chronic inflammatory response to lipid-rich material derived from the destroyed gland.

In explaining these concepts to a patient language is generally restricted to explaining that a gland in the eyelid has first become blocked and then inflamed.

Chapter 23 Dermatopathology

Case 1

1. Acute eczematous atopic dermatitis.
2. Hayfever/allergic rhinitis.
3. Chronic relapsing course, tending to improve in teenage or adult years.
4. 'Chronic dermatitis' or 'lichen simplex chronicus', the result of chronic scratching of a previous acute eczematous dermatitis lesion in the distant past.

Case 2

1. Bullous pemphigoid.
2. Yes. Age group (over 70), sites, and clinical features are typical.
3. Yes, biopsy of an early developing lesion is vital to exclude other blistering diseases, e.g. some drug reactions.

Cases 3, 4, 5

1. Yes; all three have different patterns of basal cell carcinoma.
2. Case 3, because it is a clearly defined localized lesion (nodular type).

3. Case 4 – ill-defined lesion often extending microscopically beyond visible and palpable margins (morpheic types). Case 5 – often multifocal, with minute early lesions beyond the main visible lesion (superficial type).

Complete curative excision may be difficult in both types.

4. Yes, to confirm the clinical diagnosis and assess completeness of excision.

Case 6

1. Nodular malignant melanoma.
2. Prognosis is likely to be poor with a high chance of metastatic spread because of a Breslow thickness over 1.5 mm, and the back is a high-risk location.

Chapter 24 Orthopedic and Rheumatological Pathology

Case 1

1. Osteomalacia.
2. Vitamin D deficiency due to combination of inadequate synthesis in skin (because of all-enveloping traditional dress) and poor dietary intake (because vegetarian).
3. Low serum phosphate, high serum alkaline phosphatase, probably normal serum calcium. Imaging may reveal inadequate mineralization of bone, and perhaps Looser's zones.
4. Unmineralized osteoid on outer surface of trabecular bone (see *Fig. 24.4*).
5. To exclude renal failure and renal osteodystrophy.
6. Oral vitamin D supplements.

Case 2

1. Osteosarcoma.
2. Tumor expanding lower end of femur and possibly spreading out into soft tissue. Imaging of lung requested to assess metastatic deposits in lung.
3. Malignant osteoblasts, some producing osteoid.

Case 3

1. Acute gout.
2. Serum uric acid level – should be raised.
3. Gout is due to uric acid crystal deposition in joints, as a manifestation of hyperuricemia.
4. Crystal precipitation in soft tissues (tophi) and in urinary tract (urate stones).

5. Alcohol and dietary excess may precipitate an acute attack of gout, as may some drugs, including thiazide diuretics.

Chapter 25 Important Multisystem Diseases

Case 1

1. Systemic lupus erythematosus.
2. Renal involvement in SLE is common (lupus nephropathy).
3. Urinalysis, blood urea and creatinine, creatinine clearance test, and **percutaneous renal biopsy.**

Case 2

1. The most likely diagnosis is a form of systemic sclerosis.
2. Systemic sclerosis can affect the lungs (producing progressive breathlessness) and the esophagus, producing difficulty in swallowing and heartburn due to acid reflux.
   - X-rays of hands to look for evidence of focal calcinosis in skin.
   - X-ray of lungs to look for evidence of lung fibrosis and honeycomb lung changes (see *Figs 25.6 and 25.7*).
   - Barium swallow (or esophageal manometry) – to detect esophageal involvement.
3. **CREST syndrome** is one of the patterns of systemic sclerosis, comprising **C**alcinosis, particularly in hands and fingers (see *Fig. 25.6*), **R**aynaud's phenomenon, **E**sophageal involvement, **S**clerodactyly, thickening of skin of fingers, face and other sites (see *Fig. 25.6*), and **T**elangiectasia, particularly of face and hands. The patient described in this case history may well have the CREST pattern of the disease, sometimes called 'limited scleroderma.'

Mixed connective tissue disease is a rare overlap disease in which patients have mixed features of SLE, systemic sclerosis and polymyositis.

Case 3

1. Sensory loss due to glove-and-stocking pattern of peripheral neuropathy has led to trophic ulceration.
2. Type 2 diabetes mellitus.
3. The combination of peripheral neuropathy and diabetic peripheral vascular disease (poor foot pulses) impedes healing of the ulcers.

Index

TORT LAW